SKIN GRAFTS – INDICATIONS, APPLICATIONS AND CURRENT RESEARCH

Edited by **Marcia Spear**

Skin Grafts – Indications, Applications and Current Research
Edited by Marcia Spear

Published by InTech

Janeza Trdine 9, 51000 Rijeka, Croatia

Publishing Process Manager Davor Vidic

Technical Editor Teodora Smiljanic

Cover Designer InTech Design Team

Additional hard copies can be obtained from orders@intechopen.com

Skin Grafts – Indications, Applications and Current Research, Edited by Marcia Spear
p. cm.
ISBN 978-953-307-509-9

For EU product safety concerns:
IN TECH d.o.o., Prolaz Marije Krucifikse Kozulić 3, 51000 Rijeka, Croatia,
info@intechopen.com or visit our website at intechopen.com.

Meet the editor

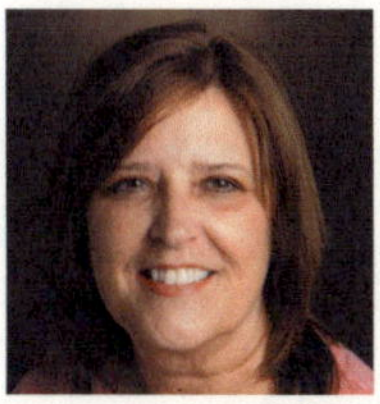

Marcia Spear is a Doctor of Nursing Practice for the Department of Plastic Surgery, Vanderbilt University Medical Center, Nashville, Tennessee, USA. She received her Masters and Doctorate degrees from Vanderbilt University, School of Nursing in 1999 and 2010, respectively. She holds faculty appointments in both the School of Medicine and School of Nursing. She has worked in the specialty of Plastic Surgery and Wound Care for over twenty years and has written numerous articles and publications on related issues.

Contents

Preface

The procedure of skin grafting has been performed since 3000BC and, with modern technology, has evolved through the years. While the development of new techniques and devices has significantly improved the functional as well as the aesthetic results from skin grafting, the fundamentals of skin grafting have remained the same, a healthy vascular granulating wound bed free of infection. Adherence to the recipient bed is the most important factor in skin graft survival and research continues introducing new techniques that promote this process. Biological and synthetic skin substitutes have also provided better treatment options as well as HLA tissue typing and the use of growth factors. Even today, skin grafts remain the most common and least invasive procedure for the closure of soft tissue defects.

It is with great pleasure that I bring you this updated collection of current concepts, the latest research, and future perspectives on skin grafting. We would like to extend a sincere thanks to the contributors of this project and encourage them to continue in their quests for solutions. We would also like to thank the entire staff at InTech for their ongoing support in the completion of this project and their dedication in bringing high-quality research and knowledge accessible across the world. It is the intent that this resource will serve as a reference for clinical decisions and generate ideas for future research, that when combined, will continue to optimize both functional and aesthetic patient outcomes.

Marcia Spear, DNP, ACNP-BC, CWS, CPSN
Doctor of Nursing Practice
Department of Plastic Surgery
Vanderbilt University Medical Center
USA

Part 1

Introduction

1

Split-Thickness Skin Grafts

Tamer Seyhan
Adana Numune Educ. & Train. Hospital
Turkey

1. Introduction

The use of split-thickness skin grafts (STSG) is the most common performed procedures to close defects unable to be closed with the simple approximation of the wound edges. The healing of a STSG donor site involves re-epithelialization from the epithelial appendages that are embedded in the dermis and subcutaneous fat.

STSGs are easy to harvest and are taken directly with a knife or with an instrument such as a dermatome. STSGs may be expanded in size using a meshing device or surgical knife.

The following topics are discussed in this chapter:

- Components of skin
- Classification of split thickness skin grafts
- Process of graft take and healing
- Indications and contraindications of split thickness skin grafts
- Preoperative considerations
- Split thickness skin graft donor sites and harvesting the graft
- Postoperative care of split thickness skin grafts and management of donor site
- Complications of split thickness skin grafts
- Preservation of split thickness skin grafts.

2. Components of skin

Skin consists of two layers derived from two different embryonic layers. The thinner, outermost layer is the "*epidermis*", which is derived from ectoderm; the thicker, innermost layer is the "*dermis*", which is derived from mesoderm. The epidermis accounts for approximately 5% of the skin thickness and the dermis comprises the remaining 95% (Vitness, 1977). The dermis contains connective tissue and skin appendages such as sebaceous glands, hair follicles and sweat glands. Although sebaceous glands are seated in the dermis, the hair follicles and sweat glands extend into subcutaneous fat.

The average thickness of human skin varies between 2 and 3 mm. Skin is thickest in the sacrum, palms, and soles of the feet and is thinnest in the eyelids and in the postauricular area. The epidermis of the face is relatively constant in thickness and measures approximately 150 microns; however, dermal thickness varies considerably. The dermis can be as thin as 200-250 μm in the eyelid and periorbital area, 900-1000 μm in the lip and forehead regions and as thick as 3 mm on the back skin (Gonzalez-Ulloa et al., 1954).

There are five distinct cellular layers of the epidermis. These layers include (from deep to superficial) the stratum basale (stratum germinativum), stratum spinosum (prickle cell layer), stratum granulosum, stratum lucidum, and stratum corneum. The *Malpighian layer* of the skin is a term that is generally defined as both the stratum basale and stratum spinosum as a unit. The cells of the epidermis arise from the stratum basale and are called keratinocytes. Keratinocytes gradually migrate superficially and fill with keratin and lipids and undergo desquamation throughout life. It has been determined that the renewal time of the Malpighian layers is about 19 days (Stal et al., 1987). Thus, each epidermal cell spends an average of 10 days in its migration to the surface. In addition to keratinocytes, melanocytes, Langerhans, and Merkel cells are also present in the epidermal layer of the skin. Melanocytes, found in the stratum basale, produce melanin, which is distributed to the epidermal cells and imparts characteristic pigmentation to the skin. Melanin also shields the skin from the deleterious effects of ultraviolet radiation by absorbing UV light and trapping photochemically activated free radicals. The Langerhans cells play a vital role in the immune response by identifying and processing the antigens for other local immunocompetent cells. The Merkel cells are found in the stratum basale clustered around hair follicles and are especially concentrated in the palms and soles. These cells also act as slowly adapting pressure mechanoreceptors.

The dermis consists of two layers: a thin outer *papillary layer* and a thick inner *reticular layer*. The papillary layer consists of randomly arranged collagen fibers, fine elastic fibers, and abundant ground substance. The ground substance consists of extracellular fluid and mucopolysaccharides, primarily hyaluronic acid, chondroitin sulfates, and glycoproteins. The proportion of ground substance and the production and turnover of collagen decreases with age and is replaced with fibrous intercellular tissue. The reticular layer is formed by dense, coarser, branching, collagenous fibers arranged in layers, mostly parallel to the surface. Fibroblasts make up the majority of cells in the dermis, along with interspersed mast cells and tissue macrophages. The structural strength of the dermal layer is provided by collagen. Collagen fibers are synthesized by dermal fibroblasts. The majority of collagen in the dermis is Type I collagen and constitutes up to 80% of the collagen in skin. Type III collagen constitutes about 15%, while Type V and Type VI account for the remainder. The typical ratio of Type I collagen to Type III collagen is 4:1(Kusuma et al., 2010).

The dermo-epidermal junction of human skin appears as an irregularly, wavy line; the ridges or rete pegs project into the dermis. With aging, these rete pegs diminish and subsequently lead to a decrease in the surface area of the dermal-epidermal junction. Branches from cutaneous arteries form a small vessel plexus within the dermis. The lymphatic plexuses are found in the papillary dermis, directly below the dermal papillary ridges. The skin possesses a rich supply of sensory nerves, which are organized as deep dermal and superficial dermal plexus. These nerves convey sensation from the skin to the brain through specialized receptors for touch (*Meissner's* corpuscles), pressure (*Pacinian* corpuscles and *Merkel* cells), temperature and pain (free nerve endings) Additionally, a network of autonomic fibers provide the primary innervation of cutaneous blood vessels, pilomotor units in the hair follicles, and the sweat and sebaceous glands (Gaboriau & Murakami, 2001).

Sweat glands, sebaceous glands and hair follicles are skin appendages. Sweat glands are found deep in the dermis and even in the subcutaneous tissue. The sweat glands are usually located deeper than the hair follicles; however, hair follicles reach in the subcutaneous fat of the bearded area of the male face. There are two types of sweat glands, apocrine and eccrine. The more numerous eccrine sweat glands are found over the general body surface of humans and open either at the sweat pores on the skin surface or above the opening of the sebaceous gland in the hair follicle walls. Apocrine sweat glands tend to be concentrated in the eyelids, axillae, periumblical area and genital area. The apocrine glands become more active at puberty secrete continuously. The secretions of apocrine glands produce a characteristic odor; however, the eccrine glands are odorless.

Sebaceous glands are derived from the pilosebaceous unit and are commonly associated with hair follicles. The sebaceous glands provide lubricant for the hair and skin and are larger and have more density in the skin of the forehead, nose, and cheeks.

Hair follicles are intradermal epithelial invaginations associated with sebaceous glands and smooth-muscle bundles called erector pili.

3. Classification of split-thickness skin grafts

Skin grafts are classified according to origin and thickness. Skin grafts are classified as *autograft, allograft (homograft), xenograft (heterograft)* and *isograft (syngenic)* according to the sources. An autograft is a graft transferred from a donor to recipient site in the same individual. An allograft (homograft) is a transplant between individuals of the same species. A xenograft (heterograft) is a graft transplanted between individuals of different species. An isograft (syngenic) is a graft transplanted between genetically matched genotypes, such as identical twins.

Split-thickness skin grafts (STSGs) are subdivided into *thin, medium* and *thick* STSGs.

- Split-thickness skin graft-thin (STSG-T; 0.008-0.012 in. or 0.2-0.3 mm)
- Split-thickness skin graft-medium (STSG-M; 0.012-0.018 in. or 0.3-0.45 mm)
- Split-thickness skin graft-thick (STSG-THK; 0.018-0.030 in. or 0.45-0.75 mm)

The STSG-T used by early surgeons such Ollier (1872) and Thiersch (1874) have been replaced by thicker split-thickness grafts (STSG-M, STSG-THK), which include all of the epidermis and a variable fraction of the dermis (Blair & Brown, 1929). Currently, the most commonly used split-thickness graft thickness is between 0.012 and 0.018 inch (0.30 to 0.45 mm) in thickness. The average STSG is cut at 0.015 inch and can be checked by inserting a No.15 blade, which approximates that thickness.

The mesh skin graft was first described by Tanner in 1964 as a method of expanding skin grafts (Tanner et al., 1964). Preparation of the meshed skin graft is performed with a skin graft mesher. The graft is placed on a template and is passed through the device. The most commonly used expansion ratio is 1:1.5, which increases the surface area by 50 percent. Mesh grafts are primarily useful in two situations: (1) when there is insufficient skin; or (2) when a very irregular surface must be covered with a graft where a sheet might not adhere well (Fig. 3c). Also, the drainage of fluid through the slit-like perforations produced by the meshing procedure prevents hematoma formation and permits the graft to be applied to an actively bleeding wound. The expanded graft must heal in between the expansion by epithelization; therefore, the underlying wound may contract significantly.

4. Process of graft take and healing

Grafts initially survive via diffusion, called *plasmatic imbibition,* and subsequently *inosculation* and *revascularization* occurs. Immediately after a skin graft is placed on the recipient bed, a fibrin network provides a scaffold for the necessary graft adherence. During the first 48 hours, the graft becomes engorged with plasmatic fluid by means of diffusion. A poorly vascularized bed requires a longer period of plasmatic imbibition before the graft is revascularized. The ingrowth of capillary buds from the recipient bed into the open vessels on the undersurface of the graft is called inosculation and occurs within 2 to 4 days. Revascularization is thought to be directed by angiogenic factors and can be restored within 5 to 7 days. Thin grafts of skin are revascularized more rapidly than thick grafts. Lymphatic circulation, which is established by the fifth day, may aid in decompressing the increased graft interstitial fluid. Within the first week the thickness of the epidermis can increase seven to eightfold. Dermal fibroblasts proliferate vigorously in healing skin grafts after an initial decrease of three days. By the seventh to eighth day there is a marked hyperplasia of fibroblasts as the graft begins to heal.

Almost all skin grafts are capable of sweating in response to stimulation of the nerves that ingrow from the recipient site. STSGs often have deficient function of sebaceous glands and therefore should be lubricated for three months. Most patients with skin grafts do not obtain completely normal sensation. The recovery of sensation in humans can begin as early as one to two months after surgery, and may be abnormal during the first year. Full-thickness skin grafts appear to achieve better sensation than split-thickness grafts, although the rate of return of innervation is faster in STSGs.

5. Indications and contraindications of split-thickness skin grafts

5.1 Indications of split-thickness skin grafts

- Immediate coverage of clean soft tissue defects and accelerated wound healing (Fig. 1a,b.)
- Immediate coverage of burn defects and reduced fluid loss from the wounds.
- Prevention of scar contracture and enhanced cosmesis in superficial wounds.

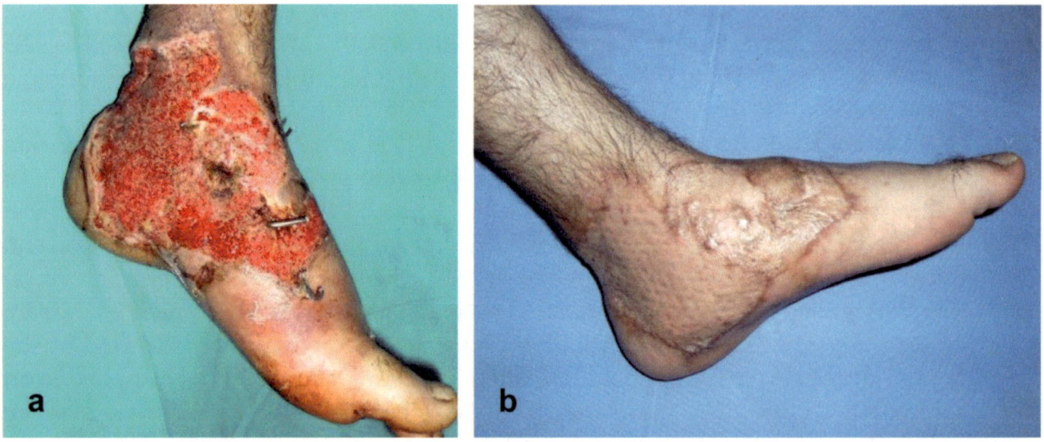

Fig. 1. (a) View of the traumatic clean soft tissue defect before split-thickness skin grafting. (b) Post-operative view of the patient after split-thickness skin grafting.

5.2 Contraindications of split-thickness skin grafts

- Infected wounds have poorly vascularized and necrotic tissue. After management of the infection and necrotic tissues, skin grafting becomes suitable (Fig. 2a,b,c; Fig. 3 a,b,c,d).

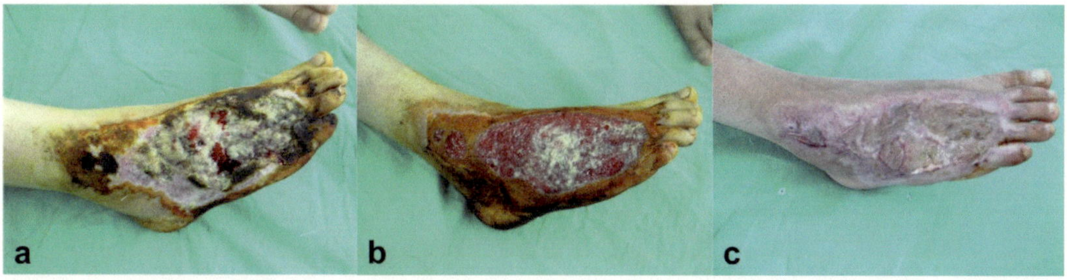

Fig. 2. (a). Preoperative view of infected, poorly vascularized wound with necrotic tissues.
Fig. 2. (b). After management of the infection and necrotic tissues of the wounds.
Fig. 2. (c). Postoperative view of the defects after split-thickness skin grafting.

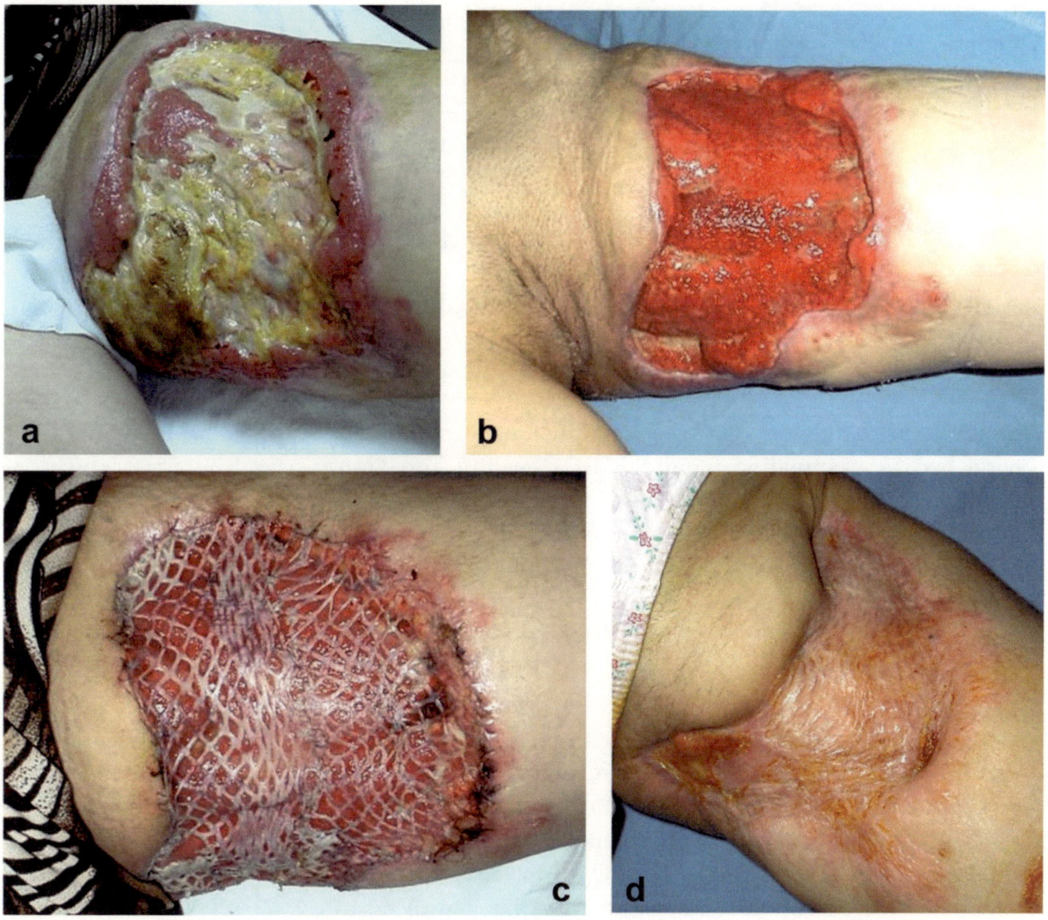

Fig. 3. (a). Preoperative view of infected, poorly vascularized wound with necrotic tissues.
Fig. 3. (b). After management of the infection and necrotic tissues of the wounds.
Fig. 3. (c,d). Postoperative view of the defects after split-thickness skin grafting.

- Exposed bone without periosteum, cartilage without perichondrium, tendon without paratenon or nerve structures (Fig. 4.).

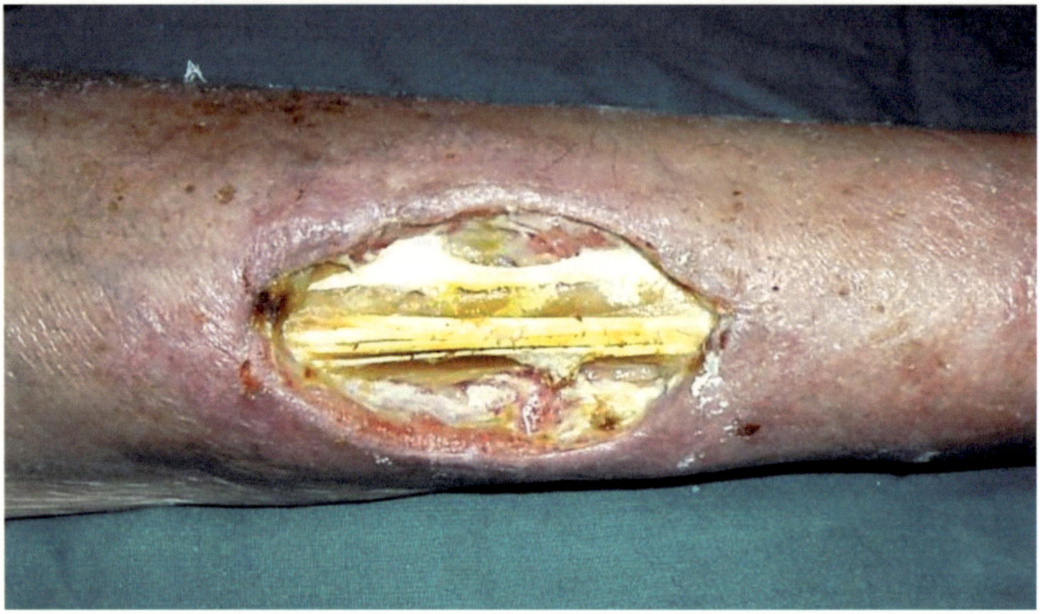

Fig. 4. View of the defect on the cruris, which is not suitable for grafting.

6. Preoperative considerations

Wounds considered for skin grafting must have a well vascularized and non-infected wound bed. A granulating wound with a healthy appearance usually denotes sufficient nutritional status and overall health of the patient (Fig. 2b, 3b). Hypertrophic granulation tissue needs to be either trimmed or flattened in order to enhance graft take and epithelial migration. Epithelial migration at the edges of the granulating surface may be a sign that the wound is ready for application of a skin graft. Serial debridements, culture-specific antibacterial therapy and frequent dressing changes continue to be the mainstay of preparing good recipient bed.

Pretreatment of a wound with vacuum-assisted closure (*V.A.C.® KCI, USA, Inc., San Antonio, TX, USA*) therapy is advisable to increase granulation tissue, tissue perfusion and decrease edema, bacterial colonization, wound exudate in chronic wounds (Fig.5 a,b,c) (Teot, 2004). VAC therapy consists of a controlled application of continuous or intermittent subatmospheric pressure to a sponge-like wound dressing to promote healing (Argenta & Morykwas, 1997). Classic VAC therapy is not advisable when the wound is infected. An alternative method for infected wounds is the use of *V.A.C. ® Instill™*, which has an additional instillation line for topical antiseptics and antibiotics and removal of topical solutions from the wound site (Bernstein & Tam, 2005). Silver-impregnated sponges (*V.A.C. GranuFoam Silver®)* provide continuous delivery of silver directly to the wound bed and may be preferred in infected wounds during VAC therapy.

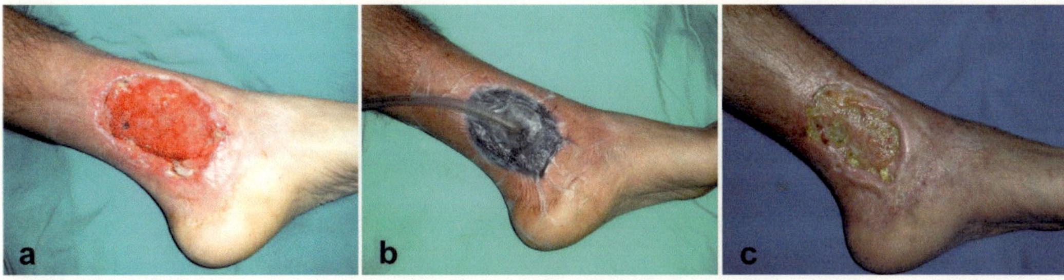

Fig. 5. (c) View of a venous ulcer on the left medial malleolus. (b) The use of VAC dressing for preparing the wound bed for grafting. (a) View of the freshly granulating venous ulcer defect after four VAC dressing changes.

6.1 Split-thickness skin graft donor sites and harvesting the graft

STSGs can be taken from any area of the body, including the scalp and extremities (Fowler & Dempsey, 1998). When possible, STSGs should be taken from hidden areas such as the anterolateral thigh and lateral buttock. If STSGs are required for the face, skin harvested from "blush zones" such as the supraclavicular area and scalp is preferable. A thin graft (0.010 inch or less) leaves the hair follicles in the donor scalp and avoids hair growth in the recipient bed. Also, an important source of STSGs is avulsed skin in trauma or surgically removed skin.

Skin graft harvesting can be performed by various tools including knives and dermatomes (Table 1, Fig. 6 a,b,c,d).

Skin graft harvesting tools
1. Free-hand knives
2. Various types of dermatomes
• Drum (manually operated)
• Powered dermatomes (Electric or air);
- Battery operated Davol dermatome
- Humeca Battery operated dermatome
- Padgett dermatome
- Zimmer air dermatome

Table 1. Skin graft harvesting tools

Free-hand knives are manual dermatomes. The large Humby-type knives and smaller Goulian type knives are used for harvesting the STSG manually but provide grafts with irregular edges and grafts of variable thickness (Fig. 6a). Of the powered dermatomes, the Padgett dermatome is lighter and is easy to handle and comes in three widths: small-3 inches wide, medium-4 inches wide, and giant-5 inches wide (Fig.6c). The thickness is determined by turning the setting dermatome knob to the appropriate thickness.

The dimensions of the graft are marked 15-20% larger than the dimensions of the defect. The skin is lubricated with sterile Vaseline ointment to facilitate graft cutting. It is essential to keep the donor area surface flat, taut and stretched, for smooth, uniform thickness during graft cutting. An assistant applies counter-tension on the skin during advancing of the dermatome and graft harvest is performed in a proximal to distal direction. An surgical assistant can pick up the ends of the skin graft with forceps while the surgeon harvests the graft with the dermatome.

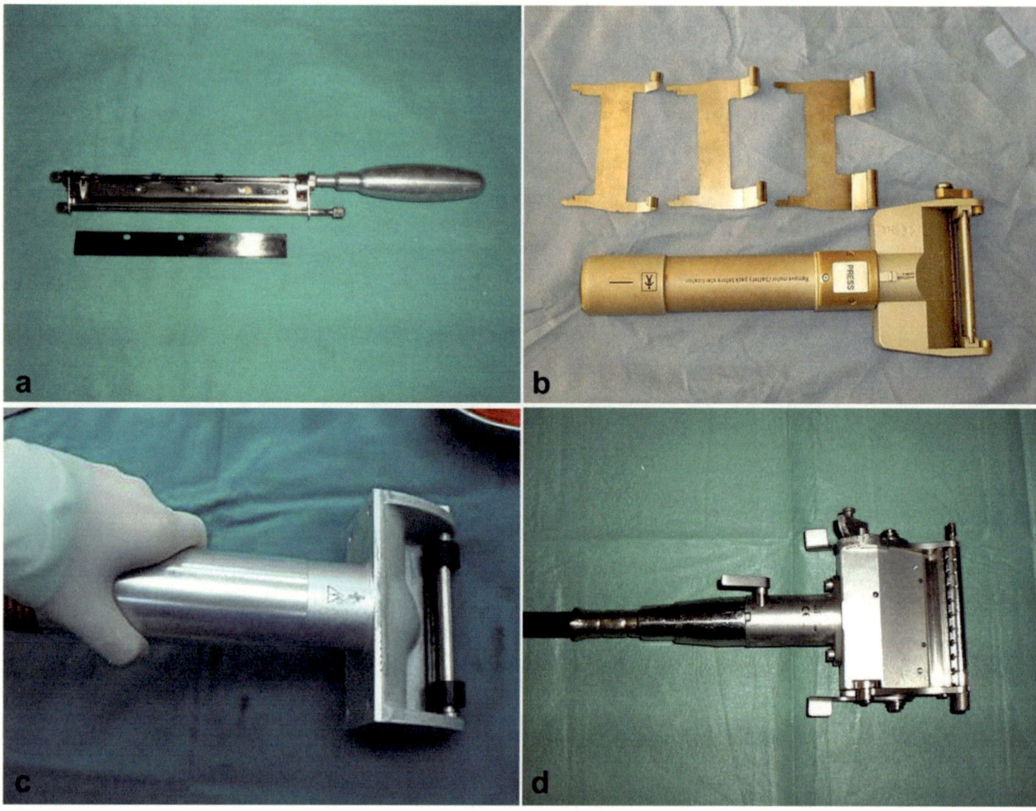

Fig. 6. The most popular tools for skin graft harvesting. (a) Watson's modification of Humby knife. (b) Humeca Battery operated dermatome. (c) Padgett Dermatome. (d) Zimmer air dermatome.

6.2 Postoperative care of split-thickness skin grafts and management of donor site

The graft is placed on the recipient bed, trimmed with scissors and fixed with sutures or metal staples. Serous fluid or blood beneath the graft can be a barrier to graft take and a source of infection that will result in graft loss. Multiple small "pie crust" incisions with a ≠11 scalpel blade or fine scissors provide drainage of the fluid or blood beneath the graft. In most cases of skin grafting, the optimal dressing is a bolus or tie-over dressing to ensure contact and immobilization between the graft and the host bed. A circumferential compression dressing and a plaster can be used for immobilization in extremity skin grafts. A tie-over dressing is fashioned by placing sutures around the periphery of the graft and is tied over a piece of fine mesh, ointment impregnated gauze, covered with cotton sheeting or cotton balls. The tied sutures gently press the dressing down onto the skin graft, which in turn is pressed onto the wound bed. This maneuver immobilizes the graft on the wound and prevents hematoma collection. Before the tie-over dressing is applied, the surgeon should ensure that there are no blood clots underneath the graft. The tie-over dressing is left in place for three or four days. After removal of the dressing, small collections of seroma may be evacuated by cutting over the top of the graft and an ointment impregnated gauze dressing applied for another 2 or 3 days. When the skin graft is stable and adherent, antibiotic ointment or another mild lubricating agent is used for three months.

Negative pressure dressing (VAC® therapy) can be used to facilitate skin graft adherence when grafting difficult wounds (e.g. radiated wounds, wounds with irregular or mobile recipient beds and in difficult anatomic locations (Schneider et al., 1998; Scherer et al., 2002) (Fig. 7a,b,c,d.). The VAC dressing is applied to the STSG at 125 mmHg "continuous" mode suction after the STSG is covered with a single layer of non-adherent Chlorhexidine or Xeroform gauze.

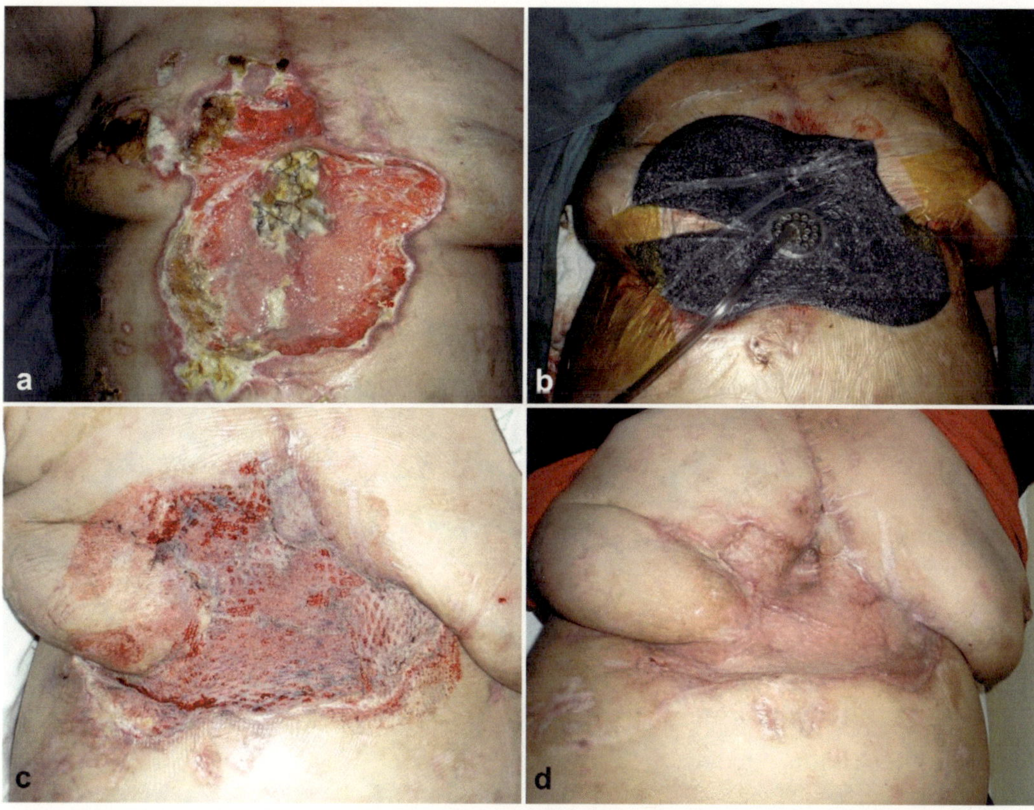

Fig. 7. (a) View of sternal wounds with irregular and mobile recipient bed. (b) Application of VAC dressing on STSG covered with a single layer of non-adherent Chlorhexidine gauze. (c) View of grafted defect after removal of VAC dressing on the fourth postoperative day. (d) Late postoperative view of the same patient.

6.3 Donor site healing and maintenance

The healing of the donor site occurs by epithelial migration from the epithelial remnants in the dermis such as hair follicles, sebaceous gland, and sweat glands. Epithelial migration also occurs at the wound margins. After harvesting a STSG, the donor site is treated with topical, epinephrine-soaked sponges to reduce bleeding and then a single layer of non-adherent Chlorhexidine or Xeroform gauze is applied to the donor site, followed by a layer of bulky gauze on top of this. The next day, the outer gauze is removed, leaving behind the Chlorhexidine or Xeroform gauze, which can be allowed to air dry; a gentle heat lamp application speeds epithelization. In an area where external contamination is likely, a closed dressing is preferable. The more superficial a STSG is cut, the faster the donor site will heal. The healing of the STSGs donor sites take place over seven to fourteen days (Fig. 8 a,b). Donor sites from which thicker split grafts are cut may not heal for several weeks

Alternatively, donor site are dressed with artificial semi-permeable transparent dressings (e.g. Biobrane®, Opsite® or Tegaderm®) or biologic dressings (e.g. cadaveric skin, sterile irradiated allograft, pig skin, amniotic membrane, cultured keratinocyte grafts) (Fedman, 1991; Voineskos, 2009). Thin STSGs usually leave minimal scarring, whereas the thicker STSGs tend to produce hypertrophic scarring in some patients.

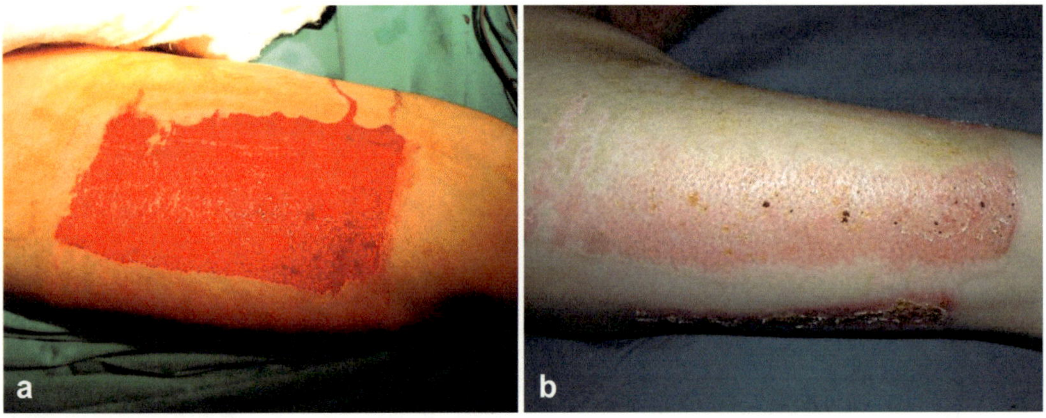

Fig. 8. (a) View of a STSG donor site on the right anterolateral thigh. (b) View of the same donor site on the fourteenth day.

6.4 Complications of split-thickness skin grafts

Graft contraction, graft failure, hyperpigmentation, itchiness and dryness of the graft, durability and growth problems are the most common complications of split- thickness skin grafting.

Primary contraction, an elastic recoil of the skin caused by retractile forces, occurs as soon as the graft is harvested. The contraction of a healing graft and wound is referred to as *secondary contraction*. Secondary contraction, a longer process and clinically more important, is probably caused by a combination of skin graft and host bed contraction. The dermal component of grafted skin appears to exert the main influence on secondary contraction. The thinner the skin graft, the less the primary graft contracture and the more marked the secondary graft contracture. Primary graft contracture is approximately 40% of graft surface for a FTSG, 20% for a medium thickness STSG, and 10% for a thin STSG (Senchenkov et al., 2009). The contraction of a wound covered by a STSG can be inhibited by splinting, which needs to be continued for four to six months to overcome the acute effect of the myofibroblasts.

The causes of split thickness skin graft failure are listed in Table 2. Most skin graft failures can be ascribed to flaws in the recipient bed. Tissue with limited blood supply, such as bone, cartilage or tendon or sites with necrosis or infection do not accept skin graft (Fig. 2a, Fig. 3a, Fig. 4). Chronic wounds must be free of pus and should have a healthy, pink to beefy-red appearance with an ideal wound pH of 7.4 or higher. All granulation tissues contain bacteria, but not all are infected. Particular attention should be paid to eliminating *Streptococcus*. Wherever possible, underlying systemic health problems causing the wound, such as venous stasis and arterial occlusion, should be corrected before skin grafting is attempted.

Causes of Split-Thickness Skin Graft Failure
• Inadequate recipient bed (poor vascularity) • Hematoma, seroma • Inadequate graft fixation and graft shearing • Infection (in particular Streptococcus, which can "eat up" a graft within 24 hours) • Technical errors (too thick or too thin graft, upside-down graft. • Systemic health problems and bad nutritional status

Table 2. Causes of Split-Thickness Skin Graft Failure

Hyperpigmentation of the skin graft is variable and depends on the amount of pigmentation present in the donor site. Generally, STSGs darken more than FTSGs. Although FTSGs maintain the best pigment match, STSGs often develop significantly dark pigmentation. Sunshine should be avoided for the first six months by use of sun-blocking agents or clothing to prevent long-lasting hyperpigmentation developing in a new skin graft. Both STSGs and their donor sites may scale and remain itchy and dry for many months because the lubricating sebaceous glands have been temporarily devitalized. Lubrication with greasy ointment such as Vaseline, lanolin or cocoa butter helps to replace the lubricating function. Thick STSGs have greater resistance to trauma. Although FTSGs grow successfully in children, the growth of STSGs may be limited.

7. Preservation of split-thickness skin grafts

In order to close skin defects, skin grafts are best stored on its donor site and harvested painless within five days (Shepard, 1972). Skin grafts may also be stored for longer periods, away from the patient, by being refrigerated. Such grafts may be moistened in sterile saline and then placed in a refrigerator at 4 °C in a sterile Petri dish labeled with the patient's name and the date of graft harvesting. It may be wise to discard grafts after 8 days, although grafts may be kept for 2 or 3 weeks (Senchenkov et al., 2009).

Long-term storage of autografts and allograft requires special techniques to protect against cell death. Freezing causes tissue death because of concentration within the cell, leaving behind a lethal concentration of salts. Protective agents such as 15% glycerol or 10% dimethyl sulfoxide (DMSO) in Ringer's solution and storage at -70 °C with liquid nitrogen help to protect against this type of injury and allow viable skin to be preserved for up to 28 days (Lawrence, 1972). Control of the rate of freezing reduces the damage caused by intracellular ice crystals. The best results were obtained when grafts were slowly frozen and rapidly thawed.

The other technique of storage is *freeze-drying* of skin for storage at room temperature. Freeze drying maintains most of the structural details of cells and presumably leaves many of the proteins and enzymes of the tissue intact. The process involves rapid freezing of the tissue by immersing it in liquid nitrogen or chilled isopentane. High-speed freezing reduces the mechanical distortion of the microscopic structure caused by the slow growth of ice crystals in and between the cells. This tissue is subsequently kept frozen while water is removed from the solid state by sublimation. The dried tissue is usually sealed in a vacuum and stored at room temperature (Yukna et al., 1977)

Specialized skin banks have been developed to store large amounts of cadaver skin for treatment of massive burns (Konstantinow, 1991). Standardized techniques for cadaver skin graft preservation use glycerol and rapid freezing with liquid nitrogen (Ninneman et al., 1978). The treated allografts are thawed and used for temporary burn dressings, to be changed every five days. Pigskin xenografts have also been used fresh or frozen for burn treatment.

8. Conclusion

STSGs constitute the most commonly performed procedures for the closure of skin defects that can not be closed with the simple approximation of the wound edges. When a patient has a full-thickness loss-of-skin defect exceeding 30% of the body area, STSGs taken from the patient are not available in sufficient quantity. Cultured autologous keratinocytes may be used to close larger open wounds in such situations. Unfortunately, the lack of dermis makes the epidermal graft rather thin and fragile. Intensive efforts to develop epidermal and dermal skin substitutes show the greatest potential, at present, for future success.

9. References

Argenta, L.C., & Morykwas, M.J. (1997). Vacuum-assisted closure: a new method for wound control and treatment: clinical experience. *Ann Plast Surg*, Vol. 38, No.6, pp.563-576, ISSN: 0148-7043

Bernstein, B.H., & Tam, H. (2005). Combination of subatmospheric pressure dressing and gravity feed antibiotic instillation in the treatment of post-surgical diabetic foot wound: a case rseries. *Wounds*, Vol.17, No.2, pp.37-48.

Blair, V.P., & Brown, J.B. (1929). The use and uses of large split skin grafts of intermediate thickness. *Surg Gynecol Obstet*, Vol.49, pp.82-97.

Fedman, D.L. (1991). Which dressing for split-thickness skin graft donor sites? *Ann Plast Surg*, Vol.27, No.3, pp.288-91, ISSN: 0148-7043

Fowler, A., & Dempsey, A. (1998). Split-thickness skin graft donor sites. *J Wound Care* , Vol.7, No.8, pp.399-402.

Gaboriau, H.P. & Murakami, C.S. (2001). Skin anatomy and flap physiology. *Otolaryngol Clin North Am*, Vol.34, No.3, pp.555-69, ISSN: 0030-6665

Gonzalez-Ulloa, M.; Castillo, A., Stevens, E., Alvarez, Fuertes, G., Leonelli, F. & Ubaldo F. (1954). Preliminary study of the total restoration of the facial skin. *Plast Reconstr Surg*, Vol.13, No.3, pp.151-161, ISSN: 0032-1052

Konstantinow, A., Mühlbauer, W., Hartinger, A., & von Donnersmarck, G.G. (1991). Skin banking: a simple method for cryopreservation of split-thickness skin and cultured human epidermal keratynocytes. Ann Plast Surg, Vol.26, No.1, pp. 89-97, ISSN: 0148-7043

Kusuma, S., Vuthori, R.K., Piliang, M., & Zins, J.E. (2010). Skin Anatomy and Physiology. In: *Plastic and Reconstructive Surgery*, Siemionow, M.Z., Eisenmann-Klein, M. (Eds) pp.161-171., Springer-Verlag, ISBN 978-1-84882-512-3, USA.

Lawrence, J.C. (1972). Storage and skin metabolism. *Br J Plast Surg*, Vol.25, No.4, pp.440-453, ISSN: 0007-1226

Ninneman, J.L., Fisher, J.C., & Frank, H.A. (1978). Clinical skin banking: a simplified system for processing, storage, and retrieval of human allografts. J Trauma, Vol.18, No.10, pp. 723-725, ISSN: 0022-5282

Scherer, L.A., Shiver, S., & Chang M. (2002). The vacuum assisted closure device: a method of securing skin grafts and improving graft survival. *Arch Surg*, Vol.137, No.8, pp.930-933, ISSN: 0004-0010

Schneider, A.M., Morykwas, M.J., & Argenta, L.C. (1998). A new and reliable method of securing skin grafts to the difficult recipient bed. *Plast Reconstr Surg*, Vol.102, No.4, pp.1195-1198, ISSN: 0032-1052

Senchenkov, A., Valerio, I.L., & Manders, E.K. (2009). Grafts. In: *Plastic Surgery: Indications and Practice*, Guyuron, B., Eriksson, E., Persing, J.A. (Eds.)pp. 95-104, Elsevier, **ISBN 13:** 978-1-4160-4081-1, USA .

Shepard, G.H. (1972). The storage of split-skin grafts on their donor sites. Clinical and experimental study. *Plast Reconstr Surg*, Vol.49, No.2, pp.115-122, ISSN: 0032-1052

Stal, S., Spira, M., & Hamilton, S. (1987). Skin morphology and function. Clin Plast Surg, Vol.14, No.2, pp.201-208, ISSN: 0094-1298.

Tanner, J.C., Vandeput, J., & Olley, J.F. (1964). The mesh skin graft. *Plast Reconstr Surg*, Vol.34, (Sep 1964), pp.287, ISSN: 0032-1052

Teot, L., (2004). The theory of negative pressure wound therapy (NPWT). *Wounds*, Vol.16, No.2, (Suppl), pp. 2-5,

Vitness, LM. (1977) Grafting of Skin. *Surg Clin North Am*, Vol.57, No.5, pp. 939-960, ISSN: 0039-6109

Voineskos, S.H., Ayeni, O.A., McKnight, L., Thoma, A. (2009). Systematic review of skin graft donor-site dressings. *Plast Reconstr Surg*, Vol.124, No.1, pp.298-306, ISSN: 0032-1052

Yukna, R.A., Tow, H.D., Carrol, P.B., Vernino, A.R., & Bright, R.W. (1977). Evaluation of the use of freze-dried skin allografts in the treatment of human mucogingival problems. J Periodontol, Vol.48, No.4, pp.187-193, ISSN: 0022-3492

2

Skin Graft Harvesting and Donor Site Selection

Yusuf Kenan Coban, Ahmet Hamdi Aytekin
and Göktekin Tenekeci
Inonu University, Medical Faculty, Plastic Reconstructive and Aesthetic Surgery Department, & Burn Unit, Malatya
Turkey

1. Introduction

Acute and chronic wounds are characterized by breakdown of the integrity of the soft tissue envelope surrounding any portion of the body. Flaps and grafts are the two main surgical procedures utilized to repair soft tissue loss. A simple skin graft applied as a thin layer harvested with a dermatome, a scalpel or a special knife may provide a durable coverage. A *free* skin graft is a piece of skin that has been completely separated from its local blood supply and transferred to a wound at another site, where it must establish new vascular connections through the recipient bed to survive. Skin grafts usually are the first consideration when primary wound closure cannot be achieved. This is true especially for deep burns of wide body areas.(Rudolph R, Ballantyne DL. Skin grafts. In: McCarthy JG, ed. *Plastic Surgery*. Philadelphia: Saunders; 1990:221–274) A skin graft would be contraindicated, if inosculation from the recipient bed is unreliable with repeated motion or trauma to the area, or in wound infection (Paletta CE, Pokorny JJ, Rumbolo P. Skin grafts. In: Mc- Carthy JG, ed. *Plastic Surgery*. Philadelphia: Saunders Elsevier; 2006:293–316.)

2. Historical perspective regarding to skin grafting

Sir Astley Cooper removed skin from an amputed thumb and used it for stump defect covarage in 1817 (Tiersch C : Über Hautverplanzung. Verh Dtsch Ges Chir 15-17, 1886). Nevertheless skin grafting was not fully accepted for clinical use untill the last quarter of the 19th century. Reverdin was first to draw attention to the technique by successfully performing small pinch grafts in 1972 (Reverdin JL: De la greffe epidermique. Arch Gen Med 19:276;555, 703, 1972.) In 1874, Thiersch extended the use of the pinch graft using large sheets of thin skin grafts to cover the wounds (Tiersch C : Über Hautverplanzung. Verh Dtsch Ges Chir 15-17, 1886.) Blair and Brown (1929) first used the term "intermediate split-thicknes graft" (Blair VP, Brown JB: Use and uses of large split skin grafts of intermediate thickness. Surg Gynecol Obstet 49: 82-97, 1929.) Afterwards, Padgett described a technique for thick skin grafting (Padgett EC. Skin grafting of the burned patient. Plast Reconstr Surg. 2(4): 368-74, 1946). Skin grafting has been the most commonly used technique for reconstruction of cutaneous defects over the last decades.

3. Techniques of harvest in different types of skin grafts

Skin grafts may be physically in one of these three forms; meshed, sheet (unmeshed), pinch/punch. Each type of skin graft has its own harvesting technique. A preoperative plan and surgical judgement is necessary for determining which type of graft will be used. Full thickness skin grafts include all skin appendages, the epidermis and full-thickness of dermis, and splitt-thickness skin graft include a superficial portion of dermis together with epidermis and some of the skin appendages. Many techniques of skin grafting require little experience and only basic surgical equipment. A classification of skin grafts according to depth is seen in Table 1.

Name		**Thickness (mm)**
Split thickness	Thin (Thiersch-Ollier)	0.15-0.3
	Intermediate (Blair-Brown)	0.3-0.45
	Thick (Padgett)	0.45-0.6
Full thickness	(Wolfe-Krause)	>0.6

Table 1. Classification of skin grafts according to depth

3.1 General principles for skin grafting

Grafting should be done only onto a well-vascularised viable wound surface, such as granulating tissue. Whether the impairments to wound healing and closure are local or systemic, they must be addressed appropriately. Proper wound preparation certainly determines the success of skin grafting. Apropriate debridement is necessary for wound bed preparation. Debridement by hydrosurgical, biological and chemical methods has been reported (Meaume S.Methods of non surgical debridement of wounds in 2011.:Soins 752:44-47; 2011). Simple metallic sponges of the sort used in the kitchens which can be sterilized easily are effective for intraoperative surgical debridement. Simple wiping of the wound surface may be adequate enough to remove debris, especilally granulation tissue and soft eschar. Optimizing the patient's medical condition before surgical closure of a wound can mean the difference between a succesfull outcome and an undesirable one. A delay in grafting a suboptimal wound is also good surgical judgment.

3.2 Splitt thickness skin graft

Split-thickness skin grafts (STSG) can be harvested rapidly by using a mechanical dermatome. The donor site will heal because the whole of this epidermis can regenerate from deeper parts of the dermis which has left behind on ground. During the harvets by using a harvesting apparatus (dermatome), the donor site should be stabilized and fixed in order to opimise the procedure. The technique of skin grafting is often learned and practiced today using electric or air-powered dermatomes the manuplation of which doesn't require any skill when compared to the harvest by free hand knives.

3.2.1 Types of dermatomes

A dermatome is a surgical instrument used to produce thin slices of skin from a donor site and is the main tool for skin graft harvesting. Dermatomes can be operated either manually or electrically. The use of different types of safety razors as a dermatome has been described by some authors. Goullian (1968) constructed a skin grafts set from a weck straight razor by adding a fixed handle and a choice of interchangeable space setters to cut different thickness of grafts.(Goullian D.A new economical dermatome Plast Reconst Surg 42: 85, 1968) Snow described the use of a shick injector razor (Snow JW. Safety razor dermatome Plast Reconstr Surg 41: 184, 1968). Shoul (1966) modified a gillette safety razor by filling out the central strut of the safety guard using another blade as a skim. (Shoul M.Skin grafting under local anesthesia using a new safety razor Am J Surg 112.959, 1966) These old- fashioned instruments and shaving blades are difficult to obtain today.

Manual dermatomes are also known as hand-held dermatomes. Occasional users are more likely to use the hand-held knife where adjustment of depth is more difficult. Though most modern graft knives, e.g. the Humby knife and the modified Watson knife, possess an adjustment facility, the appropriate setting is usually determined by eye-balling. Humby skin grafting knife is the most popular. Disadvantages of hand-held knives are harvesting of grafts with irregular edges and grafts of variable thickness. Additonally, its lenght makes many areas inaccessable to harvest skin grafts which poses another disadvantage (Figure 1). This is especially true in infants where the convexity of limbs allows grafts after only an inch wide. In fact with the narrow dermatome (modified safety razor, sober hand dermatome) one can take skin graft practically from anywhere on the body. Use of single blade for coverage of mild to moderate defects is sufficient while the very large defects may require more. The simplicity of the narrow dermatome machine is such that skin grafting can be done by every surgeon. The dermatome is hold firmly against the tightly hold skin at a predetermined angle and the graft of the desired lenght is harvested quickly. Lubrication and a tonque depressor facilitate even harvesting of STSG. Use of a semipermeable membrane in STSG donor site before harvesting has been described for minimising trauma to the graft. (Sams HH, McDonalds MA, Stasko T.Usefull adjunct to harvest split-thickness skin grafts. Dermatol Surg:30(12pt 2): 1591-1592, 2004).

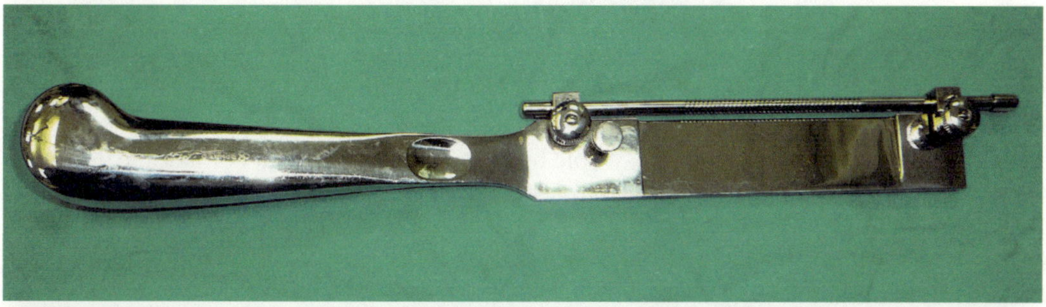

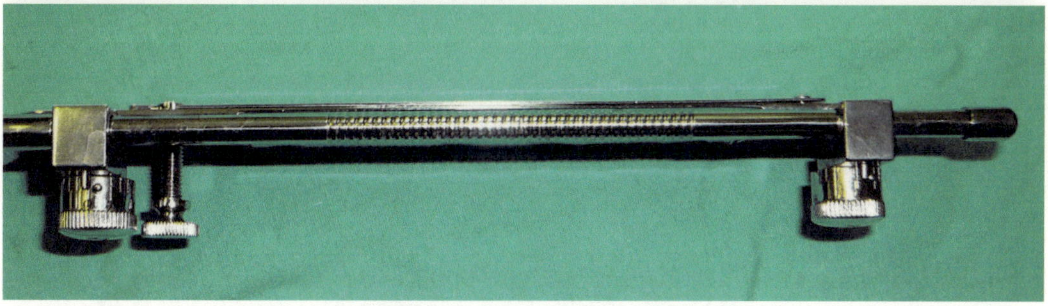

Fig. 1. An example of hand dermatome (schink type): frontal view (top) and lateral view showing Skin Graft thickness adjustment mechanism (bottom).

Electrical dermatomes are better for cutting out thinner and larger strips of skin with a more homogenous thickness. Dermatomes which were operated by air pressure, such as Brown or Zimmer dermatome, achieved higher speed and precision. Since an electrical dermatomes require electrical energy supply through an electrical cable. It is impractical to sterilize those cable during the operation. Humeca developed a new dermatome for free handed harvesting skin graft with a predetermined thickness of about 0,25 mm. (FIGURE 2).

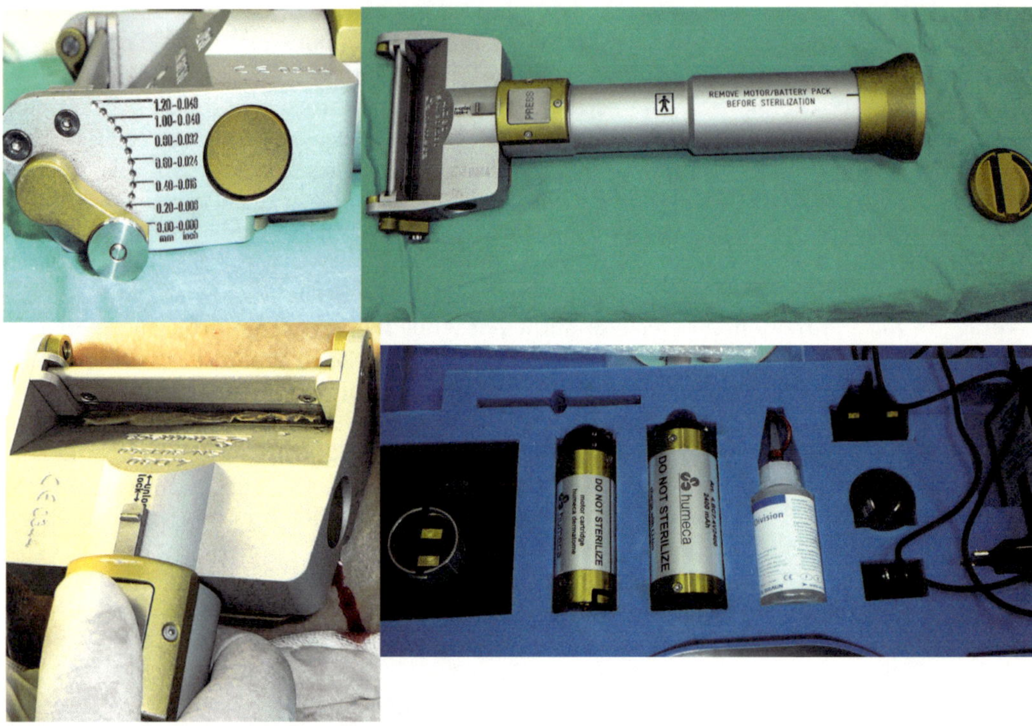

Fig. 2. Humeca electrical dermatome, whole body of cordless electrical dermatome (top right), justification site (top left), easily harvesting STSG (bottom left), and rechargeable batteries with its charging unit (bottom right).

3.2.2 Graft expansion

Expansion techniques are used to speed up the epithelialization process while diminishing the need for total amount of graft to be harvested. Various ways to expand grafts have been described including pinch grafts, meshing and micrografting (Meek technique) are among these ways. An expanded graft presents a larger cumulative perimeter through which epithelial outgrowth can proceed.

3.2.3 Meshing

Meshing is the term used for slitting a sheet graft and stretching it to open up prior to transplantation. This method of grafting has wide application in the treatment of burns and large contaminated wounds. Meshing ratios greater than 1 : 3 can be difficult to handle, as the skin curls on itself. When larger expansion ratios are desired, it is recommended to use meek micrograft technique for faster healing in body regions like thorax and abdomen. A

well-known type of mesher contains circular blades and requires the use of grooved plastic carriers (Figure 3). By using such an instrument the blades are forced under pressure to roll over the grooved carrier, thus cutting the graft at locations where the blades contact the carrier. Conventional skin graft carriers have a groove pattern of straight lines from the left to the right under a certain angle. Humeca introduced V-shaped groove pattern which prevents distortion during cutting a mesher. Advantage of these V carriers is to achieve quickly a more regular meshed grafts.
Humeca supplies two diferent expansion ratios (1:1,5 and 1 : 3) and one perforation carrier (1:1 ratio). (Humeca Mesher and V- carries.Properties and instructions for use; www.humeca.nl/humeca-mesher) Mesh grafts are expanded by a mechanical device and are used to cute multiple slits in the graft to be stretched. Grafts can be meshed at ratios of 1:1,5 - 1: 4 (FIGURE 4).

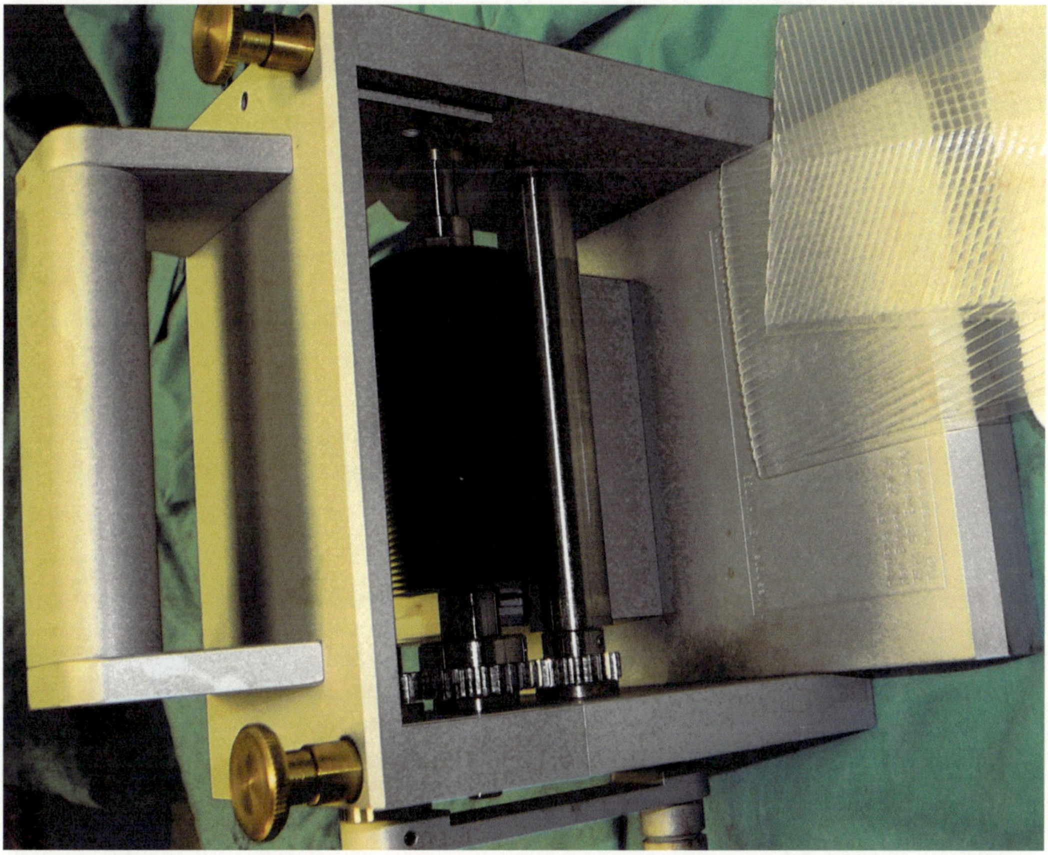

Fig. 3. Two different types of the humeca v-carries (6.V10 -1.5 and 6.V10-3.0, thickness 1.0 mm and expansion ratio 1.5 and 3).

Meshing allows the leakage of serum and blood from wound, minimizing the risk formation of hematomes or seromas that could compromise graft survival. Meshed grafts can also be useful to cover larger surface areas by means of stretching and expanding.

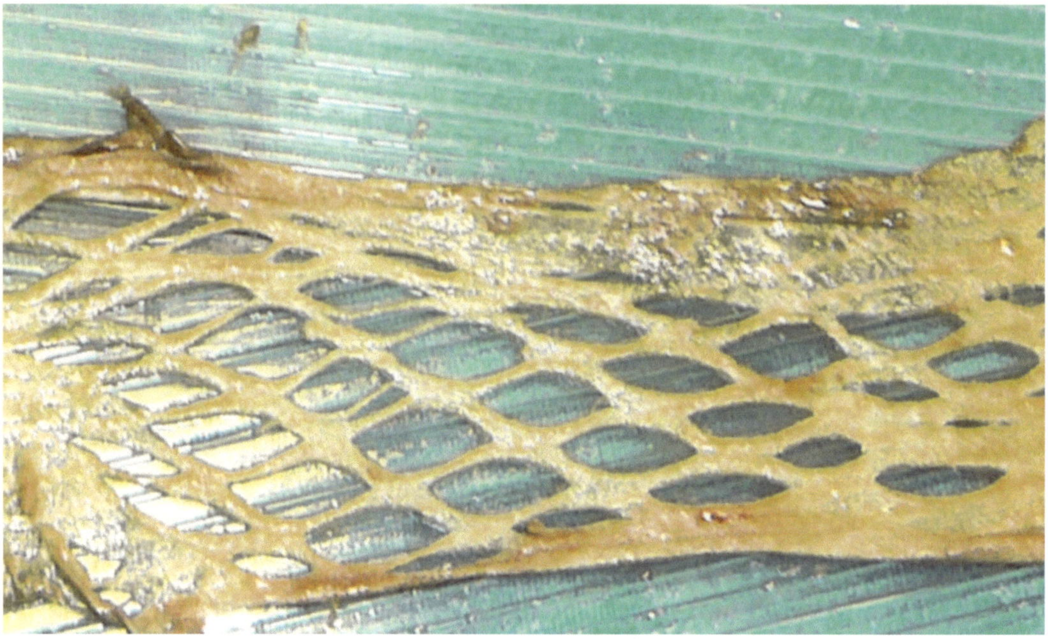

Fig. 4. Meshed skin graft at ratio of 1:3 is seen.

3.2.4 Meek technique

Meek (1958) described a technique for expanding a small piece of skin graft with a dermatome in 1958 (Meek CP, Successful microdermagrafting using the Meek-Wall microdermatome - *Am. Surg.* vol. 29, pp. 61 , 1958). This technique was later modified by other authors (Taner C, Vabdeput JF and Olley JF. The mesh skin graft, Plast Reconstr Surg 34 ; 287-292, 1964 and Kreis RW, Mackie DP, Hermans RP and Vloemans AR. Expansion technique for skin grafts: comparison between mesh and Meek island (sandwiched-) grafts, Burns 20:; 39-42, 1994) The Meek technique of skin expansion is efficient and effective in covering an open wound, particularly when there is a paucity of skin graft donor sites. Meshing of the graft was achieved by passing the carrier that housed the cork so that it was secured in a grille, when passed through the cutting machine. This device (Meek-Wall dermatome) was equipped with 13 circular blades that cut the graft into 14 strips of skin each 3 mm in width. In order to fabricate 196 pieces of micro-sized skin graft, each measuring 3 mm × 3 mm, the carrier block containing the 14 strips of skin was rotated by 90° and then passed through the cutting machine again (FIGURE 5). The the cut graft by using Meek technique was already placed on to a base which is elastic and has a speciality of preventing recoiling.

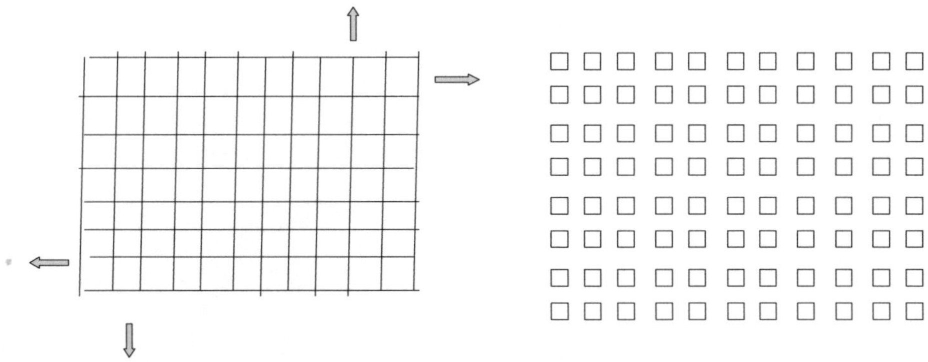

Fig. 5. Vertically and horizontally parelel cuts with following traction in two different directions expands the graft into multiple square mini skin grafts.

The cut grafts were transferred to another carrier, made of polyamide gauze with aluminum foil backing, by removing the cork plate, the epidermal surface of the graft being sprayed with adhesive. Peeters and Hubens showed that the MEEK technique the required graft donor site area is about half of that required with meshing. (Peeters R, Hubens A, The mesh skin graft - true expansion rate - *Burns*, vol. 14 (3); 239-24 , 1988). In patients with more than %50 of fullthickness body skin surface loss , the use of modified meek skin grafting technique application for body areas except face, neck and hand regions with an expansion ratio of 1:4 and 1:6 has been succesfully reported.(Raff T, Hartmann B, Wagner H, Germann G. Experience with the modified Meek technique. Acta Chir Plast. 38 (4): 142 - 146, 1996)

3.2.5 Sheet grafts

Sheet grafts where the superficial part of skin taken from another part and sliced are STSGs and harvested by a special instrument which is called as dermatome, whereas FTSGs are obtained with scalpel. Sheet grafts are applied without altering following harvest. STSG sheet grafts are usually applied to neck and face areas in where meshed grafts should not be used due to aesthetic concerns. (FIGURE 6). Sheet grafts are STSGs and they can be in there forms; thin, intermediate and thick..

3.3 Full thickness skin grafting

Full thickness grafts transfer all skin appendages and nerve endings except those sweat glands located in the subcutaneous tissue and some of Vater-Pacini corpuscles of palmar and plantar skin. (Lever WF: Histology of skin. pp 9-45. In Lever WF, Shaumburg-Lever G (eds) : Histhopathology of the skin 5th ed.JB Lippincott, Philadelphia 1975.) FTSG are especially useful for the repair of defects of the nasal tip dorsum ala lateral nasal sidewall, hands, eyelids and ear. Wound contraction is minimal and adnexal structures mostly are harvested together with the graft. An FTSG donor site should be planned in an elliptical shape to simplify direct closure. After an apropriate size has been determined, an ovoid of skin is excised from predetermined area with the axis in the direction of minimal tension. The wound is closed in a standart fashion, undermining the edges as necessary to achieve approximation. It is sometimes difficult to determine how much skin will be required. Templates can be prepared using the paper in which the glove is wrapped. FTSGs transfer all of the skin appendages and nerve endings except those sweat glands located in the subcutaneous tissue and some of the Vater-Pacini corpuscles of palmar and plantar skin. There are two techniques for harvesting FTSGs. In the meticulous technique where a sharp dissection is done, only the skin may be obtained. Second one can be described as rough technique. After the incision the predetermined graft donor site, graft can be harvested easily and rapidly by inclusion of subcutaneous fat tissue (Figure 7 and 8).

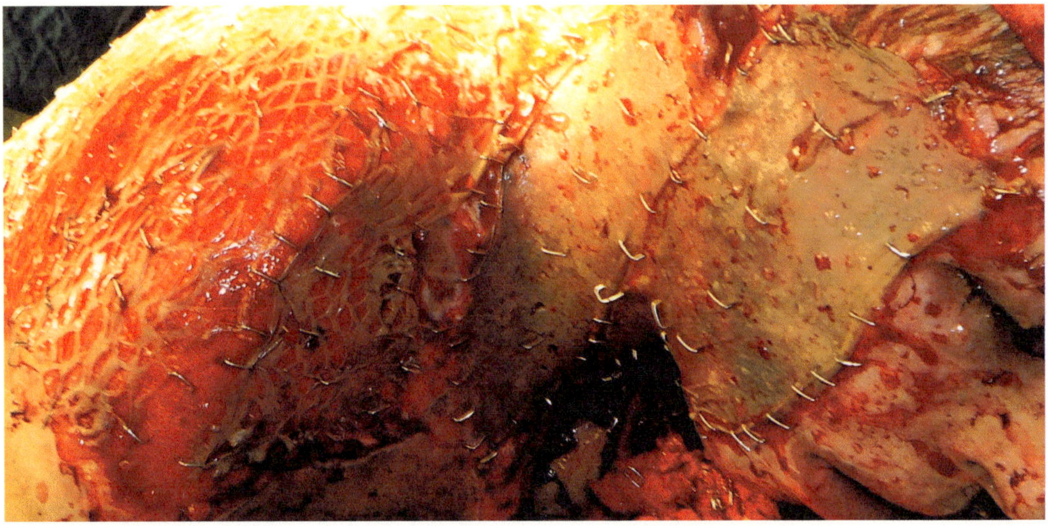

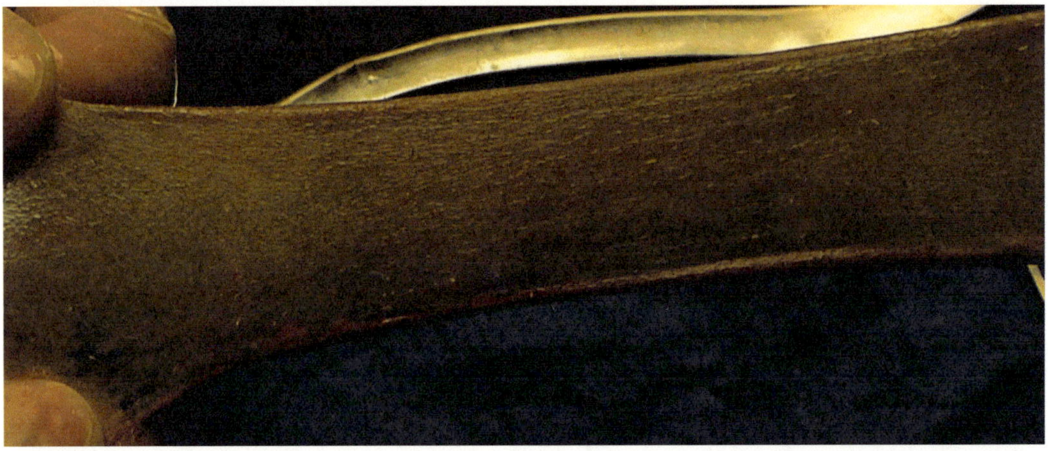

Fig. 6. Note that sheet grafts are applied to neck and face, whereas meshed grafts are other body regions where aesthetics are not primary concerns (Top). Note that some remaining elastic properties of thick STSG is clearly observed (bottom)

In the rapid technique where the skin is harvested with its subcutaneous attachments, there will be need of a following defatting process, since those structure may prevent graft vascularisation. Easily harvested with a scalpel, defatting or thinning the dermis increases the chance of "graft take."FTSGs are commonly harvested from the inguinal region, flank or from the postauricular area. These donor sites can be closed primarily, care should be taken to select a harvest site that does not contain hair.

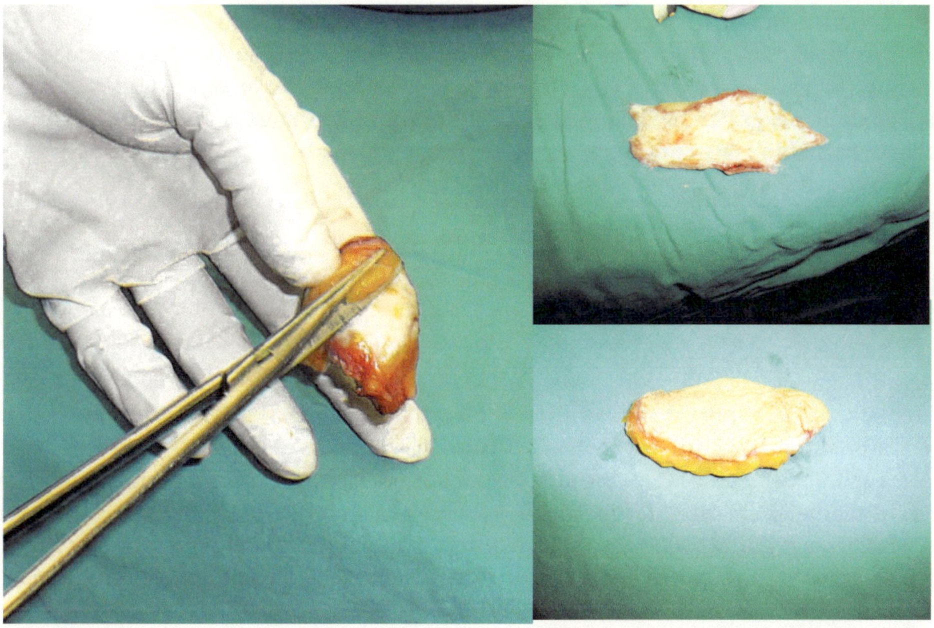

Fig. 7. Rough technique harvesting FTSG: defatting of graft (left), after the procedure (top right) and prior to the procedure the graft including subcutaneous fat (bottom, right).

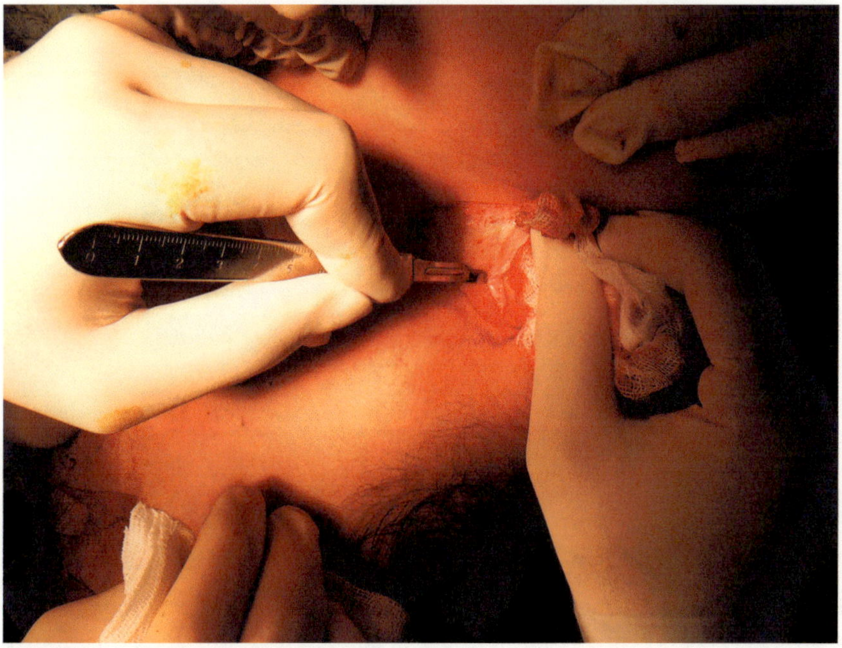

Fig. 8. Meticulouse technique for harvesting FTSG.

The most important factors affecting graft take are an inadequate recipient debridement, hematoma formation and local infection. In order to optimise these factors, Landau et. Al.

described the use of negative pressure dressing to prepare graft bed. They found FTSG take was in excess of 90%, even though a large surface area and a contour surface needed resurfacing (Landau A, Hudson DA, Adams K, Geldenhuys S, Pienaar C.Full-thickness skin grafts: Maximising graft take using negative pressure dressings to prepare the graft bed. Ann Plast Surg 60(6); 661-666; 2008)

3.4 Mini and micro skin grafting

The instruments required are 1.5 or 1.2mm punches, small jeweler's or graft holding forceps, and a small curved tip scissors for mini skin grafting. For micro skin grafting additional tools are spraying device, silver's skin grafting knife and spoon for spreading MSG. Dropper shallow stainless tray, diamond fraises and wire bushes are other useful tools. Although the micrograft technique is labour-intensive, if the expansion needed is at least 1:6, the aesthetic and functional results obtained are comparable to, or better than, those with meshed grafts. Pinch grafts should be full thickness 2-5 mm in diameter with free spaces of 5-10 mm between each of the grafts. Punch grafts are obtained by using a punch biopsy instrument, 3-5 mm in diameter (Figure 9). Pinch and punch grafts can also be called as patch or stamp grafts. Mini punch graft (MPG) may be used in transplantation forrepigmentation surgery of vitiligo, or some minor skin defects (Lahiri K.Evolution and evaluation of autologous mini punch grafting in vitiligo..Indian J Dermatol:54(2); 159-167; 2009).

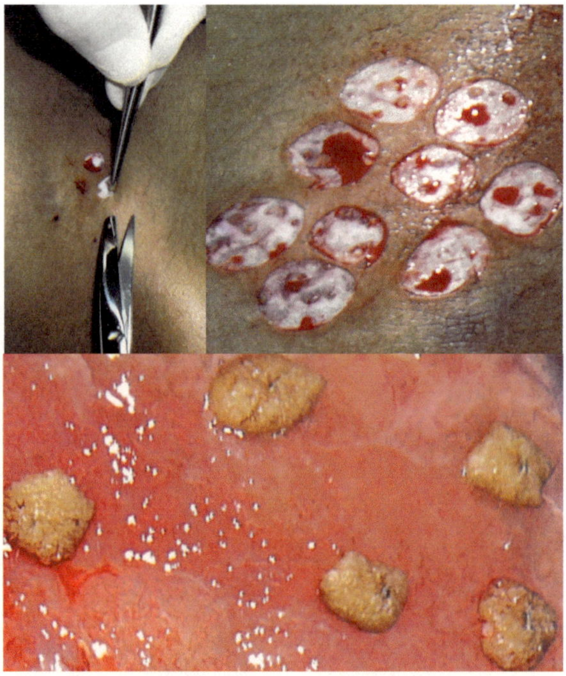

Fig. 9. Mini skin graft harvesting with simple forceps and curved tip scissors(top, , and the donor site after MSG harvesting (right).MSG that applied to a skin defect are shown (bottom).

Hair follicular graft (HFG) is like MPG but it contains a single or more hair follicles and thin sleeve of epidermis and full dermis. HFG can also be called as follicular unit grafts (FU). FU

is obtained by two methods; first is by using a special extractor and the second one is the method which elliptical harvesting of the donor strip providing more hair with less hair transection per procedure that remains the standard procedure. Although larger punch grafts and scalp flaps may play role in certain cases. FU transplantation is the culmination of decades of refinements and evolution of hair transplantation techniques. Hair naturally groups in groups of one to four individual follicles seperated by intervening soft tissue. These clumps or groups of hairs are termed follicular units.
The usual donor region is between occipital protuberance and 1 cm above the top of the ear (FIGURE 10). This donor site can easily be closed primarly.

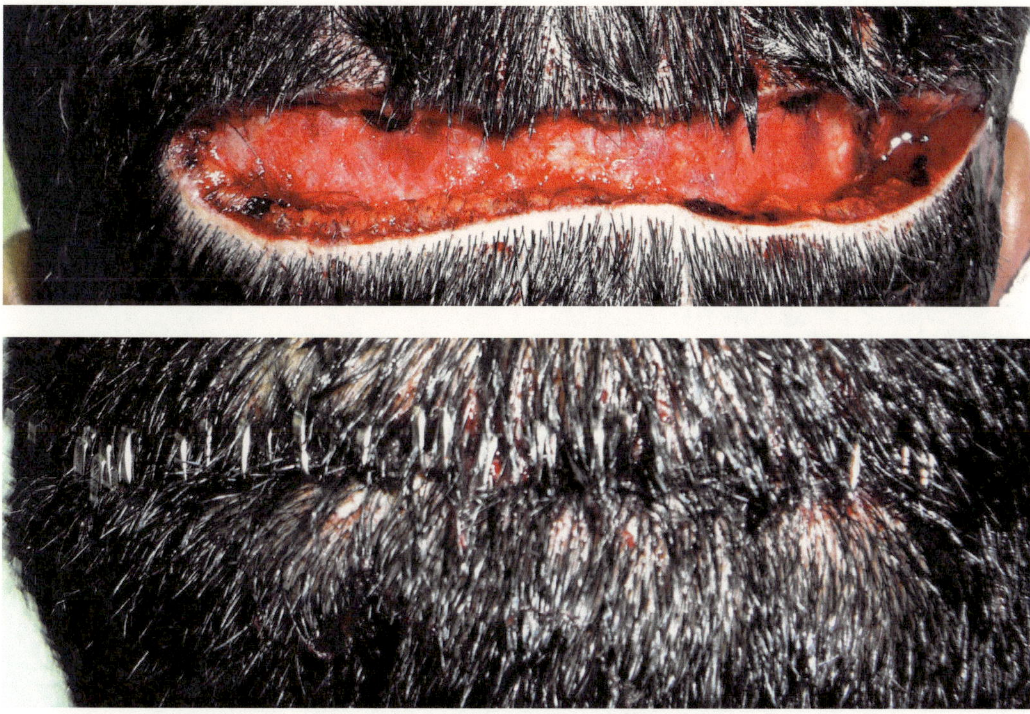

Fig. 10. Posterior occipital donor site : after the harvest (top) and closing the donor site primarly (bottom)

The average density in the posterior scalp is 65- 85 FU per cm^2. This is the safest place to harvest hair. The donor ellipse is handed by a surgical assistant and meticulous seperation of follicular goupings is begun using stereomicroscopic disssection. It is preferred greater lenght than width in a donor ellipse to achieve the desired number of follicular grouping. FUextract is the harvesting of individual FU units wtih 1 mm puches (FIGURE 11).

3.5 Composite skin grafting

Donor site selection of composite graft which is composed of multiple structures like skin and cartilage requires a more complicated approach, as defects of aesthetic subunits has its own characteristics and needs a more close attention in the repair process. Good examples of using composite graft are eyelash reconstruction with strip composite eyebrow grafts and alar rim defect repair with composite auricular graft. Strip composite eyebrow graft is the

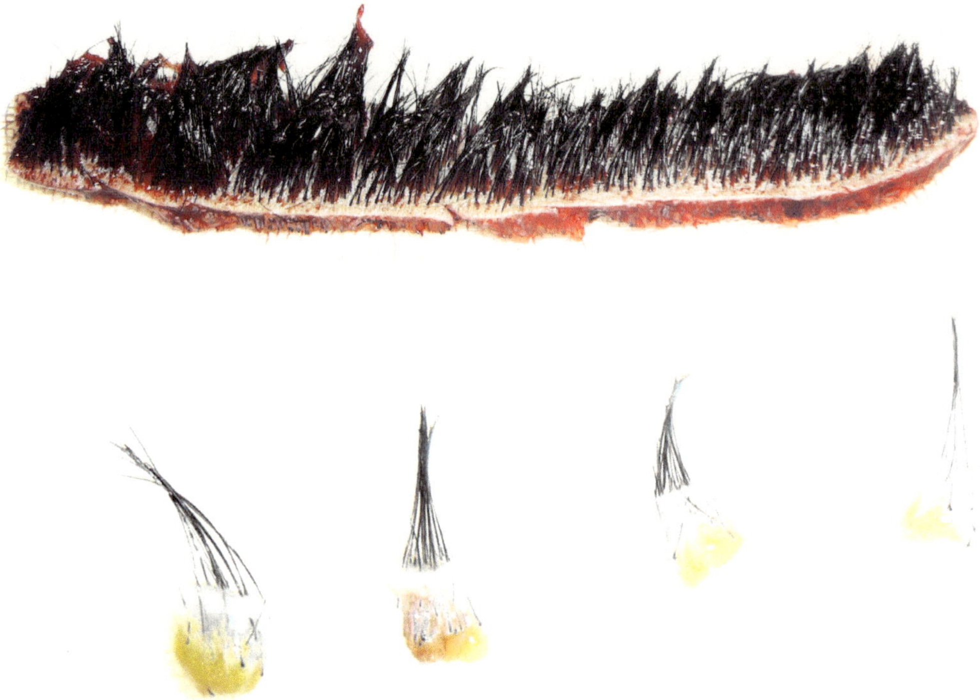

Fig. 11. A strip obtained from occipital donor site (top) and sliced FUs (bottom)

At first, the strip is divided into slices, much like slicing a loaf of bread, then each sliver is divided into individual FUs of 1, 2, 3, 4 –hair grafts (FIGURE 12). Upper limits of transplanted hair follicular unit number changes between 1500- 4500 for each session.

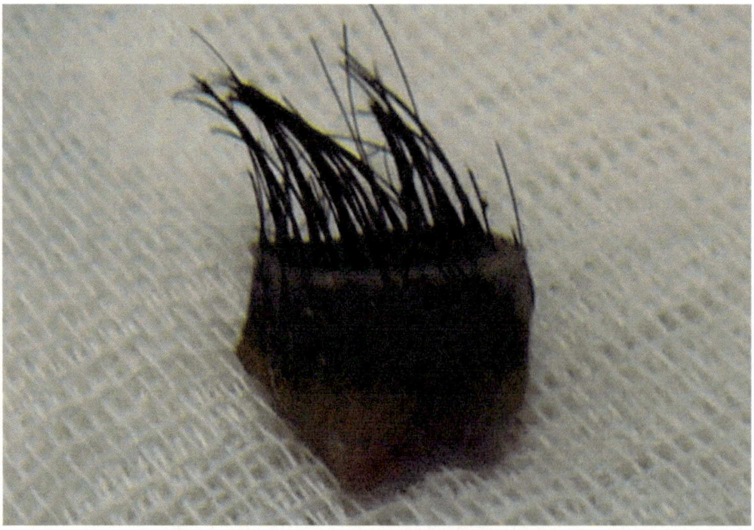

Fig. 12. This HFG is to be scliced into smaller FU grafts.

most suitable as its properties are very similiar to those of the original eyelash hairs. (Kasai K.Eyelash resonstruction with strip composite eyebrow graft. Head and Neck Surg 60(6);649-651; 2008) (Coban YK, Geyik Y.An ideal composite graft donor site for postburn alar rim deficiencies: root of helix . J Craniofac Surg: 21(4);1246; 2010)

Types of composite skin grafts	Used for	Additional content tissue
Strip eyebrow graft	Eyelash reconstruction	Subcutaneous fat
Conchal / helical composite grafts	Alar rim / columella restoration	Auricular cartilage
Scalp punch, pinch (follicular) grafts	Hair restoration	Subcutaneous fat
Strip scalp grafts	Eyebrow reconstruction	Subcutaneous fat

Table 2. Types of skin composite grafts.

4. Donor site selection criteria

The selection of donor site is essential to achieve the best possible outcome. Donor sites, from which the skin grafts are taken, can be virtually anywhere in the body. Main criteria related with donor site selection is about which kind of skin graft is to be used. The importance of clothing styles particularly those swimwear must be considered in selection of donor site. The closer the donor site is to defect, the better the color and texture match. FTSG in general, convex areas of the body are easier to harvest than concave areas. With a very thin STSG the scar at the donor site will be the least pronounced. The anterior thigh provides a large expanse of skin for larger skin grafts. Split-thickness skin graft donor sites are more numerous than those for full-thickness skin grafts, because the former heal spontaneously, mainly by reepithelialization from epidermal appendages found in the residual dermis. Whereas harvesting FTSG from any part of body leaves a donor site scar behind. So when using FTSG hidden donor areas by clothing are usually selected. A graft taken from skin adjacent to the surgical defect, known as Burrow's graft often provides an ideal match with respect to both color and texture. For example, skin taken from nasolabial fold may be used to close small nasal tip defects and may often supply a degree of sebaceous quality. Similarly clavicular skin may be used for a defect of photodamaged area, as this site provides a better color match. The ulnar border of the hypothenar area is an excellent source of small grafts for the fingertips. Preputium may be used as FTSG donor site when circumcision is also planned.(Yıldırım S, Akan M, Akoz T, Tanoglu B.Preputium: an overlooked skin graft donor site. Ann Plast Surg:46(6);&30-634; 2001).

4.1 Choice of graft

Best choice for a skin graft depends on the location of the defect. The actual principle to be cared is the similarity between the donor and recipient site characteristics. The properties that are expected from the grafted skin are the expected aesthetic appearence, the size of defect, donor availability, donor site morbidity. Palmar skin of the instep is the best replacement of the palmar skin of the digit and hand. In other way, plantar defects are usually repaired glabrous skin grafts taken from hypothenar hand regions. (Wu LC, Goutlieb LJ. Glabrous Dermal Grafting: A 12-Year Experience with the Functional and Aesthetic Restoration of Palmar and Plantar Skin Defects *Plast.Reconstr. Surg.* 116: 1679,

2005.) It has been shown that medial plantar grafts even in the form of pinch grafts are effective in resurfacing palmar wounds. (Siman R.Medial Plantar Arch Pinch Grafts Are an Effective Technique to Resurface Palmar and Plantar Wounds *Ann Plast Surg* 2004;53: 256-260.) At follow-up all those with plantar skin grafts show excellent color and texture match with adjacent palmar or plantar skin. The graft would be soft, supple, mobile and stable without any pigmentation. Walking and weight bearing has been shown to be smooth.
Another example for choice of graft is decision on glabrous or non glabrous skin grafts. Plantar defects that are to be grafted are reconstructed with split or full thickness skin grafts. If non glabrous skin grafts are used some disadvantages which includes painfull hyperkeratotic build up at the periphery of the grafts ocur. The long standing use of glabrous skin grafts for plantar defects confirms the desirability functional advantage, minimal morbidity of this technique. (Banis JC. Glabrous skin grafts for plantar defects. *Foot Ankle Clin* 2001:6(4); 827-837).

4.2 Choice of donor site and its preparation

Donor sites for full-thickness skin grafts tend to be limited to areas over joint creases or crevices where the donor site can be closed directly after graft harvest. For glabrous skin, hypothenar donor area, wrist crease and plantar arc area are good donor sites. Skin may be harvested from abdomen for facial defect repair, however the color and texture match may be less desirable. Donor sites for the harvest of skin graft include the lumbar and gluteal regions (thick skin), the thighs, and the arms (thin skin). The skin on the ventral, outer, and dorsal aspects of the thigh is classed as intermediate thickness for the purposes of skin grafting; an optimum harvest is 0.35 mm thick(Ostrovisky NV. Selection of the skin graft thickness with regard to the structure of the donor site skin. Acta Chir Plast; 27: 145-51; 1985). The usable thickness of thigh skin graft varies froma minimum of 0.25 mm to a maximum of 0.55 mm in most cases, though in elderly patients or steroid-damaged skin a thinner graft needs to be taken.

In contrast to common sites, the scalp's advantage has been seen primarily for cosmetically satisfying repair of facial defects. An additional important reason for using the scalp as a donor site for split-skin grafts is the patient's postoperative comfort and mobility. Wound healing is quick, the risk of infection is minimal, graft preparation and postoperative care are relatively easy, and the scalp as a source of meshgrafts harbors a reasonably large area for wound coverage. The site has only minimal interference with patients' rehabilitation, and later scar formation is rare. The donor site hidden under regrowing hair is invisible (Weyandt GH, Bauer B, Berens N, Hamm H, Broecker EB. Split-thicknes skin grafting from scalp: The hidden advantage.Dermatol Surg:35;1873-1879; 2009)
If possible use local anesthesia for donor site so that more likely to operate. Use plenty of very dilute local anesthetic for example, donor site is anesthesized with 1% lidocaine with epinephrine 1:100000 . In addition 10-30 cc of saline is added to produce turgor. The turgor helps with anesthesia, provides hemostasis and reduces transection of hair follicles. If possible use local anesthetic such as 0,4 % lignocaine with adrenalin and 10-30 cc of saline is added to produce turgor to graft out the skin all over the donor site. This helps hemostasis and reduces transection of hair follicles, when there is a need of hair follicle inclusion into the graft. Any medication that is not essential should be stopped at least 1 week prior to surgery. All smokers should be encouraged to cease cigarette smoking several days prior to surgery and to continue this for at least the first postoperative week. The donor skin is prepared and lubricated in the usual way, tensed using the skin graft boards and the graft taken. Proper skin tensioning is important.

4.3 Fixation techniques

Sutures, staples, or other adhesive agents can be used to affix the skin graft to the recipient bed. he use of stitches is a common method of fixation but it is quite time consuming, difficult to do in the split-thickness graft, very expensive and the stitches must be removed.A "stent" dressing and even the ubiquitous subatmospheric pressure device are intended means of preventing graft separation from the wound resulting from either shear forces or subgraft fluid accumulations. (Hallock GG. Expanded applications for octyl-2-cyanoacrylate as a tissue adhesive. *Ann Plast Surg.*;46:185–189; 2001) Human fibrin sealant (FS) has been proven effective for skin grafting after burn. FS is used as a slow clotting spray (4-5 IU thrombin / ml) (Mittermayr R, Wassermann E, Thurnher M, Simunek M, Redl H.Skin graft fixation by slow clotting fibrin sealant applied as a thin layer. Burns:32:3; 305-311; 2006).

An alternative, especially applicable for large sheet grafts, would be to leave the graft uncovered to allow frequent rolling of fluids from underneath. The use of surgical drape placed over the graft has been recognised, but must be removed at the second or third day[3]M.O. Yenidünya, E. Özdengill and I. Emsen, Split-thickness skin graft fixation with surgical drape, Plast Reconstr Surg 106 (6) (2000), pp. 1429–1430. View Record in ScopusCited By in Scopus (7) when the grafts are not well vascularized and this can lead to failure of the graft. In convex areas skin graft fixation can be done by a simple tie-over dressing (Coban YK. A novel tie-over dressing for circular defects: star tie-over .Burns:33(6);801-802; 2007)

4.4 Other parameters related to selection of donor site

Harvesting of an autograft results in a wound in healthy donor skin. Therefore several techniques have been developed to reduce the required surface area of donor skın, especially in FTSG applications of children. In order to obtain large enough FTSG and accomplish primary donor site closure, a prior tissue expansion may be applied at the donor site (Canter HI, Igde M, Vargel I, Ozgur F.Repeated tissue expansions on split-thickness skin graft in a patient with neurocutaneous syndrome.J Craniofac Surg:18(3);699-703; 2007).

Some pactical methods are also present in taking grafts like reuse skin graft patches or using freshly generated epithelium as a source of donor site. (Coban YK, Gumus N. Reuse of skin graft patches fort he coverage of skin defects.J Burn Care Res:27(2);234-236; 2006) (Gumus N, Coban YK.Freshly generated epithelium may be a donor site fort he coverage of deep skin defects in the combined skin wounds.Burns:33(5);673-676; 2007).Main logics of these applications are the presence of limited sources of donor sites and concerns on wounding a healthy donor site.Looking for an alternative donor site scalp is a suitable location to achieve STSG. If early repetetive harvesting from the same area is required such as in a burn patients, shortening of healing time and patients mobility are great advantages for this donor site .

4.5 Limitations of composite grafting

Composite grafts have limited dimentions and their usage for solving some challenging clinical conditions are also limited. Their usual dimention is about 0,5 cm (width) x 3cm (lenght). As they are dependent on recipient blood supply, grafts exceeding dimentions of these limits can not survive. If a long strip graft is to be used, its width must not exceed 0,5 cm. (Coban YK, Geyik Y.An ideal donor site for postburn alar rim deficiencies: root of helix. J Craniofac Surg: 21(4);1246; 2010).

5. Future expectations

Numerous variations such as mesh grafts, cultured epithelial autografts (CEA)and combined allo-autografts techniques have significantly enhanced the therapeutic spectrum of traditional skin graft techniques. In the absence of a dermis, mature fibroblasts secrete collagen into the altered pattern of a scar. The graft can fail to take when CEAs and autografts are applied to a wound surface in poor condition without a dermis. Moreover, there is a risk of poor epithelialization, due to the absence of a dermal component at the recipient site. Therefore, a dermal equivalent is required to overcome this problem. issue engineered skin is a significant advance in the field of wound healing. The translation from scaffolds to instructive three dimentional dermal substitues is not a simple task. New skin substitues for burn care are currently under development. They were developed due to limitations associated with the use of autografts. These limitations include the creation of a donor site which is at risk of developing pain, scarring, infection and / or slow healing.

More complex tissue-engineered skin substitues in which stroma, adipose tissue, capillaries and neurons combined with epithelium are being developed. These products are often a combination of cells, scaffolds and other factors.(Proulx S, Fradette J, Gavuin R, Larouche D, Germain L.Stem cells of the skin and cornea: Their applications in regenerative medicine. Curr Opin Organ Transplant 2010;dec 9.epub.) The application of these new products necessiate generally two-three staged operations to obtain final results.(FIGURE 13) During the past decade skin equivalents have been developed in order to reproduce epidermal and dermal elements in vivo.

A number of approaches were taken in the development of a skin substitute. One solution was to develop an acellular matrix complex that would guide the migration of fibroblasts into a pattern that had dermal-like qualities. Another approach was to expand a small piece of epidermis into a very large transplantable viable autologous-epidermal cell layer through tissue culturing. The third approach was to develop a skin equivalent composed of both a

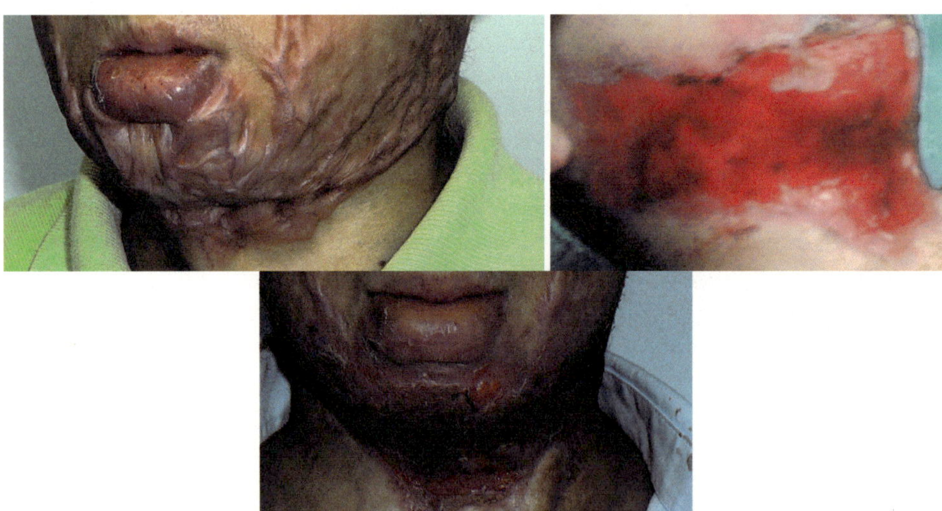

Fig. 13. Hypertrophic scarring due to flame burn injury of mandibular region (Left), well-developed granulation after the application of hyalomatrix skin substitute (esterified hyalurinic acid) for three weeks following to excision of scarred tissues (right), final result with thin STSG for epidermal replacement (centre).

collagen matrix populated with viable fibroblasts and a dermal equivalent layer that was covered with viable keratinocytes (epidermal layer). Most commercially available products are based on polymer matrices derived from both natural and synthetic sources. The majority of these products are designed to mimic the basic properties of the extracellular matrix. The use of dermal substitutes is increasingly widespread but the outcomes of substitute-asisted healing remain functionally deficient. There seems to be a long way to obtain a perfect skin equivalance that mimicks all structures of dermis and epidermis both aesthetically and functionally.

6. Conclusion

Skin grafting has become a technique that is routinely and sometimes preferentially considered as skin replacement for burns, chronic ulcers, skin defects due to other etiologies. In cases in which autologous grafts cannot be performed, skin substitutes have become an attractive alternative. Autologous skin grafts are commonly considered as the gold standard treatment. Availability of autologous grafts is a major obstacle, however, and the search for a manufactured skin replacement seems to be continued.

7. References

[1] Banis JC. Glabrous skin grafts for plantar defects. *Foot Ankle Clin* 2001:6(4); 827-837

[2] Blair VP, Brown JB: Use and uses of large split skin grafts of intermediate thickness. Surg Gynecol Obstet 49: 82-97, 1929.

[3] Canter HI, Igde M, Vargel I, Ozgur F.Repeated tissue expansions on split-thickness skin graft in a patient with neurocutaneous syndrome. J Craniofac Surg 2007:18(3);699-703.

[4] 4-Coban YK, Gumus N. Reuse of skin graft patches fort he coverage of skin defects. J Burn Care Res 2006:27(2);234-236.

[5] Coban YK. A novel tie-over dressing for circular defects: star tie-over .Burns 2007:33(6);801-802.

[6] Coban YK, Geyik Y.An ideal donor site for postburn alar rim deficiencies: root of helix. J Craniofac Surg 2010: 21(4);1246.

[7] Goullian D.A new economical dermatome Plast Reconst Surg 42: 85; 1968.

[8] Gumus N, Coban YK. Freshly generated epithelium may be a donor site for the coverage of deep skin defects in the combined skin wounds.Burns 2007:33(5);673-676.

[9] Hallock GG. Expanded applications for octyl-2-cyanoacrylate as a tissue adhesive. *Ann Plast Surg*. 2001;46:185–189.

[10] Kasai K.Eyelash resonstruction with strip composite eyebrow graft. Head and Neck Surg 2008:60(6);649-651.

[11] Lahiri K.Evolution and evaluation of autologous mini punch grafting in vitiligo..Indian J Dermatol 2009:54(2); 159-167.

[12] Landau A, Hudson DA, Adams K, Geldenhuys S, Pienaar C.Full-thickness skin grafts: Maximising graft take using negative pressure dressings to prepare the graft bed. Ann Plast Surg 2008:60(6); 661-666.

[13] Lever WF: Histology of skin. pp 9-45. In Lever WF, Shaumburg-Lever G (eds) : Histhopathology of the skin 5th ed.JB Lippincott, Philadelphia 1975.

[14] Meaume S.Methods of non surgical debridement of wounds in 2011.2011:Soins 752:44-47.
[15] Mittermayr R, Wassermann E, Thurnher M, Simunek M, Redl H.Skin graft fixation by slow clotting fibrin sealant applied as a thin layer. Burns 2006:32:3; 305-311.
[16] Ostrovisky NV. Selection of the skin graft thickness with regard to the structure of the donor site skin. Acta Chir Plast 1985; 27: 145-51.
[17] Padgett EC. Skin grafting of the burned patient. Plast Reconstr Surg 1946.1947 jul 2(4): 368-74.
[18] Paletta CE, Pokorny JJ, Rumbolo P. Skin grafts. In: Mc- Carthy JG, ed. *Plastic Surgery.* Philadelphia: Saunders Elsevier; 2006:293–316.
[19] Peeters R, Hubens A, The mesh skin graft - true expansion rate - *Burns*, vol. 14 (3), pp. 239-24 , 1988.
[20] Proulx S, Fradette J, Gavuin R, Larouche D, Germain L.Stem cells of the skin and cornea: Their applications in regenerative medicine. Curr Opin Organ Transplant 2010;dec 9.epub.
[21] Raff T, Hartmann B, Wagner H, Germann G. Experience with the modified Meek technique. Acta Chir Plast. 1996; 38 (4): 142 - 146.
[22] Reverdin JL: De la greffe epidermique. Arch Gen Med 19:276;555, 703, 1972.
[23] Rudolph R, Ballantyne DL. Skin grafts. In: McCarthy JG, ed. *Plastic Surgery.* Philadelphia: Saunders; 1990:221–274.
[24] Sams HH, McDonalds MA, Stasko T.Usefull adjunct to harvest split-thickness skin grafts. Dermatol Surg 2004:30(12pt 2): 1591-1592.
[25] Shoul M.Skin grafting under local anesthesia using a new safety razor Am J Surg 112.959,1966.
[26] Siman R.Medial Plantar Arch Pinch Grafts Are an Effective Technique to Resurface Palmar and Plantar Wounds *Ann Plast Surg* 2004;53: 256–260.
[27] Snow JW. Safety razor dermatome Plast Reconstr Surg 41: 184, 1968.
[28] Taner C, Vabdeput JF and Olley JF. The mesh skin graft, Plast Reconstr Surg 34 (1964), pp. 287–292. and Kreis RW, Mackie DP, Hermans RP and Vloemans AR. Expansion technique for skin grafts: comparison between mesh and Meek island (sandwiched-) grafts, Burns 20: 1994; 39–42.
[29] Tiersch C : Über Hautverplanzung. Verh Dtsch Ges Chir 15-17, 1886.
[30] Yıldırım S, Akan M, Akoz T, Tanoglu B.Preputium: an overlooked skin graft donor site. Ann Plast Surg 2001:46(6);&30-634.
[31] Weyandt GH, Bauer B, Berens N, Hamm H, Broecker EB. Split-thicknes skin grafting from scalp:The hidden advantage.Dermatol Surg 2009:35;1873-1879.
[32] Wu LC, Goutlieb LJ. Glabrous Dermal Grafting: A 12-Year Experience with the Functional and Aesthetic Restoration of Palmar and Plantar Skin Defects *Plast.Reconstr. Surg.* 116: 1679, 2005.

3

Indications of Skin Graft

Abdou Darwish
Minia University
Egypt

1. Introduction

The skin is the largest organ of the human body and it known as the integument or integumentary system because it covers the entire outside of the body. The skin consists of two main layers: the outer layer, or epidermis, which lies on and is nourished by the thicker inner layer, or dermis.. These two layers are approximately 0.04–0.08 in (1–2 mm) thick. The epidermis consists of an outer layer of dead cells called keratinocytes, which provide a tough protective coating, and several layers of rapidly dividing cells just beneath the keratinocytes. The dermis contains the blood vessels, nerves, sweat glands, hair follicles, and oil glands. The dermis consists mainly of connective tissue, which is largely made up of a protein called collagen. Collagen gives the skin its flexibility and provides structural support. The fibroblasts are the main cell type in the dermis and make collagen. Skin varies in thickness in different parts of the body; it is thickest on the palms and soles of the feet, and thinnest on the eyelids. In general, men have thicker skin than women, and adults have thicker skin than children. After age 50, the skin begins to grow thinner again as it loses its elastic fibers and some of its fluid content. A skin graft is used permanently replace damaged missing skin or provide a temporary wound covering. Skin is necessary because it protects the body against

Fluid loss, bacteria or virus invasion, and aids in temperature regulation. Skin that is damaged extensively by burns or non-healing wound can compromise an individual's health and well-being. Skin grafting is the next step on the reconstructive ladder for the closure of a wound that cannot be closed primarily. Skin grafts are classified as either split-thickness or full-thickness, depending on the amount of dermis included in the graft.

A partial or split-thickness skin graft (STSG) contains a variable thickness of dermis, while a full-thickness skin graft (FTSG) contains the entire dermis. Split-thickness skin grafts are further categorized as thin (0.005-0.012 in), intermediate (0.012-0.018 in), or thick (0.018-0.030 in) based on the thickness of the graft harvested. Skin grafting serves two purposes: reduce the course of treatment and improves function and appearance of the recipient area.

2. Types of skin grafts

The term "graft" by itself commonly refers to either an allograft or an auto graft. An autograft is a type of graft that uses skin from another area of the body but there has to be enough undamaged skin available and the patient has to be healthy enough to undergo surgery. An allograft uses skin obtained from another human being, Donor skin from cadavers is frozen, stored, and available for use as an allograft. Skin taken from an animal (usually a pig) is called a xenograft because it comes from a nonhuman species. Allograft and xenograft provide only a temporary covering because of rejection by the patient's immune system within seven days. The allograft or xenograft must then be replaced with an auto graft.

2.1 Split thickness grafts

The most important part of any skin graft procedure is proper preparation of the wound. Skin grafts will not survive on tissue with a limited blood supply (cartilage, bone or tendons) or tissue that has been damaged by radiation treatment. The wound must be free of any dead tissue, foreign matter, or bacterial contamination. After the patient has been anesthetized, the surgeon prepares the wound by rinsing it with saline solution or a diluted antiseptic (Betadine) and debrides any dead tissue. In addition, the surgeon stops the flow of blood into the wound by applying gentile pressure, tying off blood vessels, or administering a medication (epinephrine) that causes the blood vessels to constrict.

Following preparation of the wound, the surgeon then harvests the tissue for grafting. A split-thickness skin graft involves the epidermis and a little of the underlying dermis; (the donor site usually heals within several days). The surgeon first marks the outline of the wound on the skin of the donor site, enlarging it by 3–5% to allow for tissue shrinkage. The surgeon uses a dermatome (a special instrument for cutting thin slices of tissue) to remove a split-thickness graft from the donor site. The wound must not be too deep if a split-thickness graft is going to be successful, since the blood vessels that will nourish the grafted tissue must come from the dermis of the wound itself. The graft is usually taken from an area that is ordinarily hidden by clothes such as the buttock or inner thigh and applied on the wound. Gentle pressure from a well-padded dressing is then applied, or a few small sutures used to hold the graft in place. A sterile non adherent dressing is then applied to the raw donor area for approximately three to five days to protect it from infection.

2.2 Full thickness grafts.

Full-thickness skin grafts may be necessary for more severe burn injuries, trauma and excision of malignancy. These grafts involve both layers of the skin. Full-thickness auto grafts are more complicated than partial-thickness grafts, but provide better contour, natural color, and contract less at the grafted site. The back and the abdomen are common donor sites for full-thickness grafts. A full-thickness graft is removed from the donor site with a scalpel rather than a dermatome. After the surgeon cuts around the edges of the pattern used to determine the size of the graft, the skin is lifted with a special hood and the fatty tissue is trimmed. The graft is then placed on the wound and secured in place with absorbable sutures.

2.3 Composite skin graft

A composite skin graft is sometimes used. A composite skin graft consists of combinations of skin and fat, skin and cartilage, or dermis and fat. Composite grafts are used in patients whose injuries require three-dimensional reconstruction. For example, a wedge of ear containing skin and cartilage can be used to repair the nose.

3. Indications of skin graft

3.1 Deep fullthickness burns

Deep full thickness burns destroy the skin and damage underlying tissues and are the most common indication For split thickness skin grafts (fig. 1) where, the skin is destroyed to its full depth, in addition to damage done to underlying tissues, and Deep full thickness burns must be covered as soon as possible to prevent infection and fluid loss. Wounds that are left to heal on their own (secondary intention) can contract and result in serious and painful scarring and actually prevent normal limb movement.

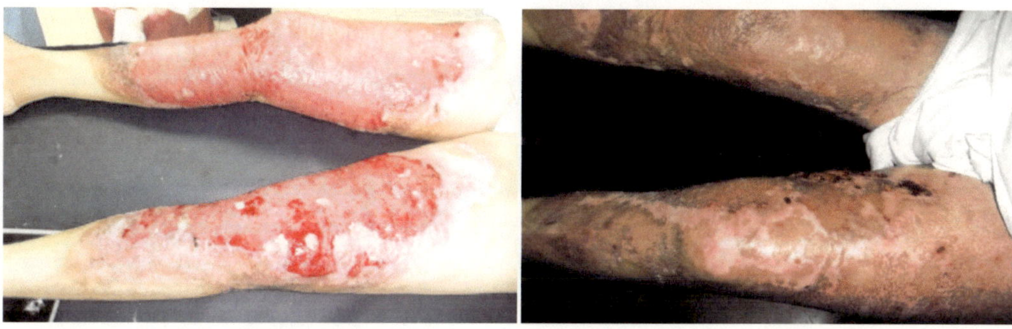

Fig. 1. Deep full thickness burns of both lower limbs and after reconstruction with STSG.

3.2 Post traumatic skin loss

Friction burns ((fig. 2) and degloving injuries (fig. 3,4) due to car accident and other traumas which leads to full thickness skin loss are indication for split thickness graft. In cases of friction burns the area of skin loss should be washed thoroughly with sterile saline to make sure that the recipient site is clean and ready for grafting. If the wound still remains contaminated, it should be dressed until complete cleanliness of the wound is obtained.

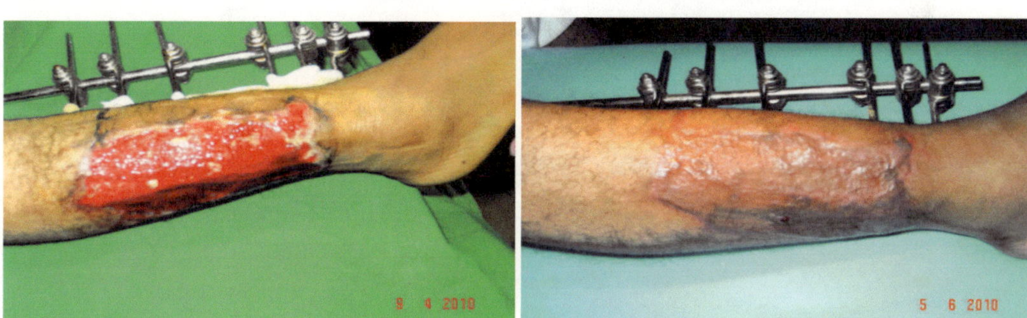

Fig. 2. Friction burns of the lateral aspect of the lower leg with full thickness skin loss and after reconstruction with STSG.

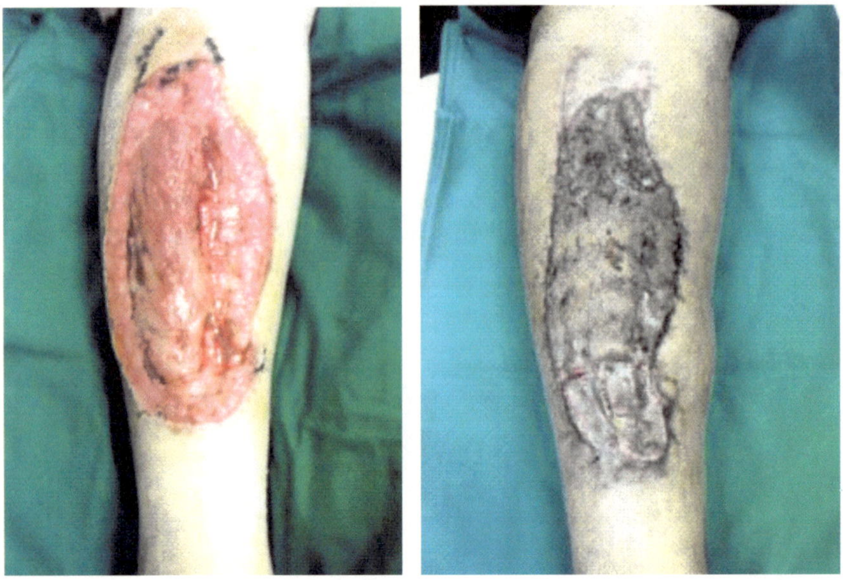

Fig. 3. Degloving injury of the right leg after debridement and after reconstruction by STSG

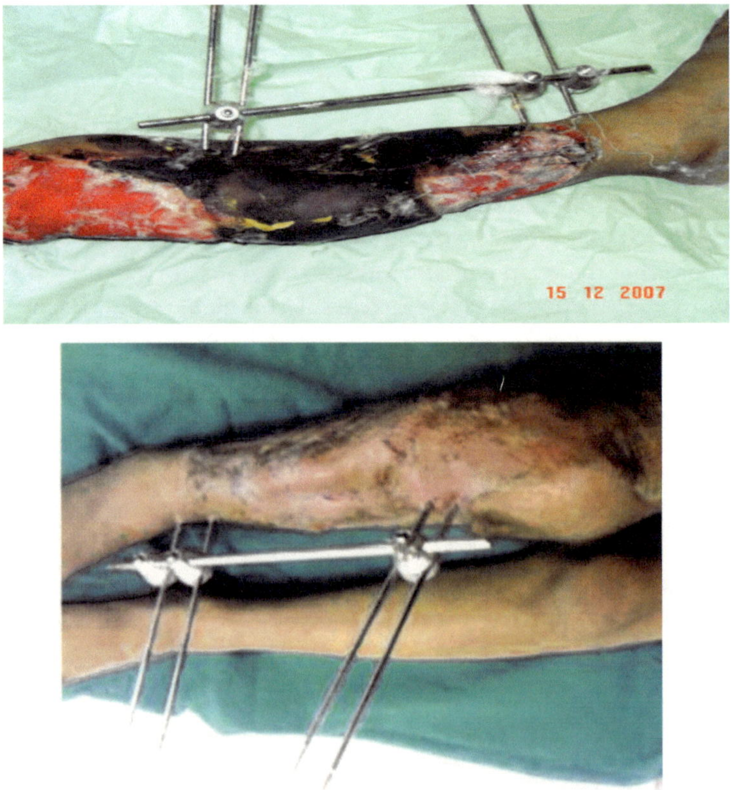

Fig. 4. Degloving injury of the right leg before and after debridement and reconstruction by STSG

3.3 During surgery

After release of post burn contractures and after reconstruction by local flaps such as a transposition or bipedicled flap requires grafting to close the donor site (fig. 5-8). Also excision of large tumor usually need skin graft to reconstruct the resultant defect.

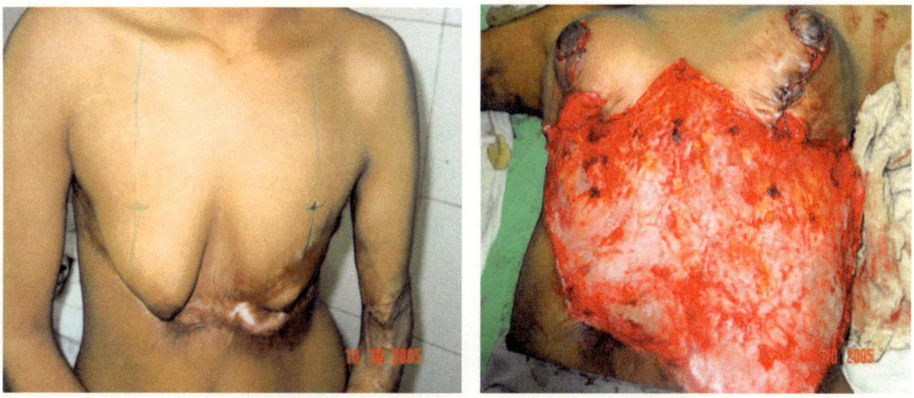

Fig. 5. A) Post burn breast contraction of both breasts and after release of breast contraction

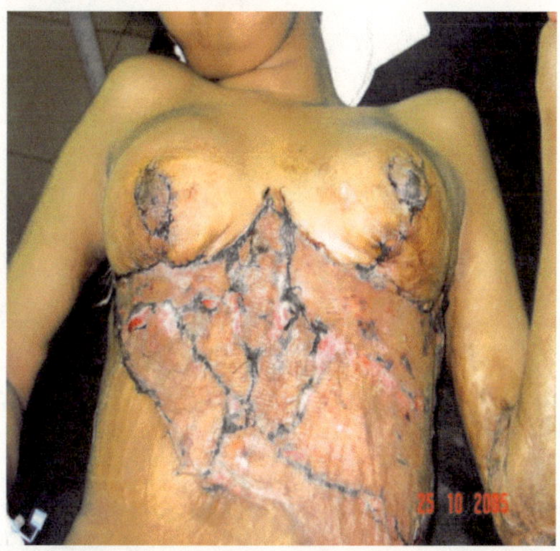

Fig. 5. B) After application of STSG to the row area of lower chest and upper abdominal wall

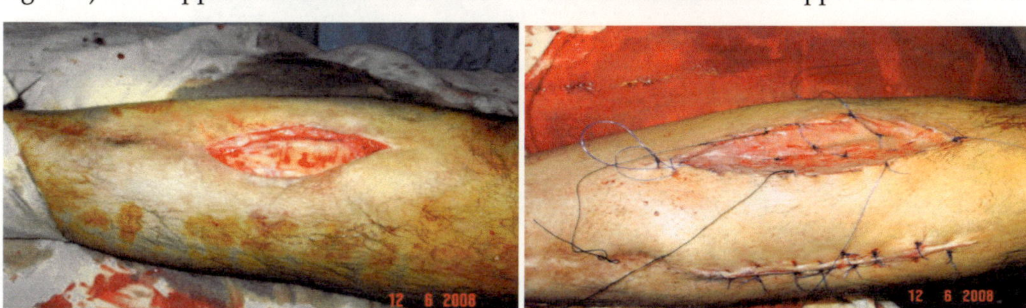

Fig. 6. Exposed tibia and after reconstruction by bipedicled flap and STSG applied to the donor site of flap

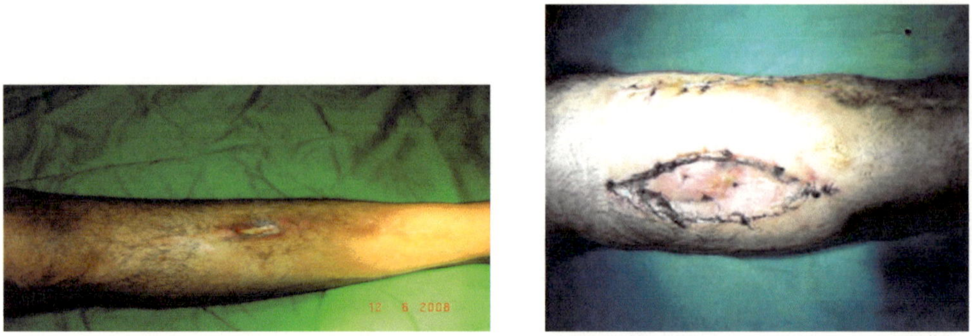

Fig. 7. Exposed tibia and after reconstruction by bipedicled flap and STSG applied to the donor site of the flap.

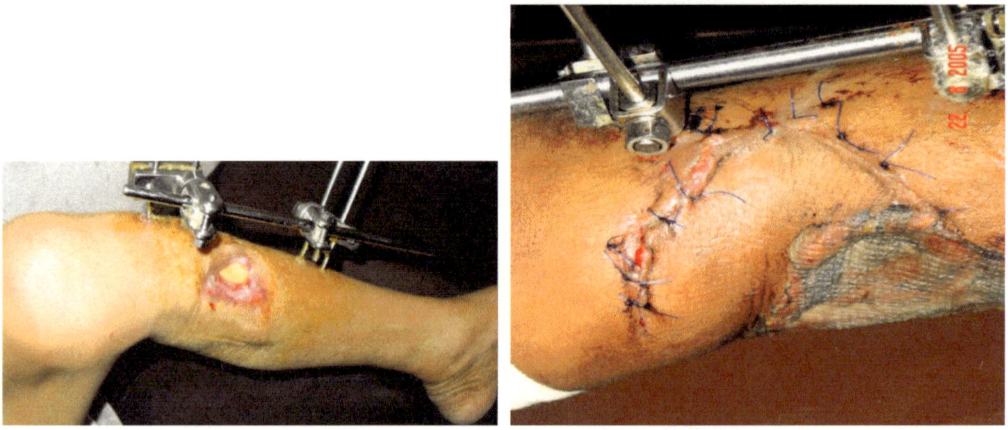

Fig. 8. A) Exposed tibia and after reconstruction by transposition flap and STSG is applied to the donor site of the flap.

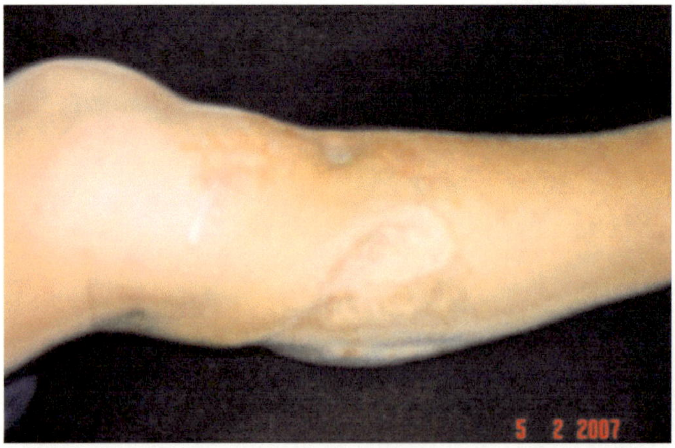

Fig. 8. B) the appearance of the graft after one year.

3.4 Post operative

Compartment syndrome of an extremity needs urgent release of the fascia (fasciotomy) to re-establish limb vasculature. The resultant fasciotomy wound usually requires reconstruction with a skin graft for closure after establishment of limb vasculature (fig. 9).

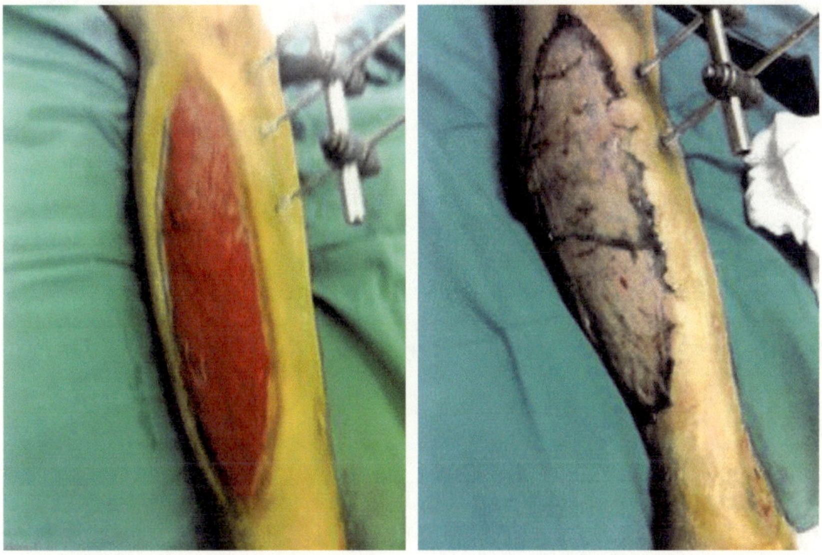

Fig. 9. Fasciotomy of the lateral aspect of the leg and after application of a STSG

3.5 Post infection skin loss

Necrotizing fasciitis is considered one of the most common indications of skin graft after a thorough debridement of the dead tissue and clearance of the infection. Diabetic infections usually need extensive debridement and the wound closed with a skin graft (fig.10).

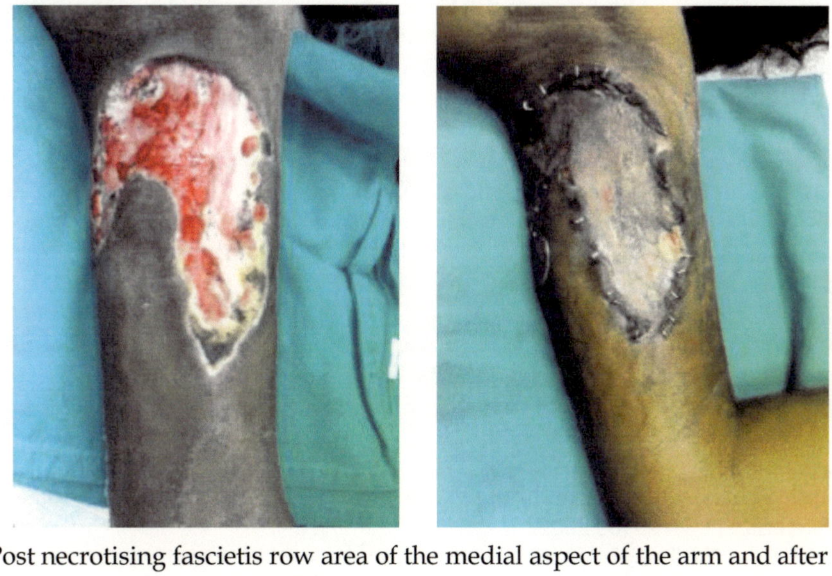

Fig. 10. Post necrotising fascietis row area of the medial aspect of the arm and after debridement and application of STSG

4. Indications of allografts and xenografts

With extensive full thickness skin loss exceeding 30% of the body surface, auto grafts are often not available in sufficient quantities. Temporary coverage can be obtained by skin allograft from volunteers, diseased free cadavers, or the patient's relatives and friends and is often a life-saving measure. It is used as a biologic dressing and can serve several functions:(1)provide clean granulating area prior to auto-grafting ,(2)protect open wound from protein and water loss until auto-grafting is available (3)decrease surface bacterial count and pain at the site of an open wound,(4) covers the vital organs and (5)facilitate early movement of affected part. In order to avoid rejection response to allo-graft, the allograft skin should be changed every three days. It can be obtained fresh from the relatives and either used immediately or stored in the live state at a temperature near or above freezing.

Skin allograft has also been recommended for coverage of second degree burns. In addition to providing pain relief and inhibition of evaporate and exudative water loss, skin allograft promote healing with an improved cosmetic results.

5. Xenografts

The functions of skin xenografts as temporary biologic dressing are similar to those outlined in the above section on allograft .Xenografts have been most extensively used in covering large burn wounds before auto-grafting .The use of xenografts have also been used for the temporary coverage of exposed vessels, tendons, large ulcers, flap donor sites and skin graft donor sites.

6. References

Bromberg,BE , Snog,IC and Mohen ,MP: The use of Pig skin as a temporary biological dressing. Plast.Reconstructive Surg. 36:80, 1965.

Bromberg,BE and Snog,IC . : Skin substitutes Homo and Hetero grafts. Am.J.Surg, 112:28, 1966.

Elliot, R A and Hoehn, J G :Use of commercial Porcine skin for wound dressing. Plast.Reconstructive Surg.52:401,1973.

Darwish A M :Bipedicled flap in reconstruction of exposed tibia.J Plast Reconstr Aesthet Surg.63, 160-163 ,2010 .

Eto, M., H. Hackstein, K. Kaneko, et al. "Promotion of Skin Graft Tolerance Across MHC Barriers by Mobilization of Dendritic Cells in Donor Hemopoietic Cell Infusions." *Journal of Immunology* 69 (September 1): 2390-2396, 2002.

Latenser, B. A. and Vern A. Kowal. "Paediatric Burn Rehabilitation." *Pediatric Rehabilitation* 5 (January-March).

Losada, F., M.D., Pedro P. Garcia-Luna, M.D., T. Gomez-Cia, M.D., et al. "Effects of Human Recombinant Growth Hormone on Donor-Site Healing in Burned Adults." *World Journal of Surgery* 26 (January): 2-8 ,2002.

Revis, Don R., Jr., , and Michael B. Seagal, . "Skin Grafts, Full-Thickness." *eMedicine* , May 17, 2002 [cited June 25, 2003].

Snyder, R. J., H. Doyle , and T. Delbridge. "Applying Split-Thickness Skin Grafts : A Step-by-Step Clinical Guide and Nursing Implications." *Ostomy Wound Management* 47 (November): 990-996 , 2002.

Woudruff M F A:The Trasplantation of tissue and organs. Springfeild,IL,Charles C.Thomas, 1960.

4

Full Thickness Skin Grafts

Saikat Ray[1] and Krishna Rao[2]
[1]*Department of Plastic and Reconstructive Surgery, Northampton General Hospital NHS Trust*
[2]*Department of Plastic and Reconstructive Surgery, Sheffield Teaching Hospitals NHS Trust*
United Kingdom

1. Introduction

Skin is the largest organ of the human body and has a number of essential functions. It forms a protective barrier against pathogens and the internal and external environment. It acts as a water resistant barrier so that essential nutrients are not washed out of the body. It provides a dry and semi-permeable barrier to fluid loss. Langerhan cells in the skin are part of the adaptive immune system . The skin plays an important role in sensation and contains a number of nerve endings that respond to heat and cold, vibration, pressure, touch and pain. Thermoregulation is another essential function of the skin. Finally, the skin also plays a vital role in the synthesis of Vitamin D. It is imperative that skin cover is preserved in humans for all the reasons mentioned above.

Skin grafts are harvested from a donor site and transferred to a distant recipient site (bed) without carrying its own blood supply. The graft relies on new blood vessels from the recipient site bed to be generated (angiogenesis).

Full thickness skin grafts consist of the entire epidermis and dermis. These grafts are a simple and reliable method of achieving closure of skin defects where primary closure or healing by secondary intention is not possible. Full-thickness skin grafts are generally used to resurface smaller defects because they are limited in size. They are invaluable for reconstruction of defects where good cosmetic outcome or a durable skin cover is necessary. Common areas include defects on the face, scalp and hand, often following excision of skin lesions. A suitable well vascularized bed is necessary for full-thickness skin graft take. 'Take' is the process which results in the reattachment and revascularization of the skin graft.

2. Mechanisms of skin graft take

There are 3 predictable stages of skin graft take which include.

2.1 Plasmatic imbibition

Initially, the skin grafts passively absorbs the nutrients in the wound bed by diffusion. Imbibition prevents the graft from desiccation and keeps the graft vessels patent. This enables the graft to survive the immediate post graft ischaemic period, which is for an undetermined period of time that varies according to the wound bed. This may be upto 24

hours for a graft placed on a bed that is already proliferative and 48 hours for a graft covering a fresh wound.
A graft can tolerate an ischemic interval when placed on a poorly vascularized bed. Thick full thickness skin grafts appear to tolerate ischemia for up to 3 days while thin full thickness skin grafts survive for up to 5 days. Split-thickness grafts take well even after 4 days of ischemia. Grafts can add as much as 40% to their pre-graft weight through fluid movement from recipient bed to graft and hence appear plump during this time.

2.2 Inosculation and capillary ingrowth

By day 3, a fine vascular network is established in the fibrin layer between the graft and its recipient bed capillary buds from the recipient bed line up with graft vessels on the underside of the dermis to form open channels. Blood flow is established and the skin graft becomes pink. Proliferation of fibroblasts and deposition of collagen to replace the fibrin maintains skin graft adhesion to its bed. Attachment strength increases rapidly, and anchorage can be provided within 4 days.

2.3 Revascularization

By day 5, new blood vessels grow into the graft and the graft becomes vascularized. The connection between graft and host vessels develops further as the graft revascularizes. Newly formed vascular connections continue to differentiate into afferent and efferent vessels. The fifth or sixth post graft day notes the presence of lymphatic drainage. The graft reduces in weight until it reaches its pre-graft weight by the ninth day.

3. Harvesting a full thickness skin graft

Different parts of the body vary greatly in terms of the appearance, colour, texture, thickness and vascularity of skin. All of these factors are taken into account when choosing a donor area appropriate to a certain defect.
Full thickness skin grafts can be harvested from a number of areas in the body that have skin redundancy. When the face is being grafted, the posterior surface of the ear extending onto the neighbouring *post auricular* hairless mastoid skin provides an excellent donor site in terms of skin colour and texture. Another useful area for facial lesions is the *preauricular area* (Figure 1). *Upper eyelid* skin is useful particularly when the defect is of another eyelid. *Supraclavicular* skin excised from the lower posterior triangle of the neck gives reasonable colour and texture to resurface facial defects. However, this is cosmetically inferior to post auricular skin. *Flexural* skin including the *ante-cubital fossa, groin* and *distal wrist crease* are also used as donor sites. The main use of groin skin is where a long, narrow piece of skin is required, such as in managing flexion contractures in the hand. The formation of a noticeable scar is a realistic possibility when closing ante-cubital fossa donor areas, often resulying in scar hypertrophy when closed under excess tension. The *medial arm* and *forearm* are other commonly used areas to provide donor skin (Figure 2). Thigh and abdominal skin are good at providing skin cover for the palm of the hand. The thicker dermis from these areas also provides a good pad to withstand pressure when used on the sole of the foot. Full thickness skin grafts undergo a significant degree of primary contraction following harvest.
It is useful to make a template of the recipient defect. This shape is then transferred to the donor area and extended to form an ellipse. The ellipse is ideally designed such that the

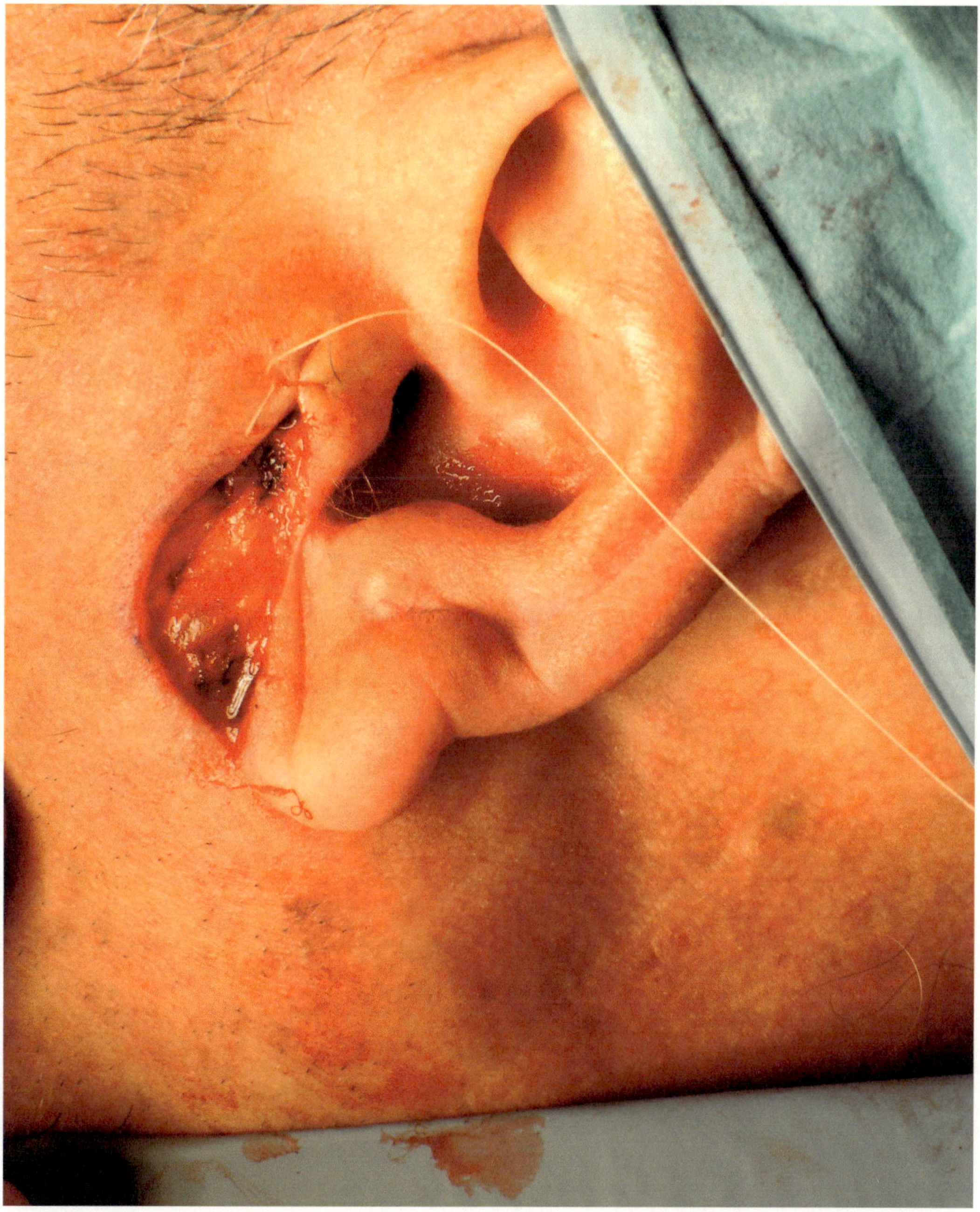

Fig. 1. Pre-auricular full thickness skin donor area. Vicryl rapide suture can be seen at the superior aspect of the ellipse to close wound

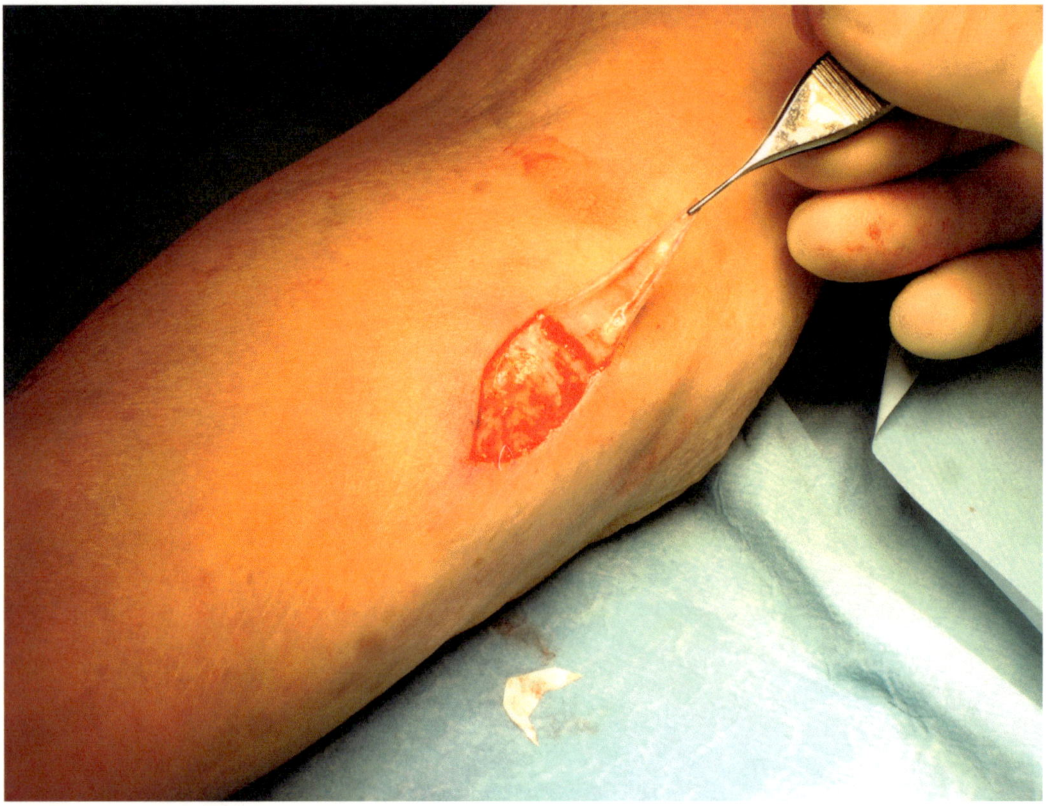

Fig. 2. Full-thickness skin graft harvest from the medial forearm donor area. Note the shiny undersurface of the graft dermis

resulting scar lies in the direction of the natural skin crease lines (Langer's lines). The graft is usually harvested with a 15 inch bladed scalpel between the dermis and the subcutaneous fat. Often, the graft is easier to cut if the area is infiltrated with fluid (1:200000 adrenaline). The full thickness skin graft leaves behind no epidermal elements in the donor site from which resurfacing can take place. For this reason, primary closure of the donor site is necessary. This is usually achieved using an absorbable suture in a single layer subcuticular stitch (Figures 3 and 4). Occasionally, a split thickness skin graft may be used to close the donor area.

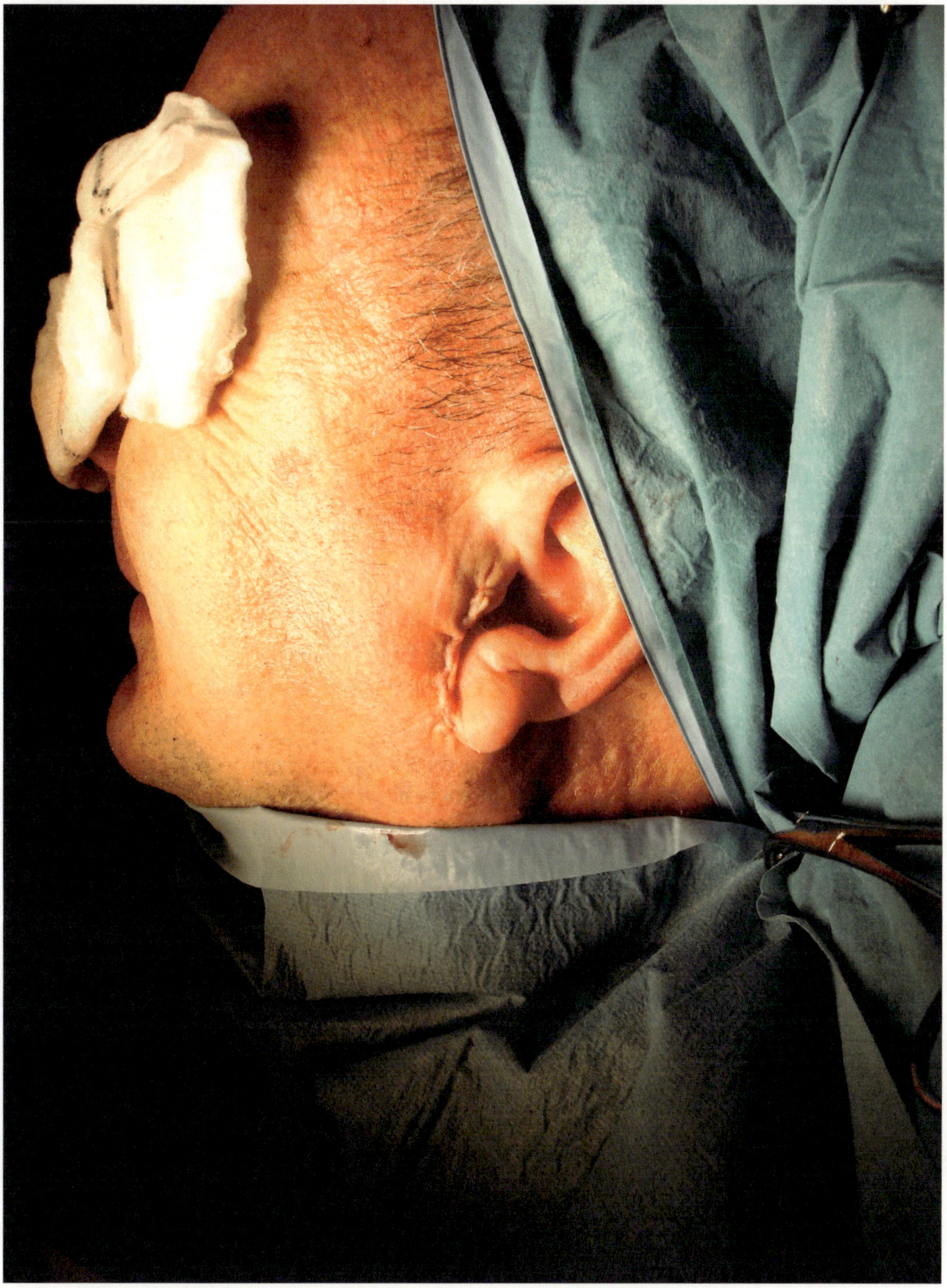

Fig. 3. Closure of pre-auricular full thickness skin donor area

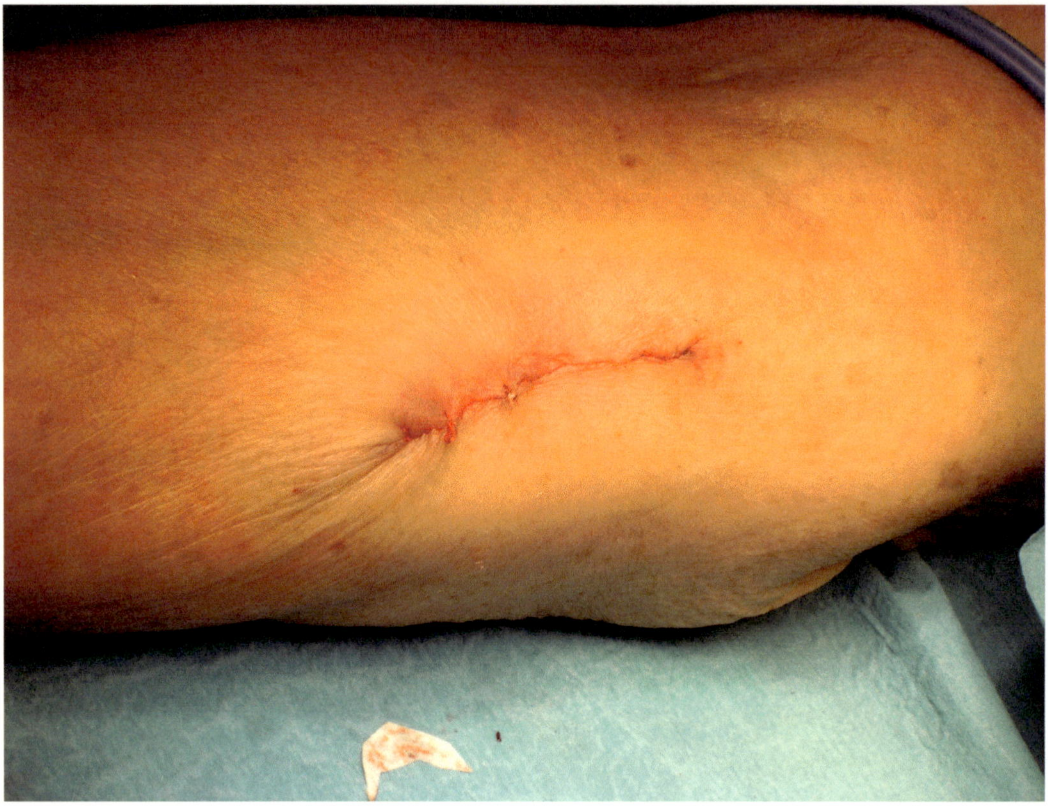

Fig. 4. Closure of medial forearm full thickness skin donor area

The graft may be further defatted, as fat is poorly vascularized and will prevent firm adherence between the graft dermis and the recipient bed. All yellow fat must be trimmed using a pair of sharp scissors until only the the shiny white undersurface of the dermis is visible.

4. Graft inset

A good graft inset is necessary to ensure immobilization of the graft on its bed and to prevent haematoma formation. The graft is secured onto the donor site by sutures with the dermis side down and trimmed to fit (Figures 5 and 6). A non-adherent layer such as a jelonet dressing is also necessary to facilitate easy separation of the dressing.

A number of techniques can be used which include tie over dressings, foam bolsters and quilting sutures. The full thickness skin graft is sutured to the wound edges circumferentially with independent sutures which are cut long. A tie-over dressing using a piece of gauze or wool soaked in proflavin is applied and the suture ends tied to secure the dressing. This helps to fix the graft and reduces shear forces (Figure 7). Alternatively, additional pressure and immobilization can be achieved using a foam bolster secured with sutures or staples (Figure 8). Quilting sutures applied between the graft and the bed ensure good contact between the graft and the wound bed, while ensuring immobilization.

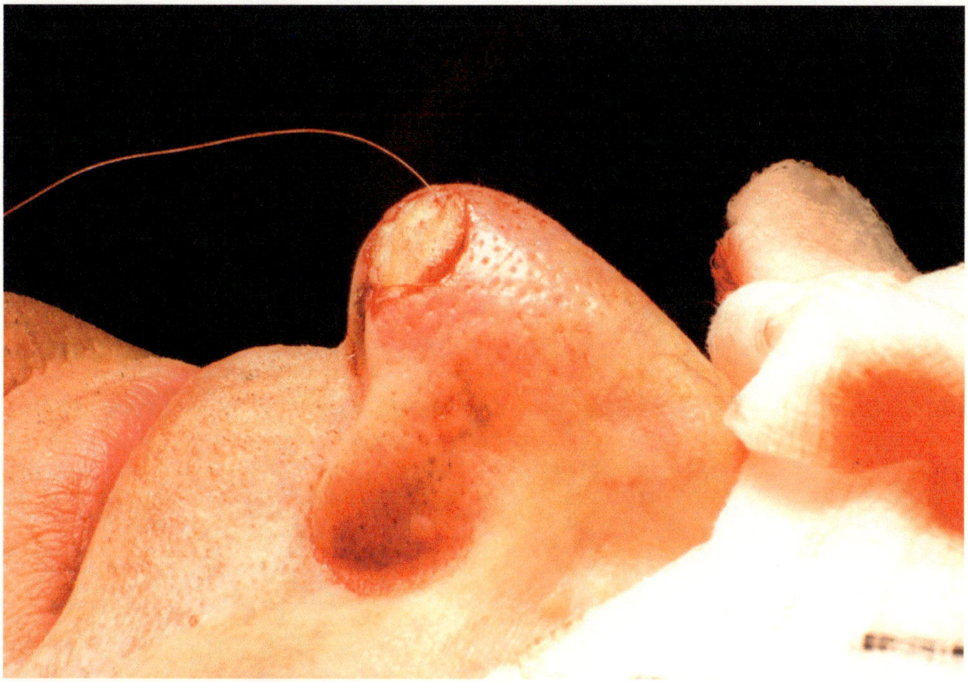

Fig. 5. Full thickness skin graft inset onto nose

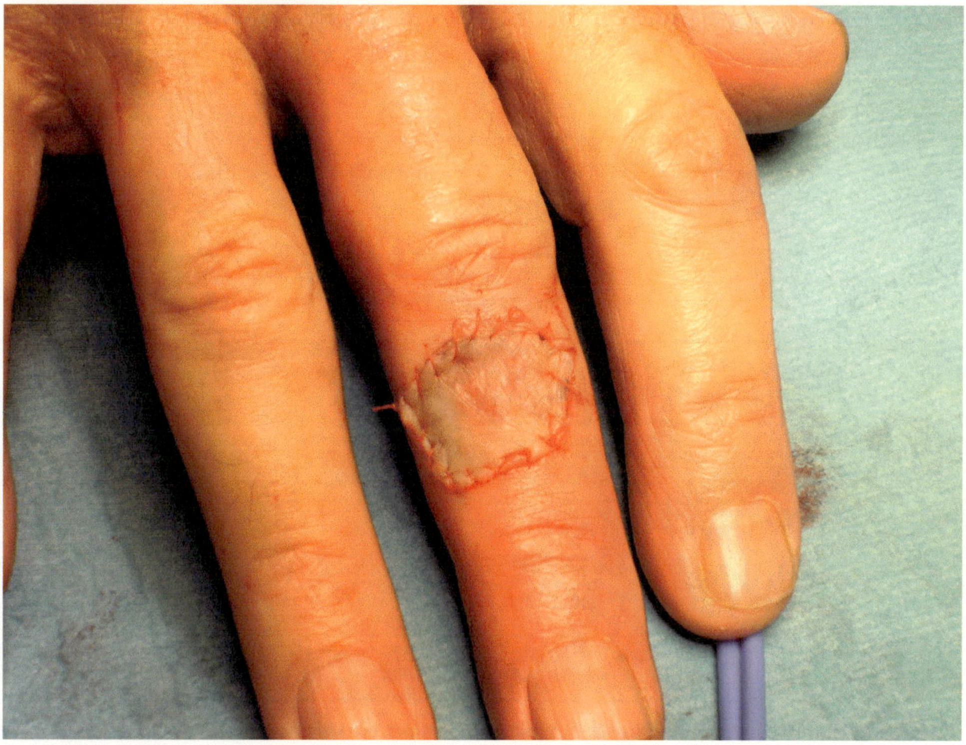

Fig. 6. Full thickness skin graft inset onto dorsum of finger

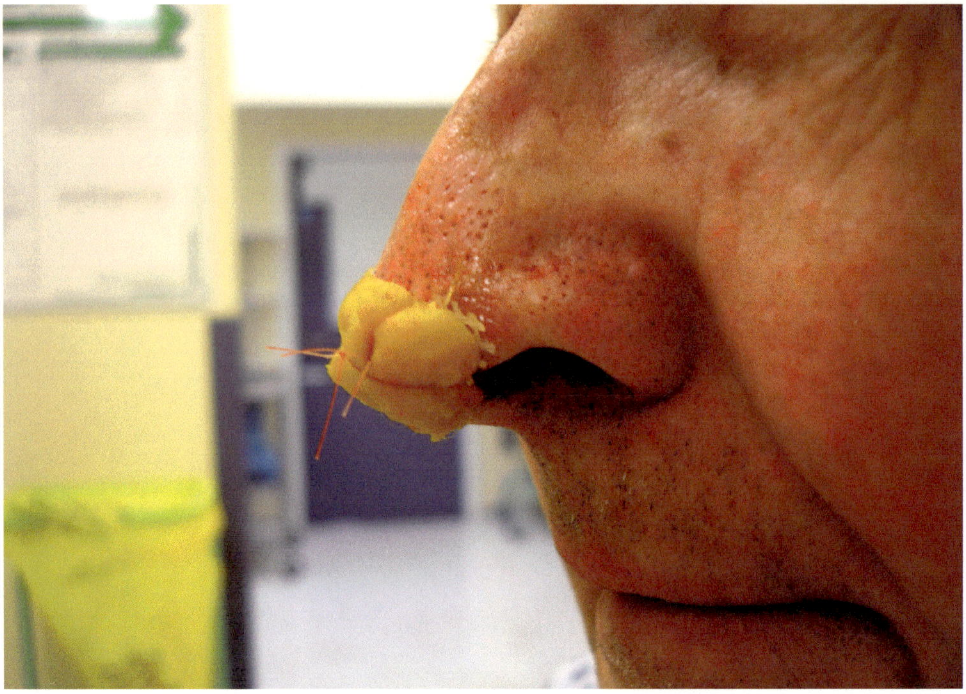

Fig. 7. Tie over dressing secured with sutures over full-thickness skin graft on nose. Note the presence of a non-adherent dressing (jelonet) between the proflavin wool and the graft

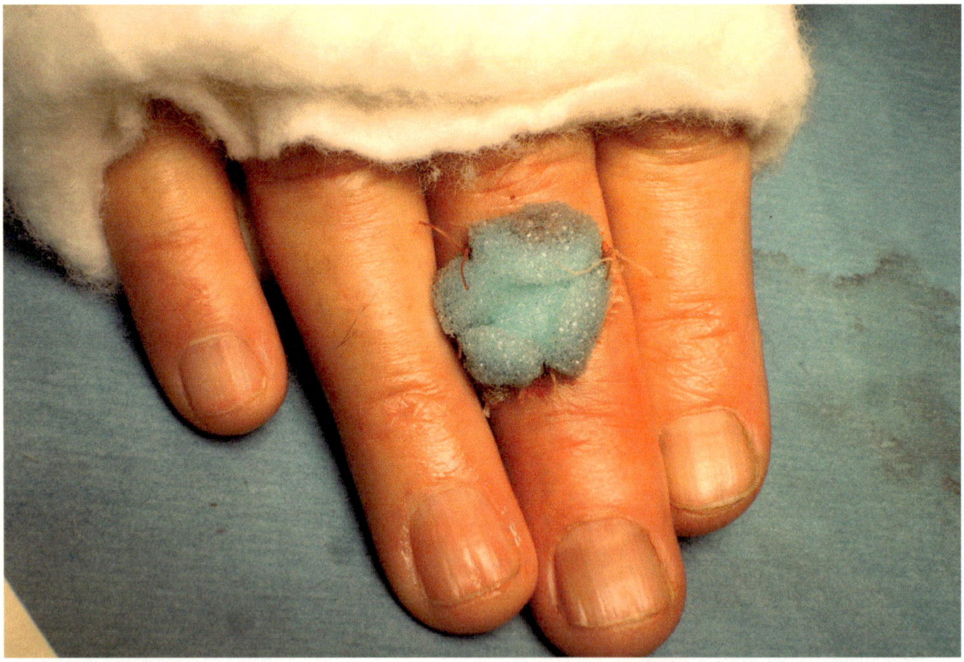

Fig. 8. Foam bolster dressing secured with sutures over full-thickness skin graft on dorsum of finger

5. Factors affecting graft survival

Before application of the graft, it is imperative that measures are taken to give the full thickness graft the best chance of survival. These include the following –

5.1 Healthy wound bed

Skin grafts rely on the underlying vascularity of the bed to maintain cellular respiration. Devascularized tissues, such as bone without periosteum, cartilage without perichondrium and tendon without paratenon, need an overlying layer of granulation tissue in order to be grafted. However, If the area is small, a graft may survive over bare cortical bone, cartilage or tendon by the phenomenon of 'bridging'. Bridging is where the blood supply of the neighbouring tissue is more than adequate to allow the graft in it vascularisation to 'bridge' the defect and successfully provide cover. Skin grafts can also survive on dermis, fascia, muscle and fat. Fat on the face is extremely vascular and grafts take readily. However the relatively poor vascularity of fat elsewhere limits its use a suitable surface to graft. Wounds which have undergone radiation have a compromised blood supply and may be unable to nourish a skin graft. Correction of underlying vascular problems is essential in vasculopaths with arterial insufficiency or venous stasis ulcers. Multiple surgical debridements may be required for a contaminated or chronic wound. Vacuum-assisted closure therapy or wet-to-dry dressing changes may occasionally be required until the recipient bed appears clean, healthy and red with punctate bleeding.

5.2 Absence of infection

Recipient sites must be healthy and free from infection. Bacterial levels greater than $10^5/cm^2$ are clinically significant. The bacterial count may be reduced by topical or systemic antibiotics. The presence of *Streptococcus pyogenes* on the wound bed is an absolute contraindication to skin grafting. The exact mechanism is unknown; however, Strep species produce fibrinolysin which lyse the fibrin attachment of the graft. In large areas which need to be grafted, e.g. following burns, routine bacteriologic swab investigation is often necessary. *Streptococcus pyogenes* must always be eliminated with antibiotics before grafting. Infection with *Pseudomonas aeruginosa* may reduce graft take by 5-10%. This can be treated by application of an antiseptic like chlorhexidine and removal of slough from the wound bed. Antibiotics for *Pseudomonas aeruginosa* are not usually necessary. Necrotic tissue must be completely debrided, as decaying tissue contains no blood supply and produces toxins that impair wound healing.

5.3 Absence of shear

Shear forces separate the graft from the bed and prevent the contact necessary for capillary link up and subsequent survival. Shear is minimised by using a foam tie dressing or proflavin cotton wool dressing to ensure good contact between the graft and the bed. This is until the initial fibrin adhesion has been converted into a strong fibrous tissue anchorage.

5.4 Hemostasis

Meticulous hemostasis is imperative during the operation in order to prevent haematoma formation (Figure 9). The operation steps should be planned to give the bed the longest time for the normal hemostatic processes to take effect. Bipolar coagulation is precise in controlling small bleeding vessels. Hematomas and seromas prevent contact of the graft to the bed and inhibit revascularization. They act as a block to link-up of the outgrowing capillaries. They must be drained by day 3 to facilitate graft survival.

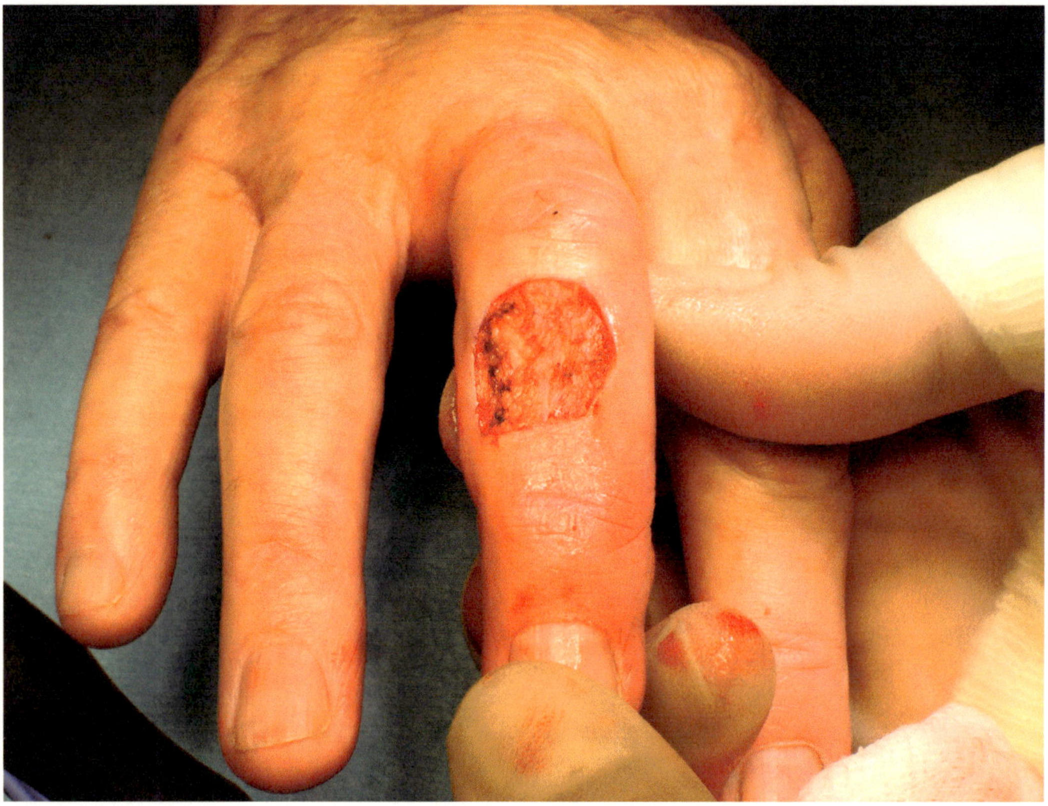

Fig. 9. Recipient 'bed' on dorsum of finger. Ensure meticulous hemostasis is achieved prior to graft

6. Advantages

Full-thickness skin grafts have a number of advantages over split skin grafts. When donor skin from the pre or post auricular region is used to resurface defects on the face, the colour match is usually excellent. Full-thickness grafts undergo minimal secondary contraction compared to split skin grafts. As a result, they maintain their characteristics well. This includes robustness of skin resulting in less likelihood of graft trauma. Also, a shapely contour is achieved compared to split skin grafts where clearly demarcated contours are often visibly seen, resulting in a sub-optimal cosmetic outcome and resultant patient embarrassment. A more uniform texture is achieved using a full-thickness skin graft. A major advantage is also the transference of dermal structures such as hair follicles if the defect is in a hair-bearing area. Finally, there is full-thickness skin graft growth potential as the patient grows.

7. Disadvantages

There are a few disadvantages in performing full-thickness skin grafting. Firstly, the presence of a well vascularized bed is necessary to ensure graft take and survival. Secondly, there is only a limited supply of donor skin that can be closed directly. An alternative way to close the donor area would be to utilise a split skin graft in addition to primary closure, however this results in another wound at the donor site which requires healing, as well as a sub-optimal cosmetic appearance. Finally, the transference of unwanted structures such as hair follicles may be disadvantageous if the grafted area is in a non hair- bearing region.

8. Conclusion

In this chapter, full-thickness skin grafts have been discussed as a simple and reliable method of skin coverage of small wounds which cannot be closed primarily. The mechanisms involved in graft take are plasmatic imbibition, inosculation and capillary ingrowth, and revascularization. There is a choice of a number of areas in the body skin grafts can be harvested from. However, the ultimate area of skin harvest is tailored to its specific destination depending on the colour match, consistency and robustness of the skin required. Particular attention must be paid to the adequate preparation of the bed to be grafted with regards to a healthy well vascularized wound bed, absence of infection, absence of shear forces and meticulous hemostasis to avoid hematoma formation.

9. References

Chen CM and Cole J (2007). Skin Grafting and Skin Substitutes In *Practical Plastic Surgery*, edited by Kryger ZB and Sisco M, pp. (145-153), Landes Bioscience, ISBN 978-1-57059-696-4, United States of America.

Giele H and Cassell O (2008). Plastic Surgery Science In Plastic and Reconstructive Surgery (Oxford Specialist Handbooks in Surgery), Oxford University Press, ISBN 978-0-19-263222-7, United Kingdom

Granzow JW and Boyd JB (2010). Grafts, Local and Regional Flaps In *Plastic and Reconstructive Surgery*, edited by John Lumley, pp. (65-87), Springer, ISBN 978-1-84882-512-3, United Kingdom.

Hackett MEJ. (1986). Restoration of skin cover : the use of free grafts In *Plastic Surgery, Rob and Smith's Operative Surgery* (4th edition), edited by Barclay TL and Karnahan DA, pp. (14-27), Butterworths, ISBN 0-407-00664-8, United Kingdom.

McGregor AD and McGregor IA. (2009). *Fundamental techniques of Plastic Surgery and their Surgical Applications* (10th edition), Elsevier Limited, ISBN 978 0 443 06372 5, United Kingdom.

Thorne CH. (2007). Techniques and Principles in Plastic Surgery In *Grabb and Smith's Plastic Surgery* (6th edition), edited by Thorne CH, pp. (3-14), Lippincott Williams & Wilkins, ISBN 978-0-7817-4698-4, United States of America.

Thornton JF (2004). Skin Grafts and Skin Substitutes, *Selected Readings in Plastic Surgery* (Vol 10, Number 1), pp. (1-23), ISSN 0739-5523.

Part 2

Applications

5

Lower Third Nasal Skin Grafting

James F. Thornton and Emily D. Rapstine
The University of Texas Southwestern
Medical Center at Dallas
United States of America

1. Introduction

Lower third nasal defects present a special challenge to reconstructive surgeons.. The unique character of the lower third of the nose, with its interwoven concavities, convexities, and varying skin thicknesses, exacerbates the difficult reconstruction of this region.

Specific flap algorithms are available for reconstruction of full-subunit alar or full-subunit tip defects (Hill, 1987). The lower third nasal defects or defects larger than 1.5 cm in diameter can be reliably reconstructed and repaired with nasolabial or forehead flaps using either a subunit or defect-only reconstruction (Barton, 1981). These techniques require multiple stages and allow for the replacement of cartilage and lining if missing.

Paradoxically, acceptable results are more difficult to achieve with smaller defects, most notably those smaller than 1 cm. Local flaps applied for these defects often result in violation of aesthetic subunits, worsening of the defect by alar notching, and frequent or unpredictable pincushioning. Likewise, the misapplication of skin grafts to large or deep lower third defects often yields a depressed patchwork with unsuitable results.

In many cases of lower third nasal reconstruction, particularly those arising from excision of neoplasms by means of Mohs' micrographic surgery, the defects are shallow and measure less than 1 cm in diameter. These defects rarely encompass greater than 50 percent of aesthetic subunits and are best treated as defect-only reconstructions (Dimitropolous et al., 2005). Such defects can be successfully and reliably treated with well-applied full-thickness skin grafting from the preauricular or more preferential forehead donor site.

The evolution of the demonstrated skin grafting techniques started with the recognition of the frustrating paradox in reconstructing small defects of the lower third. Larger defects could be easily and reliably reconstructed with the well-established algorithms (i.e., nasolabial or forehead flap reconstruction). The use of bilobed flaps from the upper third of the nose to recreate defects on the lower third commonly disappoints for two reasons. The inherent design flaw of the bilobed flap violates a second or third aesthetic unit and often completely distorts the alar groove. In addition, the final result is inherently unpredictable because of its tendency to pincushion. There is a common reluctance to advance skin from the nasal sidewall to reconstruct lower third defects, as this destroys the alar groove, an aesthetic subunit that is very difficult to reconstruct.

2. Anatomical considerations

The boundaries defining the lower third of the nose include the alar rims inferiorly, the nasolabial grooves laterally, and the alar groove, which forms the junction with the upper two-thirds of the nose (Collins & Farber, 1984; Leibovitch et al., 2006). Any distortion of the alar rim or obliteration of the nasolabial groove is exceedingly noticeable to the naked eye and difficult, if not impossible, to correct secondarily. The lower third of the nose is classically composed of six subunits: bilateral ala and soft triangles, the central tip, and columella (Baker & Swanson, 1995) (Fig. 1). Importantly, the ala and tip are biconvex structures, and maintaining and restoring the contour of these structures is essential to aesthetic nasal reconstruction. The unique nature of the lower third skin, which is often thick and richly populated with sebaceous glands, complicates reconstructions, often rendering the skin stiff and difficult to rotate and form into local flaps.

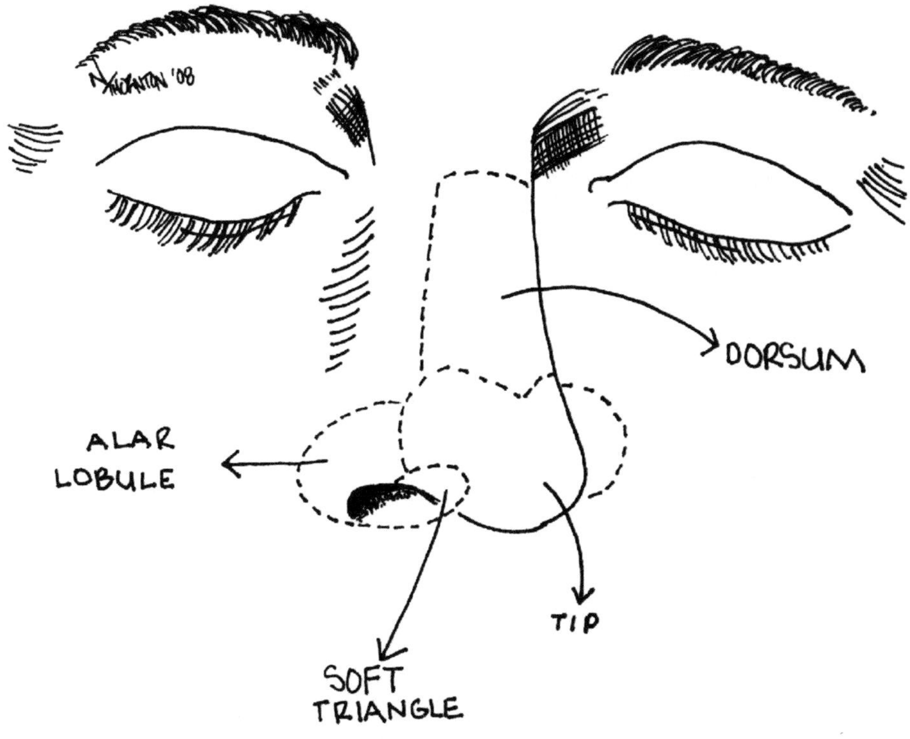

Fig. 1. Illustration of the nasal subunits of the lower third, including the dorsum, tip, and paired soft triangles and alar lobules. The columella is not shown.

3. Results

Average defect size among patients eligible for this type of grafting procedure ranges from 5 to 17 mm. Patients typically undergo one dermabrasion treatment after their procedure, with two or more dermabrasion treatments being prescribed or preferred less frequently. The aesthetic standard of a normal appearance with endpoints of good contour and color match, rather than simply a healed wound, should be used (Figs. 2 through 7). Based on postoperative photographs, some patients may present with minor contour or color defects, although a few may have more pronounced color/contour changes (Figs. 8 and 9). Active smokers are several times more likely to experience graft failure (Fig. 10).

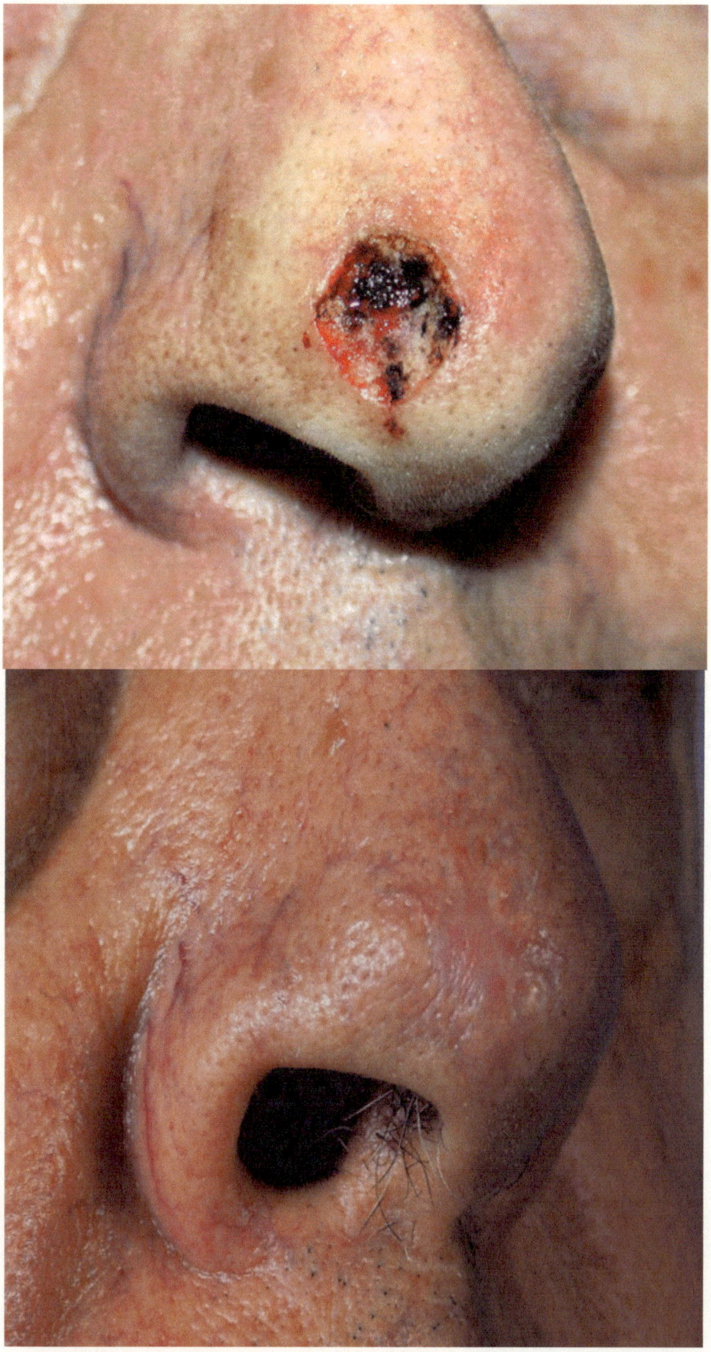

Fig. 2. A 64-year-old man presented with an 8-mm nasal defect following Mohs' excision of a basal cell carcinoma (*top*). There was exposed perichondrium in the base of the wound, although it was a relatively thin defect. Two rounds of dermabrasion were performed after the graft, which was taken from a forehead donor site, was placed. The appearance at a 3-month follow up is shown below.

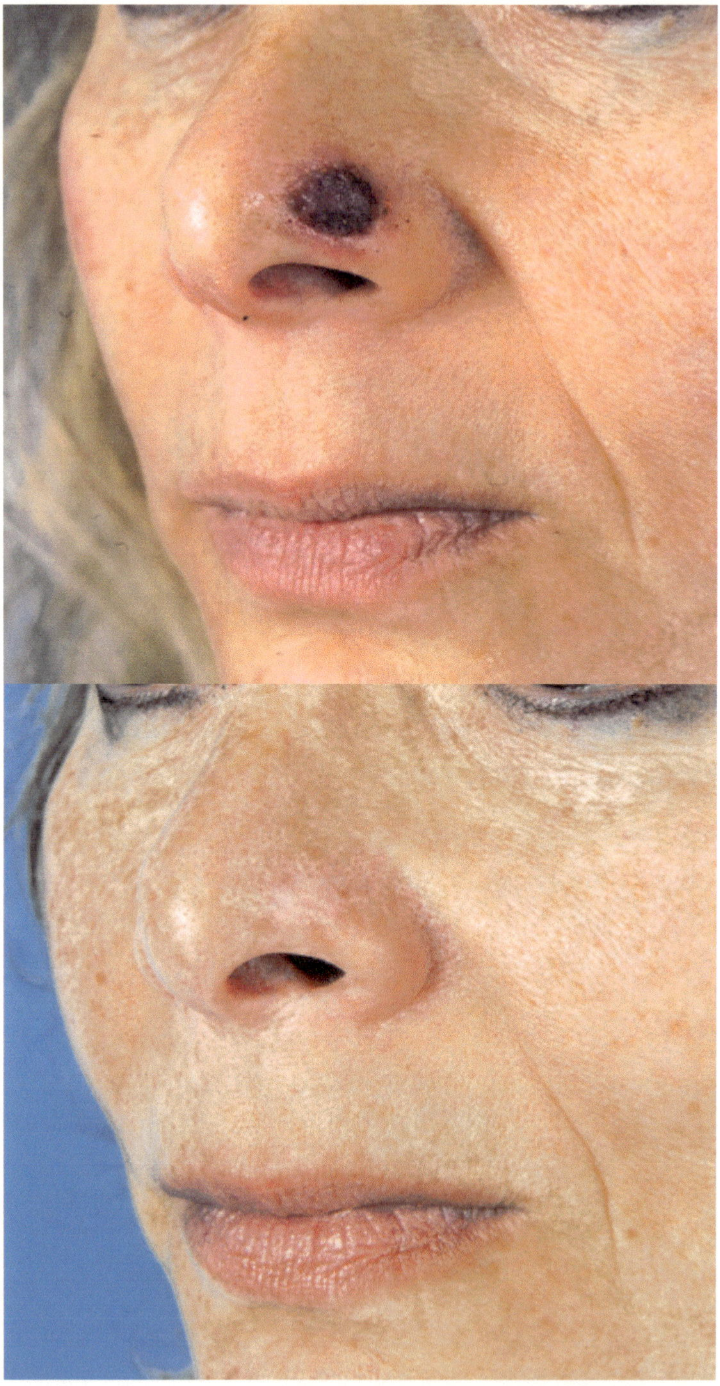

Fig. 3. A 43-year-old woman presented with a 7-mm alar defect, abutting but not crossing the alar rim. The appearance of the patient 1 week after skin grafting from a forehead donor site is shown on top. The graft appears dusky despite good take. The patient 3 months postoperatively and after two dermabrasion treatments is shown below.

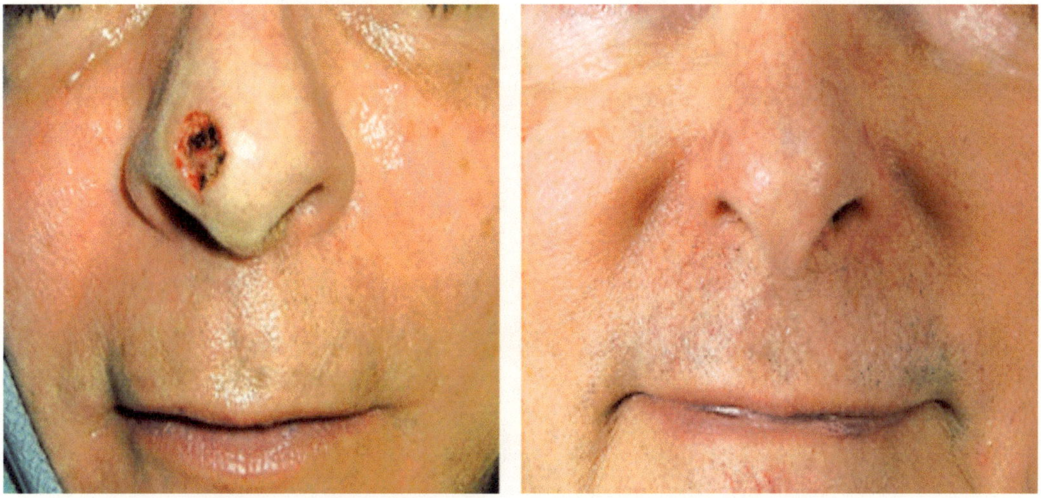

Fig. 4. A 57-year-old man with thin nasal skin underwent Mohs' excision of a basal cell carcinoma on his nasal tip (*left*). The patient's 3-month follow-up photo after full-thickness skin grafting from forehead skin and one in-office dermabrasion treatment is pictured on the right.

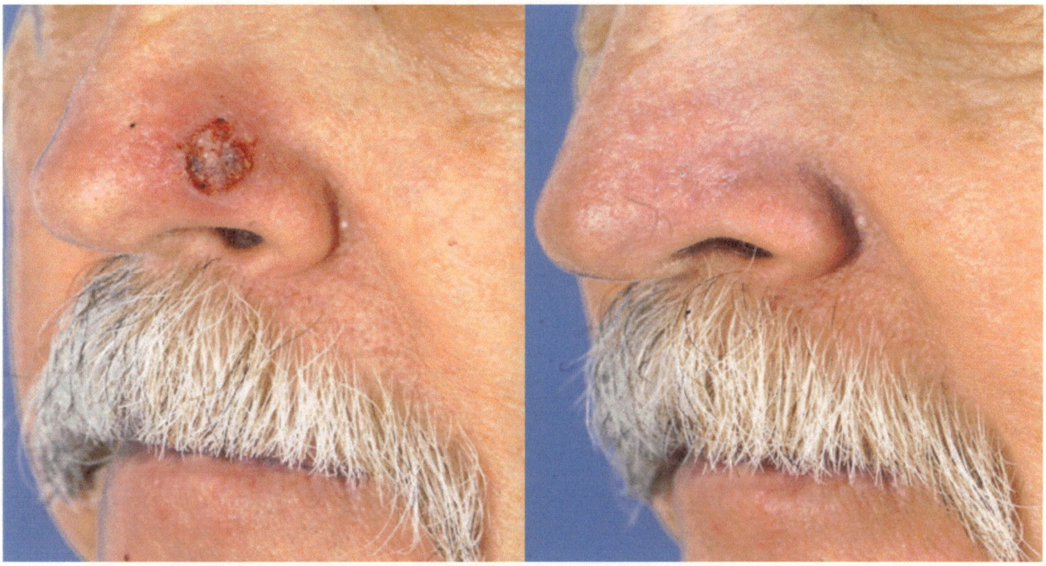

Fig. 5. A 54-year-old man had a 7-mm alar defect after excision of a basal cell carcinoma (*left*). The patient at the 3-month follow-up visit following preauricular skin grafting and one dermabrasion treatment is pictured on the right.

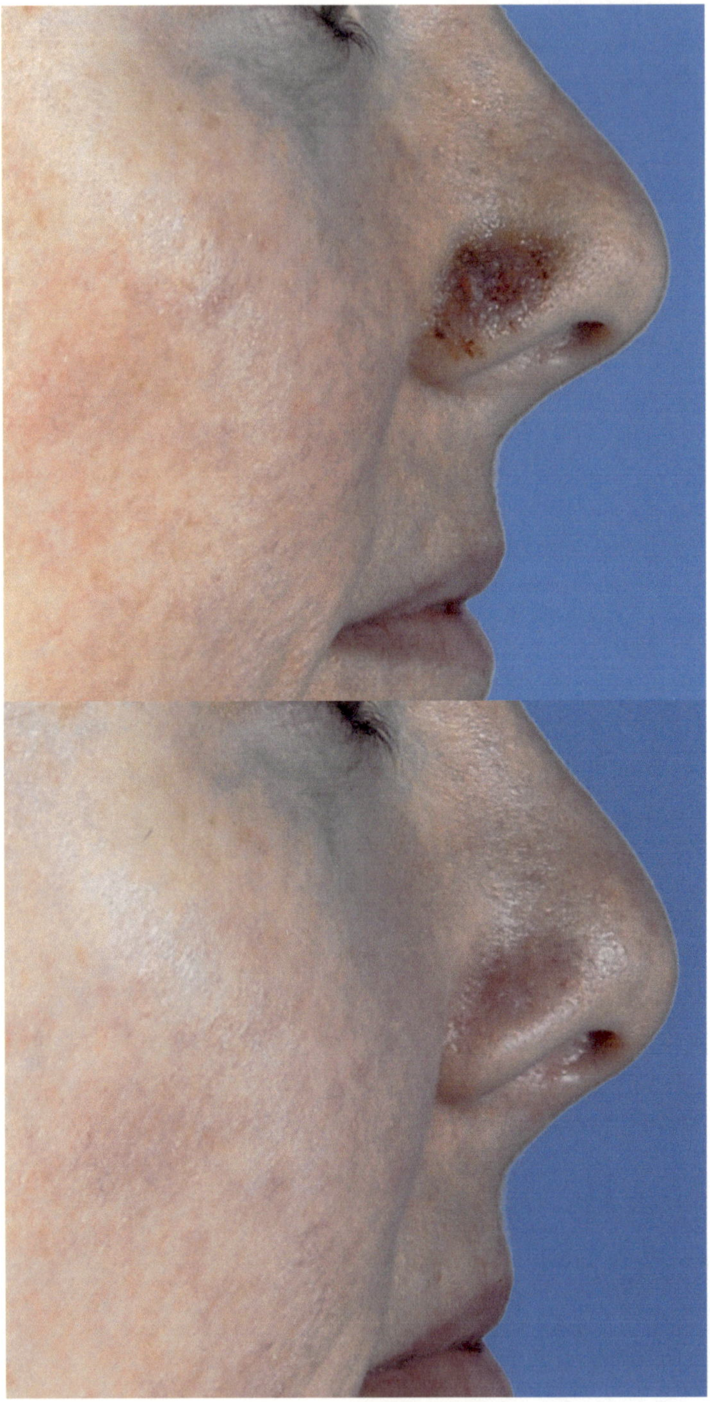

Fig. 6. A 1-cm superficial alar defect was reconstructed with a full-thickness skin graft from a forehead donor site in this 37-year-old woman (*top*). After two dermabrasion treatments, her contour and pigmentation at 3 months show a good result (*bottom*).

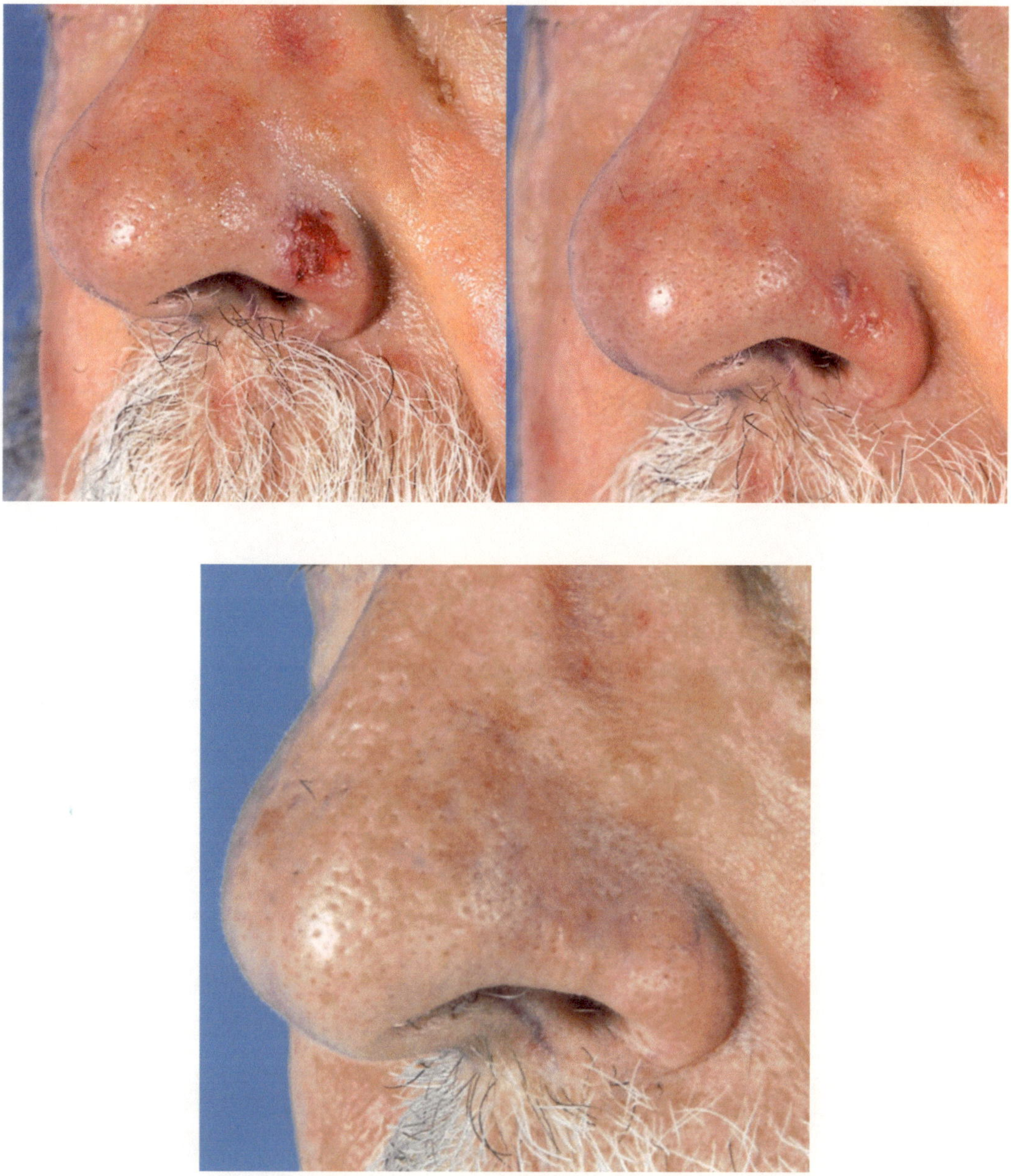

Fig. 7. The 5-mm alar rim defect was reconstructed with a full-thickness skin graft using preauricular skin (*upper left*). The degree of healing at 1-month postoperatively is pictured in the upper right. After two dermabrasion treatments, no contour or color irregularities are visible (*lower center*).

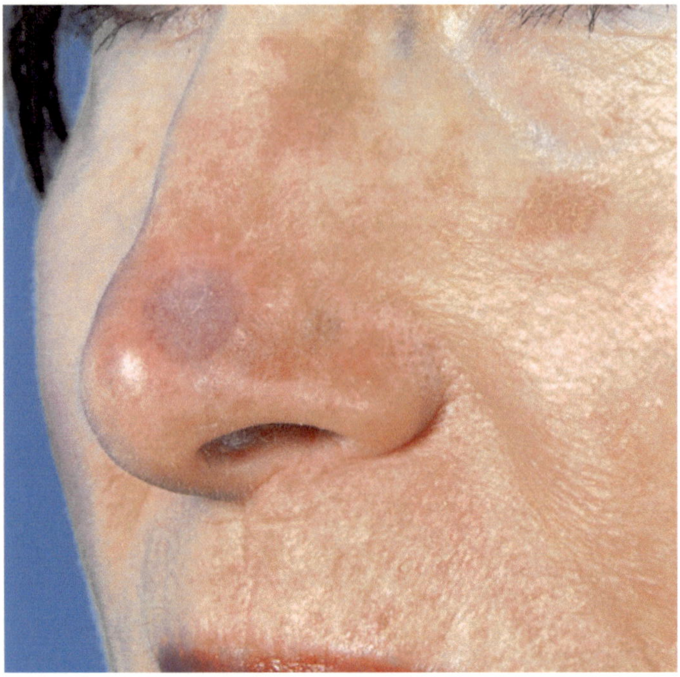

Fig. 8. A patient with a hypopigmented scar after full-thickness skin grafting from preauricular skin to the nasal tip with postoperative dermabrasion.

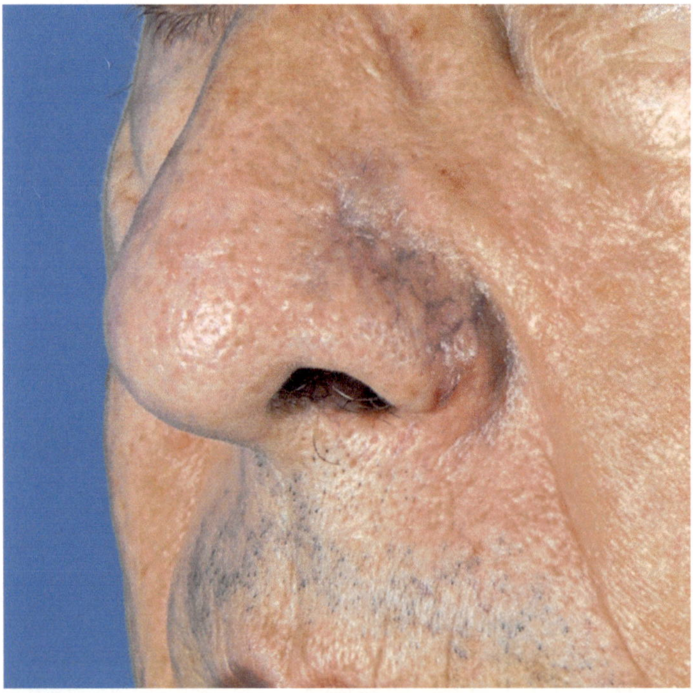

Fig. 9. This patient received a full-thickness skin graft from a preauricular donor site to his ala with postoperative dermabrasion. He has a persistent contour defect at this site.

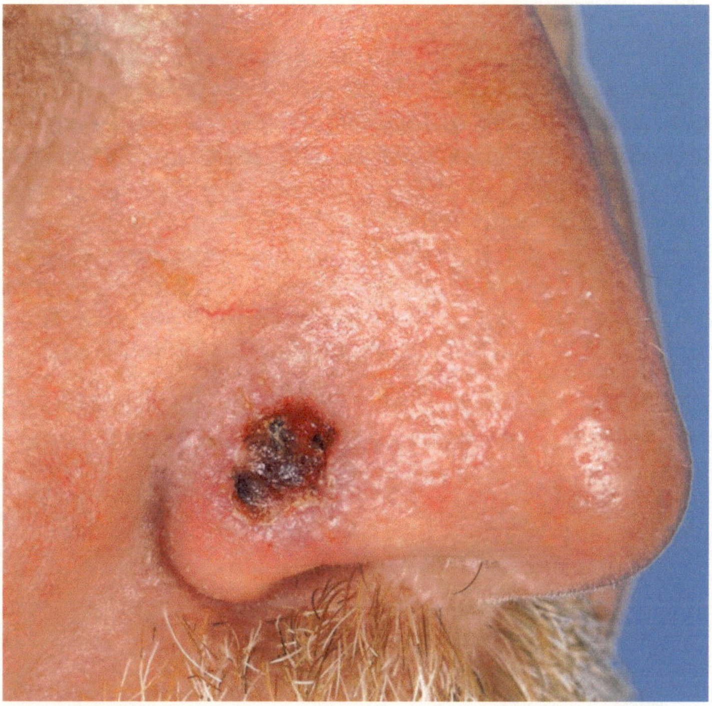

Fig. 10. An example of a failed alar graft from forehead skin in a smoker. This was successfully regrafted after the wound was débrided.

4. Technique

Procedures are performed under local anesthesia with or without intravenous sedation in an operating room setting. A 1:1 mixture of 0.25% Marcaine (Hospira, Inc., Lake Forest, Ill.) with 1% lidocaine with epinephrine (mixed 1:1000 in 30 cc of lidocaine) is used for local anesthesia, vasoconstriction, and postoperative analgesia. This mixture is injected subdermally at the site of the defect and the graft donor site. Each defect repair begins with reverticalization of the wound edges and sharp débridement of any fibrinous tissue or debris in the base of the defect. This initial step is critical for normalizing any contour abnormalities in the defect and is performed under loupe magnification with a straight, double-edged beaver blade. Further excisions are performed if required to place the borders within aesthetic subunits; however, there is not a strict adherence to aesthetic subunit reconstruction since this procedure is considered to be a defect-only reconstruction.

After reverticalization of the wound edges and normalization of the contour, a foil pattern template is used. This template should be treated as a three-dimensional construct, accounting for the relative concavity or convexity of the tissue surrounding the defect. A full-thickness skin graft from the preauricular or the preferred forehead donor site is harvested based on the foil template. The donor sites should be closed in a multilayer fashion with buried interrupted and continuous suture. The donor sites are frequently placed at the junction of the hair-bearing and non-hair-bearing scalp following the relaxed skin tension lines. Great care must be taken to ensure that the grafts harvested are matched to the identical size of the donor site. This is accomplished by using the foil pattern template and sharply scoring the harvested graft within the ellipse of the donor site to accurately reflect the size before harvesting the graft. This eliminates the distortion caused by blurry ink lines while harvesting the graft. Therefore, scoring the template before harvest represents a critical step in accurately designing the graft to be the exact size of the defect. The graft should be handled atraumatically and with great care throughout its harvest and inset.

Due to unsatisfactory inflammatory response from 4-0 or 5-0 chromic gut suture, the preferred suture material is 5-0 fast-absorbing gut. The grafts are precisely sewn into place with continuous opposing 4-0 or 5-0 plain gut sutures that run in a continuous fashion in opposite directions around the graft and are tied at the opposite side. This precisely insets the graft, providing a stable inset with no bunching or distortion, and is very time saving (Fig. 11).

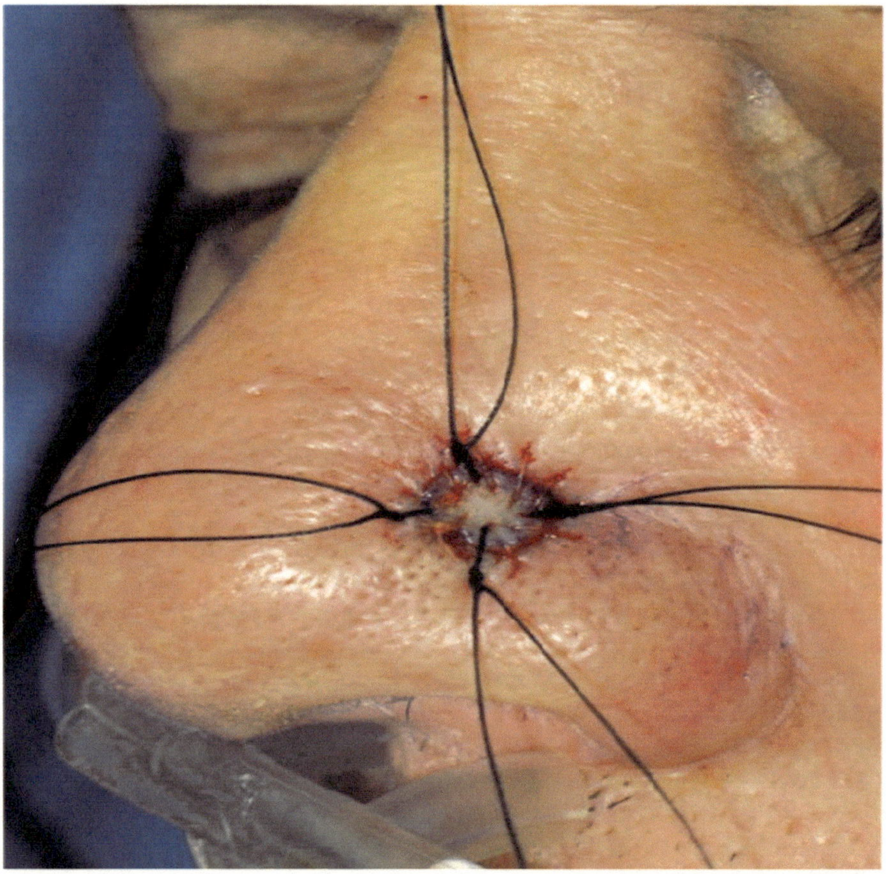

Fig. 11. An example of the fast-absorbing running suture at the graft margin, and four-corner bolster sutures.

Fabrication of the skin graft bolster completes the procedure. In the majority of cases, a double-armed 3-0 or 4-0 Prolene suture (Ethicon, Inc., Somerville, N.J.) is placed at the center through the underlying tissue and then through the center of the graft. Both arms of the suture are placed in a similar fashion and then left untied and sewn directly into the bolster (Fig. 12). Bolsters are fashioned from dry surgical preparation sponges that have been gas sterilized preoperatively and coated with antibiotic ointment away from the operative field. The surgical preparation sponge material provides adequate rebound and support. The through-and-through 3-0 Prolene sutures are placed in juxtaposition through the bolster and tied in place (Fig. 13). This technique obliterates central dead space and optimizes graft adherence. The remainder of the bolster is then secured with 5-0 silk bolster sutures placed through the graft and native skin edge, then tied at four to eight points around the graft, depending on graft size. The closed donor-site incision and the edges and exterior of the bolster should also be coated with antibiotic ointment. Donor sites are dressed with Xeroform gauze (Sherwood Medical, St. Louis, Mo.), and a set of written wound care instructions is given to the patient. The patient may begin showering on the second postoperative day with the provision that they cover the graft bolsters with a vigorous coating of antibiotic ointment before showering.

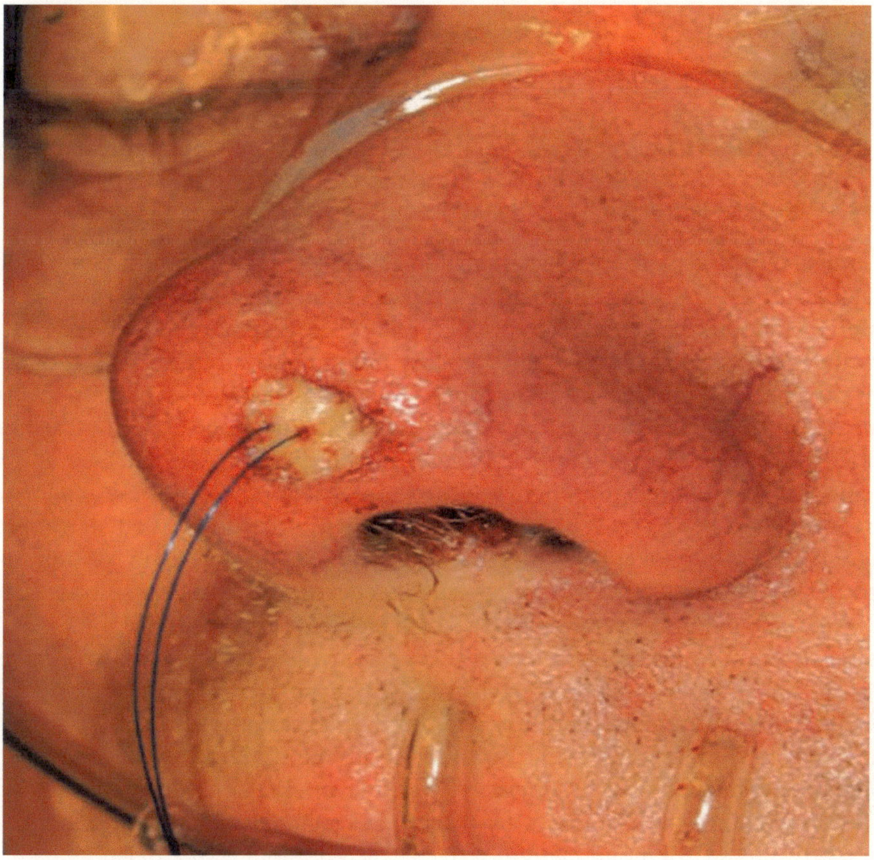

Fig. 12. The through-and-through monofilament suture used to provide additional stability and compression to the skin graft bolster. Both needles on the double-ended suture are then passed through the center of the piece of surgical sponge and tied down.

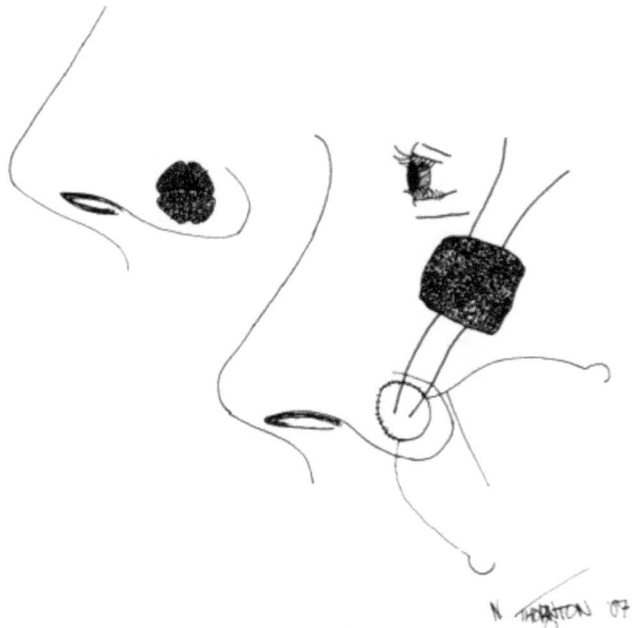

Fig. 13. Illustration of the bolster technique used by the author. Through-and-through 3-0 Prolene sutures are placed in juxtaposition through the bolster and tied in place. This technique obliterates central dead space and optimizes graft adherence.

It is not unusual for the most superficial portion of the graft to initially undergo a period of partial slough given the thickness of the forehead skin. Treatment for this is continued application of antibiotic ointment and patient reassurance. Patients should be seen at weekly intervals until full graft survival is ensured. At this point, daily application of antibiotic ointment may be discontinued and the opportunity to begin topical scar cream therapy with Mederma (Merz Pharmaceuticals, Greensboro, N.C.), Scar Zone (CCA Industries, East Rutherford, N.J.), or more recently, Transdermis scar therapy (NFI Consumer Products, Fayetteville, N.C.) is offered to patients. No clinical science supports the use of one scar cream over another; however, it has been our experience that the patients strongly prefer applying a scar care product. The Transdermis scar therapy subjectively results in a fairly rapid reduction in the inflammatory response. The opportunity to apply silicone sheeting to both the skin graft and donor-site areas could also be offered to patients.
That the postoperative recommendations for scar therapy are based not on science but on an evolving clinical practice with lessons learned from failures in scar therapy from the beginning of practice. Patients should be offered dermabrasion beginning at 6 weeks after grafting. Based on the behavior and appearance of the scar, up to three postoperative dermabrasion treatments may be offered at 6-week intervals. The dermabrasion can be carried out in the office setting with a topical tetracaine cream as an anesthetic and a rotary dermabrader using the diamond cylinder wheel. The endpoint of the dermabrasion is deep punctate bleeding. The goals of the dermabrasion procedure are to both improve the graft color and to blur or diminish the patch effect of the graft on the surrounding nasal skin by essentially improving the appearance of the surrounding scar. The procedure is confined to the graft and immediate surrounding skin. Although dermabrading entire subunits has

been advocated to provide an even contour over the subunit, we have found this practice largely unnecessary for smaller defects (Adams & Ramsey, 2005). Entire subunit dermabrasion is not frequently offered except for larger defects that encompass a majority of the subunit (Kuijpers et al., 2006). An illustration of the effects of dermabrasion is provided in sequential photographs in Figure 6.

5. Discussion

Skin grafting of defects of the lower third of the nose has historically, and often correctly, been considered to yield an inferior aesthetic result. The inappropriate placement of large, poorly color-matched supraclavicular or postauricular skin grafts to replace the thick, often convex defects of the lower third can yield results that are poor and frequently impossible to correct. Achieving a well contoured, aesthetically pleasing result begins with meticulous preoperative analysis of the nasal defect. Criteria for selecting lower third nasal defects that can be acceptably treated with full-thickness grafts include defect location, size smaller than 1 cm, and a partial-thickness defect with underlying dermis, subcutaneous tissue, or perichondrium.

The patchwork appearance caused by color mismatch and contour defects is the basic concern with using a full-thickness skin graft. Adhering to the concept of subunit reconstruction alleviates concerns for a resultant patchwork appearance, regardless of the reconstructive method. A defect-only approach is preferred to nasal reconstruction when using full-thickness skin grafts. Acceptable results are typically achieved using full-thickness skin grafts to reconstruct lower third defects smaller than 1 cm in diameter, without the need to excise an entire subunit. The decision to limit described reconstructions to less than 1 cm is not based on the inability to reconstruct larger defects; however, defects larger than 1 cm, in our experience, are reconstructed more successfully with entire subunit reconstructions using more standard reconstruction techniques (local or adjacent flap techniques). Contrasting defect-only versus subunit nasal reconstruction is beyond the scope of this discussion; however, these concepts are an important component of defect analysis and must always be considered. Again, a principle-based reconstruction, beginning with careful and meticulous defect analysis and selection, will yield an acceptable result regardless of the reconstructive method (Rohrich et al., 2004).

Adhering to the concept of replacing like with like, the individual characteristics of skin graft donor sites must be considered. After analyzing the defect and creating a like-sized template, the appropriate donor site must be selected based on texture, thickness, color, and tendency toward hyperpigmentation or hypopigmentation. Much of our current knowledge of donor-site characteristics comes from the dermatology literature (Dimitropolous et al., 2005). Preauricular and, more preferably, forehead skin are the favored candidates for lower third nasal reconstruction. Forehead sites offer thicker skin, with a relatively sebaceous, oily texture, and they suffer the same degree of daily sun exposure and actinic damage as the lower third of the nose. Other donor sites available to the reconstructive surgeon include the nasolabial fold, postauricular skin, and supraclavicular skin. Postauricular donor sites suffer very little, if any, daily sun exposure and have much thinner skin than the nasal lobule. Therefore, postauricular donor sites are prone to pigmentation changes and do not provide a good contour match for reconstructing the lower third of the nose. Likewise, the skin of the supraclavicular region contains very few sebaceous elements and is often hyperpigmented before harvest. The preauricular and forehead donor site grafts should be harvested without including terminal hairs and designed along relaxed skin tension lines, allowing for primary closure. Good results can be achieved without distorting the anterior hairline or sideburn.

Hubbard wrote a provocative article describing 33 patients who had lower third defects reconstructed with nasolabial fat and/or partially defatted skin grafts harvested from the nasolabial fold (Hubbard, 2004). The illustrated results demonstrated perfectly acceptable reconstructions, and this work serves as a useful description of a different technique using the nasolabial donor site. Although a departure from commonly preferred techniques, Hubbard's results are a testament to the concept that a skin graft can survive without being completely defatted. While the results Hubbard attained are aesthetically acceptable and associated with very few graft losses, most authors argue that leaving this fat impedes the processes of imbibition and inosculation necessary for graft survival, thereby risking high rates of graft loss. Establishing neovascularization requires contact between the graft dermis and the recipient bed. Therefore, we regard careful defatting of the graft and use of a bolster indispensable technical components to ensure survival or "take" of the full-thickness graft.

If a defect is of sufficient depth to require a graft that includes subcutaneous fat, using a full-thickness skin graft for such a defect represents a break from principle-based reconstruction. Likewise, when considering defects along or near the alar rim, one must carefully account for the potential for alar notching. Given appropriate defect analysis, reconstructing a superficial alar defect with a full-thickness skin graft may yield an acceptable result without resultant notching. Skin grafting for defects that abut the alar rim must be used with great caution. Preferentially, skin grafts on the posterior aspect of the ala or defects in male patients with very thick sebaceous skin could be grafted more safely without the risk of alar retraction secondary to the inherent stability of anatomical position on the ala (Rohrich et al., 2004). Deeper defects that extend into the subcutaneous tissue or to the perichondrium of the lateral crura demand a local flap or nasolabial flap with a nonanatomical alar contour graft.

Both the dermatologic and plastic surgery literature frequently debate whether to harvest a graft of identical size to the defect or to correct for anticipated contraction and harvest a larger graft. The technique described earlier in this discussion involves creation of a template of equal size to the defect. As previously mentioned, this template is designed in three dimensions, taking concavity or convexity into consideration. Full-thickness skin grafts primarily contract 10 to 15 percent after excision; however, insetting the graft under appropriate tension readily resolves this problem. Harvesting a larger graft to account for primary contraction presents a number of issues. First, the donor site must be larger, and in keeping with an elliptical design, increasing the diameter of the donor site necessitates an extension of its axial length. The larger donor graft, which represents an estimation of size to account for contraction, often requires trimming before inset and leads to an inexact size and shape that no longer resembles the template or the defect. Harvesting a larger graft does not improve these results but instead, presents the confounding morbidity of a larger donor site.

Graft loss is always a concern, and although results are improved by careful defatting and bolster placement with through-and-through buttress sutures, other factors such as a history of smoking come into play. It is impossible to develop and maintain a comprehensive reconstructive practice without operating on smokers; however, these patients must understand that they are at significantly higher risk of graft loss or flap necrosis, and may ultimately be left with an unacceptable result. The effect of nicotine is well documented as a potent vasoconstrictor that reduces blood flow, leading to a hypoxic cascade that impairs healing and increases platelet aggregation and adhesion. In the multicenter study of recipient-site complications of full-thickness skin grafts, authors of the Australian Mohs Database showed that "although the number of smokers was small, they had a mean graft survival of 2% on the second visit compared with 75.9% in the nonsmoking group" (Leibovitch et al., 2006). If the patients are seen preoperatively, substantial benefit has been shown in people who are able to abstain from smoking for at least 4 weeks before reconstruction.

Patients are typically well informed and understand the possibility of graft loss, as well as being highly attuned to changes in graft appearance, often presenting in the early postoperative period with concerns over a pale or overly dark graft. Indeed, full-thickness skin grafts are less predictable than nasolabial or local flaps. The healing period involves color and texture changes that can raise alarm before arriving at the final, aesthetically acceptable result. The graft is initially ischemic, appearing white and pale. As it evolves through the stages of revascularization, it will become edematous and then darken, resulting in a cyanotic or hyperemic appearance. These color changes vary from patient to patient, graft sites, and sizes in an unpredictable manner, but over weeks to months, the living graft will approximate a normal color. In some cases, especially with a thick graft, the epidermis will darken and slough. This tissue will reepithelialize, given the presence of dermal appendages, but both the patient and physician will have a justified concern that the graft has failed. Patients should be counseled to anticipate these changes in color and texture.

In keeping with the principles asserted by Rohrich et al., good contour is the aesthetic endpoint to all nasal reconstructions (Rohrich et al., 2004). To achieve this, the authors describe "complementary ablative procedures" to enhance final results. These procedures include dermabrasion, thinning of flaps, breaking up trapdoor scar lines, and steroid injections at sites of pincushioning. Primary dermabrasion is not typically performed for full-thickness skin grafts because of the risk of trauma to the delicate graft and because of the unpredictable course of healing that the graft will follow. Dermabrasion of skin grafts is instead performed at approximately 6 weeks postoperatively. Depending on the size of the graft, dermabrasion can be limited to the graft margins or can include an entire subunit(s).

6. Conclusions

The following principles make skin grafting of lower third subunits a viable reconstruction option.

1. Rigorous defect selection to include only superficial and size-limited defects. Defects larger than 1 cm will be better treated with alternative reconstructions. Defects that involve cartilage or deeper are by definition complex nasal defects that will require onlay cartilage grafting for satisfactory reconstruction. Skin grafting is not offered for these defects.
2. Caution in skin grafting defects abutting the alar rim.
3. Meticulous graft donor-site selection using the thicker and better color-matched forehead skin in the majority of cases.
4. Meticulous size matching of the graft, using a foil pattern template, and development of a bolster material from a surgical sponge that provides ideal compression and handling

qualities used in conjunction with a through-and-through central Prolene suture to minimize graft dead space.
5. Liberal use of postoperative dermabrasion to optimize the final color match.

Provided that these constraints are followed, skin grafting of the lower third of the nose is an appropriate part of the reconstructive algorithm.

7. References

Adams, D., Ramsey, M. (2005). Grafts in dermatologic surgery: Review and update on full- and split-thickness skin grafts, free cartilage grafts, and composite grafts. *J Dermatol Surg*, Vol.32, No.8 Pt 2, (August 2005), pp. (1055-1067)

Baker, S., Swanson, N. (1995). *Local Flaps in Facial Reconstruction* (1st ed.), Mosby, 0801669251, St. Louis

Barton, Jr., F. (1981). Aesthetic aspects of partial nasal reconstruction. *Clin Plast Surg,* Vol.9, No.2, (April 1981), pp. (177-191)

Collins, P., Farber, G. (1984). Postsurgical dermabrasion of the nose. *J Dermatol Surg Oncol,* Vol.10, No.6, (June 1984), pp. (476-477)

Dimitropolous, V., Bichakjian, C., Johnson, T. (2005). Forehead donor site full-thickness skin graft. *Dermatol Surg,* Vol.31, No.3, (March 2005), pp. (324-326)

Hill, T. (1987). Contouring of donor skin in full-thickness skin grafting. *J Dermatol Surg Oncol*, Vol.13, No.8, (August 1987), pp. (883-886)

Hubbard, T. (2004). Leave the fat, skip the bolster: Thinking outside the box in lower third nasal reconstruction. *Plast Reconstr Surg*, Vol.114, No.6, (November 2004), pp. (1427-1435)

Kuijpers, D., Smeets, N., Lapière, K., Thissen, M., Krekels, G., Nuemann, H. (2006). Do systemic antibiotics increase the survival of a full-thickness graft of the nose? *J Eur Acad Dermatol Venereol*, Vol.20, No.10, (November 2006), pp. (1296-1301)

Leibovitch, I., Huilgol, S., Richards, S., Paver, R., Selva, D. (2006). The Australian Mohs database: Short term recipient-site complication in full-thickness skin grafts. *Dermatol Surg*, Vol.32, No.11, (November 2006), pp. (1364-1368)

Rohrich, R., Griffin, J., Ansari, M., Beran, S., Potter, J. (2004). Nasal reconstruction--beyond aesthetic subunits: A 15 year review of 1334 cases. *Plast Reconstr Surg,* Vol.114, No.6, (November 2004), pp. (1405-1416); discussion pp. (1417-1419)

6

Penis-Sparing Surgery with Neo-Glans Reconstruction for Benign, Premalignant or Malignant Penile Lesions

Enzo Palminteri[1], Fernando Fusco[2],
Elisa Berdondini[1] and Andrea Salonia[3]
[1]Center for Urethral and Genitalia Reconstructive Surgery, Arezzo
[2]Department of Urology, University Federico II, Naples
[3]Department of Urology, University Vita-Salute San Raffaele, Milan
Italy

1. Introduction

Penile neoplasm is an uncommon malignancy affecting less than 1 out of 100000 males in Europe and in the United States. Seventy-eight percent of all tumours appear on the glans and/or prepuce [1,2]. Many of these lesions are red, moist patches which can be misdiagnosed as either a benign skin condition (i.e. Zoon's balanitis or lichen planus) or a premalignant lesion such as the lichen sclerosus (LS) that, if left untreated, has the risk of progression to invasive squamous cell carcinoma in 5 to 33% of the cases [3]. Beyond all, both benign, premalignant and malignant lesions may cause pruritus, pain, bleeding, crusting and difficulties in retracting the foreskin, and overall psychosexual disability.

The treatment of benign, premalignant and malignant penile lesions has changed over time [4,5]. Traditional penile surgery is associated with a mutilating approach, eventually characterized by a high incidence of aesthetic, dysfunctional and psychological post-operative disorders [6-8]. In this context, the use of either medical or topical surgical treatments has been supported with the specific aim to maintain a good functional and aesthetic penile shaft; topical chemotherapy, laser ablation, cryotherapy, and local excisions have been thus reported in the scientific literature [3, 4]. However, these techniques are associated with high failures rates and unsightly scarring that impacts on penile appearance and sexual activity.

Recently in patients with either premalignant or malignant superficial lesions, alternative forms of surgical therapy have aimed at preserving the phallus without jeopardizing local cancer control have been extensively suggested. These organ-sparing techniques, providing the reconstruction of an aesthetic neo-glans without any impairment of patient's survival have also been suggested for more advanced tumours [1 - 3, 9].

2. Surgical techniques

Penis-preserving surgery with cosmetic reconstruction of a neo-glans is performed via 4 different surgical techniques using a free split-thickness skin graft (STSG) harvested from the thigh.

2.1 Glans skinning and glans resurfacing

The penis is circumcised and the penile skin is degloved. The glandular epithelium is fully removed up to the coronal sulcus. After preliminary marking, skin level incisions are made distally, skirting the edges of the meatus and proximally below the coronal margin. Vertical midline incisions are made dorsally and ventrally and join these distal and proximal incisions so that the glans covering can be dissected away as separate right and left halves. The STSG is harvested from the thigh using manual dermatome, and I subsequently transplanted like an umbrella over the bed of the stripped glans. The graft is then tailored and quilted over the glans with multiple 6-zero polyglactin interrupted stitches The penile skin is sutured to the graft at the coronal sulcus (fig. 1 and 2).

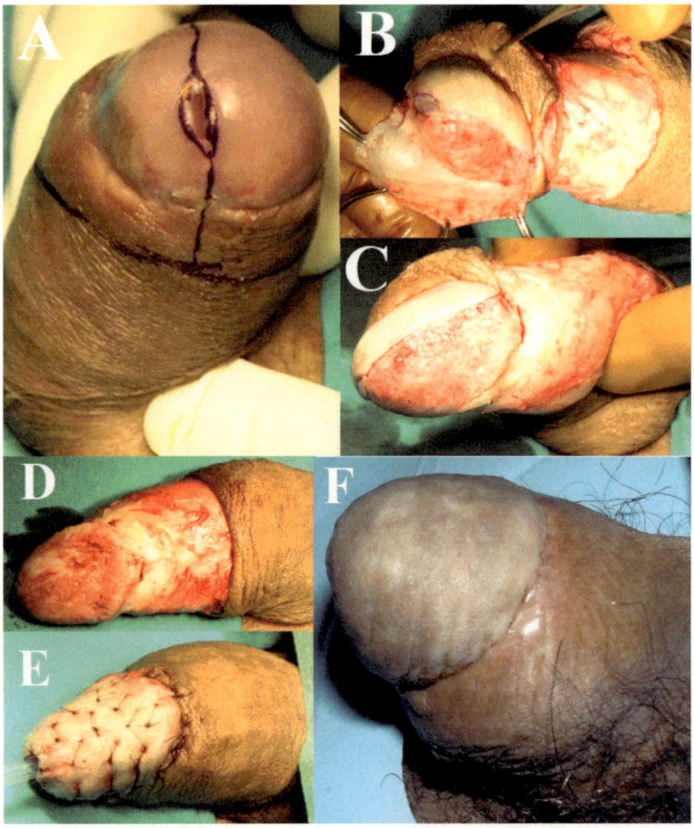

Fig. 1. Glans skinning and glans resurfacing: Squamous cell carcinoma involving glans and coronal sulcus (A).The glans epithelium is removed together with the distal foreskin (B - C - D).The skin graft is sutured and quilted over the stripped glans (E). Penile appearance 6 months after surgery (F).

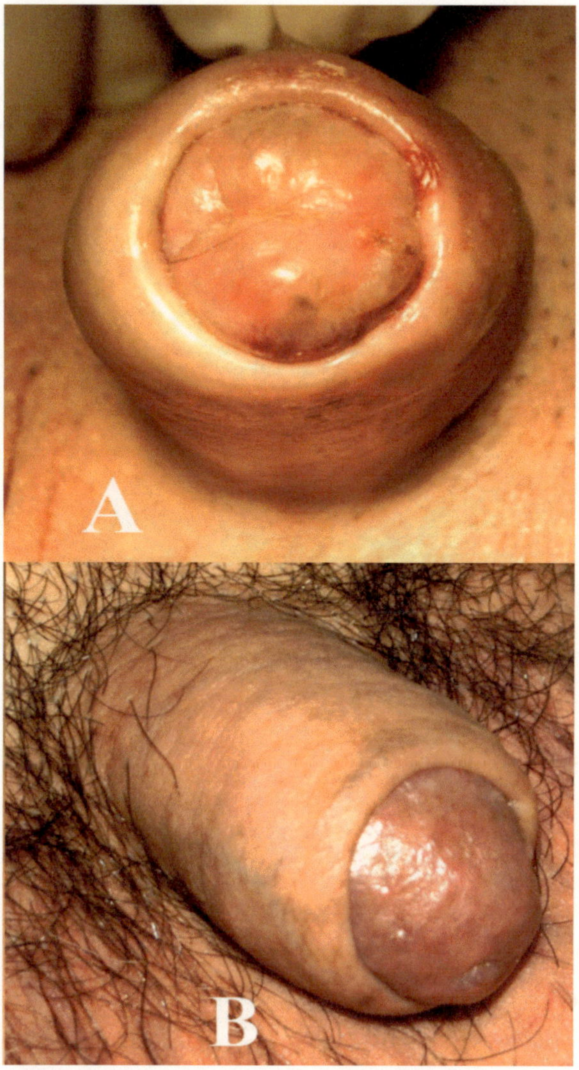

Fig. 2. Glans skinning and glans resurfacing: Lichen Sclerosus and Carcinoma in situ involving glans penis (A). Penile appearance 6 months after surgery (B).

This procedure is suitable for crippling benign and premalignant lesions, as well as malignant lesions, limited to the glandular epithelium.

2.2 Glansectomy and neo-glans reconstruction

The penis is circumcised and the penile skin is degloved. The glans is carefully segregated from the corpora cavernosa and the urethra is then distally sectioned. After removing the glans, the urethra is ventrally opened and the external urethral meatus is fixed to the tip of the corpora cavernosa. The STSG is then transplanted like an umbrella over the tips of the corpora cavernosa. The graft is tailored and quilted using interrupted stitches over the top of the corpora. Finally, the graft is fixed to the penile skin in order to recreate a neo-sulcus (fig. 3).

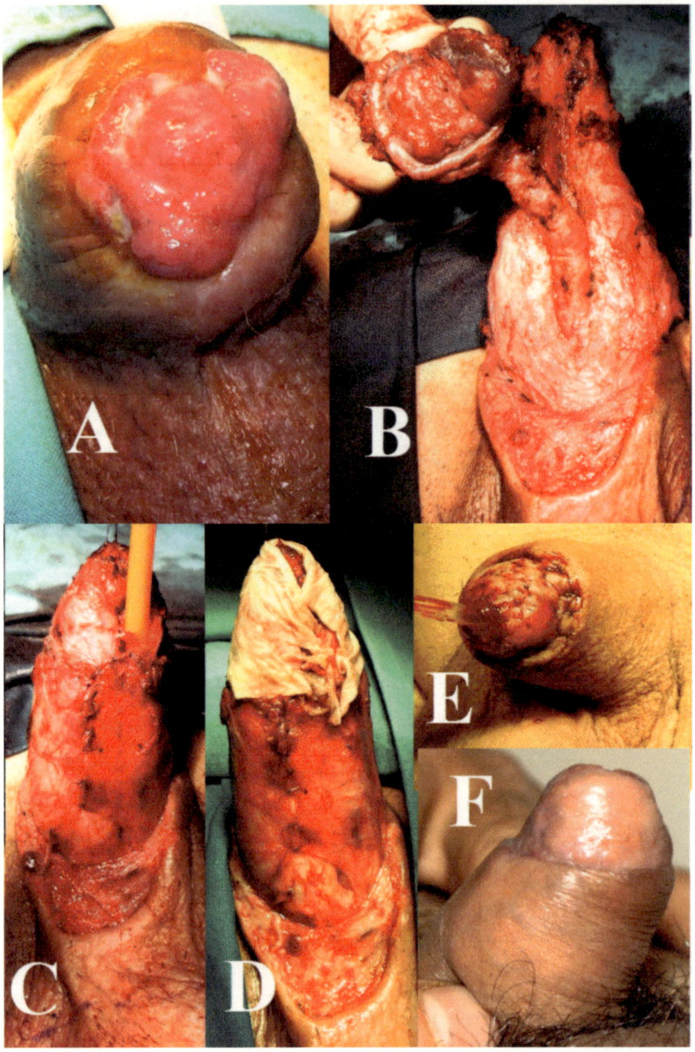

Fig. 3. Glansectomy and neo-glans reconstruction :Squamous cell carcinoma involving glans penis (A). The glans is dissected from the corpora cavernosa and the urethra is distally sectioned (B). The urethral meatus is fixed to the summit of the corpora cavernosa (C). The STSG is transplanted like an umbrella over the summit of the corpora cavernosa (D). The graft is tailored and quilted using interrupted stitches over the top of the corpora. The graft is fixed to the penile skin in order to recreate a neo-sulcus (E). Penile appearance 6 months after surgery (F).

This procedure is usually suitable for malignant lesions infiltrating the glans.

2.3 Partial penectomy and neo-glans reconstruction

The partial penectomy is performed with resection margins of only few millimetres, according to the current techniques [10].

The lateral edges of the residual corpora cavernosa are sutured together to create a hemispheric dome-shaped stump. The urethra is then spatulated and the meatus is fixed on the new tip of the corpora cavernosa. The STSG is transplanted like an umbrella over the summit of the hemispheric stump where it is quilted. The graft is eventually fixed to the penile skin with the aim to recreate a glandular neo-sulcus (fig. 4).

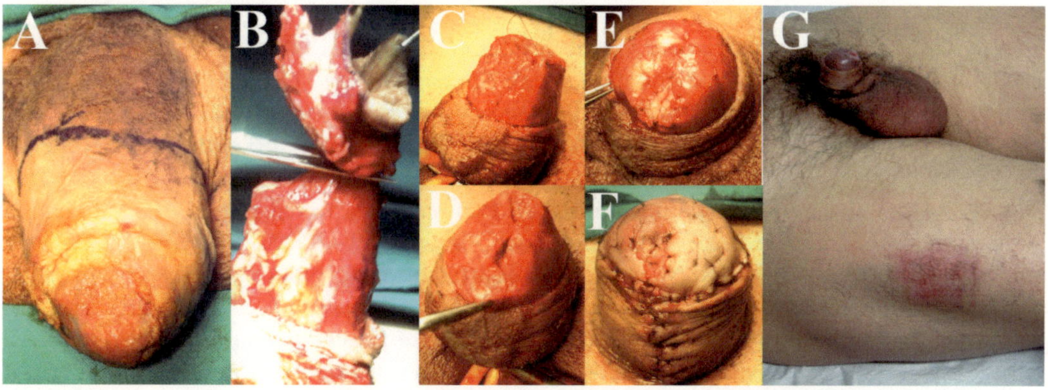

Fig. 4. Partial penectomy and neo-glans reconstruction : Squamous cell carcinoma involving glans and penile shaft (A). Foreskin degloving and partial penectomy (B).The lateral edges of the residual corpora cavernosa are sutured together to create a hemispheric dome-shaped stump (C - D). The urethra is spatulated and the meatus is fixed on the new tip of the corpora cavernosa (E). The STSG is transplanted over the summit of the hemispheric stump (F). Penile appearance 6 months after surgery (G).

This procedure is suitable for malignant lesions involving the penile shaft.

2.4 Neo-glans reconstruction following previous traditional partial penectomy

The top of the penile stump is skinned and the tip of the residual corpora cavernosa is reconverted to a hemispheric shape. The urethra is spatulated and the meatus is fixed on the new tip of the corpora cavernosa. The STSG is transplanted like an umbrella over the summit of the hemispheric stump where it is quilted. The graft is fixed to the penile skin thus recreating a glandular neo-sulcus (fig. 5).

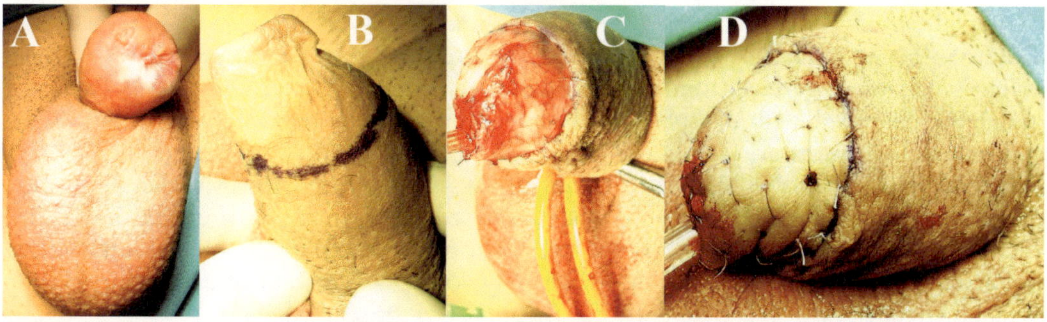

Fig. 5. Neo-glans reconstruction following previous traditional partial penectomy : Penile stump following partial penectomy (A). The top of the penile stump is skinned and the tip of the residual corpora is reconverted to a hemispheric shape (B -C). The STSG is transplanted like an umbrella over the summit of the hemispheric stump and fixed to the penile skin thus re-creating a neo-sulcus (D).

This procedure is suitable for unaesthetic residual penile stumps following previous traditional partial penectomy.

In all cases a 12-Fr silicone Foley catheter is inserted and a soft and humid dressing is applied covering the penis. The dressing is left in place for three days and the patient is requested to remain in bed. If the graft is observed to be without hematoma, seroma or infection after four days, the patient is mobilised and discharged from the hospital.

From 2002 through 2010, 21 patients (mean age 61 years; range 41-78) suffering from either benign, pre-malignant or malignant penile lesions underwent organ-sparing surgery with neo-glans reconstruction: 3 cases were treated by glans-skinning and glans-resurfacing, 10 by glansectomy and neo-glans reconstruction, 4 by partial penectomy and a neo-glans reconstruction, and 4 by neo-glans reconstruction after a traditional partial penectomy. No significant immediate post-operative complications were observed. Five (23.8%) patients showed partial graft loss and wound separation that were resolved after conservative management. No immediate or later complications were observed at the harvesting site. With a mean follow-up of 45 months, all patients were free of primary local disease. All patients were satisfied with the phallic post-operative appearance and recovered their sexual ability, although sensitivity was reduced as a consequence of glans/penile amputation.

3. Discussion

Laser ablation or other conservative therapies for penile lesions aim to remove the diseased tissue, but recurrence of the disease may eventually occur in unrecognised pre-malignant foci arising within the unstable epithelium following a partial procedure. Moreover, precancerous lesions often show recalcitrance after conservative treatments, with final evolution to a SCC in 5 to 33% of the cases [4,9,15-17]. Recently, plastic and reconstructive surgical techniques have been developed to reduce the functional and psychological morbidity in patients who have undergone mutilating penile surgery [1-3,9,11-14]. In selected patients, the use of these relatively-new plastic and reconstructive approaches provided a satisfactory aesthetic and functional outcome, without sacrificing a rigorous cancer control [1-3].

In this context, when performing a glans skinning and resurfacing, the epithelium is completely removed, thus reducing the risk of either disease recurrence or progression in different sites as compared with the primary lesion. Moreover, for lichen sclerosus which involves the male genitalia, an evolution toward a grossly scarring disease has been frequently described, with the subsequent phimosis which may promote poor local hygiene and chronic inflammatory conditions potentially being the etiological factors promoting penile malignancy. In this case, LS is frequently associated with dysplasia; therefore some authors have suggested that LS should be considered as a formal pre-cancerous lesion [15-18]. In these patients, total excision of the dysplastic glandular epithelium reduces the risk of cancer developing. Likewise, this approach may solve the problem of discomfort during sexual intercourse, which is frequently a consequence of the scarred glans.

In our series, even one patient with persistent extensive Zoon' balanitis was able to resume sexual activity after glans skinning and glans resurfacing. In patients who underwent glansectomy or partial penectomy, sensitivity was reduced as a predictable consequence of glans/penile amputation, but the cosmetic appearance of the neo-glans was similar to that of a native glans. The patients were then able to fully regain sexual functioning, with a favourable psychological impact. In these patients, the aesthetic appearance of the penis was subjectively superior when compared with patients who underwent others traditional techniques, thus promoting a positive psychological impact. This last aspect is of paramount importance since many patients with penile cancer are significantly reluctant to undergo partial or total penectomy due to the self-feeling of compromised masculinity [3]. It has been previously reported that roughly 80% of penile malignancies are probably amenable to these penis-preserving techniques, since most of the lesions occur distally and involve only the superficial epithelium of the glans [2]. In this context, it is important to highlight that in patients with superficial penile cancer associated to pre-cancerous lesions due to LS, any conservative treatment does not actually remove these lesions, thus potentially allowing cancer recurrence over time which may arise from an *unstable* epithelium bordering the primary lesion. Therefore, a rigorous patient selection is compulsory in order to technically provide an aesthetic solution with an effective long-term cancer control.

4. Conclusions

The penis-sparing surgery coupled with neo-glans reconstruction is an adequate treatment approach in rigorously selected patients with either benign, pre-malignant or malignant penile lesions. While preserving a good aesthetic appearance of the penile shaft, the goal of all these techniques is to maintain a functional penis in terms of both urination and sexual function, without jeopardizing cancer control.

5. Acknowledgement

The surgical techniques described in this article were developed and suggested to us by Dr. Aivar Bracka, without whose teaching and guidance it would not have been possible to obtain these positive results.

6. References

[1] C.T. Brown, S. Minhas and D.J. Ralph, "Conservative surgery for penile cancer: subtotal glans excision without grafting,". *British Journal of Urology International*, vol. 96, pp. 911-912, 2005.

[2] P. Pietrzak, C.M. Corbishley and N. Watkin, "Organ-sparing surgery for invasive penile cancer: early follow-up data," *British Journal of Urology International* , vol. 94, pp. 1253-1257, 2004.

[3] P. Hadway, C.M. Corbishley and N.A. Watkin, "Total glans resurfacing for premalignant lesions of the penis: initial outcome data,"*British Journal of Urology International* , vol. 98, pp.532-536, 2006.

[4] P.K. Hegarty, R.W. Rees, N.C. Borley, et Al. "Contemporary management of penile cancer,"*British Journal of Urology International*, vol. 102, pp.928-932, 2008.

[5] A. Bracka,"Glans resection and plastic repair,"*British Journal of Urology International*, vol. 105, pp. 136-144, 2009.

[6] S. Opjordsmoen and S.D. Fossa,"Quality of life in patients treated for penile cancer. A follow-up study," *British Journal of Urology*, vol. 74, pp. 652-657.

[7] C.A. D'Ancona, N.J. Botega, C. De Moraes, et Al.. "Quality of life after partial penectomy for penile carcinoma,"*Urology*, vol. 50, pp. 593-596, 1997.

[8] F.R. Romero, K.R. Pereira Dos Santos Romero, M.A. Elias De Mattos, et Al."Sexual function after partial penectomy for penile cancer,"*Urology*, vol. 66, pp. 1292-1295, 2005.

[9] E. Palminteri E, E. Berdondini, M. Lazzeri, et Al."Resurfacing and reconstruction of the glans penis,"*European Urology*, vol. 52, pp. 893-900, 2007.

[10] S. Minhas, O. Kayes, P. Hegarty, et Al."What surgical resection margins are required to achieve oncological control in men with primary penile cancer ?",*British Journal of Urology*, vol. 96, pp. 1040-1043, 2005.

[11] A.G. Fonseca, G.N. Rabelo, K.S. Vidal et Al. "Glandectomy with preservation of corpora cavernosa in the treatment of penile carcinoma,"*International Brazilian Journal Urology*, vol. 29, pp. 437-440, 2003.

[12] N. Bissada,"Organ-sparing surgery for invasive penile carcinoma,"*British Journal of Urology*, vol. 95, pp. 1118-1119, 2005.

[13] M.L. Greenberger and B.A. Lowe BA, "Penile stump advancement as an alternative to perineal urethrostomy after penile amputation,"*Journal of Urology*, vol. 161, pp. 893-894, 1999.

[14] S. Parkash, N. Ananthakrishnan and P. Roy, "Refashioning of phallus stumps and phalloplasty in the treatment of carcinoma of the penis,"*British Journal of Surgery*, vol. 73, pp. 902-905, 1986.

[15] A.L. Cubilla, E.F. Velazquez and R.H. Young, "Epithelial lesions associated with invasive penile squamous cell carcinoma: a pathologic study of 288 cases,"*International Journal of Surgical Pathology*, vol. 12, pp. 351-364, 2004.

[16] M.R. Nasca, D. Innocenzi and G. Micali, "Penile cancer among patients with genital lichen sclerosus," *Journal American Academy Dermatology*, vol. 41, pp. 911-914, 1999.

[17] J. Powell, A. Robson A, D. Cranston, et Al, "High incidence of lichen sclerosus in patients with squamous cell carcinoma,"*British Journal of Dermatology*, vol. 145, pp. 85-89, 2001.

[18] G. Barbagli, E. Palminteri, F. Mirri, et Ali,"Penile carcinoma in patients with genital lichen sclerosus: a multicentric survey,"*Journal of Urology*, vol. 175, pp. 1359-1363, 2006.

7

Skin and Soft Tissue Injuries in Congenital Vascular Malformations

Kyung-Bok Lee[1] and Dong-Ik Kim[2]
[1]*Department of Surgery, Seoul Medical Center*
[2]*Division of Vascular Surgery, Samsung Medical Center, Sungkyunkwan University School of Medicine, Seoul*
South Korea

1. Introduction

Congenital vascular malformation (CVM) refers to malformed vessels resulting from arrested development during various stages of embryogenesis and presents in about 1.5% of the population (Belov, 1989; Malan & Pulionisi, 1965; Villavicencio et al, 2002). The CVMs may originate from multiple vascular systems, including arterial, venous, and lymphatic, and represent as either a predominant form (e.g., arterial malformation) or as a mixed condition (venolymphatic malformation). As such, CVM has various clinical manifestations depending on vascular structural architecture, involved site(s), and type of malformed vessels present. In general, most CVMs are sporadic, but some are heritable in an autosomal dominant fashion (Arneja & Gosain, 2008). In spite of advances in the field of vascular biology, the pathogenesis, natural history, and treatment principles of CVMs have yet to be understood or developed.

Occasionally, CVMs can be confused with infantile hemangiomas (Figure 1). Even though both anomalies represent cutaneous vascular manifestations, their histologic findings and clinical courses are completely different. Most hemangiomas appear at birth, are self-limited, and resolve spontaneously before 12 years of age. However, CVMs may be identified at birth, progress during childhood, and never regress during the lifespan (Figure 1).

Clinical manifestations of the CVM are determined by its embryologic characteristics, especially the stage of embryogenesis in which development was arrested. Thus, it represents a wide range of clinical symptoms from a simple birthmark to a life-threatening condition (Lee, 2005). A small, localized venous malformation may cause a simple cosmetic problem such as a birthmark; however, a diffuse type of arteriovenous malformation in a major organ may result in a life-threatening condition, such as congestive heart failure, intractable bleeding, or airway obstruction, in addition to serious disfigurement.

Despite diagnostic advances over the last three decades, it is very difficult to diagnose the CVM for a sole physician because the CVM may involve multiple vascular systems and manifest variable clinical presentations. Therefore, multidisciplinary collaboration of physicians from special departments is necessary for accurate diagnosis and successful treatment of CVM.

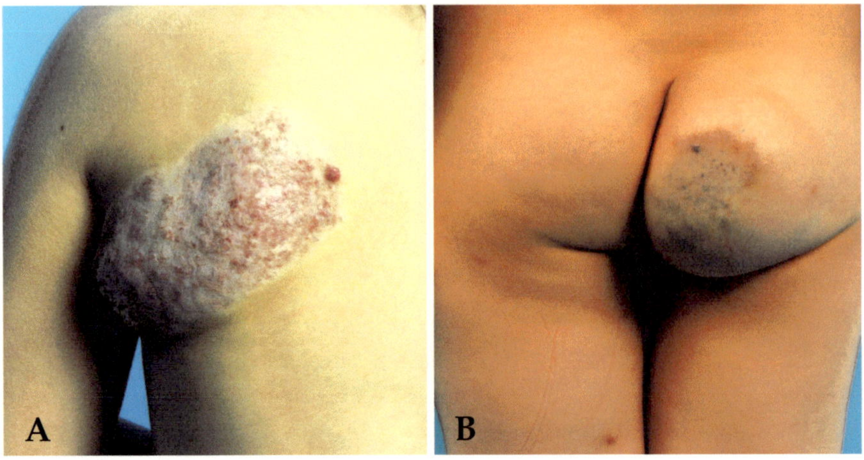

Fig. 1. Hemangioma and congenital vascular malformation. A, hemangioma in left back. B, venous malformation in right buttock.

Currently, complete excision of the nidus has been known as the only therapeutic modality for a cure of the CVM. However, complete surgical removal is nearly impossible because most CVMs are diffuse and of an infiltrative nature.

As an alternative treatment method, embolo/sclerotherapy may be an effective modality and successful in most CVMs, in particular the diffuse and infiltrative types. We previously reported that the incidence, the susceptible types, and the outcomes for skin and soft tissue injuries of embolo/sclerotherapy in CVMs (Lee et al., 2008).

This chapter reviews the general aspect of the CVMs and, based on our study, expands the incidence and treatment methods, including skin graft, in addition to the prognosis of skin and soft tissue injuries developed after embolo/sclerotherpay in patients with CVMs.

2. Congenital vascular malformations: General aspect

2.1 Classification

A proper classification of CVMs is very difficult since they develop as a result of arrest during various embryologic stages and represent a variety of clinical manifestations.

Over the centuries, various CVMs have been labeled with name-based eponyms, such as Klippel-Trenaunay or Parkes Weber syndromes. However, these eponyms were defined by only clinically relevant manifestations (e.g., birthmark, swelling, disfigurement) and did not identify the primary vascular lesion and/or other nonvascular anomalies. Although these old name-based eponyms have been replaced by new classifications based on anatomic and pathophysiologic status as well as clinically relevant manifestations, these are still valuable for understanding the cutaneous lesions of CVM, as well for the historical significance. For instance, Klippel-Trenaunay syndrome, which is characterized by cutaneous hemangiomas, soft tissue hypertrophy, and varicosities, can be replaced with hemolymphatic malformation in the Hamburg classification (Figure 2). However, as its historical eponym is well known, it can still be used to represent the cutaneous manifestations.

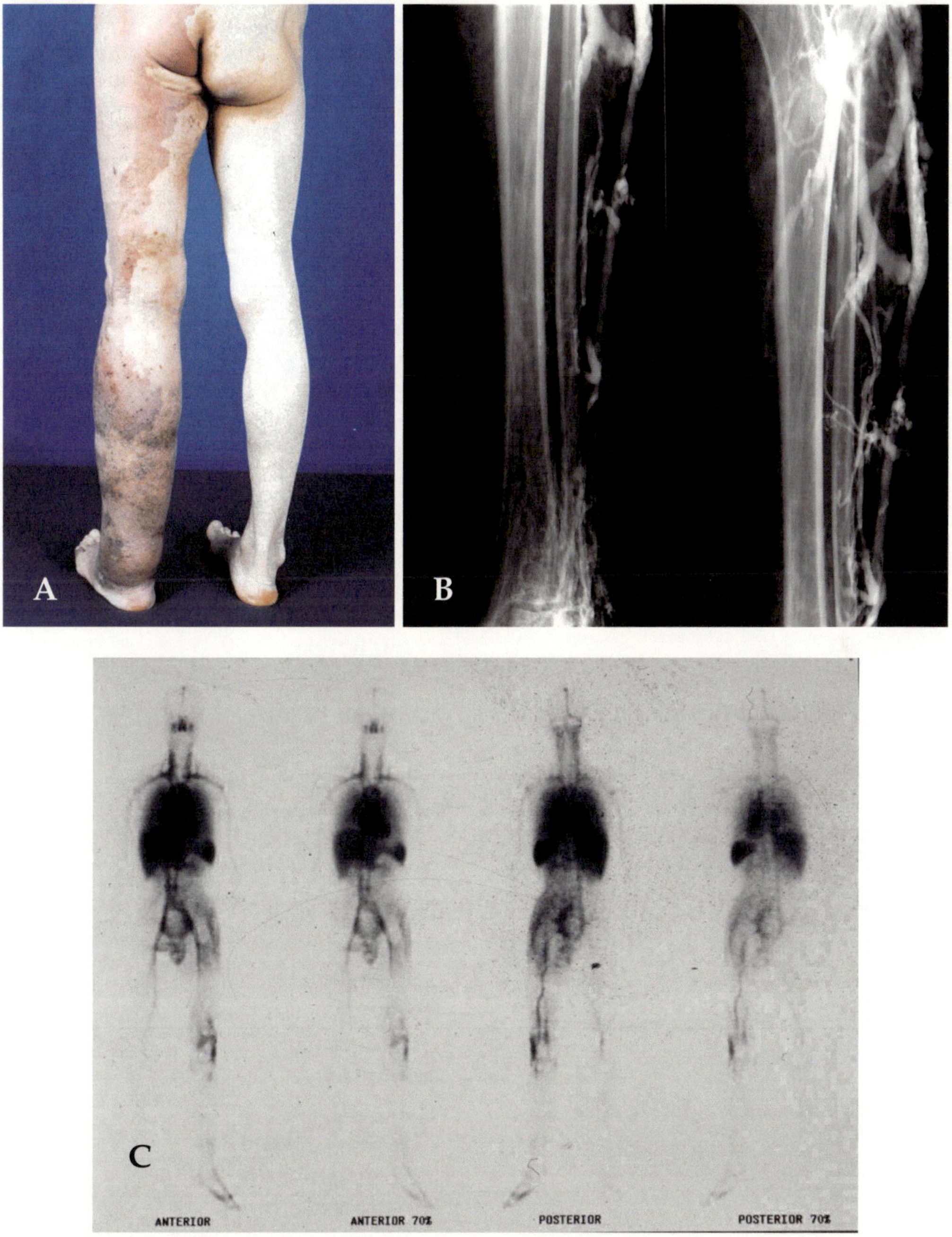

Fig. 2. Klippel-Trenaunay syndrome. A, Gross appearance. B, Ascending venogram. C, Whole body blood pool scan.

2.1.1 Hamburg classification

In 1988, the ISSVA (International Society for the Study of Vascular Anomalies) that was held in Hamburg, Germany, has adopted the new classification of CVMs based on the underlying anatomic, histologic, pathophysiologic, and hemodynamic status (Belov, 1989, 1990; Lee et al., 2007). This classification has been considered to be clinically applicable and is regarded as a modern system. In the Hamburg classification, CVMs are divided into five types based on the predominant vascular defect: arterial, venous, arteriovenous shunting, lymphatic, and combined (Table 1). Each type was subclassified into a truncal form and extratruncal form depending on the embryonic stage of developmental arrest (Lee, 2005). The initial classification system did not contain the capillary malformation, since their clinical significance had been considered uncertain. However, the addition of capillary malformation was subsequently proposed and supported.

Types	Embyologic subtypes
Predominantly arterial defects	Truncular forms
	Aplasia or obstruction
	Dilatation
	Extratruncular forms
	Infiltrating
	Limited
Predominantly venous defects	Truncular forms
	Aplasia or obstruction
	Dilatation
	Extratruncular forms
	Infiltrating
	Limited
Predominantly AV shunting defects	Truncular forms
	Deep
	Superficial
	Extratruncular forms
	Infiltrating
	Limited
Predominantly lymphatic defects	Truncular forms
	Aplasia or obstruction
	Dilatation
	Extratruncular forms
	Infiltrating
	Limited
Combined vascular defects	Truncular forms
	Arterial or venous
	Hemolymphatic
	Extratruncular forms
	Infiltrating hemolymphatic
	Limited hemolymphatic

Table 1. Hamburg classification for congenital vascular malformations (AV, arteriovenous)

Although the Hamburg classification is currently used worldwide and accepted in most clinical settings, further improvements in the CVM classification system will be needed to completely replace the old name-based eponyms.

2.1.2 Muliken classification

The Muliken classification is a widely used alternative system which is based on the hemodynamic status of the CVM and also provides guidelines for clinical management (Mulliken, 1993; Mulliken & Glowacki, 1982). In this classification, all CVMs are divided into two types depending on blood flow: fast-flow and slow-flow. It supplies a simple understanding for the complex nature of CVM and helps to determine whether treatment is needed, as well as treatment modality. Currently, the Muliken classification has been used in conjunction with the Hamburg classification in the clinical field.

2.2 Pathophysiology

2.2.1 Extratruncular types

Extratruncular CVMs present by arrest during early embryonic life while the vascular system is in the reticular stage (Bastide & Lefebvre, 1989). As such, extratruncular CVMs contain the characteristics of mesenchymal cells and have proliferative potential. Therefore, all extratruncular CVMs show high risk for exacerbation or recurrence when stimulated or treated improperly and can infiltrate and invade the surrounding tissues and show a secondary impact, as well as the hemodynamic effect.

Almost all extratruncular CVMs present with mechanical and hemodynamic effects. For example, if the CVM is located in the neck, it may cause airway or esophageal obstruction due to the mechanical characteristics of CVM progression. Moreover, the hemodynamic effect, particularly the arteriovenous malformation of extratruncular CVM, may result in serious complications of the cardiovascular system because the arterial flow directly enters the venous drainage system without the resistance of the capillary system.

2.2.2 Truncular type

Truncular CVMs occur when developmental arrest happens later during the vascular trunk formation stage of embryonic development (Bastide & Lefebvre, 1989). These CVMs have a significant risk for hemodynamic complications because the lesions lose their embryonic characteristics. If the truncular type of CVM is located in a lower extremity, it may show clinical manifestations of lymphedema or chronic venous insufficiency. In addition, if arteriovenous malformation presents as the truncular type, life-threatening cardiovascular complications, including congestive heart failure, could develop.

2.3 Diagnosis

It is impossible for one expert to diagnose the CVM because it has numerous clinical manifestations and various diagnostic modalities. For these reasons, a multidisciplinary team, composed of a vascular surgeon, a plastic and reconstructive surgeon, an orthopedic surgeon, a dermatologist, and an interventional radiologist, is needed to diagnose and classify the CVM. In addition to the diagnosis and classification, the CVM treatment plan must also be developed by the consensus of the multidisciplinary team.

2.3.1 CVM *versus* hemangioma

Both CVM and hemangioma are grouped as vascular anomalies; however, each anomaly presents with completely different behaviors (Lee, 2005).

By definition, a hemangioma is a vascular tumor that mainly appears at birth and is characterized by rapid growth and spontaneous regression. Hemangioma growth starts after birth, and spontaneous regression usually occurs before 12 years of age. In comparison

to CVM, a rapidly growing hemangioma represents mature endothelium that shows normal mitotic activity.
In general, the differential diagnosis between CVM and hemangioma depends on the clinical manifestations and physical examinations. However, if a vascular lesion is the only diffuse mass located in the subcutaneous tissue or the muscle layer, diagnosis may be impossible and needs to be differentiated. Therefore, tissue confirmation is sometimes required in a specific case for the differential diagnosis.

2.3.2 Clinical manifestations

CVMs can show a wide range of clinical forms depending on the predominant type and location. Most capillary malformations may present as a port-wine stain and can appear anywhere in the body as a localized or extensive form. In addition, cutaneous manifestations of capillary malformations are associated with anomalies of the soft tissue or the skeletal system. For example, hypertrophy of soft tissue and leg bone is expressed with cutaneous manifestations in patients with Klippel-Trenaunay syndrome.
Venous malformations also may present at birth and can be distinctively compressed. Some venous malformations located in the skin and the subcutaneous layer of the face or neck may cause cosmetic problems, such as disfiguration or asymmetry. Venous malformation in the bone can cause a leg length discrepancy due to bone growth disturbances and pathologic fractures due to bone destruction. However, if the malformation is located near the airway, it has a potential life-threatening risk due to the secondary compression effect and intractable bleeding (Figure 3).
Most lymphatic malformations are asymptomatic except for skin manifestations. Lymphatic malformations present as a primary lymphedema (diffuse swelling) or a lymphangioma (localized swelling). Complicated lymphatic malformations may lead to non-vascular consequences rather than vascular complications, such as the compression of surrounding organs, pathologic fractures, or infection.
Arteriovenous malformations are often indistinct unless complications have developed. The direct fistulas between the arteries and the veins are formed in the lesion, and these fistulas are represented as the thrill and bruit. Arteriovenous malformation frequently manifests several serious complications, including distal ischemia and gangrene due to the shunt, intractable bleeding, or high-output cardiac failure.

2.3.3 Non-invasive tests

Clinical suspicion is most important for the diagnosis when the baby or child shows the skin manifestation or disfigurement. If a CVM is suspected, a detailed history and a physical examination are taken. In patients with suspected CVM, non-invasive tests, such as duplex ultrasonography, CT or MR angiography, or Tc-99m RBC whole body blood pool scintigraphy (WBBPS), can lead to a definite diagnosis in most circumstances.
Duplex ultrasonography can be examined initially because it provides excellent hemodynamic as well as anatomic information. CT or MR angiography shows the exact location and the relationship with adjacent tissue, the feeding artery, and the draining vein, so it helps to determine the treatment plan. WBBPS can detect another lesion in the body, assess the treatment efficacy, and rule out lymphatic malformation (Figure 4). In addition to these basic tests, if the patient has a leg-length discrepancy, a bone X-ray should be

performed to rule out osseous CVM. When lymphatic malformation is suspected, radioisotope lymphoscintigraphy could be added. In arteriovenous malformation, transarterial lung perfusion scintigraphy can provide useful information for the general impact of an arteriovenous shunt.

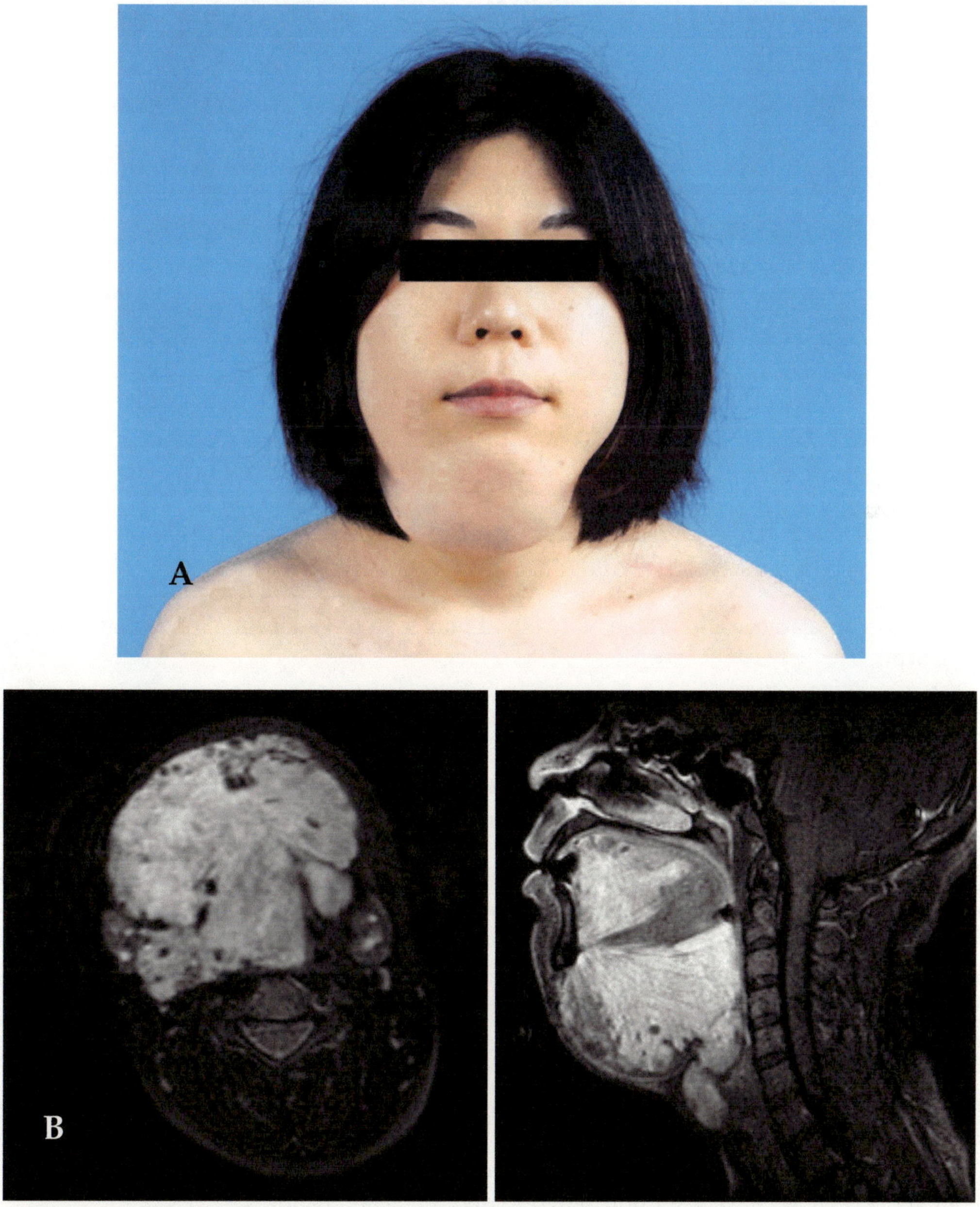

Fig. 3. Venous malformation affecting the airway A, Huge venous malformation presents as diffuse swelling below the chin. B, T2-weighted MRI images show the airway involvement of venous malformation.

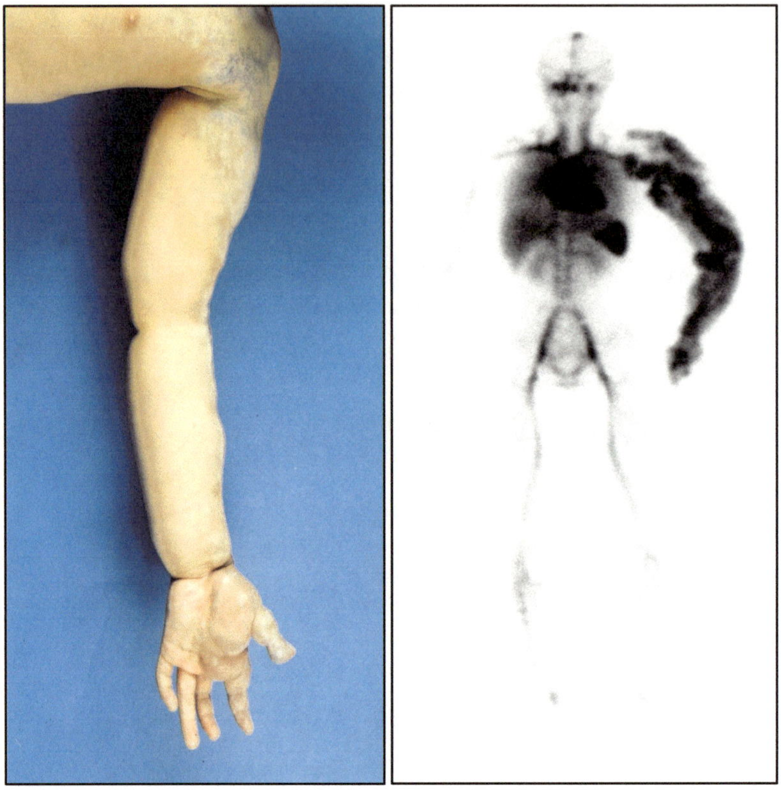

Fig. 4. Gross appearance and whole body blood pool scan of venous malformation involving entire arm.

2.3.4 Invasive tests

Currently, most invasive diagnostic tests have been replaced by noninvasive studies because the majority of CVMs can be definitely diagnosed by the latter. However, invasive tests, such as digital subtraction angiography and venography, remain as a standard and useful modality for diagnosing and determining the treatment plan.

A selective angiography provides a guideline for a treatment method in patients with arteriovenous malformations. A venography in conjunction with direct-puncture phlebography simultaneously enables the diagnosis and treatment in venous malformations. However, traditional percutaneous direct-puncture lymphangiography is rarely needed in patients with lymphatic malformations.

2.4 Treatment

Until the pathophysiology and biological behavior of CVMs had been characterized, most treatment approaches failed to relieve the hemodynamic consequences and secondary complications or to cure the CVM itself. Overaggressive treatment due to lack of knowledge about various CVMs have also contributed to poor clinical outcomes.

In the treatment of CVMs, the complete eradication of the nidus provides complete curability, but it is rarely possible because most CVMs are infiltrative and located in deeper and surgically inaccessible regions.

Two decades ago, the Hamburg classification provided a better understanding of the anatomy, the pathophysiology, and hemodynamic status of CVMs. Based on this classification, new treatment approaches have been developed.

Previously, we proposed a multidisciplinary team approach composed of 15 clinical specialists for diagnosis and treatment. Surgeons and clinicians in vascular surgery, plastic and reconstructive surgery, pediatric surgery, interventional and diagnostic radiology, nuclear medicine, orthopedic surgery, head and neck surgery, oral-maxillary surgery, anesthesiology, vascular medicine, pathology, physical medicine and rehabilitation, psychiatry, and dermatology should all be represented (Lee, 2005). This team has been operated effectively by a 'referral system' to diagnose, develop a treatment plan, and manage the consequence after treatment.

All CVMs may not require treatment and a poorly planned treatment could awake the quiescent stage of CVM. In particular, aggressive treatment for CVM should be considered when the CVM is associated with symptoms such as hemorrhage, high-output heart failure, disabling pain, cosmetically severe deformity, etc.

2.4.1 Surgical treatment

Although surgical resection provides the only complete curable option, it is rarely indicated because of the extensive nature and high morbidity and recurrence of CVMs. Complete resection is limited to superficially isolated lesions without invasion into deeper structures, such as muscle, nerve, and bone. Incomplete resection of the nidus or ligation of the feeding artery without removal of the nidus may result in the faster growth of quiescent malformations (Kim et al., 2006). Therefore, only selective cases have been recommended for surgical removal.

If a surgical resection is planned, preoperative embolization using ethanol, ethanolamine oleate, or N-butyl cyanoacrylate (NBCA) helps to delineate the extent of surgery and reduce intra-operative bleeding.

In conclusion, surgical approach for CVM should be considered carefully and planned perfectly because it has a potential to exacerbate the manifestations of CVM, as well greatly increasing risk for complications and recurrence.

2.4.2 Endovascular treatment

As previously described, surgical intervention for most CVMs is not an option due to location and infiltrative nature. The new concepts of "endovascular treatment" to treat CVMs or to control symptoms have been developed by the multidisciplinary team approach. Endovascular treatment, composed of embolization and sclerotherapy, is now well accepted as an effective treatment modality for CVMs, the diffuse type of extratruncular form in particular.

Several sclerosing agents have been used in the clinical setting. First, absolute ethanol is the most effective sclerosing agent to treat the CVM itself or to control the secondary consequences caused by the CVM. Ethanol can be delivered by an endovascular approach or administered by a direct puncture technique (Figure 5). However, acute caution is required when the ethanol is delivered into circulatory system via malformed vessels. The ethanol increases pulmonary arterial pressure and can, in the worst case, cause a pulmonary artery spasm and subsequent cardiopulmonary arrest. In addition, it can directly damage the surrounding tissues, including skin, soft tissue, nerve, tendon, muscle, and bone, and cause cosmetic problems and functional complications. Therefore, close monitoring of the cardiopulmonary system, including the pulmonary artery wedge pressure, is absolutely necessary during and immediately after the embolo/sclerotherapy. Embolo/sclerotherapy using ethanol should be performed only when the therapeutic benefits are considered to outweigh the risks.

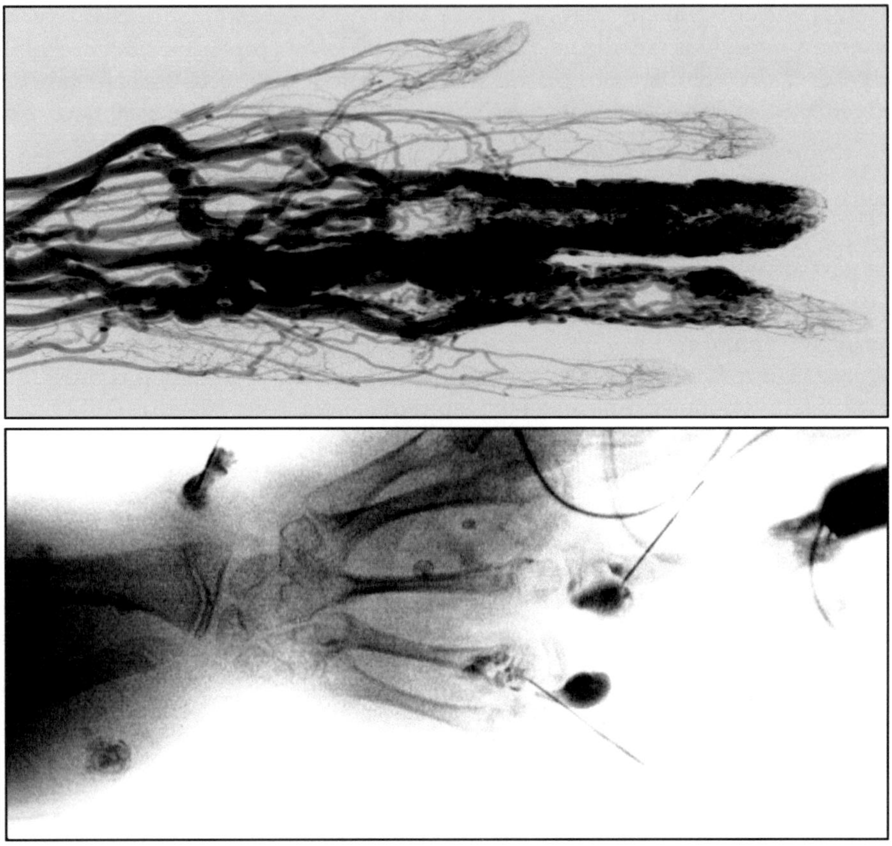

Fig. 5. Embolo/sclerotherapy by direct puncture technique in patient with arteriovenous malformation in the hand.

NBCA as an independent agent is not an ideal treatment for the diffuse and infiltrative types of CVM, but preoperative NBCA embolo/sclerotherapy assists in hemorrhage minimization during the surgical excision of CVM. Safer alternative agents, such as ethanolamine, polidocanol, and sodium tetradecyl sulfate, are currently being used and assessed in the control of CVM symptoms, particularly venous malformation

3. Congenital vascular malformations: Skin and soft tissue injuries

Embolo/scleotherapy may be an effective treatment modality for most CVMs, especially the diffuse infiltrating type of extratruncular CVM, due to the low recurrence and acceptable morbidity. Thus, the embolo/sclerotherapy is the main strategy utilized to treat the CVM itself and control secondary symptoms when complete surgical excision is not a viable option.

However, few reports exist for the incidence and treatment of skin and soft tissue injuries developed after embolo/sclerotherapy in patients with CVMs. In addition, it is unknown which types of CVMs are more susceptible to skin and soft tissue injuries and which treatment methods are the most successful for these injuries.

We previously reported the incidence of skin and soft tissue injury after embolo/scleorotherapy for CVM and reviewed the prognosis according to the treatment modalities in patients with skin and soft tissue injuries (Lee et al., 2008). This chapter, based on our study, has described the outcomes according to treatment methods in patients with skin and soft tissue injuries developed after embolo/sclerotherapy.

3.1 Incidence

A retrospective review of 1,823 patients with a CVM, 573 of whom were managed by a multidisciplinary approach of embolo/sclerotherapy, was performed. Absolute or 80% ethanol, ethanolamine oleate, NBCA, or various types of coils or contour particles were used as the embolo/sclerosing agents based on the location, the severity, and the extent of the CVM.

Our study indicated that skin and soft tissue injuries occurred in 11.9% of patients (n = 68). Yun et al. (2009) also demonstrated that the incidence of skin necrosis after percutaneous ethanol sclerotherapy in venous malformations was 8%. However, Jin et al. (2008) reported that only 6 sessions of tissue necrosis (1%) among 592 sclerotherapy sessions. The necrosis developed in the finger tips after 5 treatment sessions and in the chin area after 1 treatment session. They reported that all lesions were spontaneously healed. We thought that lower incidence of tissue necrosis was due to ethanol usage only for sclerosis of the draining vein of venous malformations.

In our study, skin and soft tissue injuries occurred in 15.6% of those that used ethanol, in 6.3% of those that used ethanolamine oleate, and in 8.3% of those that used glue (Lee et al., 2008). The incidence of skin and soft tissue injuries after embolo/sclerotherapy according to the Hamburg classification is described in Table 2.

First of all, our study indicated there were no skin and soft tissue injuries in patients with the truncular forms of CVMs (Lee et al., 2008). Moreover, embolo/sclerotherapy for extratruncular forms of arterial and lymphatic malformations did not lead to skin and soft tissue injuries. In addition, embolo/sclerotherapy in patients with extratruncular type of arteriovenous shunting types was correlated with the largest portion of skin and soft tissue injuries (n = 42/142) and these injuries showed similar rates for both the infiltrating and the limited types (30.6% vs. 26.7%). Skin and soft tissue injuries were more common in the infiltrating type than in the limited type of the extratruncular form (13.2% vs. 9.7%) of the CVMs. Based on the location of the CVMs, the incidence of skin and soft tissue injuries was 20.4% in the upper extremities, 14.3% in the lower extremities and the perineum/genitalia, 9.1% in the pelvis, 7.5% in the head and neck, and 6.4% in the thorax. Among all skin and soft tissue injuries, only one occurred in a patient with a venous malformation which involved the tongue and lip.

In conclusion, our study suggested that the extratruncular form of arteriovenous shunting malformation and the extratruncular form of venous malformation were more susceptible to skin and soft tissue injuries after embolo/sclerotherapy in patients with CVMs.

Types of CVM (n=573)	Forms of CVM (n=573)	Skin and soft tissue injuries (n=68)
Arterial (n=1)	Truncular (n=0)	0 (0%)
	Extratruncular (n=1)	0 (0%)
	Limited (n=1)	
	Infiltrating (n=0)	
Venous (n=273)	Truncular (n=1)	0 (0%)
	Extratruncular (n=272)	22 (32.4%)
	Limited (n=57)	6
	Infiltrating (n=215)	16
Lymphatic (n=102)	Truncular (n=4)	0 (0%)
	Extratruncular (n=98)	0 (0%)
	Limited (n=80)	
	Infiltrating (n=18)	
AV shunting (n=143)	Truncular (n=1)	0 (0%)
	Extratruncular (n=142)	42 (61.8%)
	Limited (n=45)	12
	Infiltrating (n=97)	30
Combined (n=54)	Truncular (n=1)	0 (0%)
	Extratruncualr (n=53)	4 (5.9%)
	Limited (n=13)	1
	Infiltrating (n=40)	3

Table 2. Patients with skin and soft tissue injuries after embolo/sclerotherapy according to Hamburg classification in patients with congenital vascular malformations. (CVM, congenital vascular malformation; AV, arteriovenous)

3.2 Treatment and outcome

The treatment strategy for skin and soft tissue injuries was developed after embolo/sclerotherapy was decided by multidisciplinary team and was determined by the extent, the depth, and the severity of the injury. First, conservative management such as a simple dressing was applied, but the infected wound was managed by antibiotics, surgical debridement, and drainage. If the eschar led to the contracture, then escharectomy has been performed to relieve the contracture and recover the joint motion. The skin and soft tissue injuries did not heal with conservative management or those that involved deeper structures, such as muscles or tendons, have subsequently required plastic reconstructive surgery. In the extremities, severe injuries with extensive necrosis in deeper tissue, severe deformity or pain, or functional disabilities were amputated (Figure 6).

As a result, 40 of 68 patients (58.8%) with skin and soft tissue injuries have been healed by conservative management and 18 escharectomies (26.5%) and 4 amputations (5.9%) were performed (Lee et al., 2008). As a result of embolo/sclerotherapy, all patients who needed amputation had the infiltrating arteriovenous shunting extratruncular type.

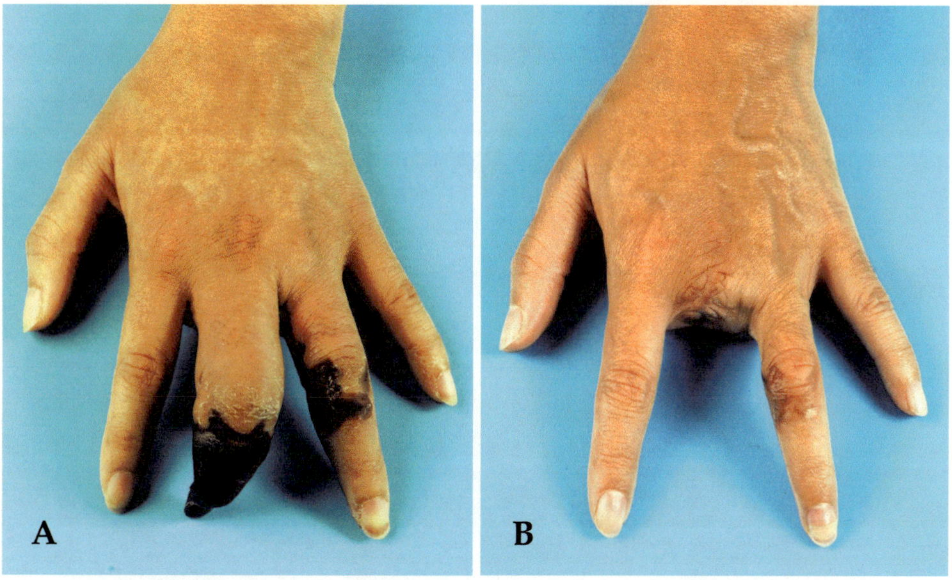

Fig. 6. A, Necrosis of 3rd fingertip after embolo/sclerotherapy in patient with arteriovenous malformation. B, After 3rd finger amputation.

In our study, plastic reconstructive surgeries, including split-thickness or full-thickness skin grafts, were performed in 6 of 68 patients (8.8%) with skin and soft tissue injuries (Lee et al., 2008). The characteristics of the patients who underwent skin grafts and the clinical outcomes are described in Table 3.

No.	Type of CVM	Form of CVM	Type of sclerosant (ml)	Location of injury	Method of skin graft	Outcome
1	AV shunting	ET	Pure ethanol(12)	Ear	FTSG	Completely healed
2	AV shunting	ET	Pure ethanol(40.5)	Knee	STSG	Completely healed
3	AV shunting	ET	Pure ethanol(6.75)	Hand	STSG	Completely healed
4	AV shunting	ET	NBCA(12)	Occiput	STSG	Completely healed
5	Venous	ET	Pure ethanol(18)	Arm	STSG	Completely healed
6	Venous	ET	Pure ethanol(20.5)	Arm	STSG	Completely healed

Table 3. The characteristics and the outcome for 6 skin and soft tissue injuries that were performed skin graft. (CVM, congenital vascular malformation; AV, arteriovenous; ET, extratruncular; NBCA, N-butyl cyanoacrylate; FTSG, full-thickness skin graft; STSG, split-thickness skin graft)

Two plastic surgeries were performed in the injuries that developed as a result of embolo/sclerotherapy for the infiltrating venous extratruncular types, 1 for the limited arteriovenous extratruncular type, 3 for the infiltrating arteriovenous shunting extratruncular type. All plastic reconstructive surgeries were performed only if the injured wound had not healed with conservative management or involved deeper structures and all skin grafts could be successfully performed (Figure 7).

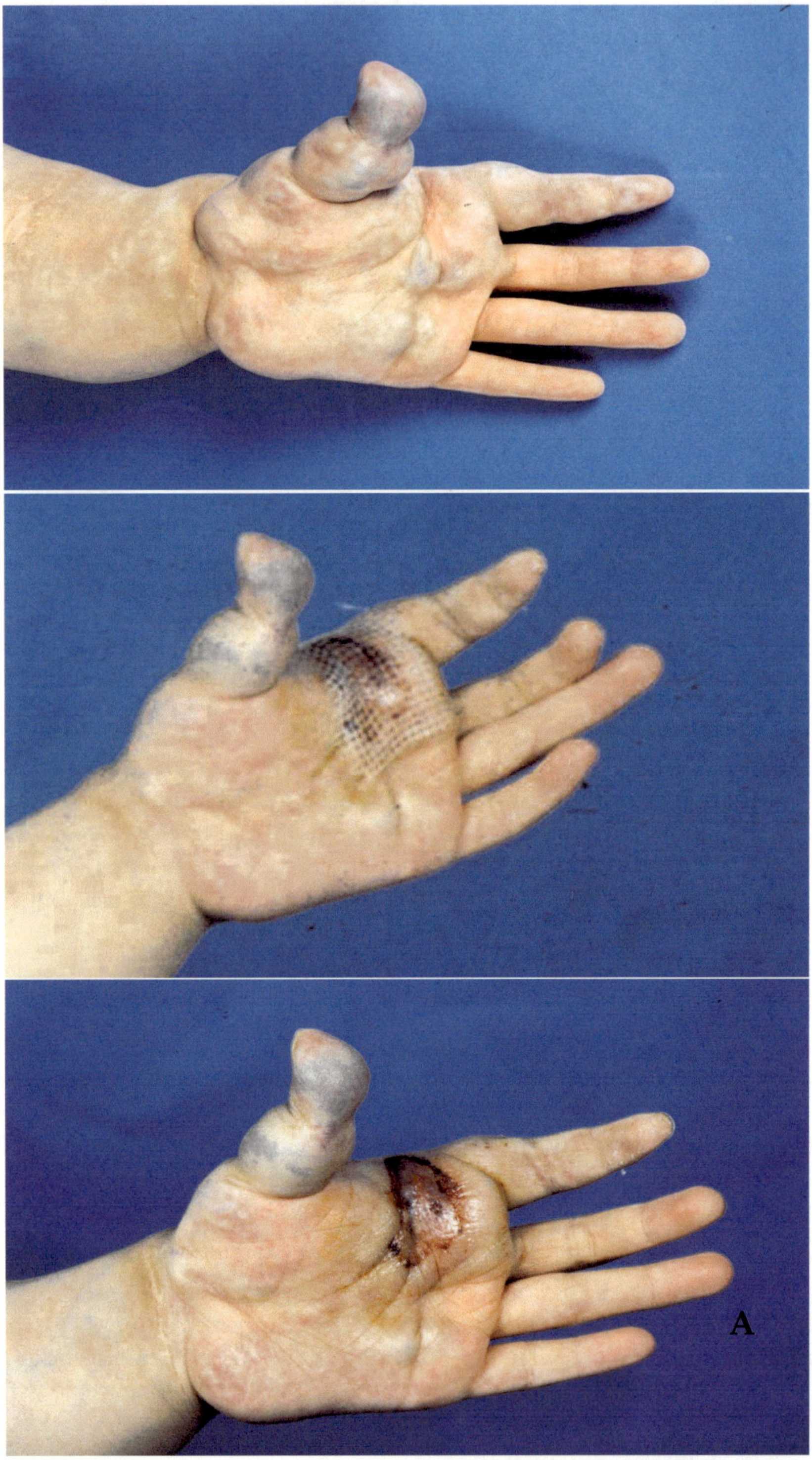
A

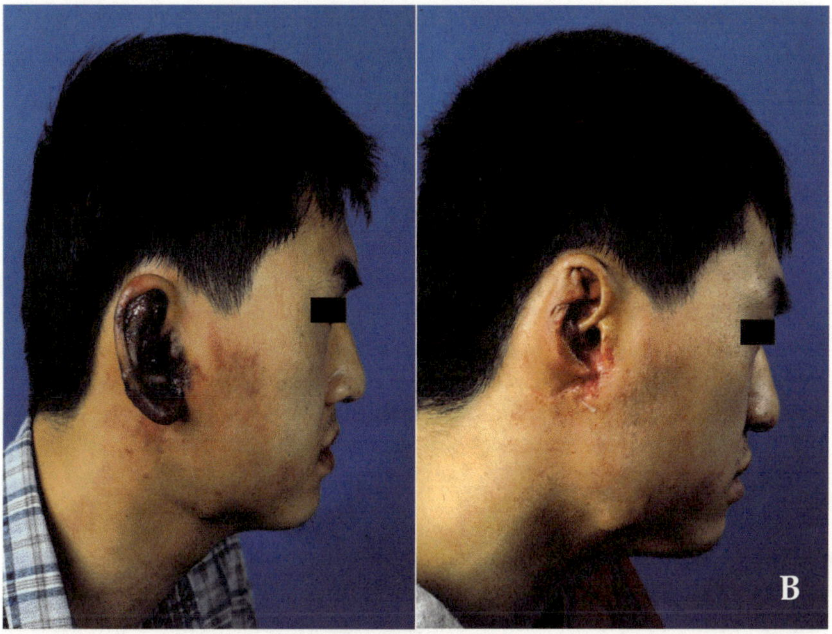

Fig. 7. A, Split-thickness skin graft in patient with skin and soft tissue injury in the palm after pure ethanol embolo/sclerotherapy. B, Full-thickness skin graft in patient with necrosis of the ear after pure ethanol embolo/sclerotherapy.

4. Conclusions

CVMs are relatively uncommon congenital anomalies and difficult to be distinguished from other vascular conditions, such as a simple birthmark or a hemangioma. In addition, the CVMs show numerous clinical manifestations according to the involved vascular system, the location, and the extent, and additionally require variable clinical responses depending on the manifestation.

Although much effort has been made to accurately diagnose and completely treat CVMs, they still remain challenging even to a specialist. Therefore, a multidisciplinary team composed of specialists from many surgical and clinical disciplines is absolutely needed to develop a successful strategy for the treatment modality and management of complications after treatment.

As a current treatment method for CVMs, embolo/sclerotherapy has become a mainstay because in most CVMs it is impossible to completely remove the nidus. Even if embolo/sclerotherapy has been proven a relatively safe and effective treatment modality in most patients with CVM, our study indicated that skin and soft tissue injuries occurred with relatively high frequency in patients undergoing embolo/sclerotherapy. In particular, our results suggested that the extratruncular forms of the arteriovenous shunting malformation and the venous malformation require acute vigilance for signs of skin and soft tissue injuries in patients undergoing embolo/sclerotherapy, even though most injuries were completely healed with conservative management.

Additionally, skin grafts may be the best treatment option for most skin and soft tissue injuries unable to be healed by conservative management or involved beyond the muscle layer after embolo/sclerotherapy in patients with CVMs.

5. Acknowledgment

We gratefully appreciate the efforts of Byung-Boong Lee, M.D., PhD, FACS, who established the Congenital Vascular Malformation Clinic in Samsung Medical Center. In addition, we specially thank to Na-Ri Kim, RN, APN and Shin-Young Woo, RN for collecting and organizing the data of the patients with CVMs.

6. References

Arneja, JS. & Gosain, AK. (2008) Vascular malformations. *Plast Reconstr Surg.*, Vol.121, No.4, pp. 195e-206e, ISSN 0032-1052

Bastide G. & Lefebvre D. (1989) Anatomy and organogenesis and vascular malformations. In: *Vascular Malformations*, Belov S, Loose DA, Weber J, ed., pp. 20-22, Einhorn-Presse Verlag GmbH, Reinbek, Germany

Belov S. (1989) Classification, terminology, and nosology of congenital vascular defects. In: *Vascular Malformations*, Belov S, Loose DA, Weber J, ed., pp 25-30, Einhorn-Presse, Reinbek, Germany

Belov S. (1990) Classification of congenital vascular defects. *Int Angiol.*, Vol.9, No.3, pp. 141-146, ISSN 1061-1711

Jin Y.; Lin X; Li W.; Hu X.; Ma G. & Wang W. (2008) Sclerotherapy after embolization of draining vein: a safe treatment method for venous malformations. *J Vasc Surg.*, Vol.47, No.6, pp. 1292-1299, ISSN 0741-5214

Kim JY.; Kim DI.; Do YS.; Lee BB.; Kim YW.; Shin SW.; Byun HS.; Roh HG.; Choo IW.; Hyon WS.; Shim JS. & Choi JY. (2006) Surgical treatment for congenital arteriovenous malformation: 10 years' experience. *Eur J Vasc Endovasc Surg.*, Vol.32, No.1, pp. 101-106, ISSN 1078-5884

Lee BB. (2005) New approaches to the treatment of congenital vascular malformations (CVMs)--a single centre experience. *Eur J Vasc Endovasc Surg.*, Vol.30, No.2, pp. 184-197, ISSN 1078-5884

Lee BB.; Laredo J.; Lee TS.; Huh S. & Neville R. (2007) Terminology and classification of congenital vascular malformations. *Phlebology*, Vol.22, No.6, pp. 249-252, ISSN 0268-3555

Lee KB.; Kim DI.; Oh SK.; Do YS.; Kim KH. & Kim YW. (2008) Incidence of soft tissue injury and neuropathy after embolo/sclerotherapy for congenital vascular malformation. *J Vasc Surg.*, Vol.48, No.5, pp. 1286-1291 ISSN 0741-5214

Malan E. & Puglionisi A. (1965) Congenital angiodysplasias of the extremities, note II: arterial, arterial and venous, and hemolymphatic dysplasias. *J Cardiovasc Surg (Torino).*, Vol.6, No.4, pp. 255-345, ISSN 0021-9509

Mulliken JB. (1993) Cutaneous vascular anomalies. *Semin Vasc Surg.*, Vol.6, No.4, pp. 204-218, ISSN 0895-7967

Mulliken JB. & Glowacki J. (1982) Hemangiomas and vascular malformations in infants and children: a classification based on endothelial characteristics. *Plast Reconstr Surg.*, Vol.69, No.3, pp. 412-420, ISSN 0032-1052

Yun WS.; Kim YW.; Lee KB.; Kim DI.; Park KB.; Kim KH.; Do YS. & Lee BB. (2009) Predictors of response to percutaneous ethanol sclerotherapy (PES) in patients with venous malformations: analysis of patient self-assessment and imaging. *J Vasc Surg.*, Vol.50, No.3, pp. 581-589, ISSN 0741-5214

Villavicencio JL.; Scultetus A. & Lee BB. (2002) Congenital vascular malformations: when and how to treat them. *Semin Vasc Surg.*, Vol.15, No.1, pp. 65-71, ISSN 0895-7967

8

Oral Mucosa Graft

Ismaila A Mungadi and Ngwobia P Agwu
Urology Unit, Department of Surgery, Usmanu Danfodiyo University Teaching Hospital. Sokoto Nigeria

1. Introduction

Oral mucosa has been used for reconstructing oral and maxillofacial defects for many years (Payne et al., 1998); in repairing the conjunctival mucosa of the eye (Donoff, 1976), in oral pharyngeal reconstructive surgery (Leone, 1995) and in reconstructing vaginal defects (Lin et al., 2003). Since the initial introduction by Humby (1941) and then the re-introduction by Burger, oral mucosa graft has gained widespread use in urethral reconstruction of long segment anterior urethral strictures, hypospadias, epispadias and bladder exstrophy (Barbagli et al., 2006, Martins et al., 2006, Xu et al 2007). Oral mucosal graft, as a free graft for urological reconstruction, has numerous advantages including constant availability, favourable immunological properties, easy harvesting, excellent tissue characteristics; easy handling properties, minimal contracture formation and adaptation to a moist environment (Hensle et al., 2002, Simonato et al.,2006; Chi-Chi & Chi-Yang, 2007)

The purpose of this overview is to provide the reader with an understanding of the biologic characteristics of the oral mucosa and the anatomic features that make it such a versatile tissue for urethral reconstruction. In addition, to report on the technique for oral mucosa graft harvest using sound biologic principles, its clinical applications in urologic reconstruction as well some observed donor site complications will be reviewed.

2. Biology of the oral mucosa

The entire oral cavity is lined by a protective epithelial membrane, the ***oral mucosa.*** Anatomically, the oral mucosa is located between the skin of the outer face and the mucosal lining of the gastrointestinal tract displaying properties of both tissues (Markiewicz et al., 2007). According to standard and accepted dental terminology, the buccal mucosa refers to the oral mucosa overlying the inner cheek of the oral cavity. The labial mucosa refers to the alveolar mucosa of the inner lower lip. The lingual mucosa refers the mucosa overlying the tongue. These are collectively referred to as oral mucosal grafts.

The epithelium of the oral mucosa is stratified squamous and becomes keratinized in areas subject to considerable friction such as the palate. The oral epithelium is supported by a dense collagenous tissue, the lamina propria. In highly mobile areas, such as the soft palate and floor of the mouth, the lamina propria is attached to the underlying muscle by loose submucosal supporting tissue. In contrast, in areas where the oral mucosa is spread over the surface bone, such as the hard palate and tooth-bearing ridges, the lamina propria is firmly bound to the periosteum by a relatively thick fibrous submucosa. Throughout the oral mucosa, abundant small accessory salivary glands of both mucous and serous varieties are distributed in the submucosa (Burkitt et al., 1993). The oral mucosa is architecturally comparable to the stratified squamous epithelium of the penile and glanular urethra, making it remarkably adaptable for urethral substitution. Oral mucosa consists of a thick non-keratinized stratified squamous avascular epithelium ,slightly vascular underlying lamina propia. These properties contrast with the bladder mucosa and the penile skin, both of which have a thin epithelium and a thick lamina propria. Oral mucosa is approximately 5.0 mm in depth and the thickness is directly associated with male gender and varies indirectly with age (Vandana et al., 2005).

Oral epithelial cells are infused with polymicrobial intracellular and extracellular flora, mainly streptococci, but include other species such as Actinobacillus actinomycetemcomitans, Tannerella orsythensis, Fusobacterium nucleatum, Prevotella intermedia, Porphyromonas gingivalis, Oral Campylobacter species , Eikenella corrodens and Treponema denticola (Rudney, 2005). Despite these harsh microbial exposures, inflammatory infiltrate is seldom witnessed under histological examination of oral mucosa in healthy individuals and the reasons for this are the suppressing activity mediated between polymicrobial flora, production of antimicrobial peptides by the epithelia (defensins, cytokines, etc). Mucosal epithelial cells of the oral cavity impede microflora colonization by sustained exfoliation and by a specialized immune system, the mucosa-associated lymphoid tissue (MALT) (Michael et al., 2007). The lamina propria of a well-defatted oral mucosa graft can be considered a secondary barrier preventing microorganisms from entering adjacent tissue layers and exhibits noteworthy antimicrobial properties including lymphocytes, immunoglobulin-synthesizing plasma cells, monocytes/macrophages ,polymorphonuclear neutrophils , mast cells. Sebaceous glands, where present, are located in the lamina propria and are more widespread in labial than buccal mucosa. It can be demonstrated through immunohistochemical staining that nerve fibers and blood vessels from the submucosa infiltrate into the lamina propria, therefore providing a mechanism for angiogenesis and revascularization of the tissue whilst grafting. Oral mucosa is highly resilient and resistant to recurrent exposure to compression, stretching, and shearing forces. This resilient and resistant can be partially credited to the lamina propria-oral epithelium interface, which consists of widespread projections of connective tissue into the epithelial layer, increasing the surface area of the epithelial-lamina propria interface, and providing the oral mucosa's capacity to resist overlying forces. In contrast to the mucosa of the gastrointestinal tract, oral mucosa has no muscularis mucosae layer between its epithelial and lamina propria layers.

3. Surgical anatomy of the oral mucosa

The morphology of oral mucosa varies from region to region, and is related to the functional demands placed upon it. These regional differences exist in the nature of the submucosa, the morphology of the epithelial-connective tissue boundary the composition of the lamina propria, the thickness of the epithelium and the type of keratinization (Mungadi & Ugboko, 2009).

3.1 Anatomy of the labial mucosa

The upper and lower borders of the mandibular labial mucosal are designated by the vermillion border of the lower lip and the vestibular fold between the lower lip and the anterior border of the mandible, respectively. The lateral borders are a made up by the outer commissures of the lower lip. Mental nerve, a terminal branch of the inferior alveolar nerve of the mandibular division of the trigeminal nerve, innervates the mandibular labial alveolar mucosa. The mental nerve exits the mandible between the first and second premolar teeth through the mental foreman. The surgeon should plan the incision for a labial mucosa harvest medial to the middle of the canines to evade injuring the mental nerve and compromising sensation to the lower lip. The mandibular labial alveolar mucosa receives its blood supply from the inferior labial artery (a branch of the facial artery), the mental artery (a continuation of the inferior alveolar artery), as well as anastomoses from the buccal artery. The mental and buccal arteries are both branches of the maxillary artery. Both the facial artery and the maxillary artery are divisions of the external carotid artery. The labial mucosa is elastic, thin, resistant and technically easy to harvest and requires no suturing of the harvest site, but the buccal mucosa provides a wider graft and has a more robust quality oral mucosa.

3.2 Anatomy of the buccal mucosa

The vertical boundary of buccal mucosa is the maxillary and mandibular vestibular folds, whereas its anterior and posterior borders are shaped by the outer commissure of the lips and the anterior tonsillar pillar, respectively. The buccal mucosa is primarily innervated by the long buccal nerve and by the anterior, middle, and posterior superior alveolar nerves of the second division of the trigeminal nerve. Additionally there is limited sensory innervation from the facial nerve(Michael et al.,2007). The blood supply of the buccal mucosa has multiple arteries of origin including the buccal artery(a branch of the maxillary artery), the anterior superior alveolar artery of the infraorbital artery(a branch of the third part of the maxillary artery), the middle and posterior superior alveolar arteries(branches of the maxillary artery) and accessory vessels from the transverse facial artery (branch of the superficial temporal artery). The buccal mucosa is tough, resilient, easy to harvest, easy to handle and **leaves** no visible donor-site scar (Epply et al., 1997; Mahdavi et al.,2006).

3.3 Lingual mucosa

The mucosa covering the inferior lateral surface of the tongue is indistinguishable from that of the lining of the rest of the oral cavity. The mucosal covering the lateral and under surface of the tongue are the same in structure with that lining the rest of the oral cavity(Song et al., 2007). The mucosa covering the tongue has no particular functional features, and like buccal mucosal, lingual mucosa has constant availability, is easy to harvest and has favorable immunological properties (resistance to infection) and tissue characteristics (a thick epithelium, high content of elastic fibers, thin lamina propria and rich vascularization) (Simonato et al., 2006). As the lining of the oral cavity is limited, buccal mucosal graft(BMG) might not be adequate for treating complicated lengthy urethral strictures that require a larger supply of graft tissue. An ideal donor site for substitution urethroplasty will have characteristics comparable to buccal mucosa, but be easier to harvest and provide grafts of sufficient dimensions. Potential complications, although low or absent, in the using buccal mucosal grafts include numbness, difficulty with mouth opening, deviation or retraction,. The lateral aspect of the tongue offers mucosal tracts that are up to 7 to 8 cm long. Two grafts may be available in all patients. The harvesting technique is simple, quick and does not require nasal intubation or special retraction and, in addition, leaves a concealed donor site scar. The lingual mucosa grafts are similar to the labial grafts. In patients with a small mouth or difficult mouth opening, the tongue represents a good alternative for oral mucosa graft harvest site(Song et al.,2007). Our patients reported only slight oral discomfort at the donor site. For all of these reasons the tongue seems to be a good alternative donor site for graft harvest; however, lingual mucosal grafts are thin and are not as widely used as buccal mucosal grafts.

4. Mucosa graft harvest

4.1 Buccal grafts

The donor site is prepared, and cleaned using solution containing 10% povidone-iodine. Stay sutures are applied to the external edge of the cheek or lip to keep the oral mucosa stretched. The Stensen's duct, located at the level of the second molar, is identified and the desired graft size measured and marked in an ovoid shape(figure 1). Lidocaine HCl, 1% in adrenaline (1:100,000) is injected along the lateral borders of the graft site, to enhance haemostasis(figure 2). Oral mucosa graft is harvested by dissecting the mucosa off the buccinator muscle(figure 3). The oral mucosal donor site was inspected for bleeding and the defect closed with chromic 3/0 suture. This closure is optional(figure 4). When necessary (for longer stricture or extensive graft need) graft is taken from the lip or the other cheek, figure 5. The donor site is packed with a piece of gauze which is removed in the ward.

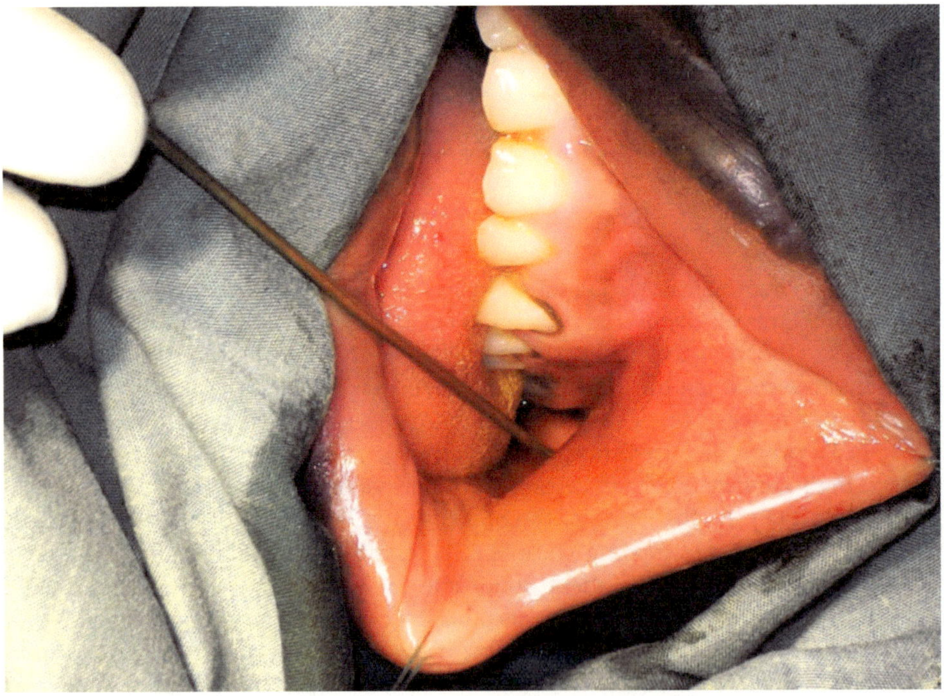

Fig. 1. Exposure of the buccal mucosa graft donor site. The Stensen's duct has been identified by the probe.

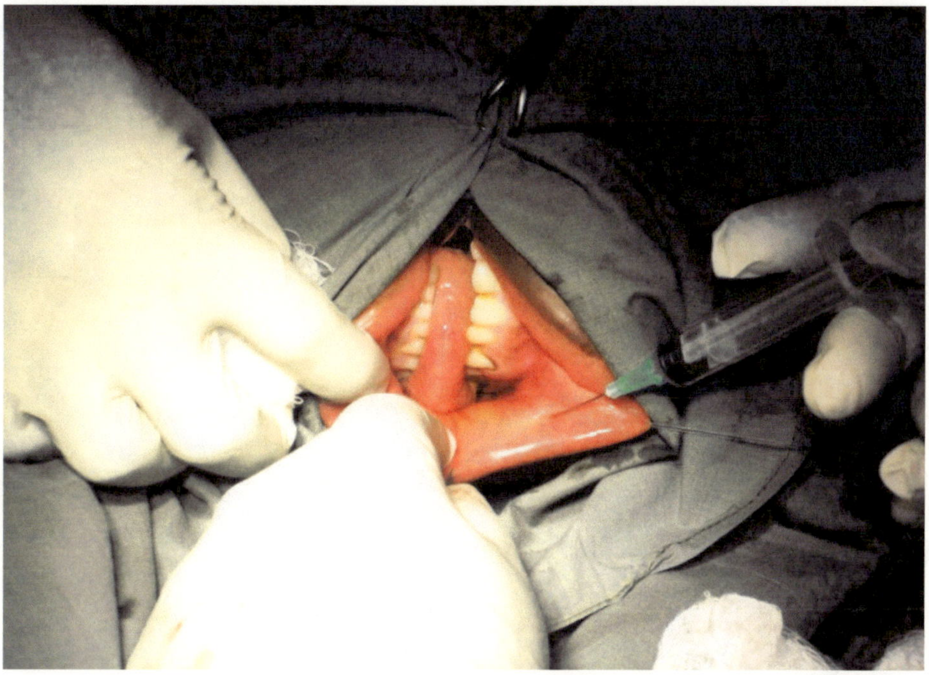

Fig. 2. Submucosal infiltration of donor site with 1% lignocaine in adrenaline to elevate graft and reduce bleeding.

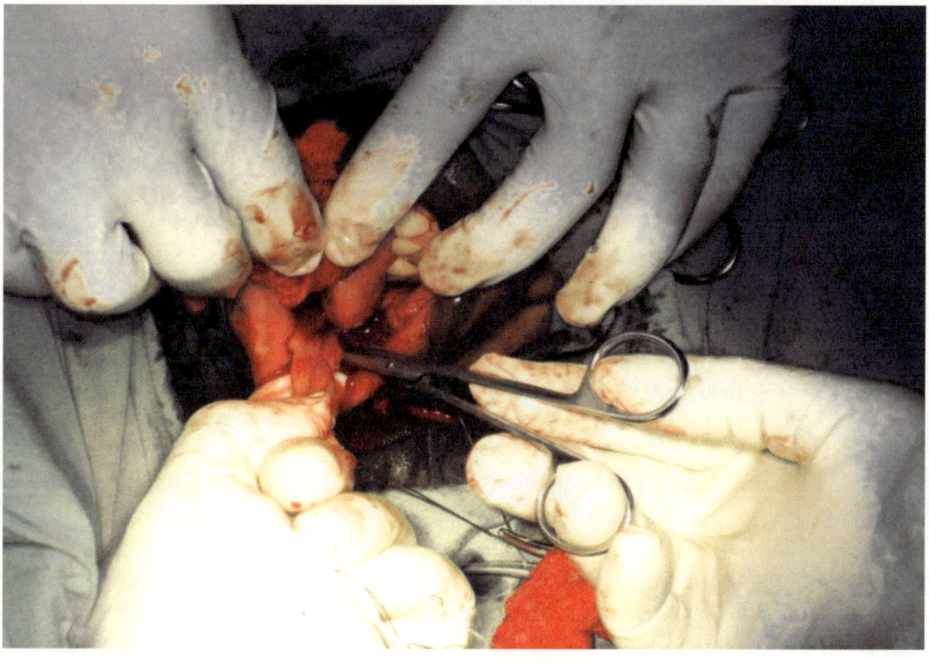

Fig. 3. Buccal mucosa graft being dissected off the cheek.

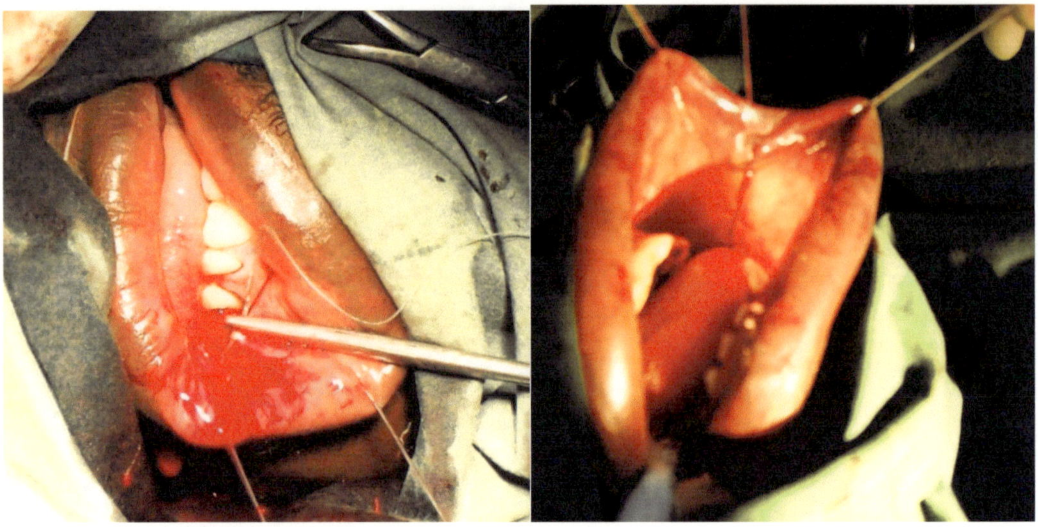

Fig. 4. Closure of buccal mucosa donor site. This is optional

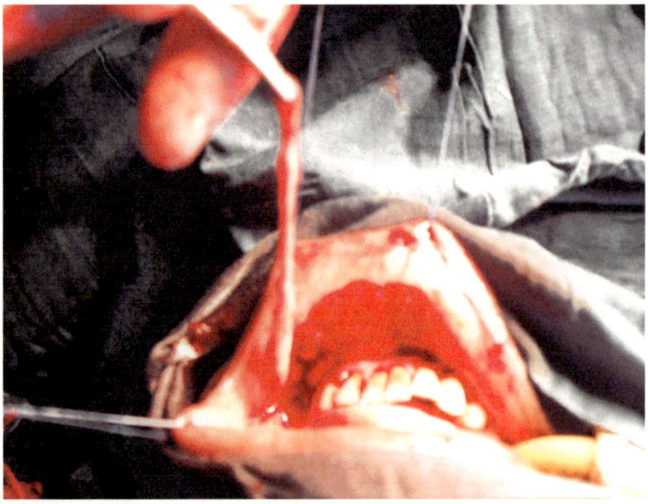

Fig. 5. Oral mucosa harvest from the lower lip

4.2 Lingual mucosa graft harvest

The mucosa covering the inferior lateral surface of the tongue is identical to the lining of the rest of the oral cavity.

For lingual graft harvest, the mouth is opened with a mouth opener. The apex of the tongue is passed through with a suture for traction or direct traction with a Babcock clamp to expose the ventrolateral surface of the tongue. The location of the harvest graft is the ventrolateral mucosal surface of the tongue, below the lining that separates the dorsum, where the papillae are situated, from the sublingual mucosa. The required graft (which may be infiltrated with lignocaine in adrenaline solution) is measured and marked with a surgical pen after identification of the opening of the parotid duct. The graft edges are incised with a scalpel and a full-thickness mucosal graft is harvested using sharp instruments beginning at the anterior land mark of the graft, figures 6 and 7. A 4-0 traction stitct may be useful to better handle the graft. The donor site is carefully examined for bleedinsg and easily closed with interrupted polyglactin 3-0 sutures

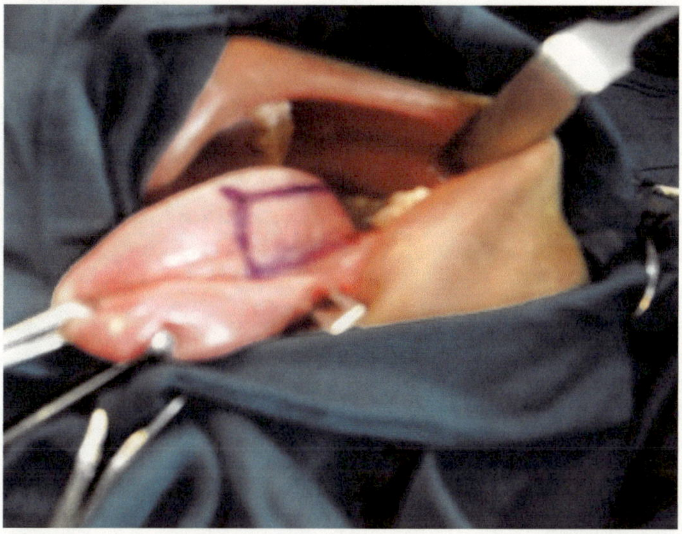

Fig. 6. Lingual mucosa donor site exposed.

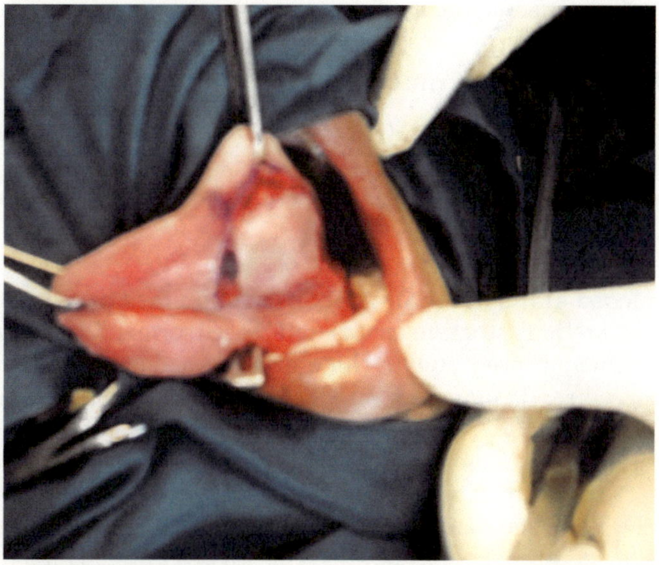

Fig. 7. Limgual graft being havested

4.3 Handling of the oral mucosa grafts

The harvested graft is immediately placed in isotonic saline and kept wet, thus preventing dessication especially in our tropical hot climate.The graft is then defatted to remove any remnants of fatty tissue and strands of muscle. The fatting process can be accomplished after pinninig the graft on a board or can be done while rolling it on the finger as illustrated(Figure 8). We find this defatting easy to accomplish on the finger using tenotomy scissors. The graft is fenestrated so as to create openings that may allow egress of serum after the graft has been fixed on the recipient site.

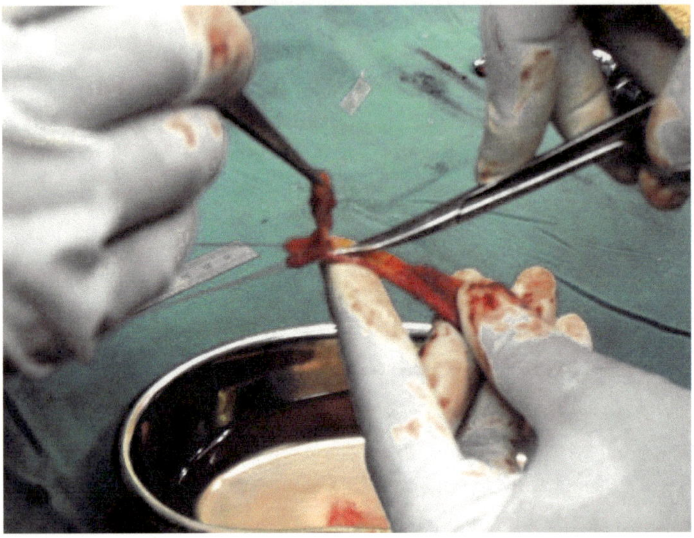

Fig. 8. Oral mucosa is defatted before application

5. Clinical applications of oral mucosa grafts in urology

Clinical application of oral mucosa grafts consists of autologous transplantation of non-keratinized oral mucosa for
repair of a variety of acquired and congenital urethral defects such as urethral strictures, hypospadias and epispadias.

5.1 Use of oral mucosa grafts in urethral reconstruction for stricture disease

Surgical options for urethral stricture disease are based primarily on the location of the stricture and the technique used and include excision and primary anastomosis, on-lay repairs, stricture excision and augmented anastomosis, flap based repairs and staged repairs (McAninch et al., 2008).
In situations where simple excision and primary anastomosis is not appropriate to maintain urethral continuity, some form of substitution urethroplasty will be necessary. Substitution urethroplasty is the gold standard for treatment of strictures of the male urethra not amenable to excision and primary anastomosis. This involves augmentation or replacing the circumference of the urethra using a patch or tube respectively of suitable material which may be genital or extra- genital tissues (Andrich & Mundy 2001; Turner-Warwck 1989). This involves the transfer of tissues in the form of a free graft or flaps (Weasells & McAninch 1996; Fischer,1997). The term graft implies that tissue has been excised and transferred to a graft host bed where a new blood supply develops by a process of take. This requires about

96 hours and occurs in two phases: The initial phase is imbibitions and during this phase the graft survives by absorbing nutrients from the host bed. The second phase is termed inosculation and this is when the microcirculation is established in the graft (Fischer, 1997).
On the other hand, a flap implies that a tissue is excised and transferred with the blood supply either preserved or surgically re-established at the recipient site. Until recently, flaps have been favoured to grafts for substitution urethroplasty because of the theoretical benefit that they carry their blood supply, and therefore , their viability is more secure (Andrich & Mundy, 2001). Flap construction is time- consuming with extensive dissection and redeployment of dartos fascia and have a tendency to cause penile deformity and scarring (Mungadi & Mbibu, 2006).
There has been a recent surge in the use of grafts for urethral reconstruction in the last decade because of the outstanding success of free grafts (especially oral mucosa) which are technically more efficient (Myers & Morey, 2008). The types of grafts used for urethral reconstruction include full thickness skin grafts, the split- thickness skin graft from the scrotum, penis and extra-genital sites, bladder epithelial grafts and oral mucosal grafts (Bhargava & Chapple, 2004; Weasells & McAninch, 1996). Other graft materials that have been used for substitution urethroplasty and include tunica vaginalis (Foinquinos et al., 2007), tunica albuginea (Mathur et al., 2009), colonic mucosa (Xu et al., 2009), small intestine submucosa (Donkov et al., 2006) and human dura matter (Maverich et al., 1998)
The scrotal skin has been used for two-stage urethroplasty as it provides a large quantity of easily accessible graft but its keratinized epithelium and split- thickness depth increases susceptibility to post-operative contracture, hyperkeratosis leading to graft failure in the wet environment of the urethra and the increased risk of diverticulum formation . In addition, scrotal skin is usually hair -bearing and may form hair balls in the urethra.
Non- hirsute full thickness grafts from the penis were initially found to provide satisfactory results in urethral reconstruction for stricture, but donor- site problems such as penile scarring , torsion of the penis, stricture recurrence and the high likelihood of failure in the presence of balanitis xerotica obliterans led to the hunt for a better urethral substitute (Greenwall et al., 1999)
Bladder mucosa grafts theoretically may be well suited for contact with urine but its use has been associated with many complications including meatal stenosis, prolapse and granulomatous reaction at the urethral meatus. Besides, bladder mucosa is difficult to harvest especially in patients who had previous bladder surgery, extrophy, chronic cystitis or neurogenic dysfunction and is weak to handle and liable to shrinkage (El- Sherbny et al., 2002)
Unlike bladder mucosa and skin, oral mucosa has a thick, non- keratinized epithelial layer and a well vascularised thin lamina propria favouring early inosculation (Duckett et al., 1995; Weasells and McAninch,1996; Duckett et al.,1995). Among reconstructive urologists, oral mucosa is emerging as the ideal substitute for the urethra with medium term results comparable to penile skin flaps.

5.1.1 One-stage oral mucosal graft meatoplsty

This technique is used in patients with hypospadias or ischaemic urethral stricture within the glans. The external urethral meatus and fossa navicularis are fully opened. The oral mucosa graft is sutured to the left side of the opened urethra. The graft is rotated over the urethral plate and sutured to the right of the urethra. The glans is closed over the graft and a Foley silicone catheter left in place for one week (Barbagli et al 2003b).

5.1.2 Dorsal oral mucosal graft urethroplasty

Dorsal oral mucosal grafts are suggested for repair of penile urethral strictures only in patients with normal corpus spongiosum. A circumcoronal foreskin incision is made with complete degloving of the penis, the penile urethra is exposed and the strictured tract fully opened by a ventral midline incision. The oral mucosa graft is sutured and quilted on the bed of the dorsal urethral incision with interrupted 6/0 sutures (Figure 9). The urethra is closed and tubularized. A dartos fascial flap is obtained to cover the urethral repair.

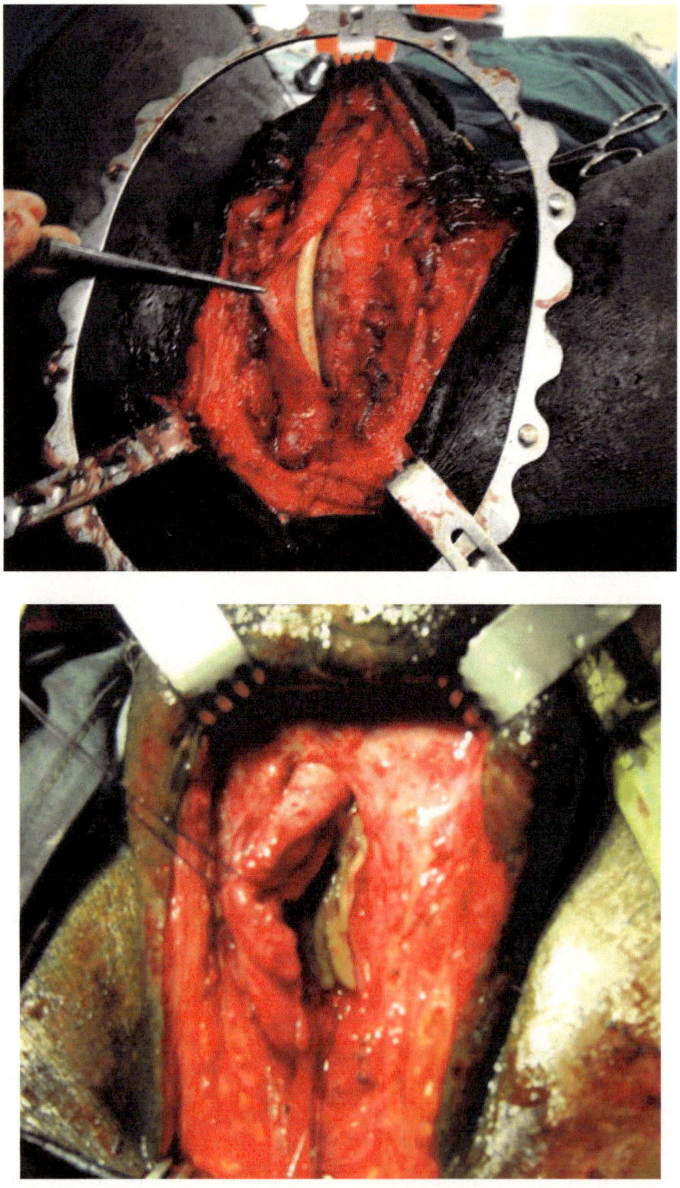

Fig. 9. Buccal mucosa applied for dorsal onlay urethroplasty

5.1.3 Staged oral mucosal graft urethroplasty

Staged oral mucosa graft urethroplasty is advocated for patients with complex penile or bulbar strictures in which a long stricture is associated with adverse local conditions such as fistula, periurethral inflammation, perineal abscess and extensive local scarring, balanitis xerotica obliterans(BXO) or previous failed urethroplasties (Bhargava & Chapple,2004; Greenwall et al.,1998; Barbagli et al.,2003;Joseph et al., 2002; Palminteri et al.,2002; Pansadoro et al.,1999) . Such adverse local tissue conditions will not favour graft take, thus requiring staging of the operation. In the first stage, the urethral plate is removed, the glans fully opened and oral mucosa graft splayed and quilted over the tunica albuginea. Six months later, after the graft has fully taken, the urethra is tubularized.

5.1.4 Augmented anastomotic urethroplasty

Augmented anstomotic urehroplasty combines stricture excision and urethral floor (or roof) strip re-anastomosis with augmentation of the anastomotic area using either a penile skin flap or a full- thickness graft (oral mucosa). The urethra is approached as for a standard anastomotic repair, being transected at the distal limit of the stricture and the strictured portion of the urethra is opened proximally on its dorsal surface (MacDonald et al., 2005; Datta et al., 2007). Strictures amenable to augmentation anastomotic repair are long bulbar strictures (>2cm) in which excision and primary anastomosis may result in a short urethra and chordee formation(figure 10).

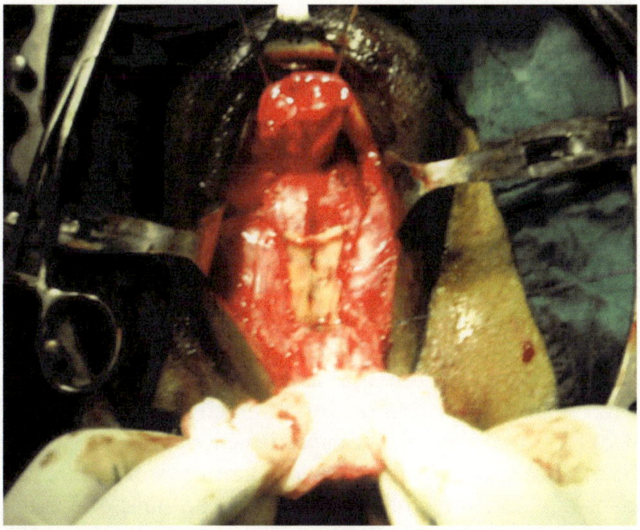

Fig. 10. Buccal mucosa applied for augmented anastomotic urethroplasty

5.1.5 Onlay graft orientation

There is controversy over placement of oral mucosa grafts- either dorsally, ventrally or laterally on the urethra (Morey, 2005; Datta et al.,2007; Barbagli et al., 1998; Morey 2005). Traditionally, grafts have been placed on the ventral aspect of the urethra because it allows easier access to the urethra and a better visualization of the stricture. Some authors have espoused that use of oral mucosa grafts as ventral onlay grafts and gives good outcomes (Gupta et al., 2004; MacLaughlin et al., 2006)

Barbagli et al (2003a) championed dorsal placement of the buccal mucosa grafts adducing that the dorsal approach to strictures of the bulbar urethra to be anatomically superior to ventral, requiring less extensive opening of the spongy tissue and reducing significant bleeding from the corpus spongiosum and mechanical weakening of the graft with better outcome. Dorsal placement of the graft on the urethra is simpler and safer in the distal part of the bulbar urethra whereas ventral placement of the graft is more efficacious in the proximal part of the bulbar urethra, where the spongiosum tissue is thicker and has better vascularise. In addition, a dorsally placed graft is more stable and is mechanically supported (by the corporal bodies) than a ventral graft. The take is reliable and out-pouching of the graft with increased intra-urethral pressure on voiding is prevented (Heinke et al., 2003).

5.1.6 Combined tissue transfer

Extensive, focally dense or panurethral strictures involving more than one segment of the anterior urethra, present a very challenging condition because sufficient oral mucosa may not be present to complete the repair. One of the reconstructive options in this case is the use of a combination of oral mucosa and a genital skin island flap to reconstruct the long urethral defect. Thus, dorsal on-lay oral mucosa grafts may be combined with various substitute materials like preputial skin, pedicled flaps, labial mucosa and human urethral mucosa from corpse (Rajiv et al., 2002). This makes it possible for one-stage reconstruction of urethral strictures avoiding the problems associated with hair bearing flaps and two-stage procedures (Elliot et al 2003)

5.1.7 Oral mucosa as tube graft

Tubularized grafts in urethral reconstruction failed mainly due to inadequate graft take as they are circumferentially surrounded by vascularised tissue. The use of oral mucosa onlay grafts are superior to tubularized grafts(El-Sherbny et al.,2002)

5.2 Use of oral mucosa grafts in hypospadias repair

Surgical treatment of hypospadias remains a challenge to the paediatric urologist due to the variation in the nature of the anomaly and availability of a multitude of techniques for repair. The surgical techniques have continued to evolve over the years. The goals of hypospadias repair include creating a straight penis, reconstructing a slit-like meatus at the tip of the penis, a urethra of adequate length and uniform calibre, symmetry in appearance of the glans and penile shaft and normalization of erection thereby restoring confidence on the child; (Bhat, 2008). The majority of hypospadias cases are mid shaft or distal. Here the axial integrity of the urethral plate can be conserved and hypospadias can be corrected with native tissue by means of either the well established techniques of tubularized incised plate urethroplasty or meatal advancement with glanuloplasty (Snodgrass, 2008; Goyal et al.,2010; Braga et al., 2008). In a number of patients there is a scarcity of local tissue to utilize for reconstruction, usually due to complications from earlier hypospadias surgery. In these patients a source of extra-genital tissue is frequently necessary for urethral reconstruction, and a number of tissues have typically been used (Hensle et al., 2002; Catti et al., 2008). Oral mucosa graft is a versatile substitute and a useful alternative in salvage situations. Whether harvested from the cheek, lip or tongue, it is currently the most widely used alternative to the inner prepuce skin and is an excellent urethral substitute as it leaves no visible scar with no significant donor- site morbidity and no danger of intra- urethral hair growth (Bracka, 2008).

Oral mucosa can be used for either urethral plate augmentation as a ventral or dorsal graft, or complete substitution (1-stage tube graft or 2-stage Bracka repair). Conventionally. OMG has been used as a ventral onlay graft with the advantage of easier placement. Barbagli (1998), introduced the dorsal onlay OMG for stricture urethroplasty with proposed advantages of better mechanical support, better blood supply to the graft, and hence, better chances of take and less chance of urethral diverticula. The dorsal placement of the oral mucosa graft can be applied in hypospadias repair can be used as one or two- stage procedure depending on the prevailing penile tissue.
Outcome following use of oral mucosa graft for hypospadias repair has been good with durable results; although, some complications may be observed. Hensle and colleagues (2002), reported complication rate of 32% in their series and observed that oral mucosa grafts do not have higher success rate than vascularized pedicle flaps.

5.3 Use of oral mucosal grafts for ureteral replacement.

Surgical correction of complicated, long-segment ureteral defects resulting from congenital malformations, retroperitoneal fibrosis, specific and non- specific inflammation, trauma, iatrogenic injuries and malignancy can be challenging (Selzman et al., 1996). Options for ureteral replacement traditionally include psoas hitch, boari flap, the Monti tube, use of the appendix, reconfigured colon or ileal segment (Brandes et al., 2004; Mathews &Marshal,1997; Ali-El-Dein&Ghoneim,2003; Jeffrey et al.,2000; Armatys et al.,2009; Pope&Koch,1996). Ureteral defects too long to be treated by excision and spatulated end-to-end anastomosis can be treated by use of oral mucosa grafts. Naude (1999) treated 4 patients with long segment ureteral loss using oral mucosa grafts applied as a patch wrapped with omentum. However, Badawy and co-workers(2010) reported a series of five patients who presented with extensive ureteral strictures who had oral mucosa grafts laid and fixed to the ureteral adventitia and tubularized over a double -J stent (Badawy et al., 2010). Although there is paucity of this application of oral mucosa grafts in the literature at the present, increasing use of this will increase.

5.4 Use of oral mucosa grafts for vaginal reconstruction

Vaginal reconstruction is indicated in congenital absence of the vagina as found in Mayer-Rokitansky- Kuster- Hauser syndrome, isolated vaginal agenesis in children, in adults following pelvic exentration for malignancy, patients who had undergone sex re-assignment and in those undergoing feminizing genitoplasty for congenital adrenal hyperplasia (Gupta et al., 2002; Hensle&Reily, 1998; Fleighner, 1994; Leslie et al, 2009; Gollu et al,2007).
Surgical techniques for vaginal reconstruction include use of myocutaneous flaps, partial and full thickness skin grafts and use of intestinal segments (Leslie et al., 2009; Johnson et al., 1991; Michal et al 2007; Rajimwale et al., 2004; Franz, 1996). The neo-vagina created by flap and graft vaginoplasty call for constant dilatation and are prone to stenosis but the intestinal neo-vaginas do not require frequent dilatations but generate mucus which may be plentiful to make patients put on sanitary pads. However, all these techniques entail abdominal procedures and visible scars. Oral mucosa grafts have been applied for vaginal reconstruction in selected patients. Samuelson et al (2006) performed autologous buccal mucosa graft vaginoplasty in a post-pubertal patient with adrenogenital syndrome who had excellent functional and cosmetic outcome. Muxin and colleagues (2009) reported of a

series of 9 patients presenting with vaginal agenesis who had construction of neo-vagina that was lined with autologous micromucosa . Both reports corroborate the advantages of oral mucosa grafts in vaginoplasty which include wet, non-keratinized neo-vaginal mucosa with excellent color and texture matching to the genital and vaginal skin. In addition, OMGs leaves no visible surgical scars, avoids abdominal bowel surgery and do not produce excess mucus. Buccal mucosa may be a replacement for the female vulva and vaginal glabrous skin and be an excellent adjunct or alternative in challenging reconstruction.

6. Donor-site morbidity in oral mucosa graft harvest.

Serious complications from oral mucosal graft harvest are uncommon. Possible adverse effects of harvesting oral mucosa include intra-operative haemorrhage, post-operative infection, pain, swelling, injury to the parotid duct, limitation of oral opening and loss of or altered sensation of the cheek or lower lip through nerve damage (Dublin &Stewart, 2004; Markiewcz et al., 2007)

Wood et al (2004) noted reduction of sensation in the oral cavity in the region of the site of graft harvest in 68% of patients which persisted in 26% at, or further than, six months follow-up. This complication is more frequent when the graft is harvested from the lower lip (Kamp et al., 2005). The neurosensory deficit of the long buccal and mental nerves could be explained by individual variations in the location and nature of branching of these two nerves. This may happen with short and thin patients especially when the amount of available buccal mucosa tissue is small or a larger graft is harvested.

Tulstunov et al (1997) in a more detailed study of twelve patients reported that all patients had only mild oral discomfort at the end of the first week and by the third week, no patient had oral discomfort. Dublin et al (2004), found that 10% of the patients had moderate-to-severe pain on discharge but after about three weeks the pain resolved. Wood et al(2004) found that the daily pain score was higher in those patients with donor- site closure than in those in whom the donor-site was left open·

Damage to surrounding structures can be avoided by careful marking of the cheek mucosa before harvesting. It is recommended that the dissection should be at least 1 cm from the opening of the parotid duct and care should be taken during suturing of the wound. Parasthesia after harvesting a buccal mucosal graft is the most common complication in our patients.

7. Role of tissue engineering in urethral reconstruction.

The main constraint in use of oral mucosa grafts for extensive urologic reconstruction is the limited amount of graft available for harvest in patients as a result of previous dental procedures, trauma, infection, malignancy or prior oral mucosa grafts.

Tissue engineering encompasses a multidisciplinary approach that applies the principles and methods of engineering and life sciences geared for the development of tissue and organs as biological substitutes to restore and preserve normal function in diseased or injured tissues (Cross et al., 2003). Tissues that are engineered using the patient's own cells or immunologically inactive allogenic or xenogenic cells have the potential to overcome current problems of replacing function (Saxena, 2005). Bhargava and colleagues (2004) developed a technique to increase the amount of tissue available for harvest called tissue-engineered buccal mucosa (TEBM). Izumi and colleagues (2003) reported clinical study using ex vivo produced human oral mucosa composed of both epithelial dermal component for intraoral grafting procedures. Tissue engineering has a principal advantage over organ transplantation and circumvents organ shortage. Tissues that match the patient's requirements can be reconstructed from readily available biopsies and then re-implanted with minimal or no immunogenicity.

Tissue engineering in urology is a rapidly emerging field with researchers and clinicians world-wide in search of 'off- the- shelf' replacements for the bladder and urethra. Buccal mucosa has been successfully tissue-engineered by culturing oral keratinocytes and fibroblasts. These cells were applied to de-epidermised dermis to obtain full-thickness tissue-engineered oral mucosa for substitution urethroplasty (Bhargava et al., 2004, Lavick & Langer, 2004; Li et al., 2008). De Fillipo et al (2002) demonstrated in rabbit models that collagen matrices seeded with cells from normal urethral tissue can be used for tubularized replacement.

The success of tissue engineered grafts is dependent on the ability to provide a suitable environment for regulating cell behaviour such that adhesion, proliferation, migration and differentiation eventually result in a graft composed of a population of cells similar in morphology and phenotype to the desired tissue(Fransis et al., 2009). Engineered buccal mucosa will offer a useful addition in urethral reconstruction, thus creating sufficient tissue for urethroplasty with minimal donor-site morbidity and quicker surgery for longer and complex procedures such as those associated with balanitis xerotica obliterans and two-stage circumferential urethral replacements (Lavick et al., 2004).

8. Conclusion

Oral mucosa is an excellent substitute to skin whenever reconstruction is required with a non hirsute and non keratinized skin. This requirement had previously posed an immense challenge to urologic, pediatric and plastic surgical reconstruction. As skin substitute, oral mucosal grafts are reliable with long term results comparable to that of penile skin flaps. Oral mucosa is more resistant to infection and has a micro-vasculature that encourages inosculation. Oral mucosa grafts are easier to harvest compared with penile flaps and are not attended with potential complications of scaring, cordee and torsion. This is also an ideal substitute in patients with Lichen sclerosis. In addition to urethral reconstruction in adult and children, OMGs can be used for glans reconstruction and resurfacing, clitoral reconstruction, ureteral repair and vaginal reconstruction. The graft volume can be improved with tissue engineering making it potentially available for wider coverage

9. References

Ali-El-Dein B & Ghoneim M. Bridging long ureteral defects using the Yang-Monti princilpe. *J Urol 2003*; 169: 1074-1077.

Andrich DE & Mundy AR. Substitution with Buccal Mucosa- Free Grafts. *J Urol* 2001; 165: 1131 - 1134.

Armatys SA, Mellon MJ, Beck DW, Koch MO, Foster RS & Bihrle R. Use of ileum as ureteral replacement in urological reconstruction. *J Urol* 2009; 181: 177-188.

Badawy AA, Abolysor A, Saleem MD & Abuzeld AM. Buccal mucosa grafts for ureteral stricture substitution: Initial experience. *Urology* 2010; 76: 971-976.

Barbagli G & De Stefani S. Reconstruction of the bulbar urethra using dorsal onlay buccal mucosal graft: New Concepts and surgical tricks. Indian *J Urol* 2006; 22: 113-117.

Barbagli G , Palminteri E, Guazzoni G & Cavalcanti A. Bulbar Urethroplasty Using the Dorsal Approach: Current Techniques. Int. *Braz J Urol* 2003a; 29: 155-161.

Barbagli G, Palminteri E, Lazzeri M et al. Anterior Urethral Strictures. *BJU Int* 2003b; 92: 497-505.

Barbagli G, Palminteri E & Rizzo M. Dorsal Onlay Graft Urethroplasty Using Penile Skin or Buccal Mucosa in Adult Bulbourethral Strictures. *J Urol* 1998; 160: 1307-1309.

Bhargava S & Chapple CR. : Is Buccal Mucosa Urethroplasty the new gold standard? *BJU. Int* 2004; 93:1191-1192/

Bhargava S, Chapple CR, Bullock , Layton C & Macneil S. Tissue-Engineered Buccal Mucosa For Substitution Urethroplasty. *BJU Int* 2004; 93:807-811.

Bhat A. General Considerations in Hypospadias Surgery. *Indian J Urol* 2008; 24: 188-194.

Bracka A. The role of two-stage repair in modern hypospadiology. *Indian J Urol* 2008; 24: 210-218.

Braga LHP, Lorenzo AJ & Pippi Salle JL. The Use of Tubularized incised plate urethroplasty for distal hypospadias. Indian *J Urol* 2008; 24: 221-225.

Brandes S, Coburn M, Armenakas N & McAninch J. Diagnosis and management of ureteric injury: an evidence-based analysis. *BJU Int*2004: 94: 277-289.

Burkitt GH, Young B & Heath JW. Oral Tissues. *Wheaters Functional Histology: a textbook and color atlas.* 3rd Edition. Churchill Livingstone; Edinburgh 1993. P. 235.

Catti M, Demede D, Valmalle A-F, Mure P-Y, Hameury F & Mouriquand P. Management of Severe Hypospadias. *Indian J Urol* 2008; 24: 233-240.

Cross WR, Thomas DFM & Southgate J. Tissue Engineering and Stem Cell Research in Urology. *BJU Int* 2003; 92:166-171.

Datta B, Rao M P , Acharga RL, N. Goel,N , Saxena V , Trivedi S, Dwivedi US &.Singh PB. Dorsal Onlay Buccal Graft Urethroplasty in Long Anterior Urethral Stricture. *Int. Braz J Urol*. 2007; 33: 181- 187.

Desanti A, Iannuccelli M, Ginesu G & Feo C. Reconstruction of Hypospadias and Epispadias with buccal mucosa free grafts as primary surgery: 10 years experience. *J Urol* 2003; 170: 1600-1602.

Donkov II, Bashir A, Elenkov CHG, & Panchev PK. Dorsal onlay augmentation urethroplasty with small intestinal sub-mucosa: Modified Barbagli technique for strictures of the bulbar urethra. *Int J Urol* 2006; 13: 1415- 1417.

Donoff RB. Biological basis for vestibuloplasty procedures, *J Oral Surg* 1976;34 : 890

Dubey D, Kumar A, Mandhani A, Srivastava A, Kapoor R & Bhandari M. Buccal Mucosal Urethroplasty: A Versatile Technique for urethral segments. *BJU Int. 2005;* 95(4): 625-

Dublin N & Stewart L H. Oral Complications after buccal mucosal graft harvest for urethroplasty. *BJU Int.* 2004; 94: 867-869

Duckett JW, Coplen D, Ewalt D et al. Buccal Mucosa Urethral Replacement. *J Urol* 1995; 153: 1660-1663

Elliott SP, Metro MJ & McAninch JW. Long-Term Follow-up of ventrally placed Buccal Mucosal Onlay Graft in Bulbar Urethral Reconstruction. *J.Urol* 2003; 169 : 1754-1757.

El-Sherbny MT, Abol-Eneim H, Dawaba MS & Ghonein M. Treatment of Urethral Defects: Skin, Buccal or Bladder Mucosa, Tube or Patch? An Experimental Study in Dogs. *J Urol* 2002; 167: 2225 - 2228.

Epply BL, Keating M & Rink RA. A Buccal Mucosal Harvesting Technique For Urethral Reconstruction. *J Urol* 1997;157:1268-1275.

Fischer JC. Skin Grafting. In: *Georgiade Plastic, Maxillofacial and Reconstructive Surgery*, 3rd Ed. Georgiade, GS, Riefkolil, Levin SL (Eds). William and Wilkins Baltimore 1997. p17.

Fleigner JRH. Vaginal agenesis and embryology of vaginal epithelium. *Aust NZ Obster Gynaecol* 1994; 34: 562-566.

Foinquinos RC, Calado AA, Janio R, Griz A., Macedo A & Ortiz V. The tunica vaginalis dorsal graft urethroplasty: Initial experience. *Int Braz J Urol* 2007; 33:523-531.

Fransis K, Eeckt K V, Poppel HV & Joniau S. Results of buccal mucosa grafts for repairing long bulbar urethral strictures *BJU Int* 2009; 105: 1170-1172.

Franz RC. Sigmoid colon vaginoplasty: a modified method. *BJOG* 1996; 103: 1148-1155.

Gollu G, Yildiz RV, Bingol-Kologlu M et al. Ambiguous genitalia: an overview of 17 years' experience. *J Pediatr Surg* 2007; 42: 840-844.

Goyal A, Singh MV & Dickson AP. Oral Mucosa Graft for Repair of Hypospadias: Outcome at Puberty. *J Urol* 2010; 184: 2604-2609.

Greenwall TJ, Venn SN & Mundy AR. Changing Practice in Anterior Urethral Strictures. *BJU Int.* 1999;83:631-635.

Gupta NP & Ansari MS. Mayer- Rokitansky- Kuster- Hauser (MRKH) Syndrome- a review. *Indian J Urol* 2002; 18: 111-116.

Gupta NP, Ansari MS, Dogra PN & Tandon S. Reconstructive Urology. Dorsal Buccal Mucosal Urethroplasty by a Ventral Sagital Urethrotomy and Minimal- Access Perineal Approach For Anterior Urethral Stricture. *BJU Int* 2004; 1287-1290.

Heinke T, Elmar W, Bonfig GR & Riedmiller H. Ventral Onlay Urethroplasty using Buccal mucosa for Complex Stricture Repair. *Urology* 2003;61:1004-1007.

Hensle TW & Reily EA. Vaginal replacement in children and young adults. *J Urol* 1998; 159: 1035-1038.

Hensle TW, Kearney MC & Bingham JB. Buccal Mucosa Grafts for Hypospadias Surgery: Long Term Results. *J Urol* 2002; 168: 1734-1737.

Weasells H & McAninch JW. Use of Free Grafts in Urethral Stricture Reconstruction. *J Urol.* 1996: 1912-1915.

Jeffrey FR, Stock JA& Hanna MK. The appendix as right ureteral substitute in children. *J Urol* 2000; 163: 1908- 1912.

Johnson N, Lilford RJ & Batchelor A. The free flap vaginoplasty; a new surgical procedure for the treatment of vaginal agenesis. BJOG 1991; 98: 184-188.

Joseph JV,. Andrich DE, Leach CJ and Mundy A R. Urethroplasty for Refractory Anterior Urethral Stricture. *J Urol* 2002 ; 167: 127-129.

Kamp S, Knoll T, Osman M, Hacker A, Michel M S & Alken P. Donor-site Morbidity in Buccal Mucosa Urethroplasty Lower lip or Inner Cheek. *BJU Int.*2005; 96: 619-623.

Kumar A, Goyal, NK, Das SK , Trivedi S , Dwivedi U S, & Singh P B. Oral Complications After Lingual Mucosal Graft Harvest For Urethroplasty. *Anz J. Surg*. 2007; 77:970-973.

Lavick E & Langer R. Tissue Engineering: Current State and Perspectives. *Appl Microbiol Biotechnol* 2004; 65(1): 1-8

Leone CR. Conjunctivodacryocystorhinostomy with buccal mucosal graft. *Arch Ophthalmol* 1995; 113: 113.

Leslie JA, Cain MP & Rink RC. Feminizing genital reconstruction in congenital adrenal hyperplasia. *Indian J Urol* 2009; 25: 17-25.

Lin WC, Chang CYY, Shen YY & Tsai HD, Use of autologous buccal mucosa for vaginoplasty: a study of eight cases, *Hum Reprod* 2003;18: 604

MacDonald M F & Santucci R. Review and treatment algorithim of open surgical techniques for management of urethral strictures. *Urology* 2005; 65: 9-15.

Mahdavi ZR, Yazdani KM, Arab D, Ahanian A & Mahdavi M. Dorsal onlay graft urethroplasty using buccal mucosa in extensive anterior urethral strictures. *Urology* 2006; 68 (Suppl. 1): 247-248. 25.

Markiewicz MR, Lukose MA, Margarone III JE, Barbagli G, Miller KS & Chuang SK. The Oral Mucosa Graft: A Systematic Review. *J Urol* 2007; 165:1131-1134.

Martins F, Badona J, Rodrigues R , Marcelino R , Varela J & Lopes T. Buccal Mucosa: Versatile Graft in anterior urethroplasty. *Urology* 2006; 68: (Suppl.) : 220.

Mathews J & Marshal FF. Versatility of the adult psoas hitch ureteral ureteral reimplantation. *J Urol* 1997; 158: 2078-2082.

Mathur RK, Sharma AK & Odiya S. Tunica albuginea urethroplasty for anterior urethral strictures : A urethroscopic analysis. *Int J Urol*. 2009; 16: 751-755.

Maverich HV, Moreno RP, Soriol JC, Briones JR, Bordes AR & Rodriguez JV. Experience with human dura matter for urethral strictures. *J Urol* 1998; 160: 1310 -1311.

McAninch JW. Disorders of the Penis and male Urethra. In Tanagho EA.McAninch JW eds. Smiths Urology, 2008, 17th Ed. McGraw Hill, Lange, p 626.

McLaughlin MD, Thrasher JB, Celmer A & Bruegger D. Buccal Mucosal Urethroplasty In Patients who had Multiple Previous Procedures. *Urology* 2006; 68:1156-1159.

Michael R. Markiewicz MR ,Joseph E, Margarone III JE, Barbagli G & Scannapieco FA. Oral Mucosa Harvest: An Overview of Anatomic and Biologic Considerations. *EAU- EBU Updates* 2007; 5: 179-187.

Morey AF. Buccal Mucosal Urethroplasty: A Versatile Technique for All Urethral Segments. *J Urol* 2005; 174: 2265-2266.

Mungadi I A & Mbibu N H. Current Concepts in the management of anterior urethral strictures. *Nigerian Journal of Surgical Research;* 8 (3-4): 103-110

Mungadi IA & Ugboko VI. Oral Mucosa Grafts for urethral Reconstruction. *Annals Afr Med* 2009; 8: 203-209.

Muxin Z, Li P, Li S & Li Q. Use of autologous micromucosa graft for vaginoplasty in vaginal agenesis.*Ann Plast Surg* 2009; 63: 645-649.

Myers JB & Morey A. Anterior Urethral Reconstruction: Penile Island flaps. *In: Montague DK et al (Eds). Reconstructive Urologic Surgery.* 2008, Informs UK Ltd London, p473.

Naude JH. Buccal Mucosal grafts in treatment of ureteric lesions. *BJU Int* 1999; 83: 751-754.

Palminteri E, Lazzeri M , Guazzoni G, Turini D & Barbagli G. New 2-Stage Buccal Mucosal Graft Urethroplasty. *J Uro* 2002; 167: 130 - 132.

Pansadoro V, Emiliozzi P, Gaffi M and Scarpone P. Buccal Mucosa Urethroplasty for the Treatment of Bulbar Urethral Strictures. *J Urol* 1999; 160: 1501-1503.

Payne CE, Sumfest JM & Deshon Jr GE, Buccal mucosal graft for hypospadias repairs, *Tech Urol* 1998; 4: . 73.

Pope J & Koch MO. Ureteral replacement with reconfigured colon substitute. *J Urol* 1996; 155: 1693- 1695.

Rajimwale A, Furness III PD, Brant WO and Koyle MA. Vaginal construction using sigmoid colon in children and young adults. *BJU Int* 2004; 94: 115-1159.

Rajiv G, Deepak D, & Aneesh S. Bulbar urethroplasty mucosa graft placed on the ventral, dorsal or lateral surface of the urethra: Are results affected by the surgical technique? *Uroscan* 2002; 22: 165-166.

Rudney D, Chen R, & Sedgewick G.J. Actinobacillus actinomycetemcomitans, Porphyromonas gingivalis, and Tannerella forsythensis are Components of a Polymicrobial Intracellular Flora within Human Buccal Cells. J Dent Res. 2005; 84: 59-63.

Samuelson ML & Baker LA. Autologous buccal mucosa vulvovaginoplasty for high urogenital sinus. J Pediatr Urol 2006; 2: 486-488.

Saxena AK. Tissue engineering: Present concepts and strategies. Indian Assoc Paedatr Surg 2005; 10:

Selzman AA & Spirnak JP. Iatrogenic ureteral injuries: A 20 year experience in treating 165 injuries. J Urol 1996; 155: 878- 881.

Simonato A, Gregori A, Lissiani A, Galli S , Ottaviani F ,Rossi R ,Zappone A & Carmignani G . The Tongue as an Alternative Donor Site for Graft Urethroplasty: Pilot Study. J Urol 2006; 175: 589-92.

Simonato A, Gregori A. Lissiani A, Galli S, Ottaviani F, et al. The tongue as an Alternative donor site for Graft Urethroplasty: A Pilot Study. J Urol 2006; 175: 589- 592.

Snodgrass WT. Utilization of urethral plate in hypospadias Surgery. Indian J Urol 2008; 24: 195-199.

Song L J, Xu YM, Lazzeri M & Barbagli G. Lingual mucosal graft for anterior urethroplasty: a review. BJU Int 2009; 104: 1052-1056.

Song L-J, Xu Y-M, Hu X-Y & Zhang H-Z. Urethra substitution using autologous lingual mucosal grafts: an experimental study. BJU Int 2007; 101: 739-743.

Tolstunov L, Pogrel MA & McAninch JW. Intraoral Morbidity following free buccal graft harvesting for urethroplasty. Oral Surg Oral Med Pathol Oral Radiol Endod 1997; 84: 480-482.

Turner- Warwick R. Urethral Strictures Repair: General Considerations. In: Atlas of Urologic Surgery. Frank Hinman Jr (Ed). WB Saunders Company Ltd. Philadelphia 1989. p 166 .

Vandana KL & Savitha B. Thickness of gingiva in association with age, gender and dental arch location. J Clin Periodontol 2005; 32: 828–830.

Wood DN, Allen SE, Andrich DE, Greenwell T J & Mundy AR. The Morbidity of Buccal Mucosal Graft Harvest for Urethroplasty and the Effect of Non- closure of Graft Harvest -Site on Post-operative Pain. J Urol 2004; 172: 580- 583.

Xu Y-M, Qiao Y , Sa Y-L, Wu D-L, Zhang X-R, Zhang J, Gu B-J & Jin S-B. Substitution Urethroplasty of Complex and Long- Segment Urethral Strictures: A Rationale for Procedure Selection. Eur. Urol 2007; 51: 1093-1099.

Xu YM, Qiao Y, Sa YL, Zhang J, Fu Q & Song LJ. Urethral Reconstruction using colonic mucosa graft for complex strictures. J Urol 2009; 182: 1040-*1043*.

9

Full-Thickness Skin Grafts in Reconstructive Dermatologic Surgery of Nasal Defects

Carmen Fernández-Antón Martínez
and Ricardo Suárez-Fernández
Gregorio Marañón Hospital, Madrid
Spain

1. Introduction

The nose is one of the most important facial features and any change in its shape, colour or skin cover may be very obvious. Nasal defects are a common challenge for dermatologists and plastic surgeons in daily practice. Many benign and malignant lesions are located in the nasal region. Basal cell carcinoma is the most common skin cancer and is found frequently in this anatomical region. The size of defects secondary to excision of these lesions may not allow primary closure or reconstruction using skin flaps and requires the use of skin grafts. Skin grafts are particularly suitable for large defects occupying almost entire cosmetic units, and especially in elderly patients with acceptable cosmetic results in many cases.

A precise knowledge of the anatomy of the nasal region is essential, before considering reconstructive options. Like the underlying bony-cartilaginous framework of the nose, the overlying skin may also be divided into vertical thirds. The skin of the upper third is fairly thick but tapers into a thinner mid-dorsal region. The inferior third regains the thickness of the upper third owing to the more sebaceous nature of the skin in the nasal tip. The dorsal skin is usually the thinnest of the 3 sections of the nose. The nasal muscles are deep in the skin and include four main groups: the elevators, depressants, compressor, and the dilators. The elevators are the procerus and levator muscle of upper lip and nasal ala. Depressants are composed of the nasal alar and nasal septum depressor. The muscles are interconnected by a fascia called the nasal superficial musculoaponeurotic system (SMAS).

The soft outer tissue of the nose can be divided into subunits. The purpose of the subunits is to divide the nasal anatomy into segments useful for reconstruction. If more than 50% of a subunit is lost, it may be necessary to replace the entire unit with regional tissue or tissue from a donor. The subunits include the nasal dorsal segment, lateral wall segments, the hemi-lobe soft tissue triangle segment, and alar columellar segments.

The nose, like the rest of the face, has a rich blood supply. The arterial supply to the nose can be divided principally into the internal carotid branches, ie branches of the anterior and posterior ethmoidal arteries of the ophthalmic artery and the external carotid branches, namely the sphenopalatine, greater palatine arteries, upper lip, and angular. The external nose is supplied by the facial artery, which becomes the angular artery attending on the superomedial side of the nose. Sellar and dorsal regions of the nose are supplied by branches of internal maxillary artery (ie, the infraorbital) and ophthalmic arteries (corresponding to the internal carotid system). Internally, the lateral nasal wall is supplied by the sphenopalatine artery and posterior ethmoidal arteries. The nasal septum is also derived from the blood supply from the sphenopalatine and anterior and posterior ethmoidal arteries with additional input from the superior labial artery (above) and the greater palatine artery (posterior). The Kiesselbach plexus or Little's area, represents a region in the anterior third of the nasal septum, where all three of the main arteries convergence in the inner nose.

The veins of the nose essentially follow the arterial pattern and are important for direct communication with the cavernous sinus. The vein of the cavernous sinus lacks valves, which enhances the spread of intracranial infection.

Nodes arise from the superficial mucosa and drain in retropharyngeal and upper deep cervical lymph nodes and / or submandibular glands. The sensation of the nose is derived from the first two branches of the trigeminal nerve. The parasympathetic innervation arises from the greater superficial petrosal (GSP) branch of cranial nerve VII. The GSP joins the deep petrosal nerve (sympathetic innervation), which comes from the carotid plexus to form the nerve in the canal vidian. Vidian nerve travels through the pterygopalatine ganglion (only the parasympathetic nerves synapse here) to the lacrimal gland and glands of the nose and palate by the maxillary division of trigeminal nerve.

The nose can also be divided into the superior cosmetic unit, in which skin is usually thin, elastic, loose and frequently not sebaceous, and the inferior cosmetic unit in which the skin is usually thick, less elastic, tightly attached to the underlying structures and much more sebaceous. The inferior cosmetic unit is much more complex because the cartilages of the lower unit attach to each other and to the nasal septum by fibrous aponeurotic bands. Distortion of this lower segment can lead to both cosmetic and functional defects.

2. Full-thickness skin grafts to repair nasal defects

Full-thickness skin grafts (FTSGs) contain the entire epidermis and dermis and preserve adnexal structures, so they are very useful in the reconstruction of nasal defects. Grafts offer great variability in size and shape and allow for the closure of a wide variety of defects.

Multiple donor sites are available, enabling selection of the closest tissue match. Disadvantages include the creation of a second surgical site and suboptimal tissue colour and texture match if an improper donor site is selected. Additionally, complete denervation of the graft occurs such that patients rarely experience full sensation at the recipient site even after prolonged periods. Currently skin grafting continues to be a viable, useful, and versatile closure option, and in some instances, is the best choice. FTSGs are indicated as a repair consideration for surgical defects that cannot be opposed primarily or with a flap, and where healing by second intention is likely to result in poor cosmetic or functional deficits.

The use of FTSGs enables better cosmetic and functional results and preserves the basic skin functions such as sweating, and pigment production. In addition, the increased thickness of FTSGs results in a more complete filling of deeper surgical defects and less wound contracture.

2.1 Performance of nasal full-thickness skin grafts

Tumour-free margins prior to reconstruction are the most important challenge. In the case of well-defined malignant lesions, excision should be performed with an adequate margin for curative oncological outcome (figure 1). When the lesions have vague or unclear boundaries, Mohs micrographic surgery with surgical pathology frozen sections, or delayed reconstruction after securing margins are free from tumour are good alternatives.

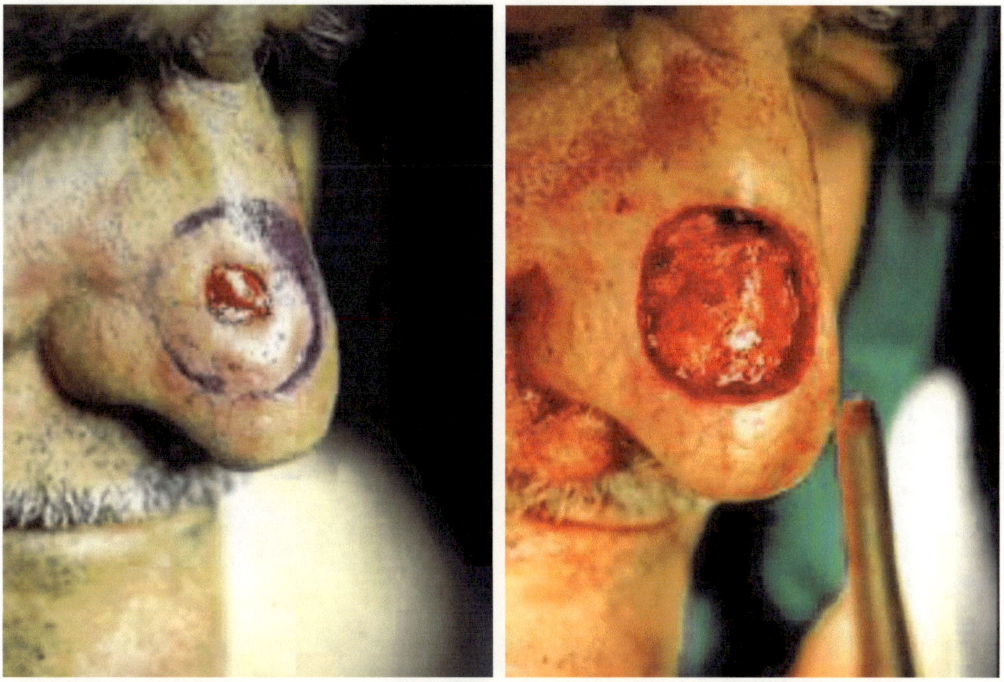

Fig. 1. Basal cell carcinoma excised with an adequate margin in order to achieve oncological cure. On the left, before excision and on the right after it.

When selecting the donor area, the first key point is to choose the donor skin area in such a way that it resembles as much as possible the skin of recipient area. A donor site must be selected in order to achieve direct closure with a minimally visible scar. Among the factors to consider for a successful donor site selection, include the colour of the skin, the texture of the tissue, the amount of sun damage, and the presence or absence of hair. The most frequent donor sites used for the reconstruction of nasal defects that meet the above requirements are preauricular skin and skin of the glabella (figures 2 and 3). If the patient has hair on the glabella, which is quite common in males, glabella will not be a good donor site.

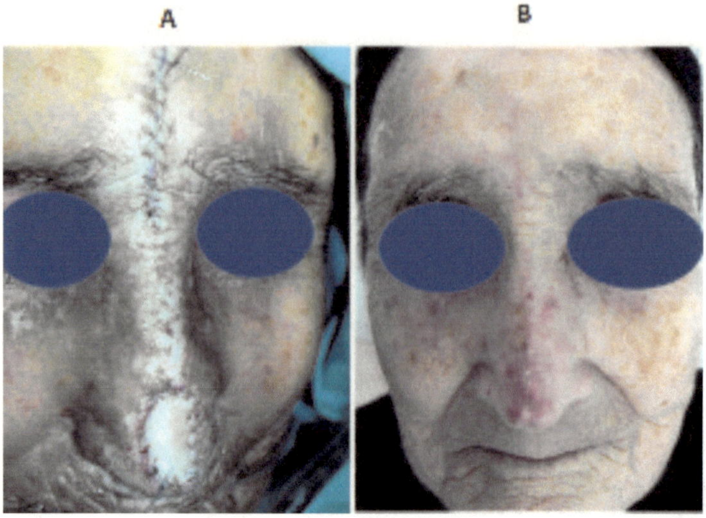

Fig. 2. Full-thickness skin graft to cover a big defect on the nasal tip. The donor site chosen was the glabella. A: In the immediately postoperative moment; B: Four month later.

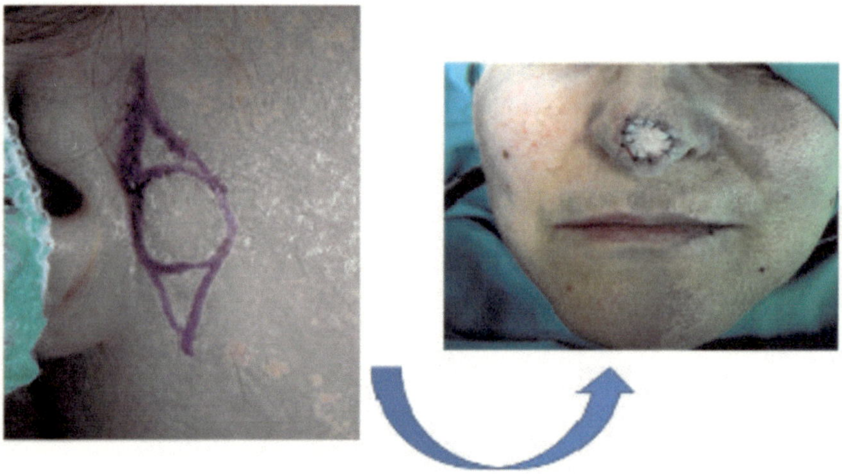

Fig. 3. Full-thickness skin graft to cover a big defect on nasal tip. The donor site in this case was the preauricular skin. A: Design of the graft at the donor area; B: Immediately postoperative moment.

After selecting the donor area, the defect is measured accurately and those measures are moved and drawn with a surgical marker on the donor skin. It is recommended that the dimensions of the graft are a 10-20% larger, to avoid obtaining a final graft too small. The split graft donor site with oval morphology, although the defect may be circular, ensures sufficient tissue for grafting. However it is preferable that the graft is well stretched, once fixed, as an excess of tissue impedes adequate diffusion of nutrients. Thus once set, the redundant tissue should be trimmed

Atraumatic handling of the skin graft should not be forgotten at any time, to avoid complications due to damage to the vascular network. Management of the graft is preferred with toothed forceps, without exerting excessive pressure, taking the ends of the ellipse, and preferably only the dermis.

Once the graft is removed, it should be quickly transferred to a sterile container with saline solution. It is important to work efficiently to prepare the graft for placement as soon as possible on its recipient bed to permit that diffusion of nutrients can begin. To facilitate this, it is recommended only essential haemostasis at the donor site. Excessive haemostasis may prevent grafted skin from adequate nourishing from the receptor bed, while inadequate haemostasis can cause bleeding and development of hematoma under the graft, creating a gap between it and the bed, leading to the same problem.

Defatting of the graft is performed effectively with scissors, preferably if they have a curved tip, even though straight scissors are also appropriate (figures 4 and 5). It is important to make this process as soon as possible to avoid the lack of perfusion of the graft over time. The shorter the time that the graft is immersed in saline, without oxygen, the greater the likelihood of success. The fat globules are removed carefully by tangential cuts with scissors. All fat should be removed, until only the dermis, with its distinctive glistening white colour, is visibly (figure 6). If this process is not properly managed, there is a greater likelihood of necrosis, as any adipose tissue acts as a barrier to the diffusion of nutrients between the recipient bed and graft dermis. If the process continues it is recommended to periodically wet the graft with saline.

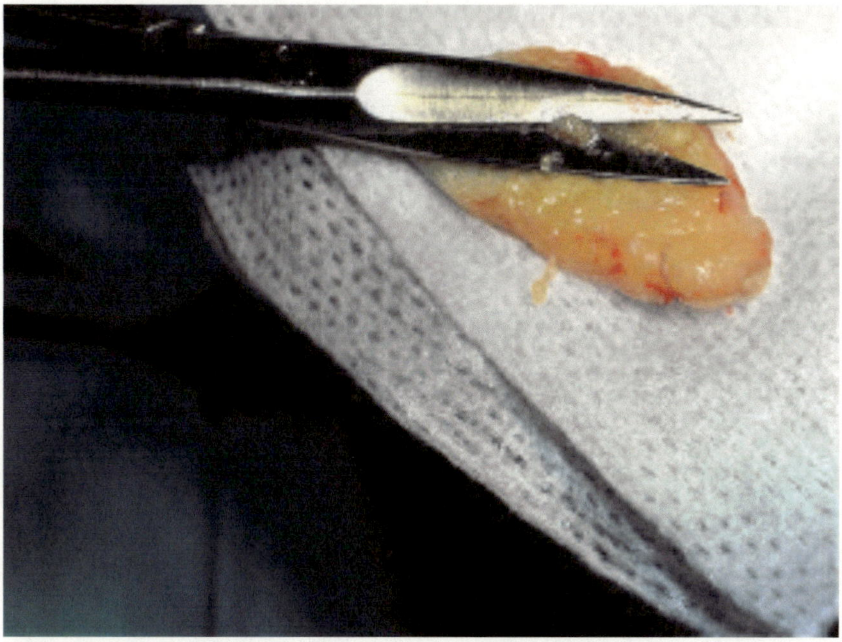

Fig. 4. Defatting of the graft performed with straight scissors.

The skin around the defect should be undermined several millimetres, before the suture of the graft, to prevent an excessive traction of the surrounding skin and a retraction of the scar. This minimizes potential postoperative pin-cushioning and allows a uniform wound contracture.

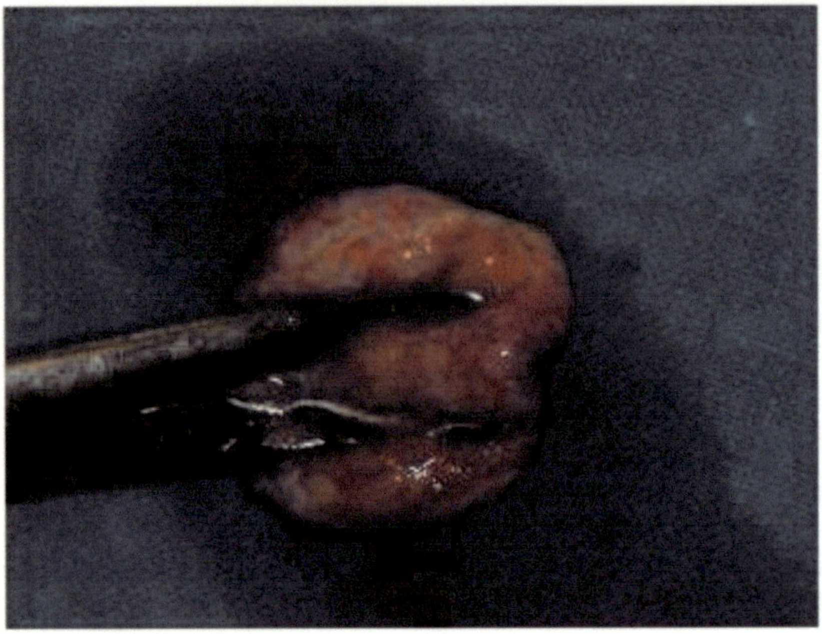

Fig. 5. Defatting of the graft performed with curved scissors.

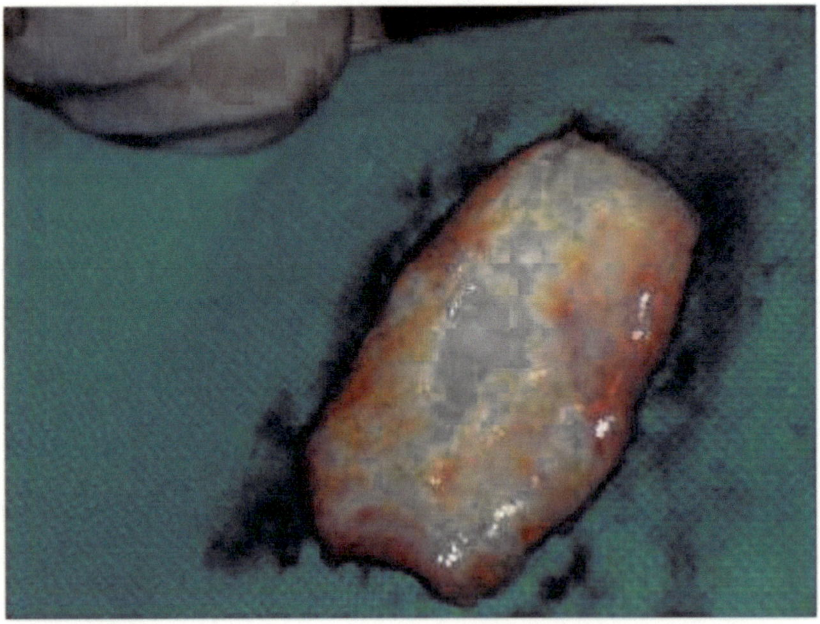

Fig. 6. Final appearance of skin graft after deffating. Notice the characteristic glistening white colour of dermis

Once the graft is ready for transfer to the receiving area, it is placed over the recipient area with the dermis side down. It is helpful to make a single central suture to fix the graft to the dermis to the recipient bed. This is done with an absorbable suture, preferably 4 / 0 thick. This promotes proper graft fixation to the recipient site with minimal risk of injury to the bed and subsequent bleeding (figure 7).

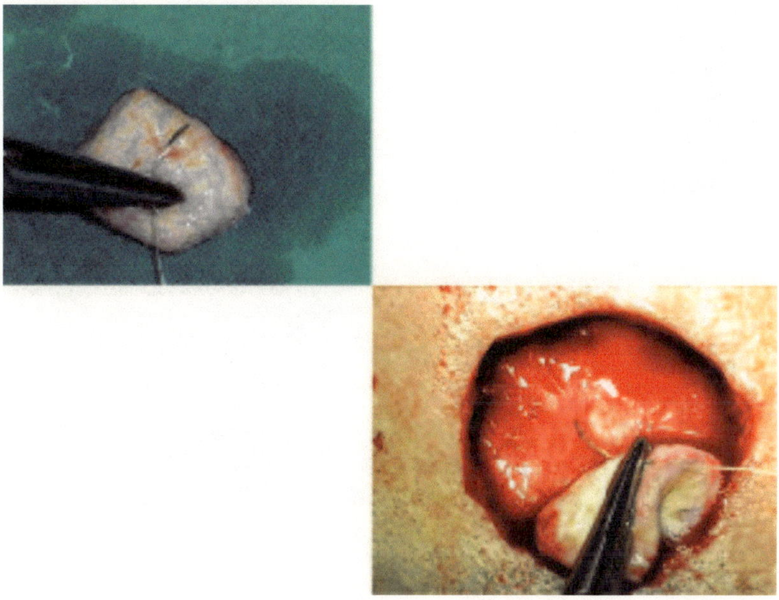

Fig. 7. Fixation of the graft to the recipient bed.

The optimal suture technique is first entering in the graft, 2-3 mm from the edge and exiting at the skin site adjacent to the defect, spacing stitches usually 4-5 mm in the adjacent recipient site skin and subsequently tied with 3–4 throws of a square knot. Simple interrupted sutures are generally used, even though a running stitch can also be used (figure 8). Simple interrupted sutures are recommended as we feel these allow for more precise apposition of the epidermal edges, although a running stitch can be used.

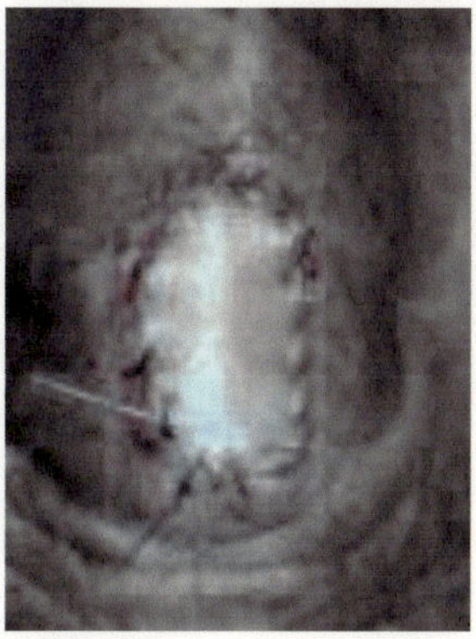

Fig. 8. Nasal graft showing a running stitch

While in other locations, tie-on bolsters remain good options to promote adherence of the graft, however, on the nose it is preferable to avoid bolsters because they are much more uncomfortable for the patient and are often not accurate (figures 9 and 10) . Hydrocolloid dressings applied directly on the graft are much more useful and provide for adequate gas exchange of grafted skin (figure 11).

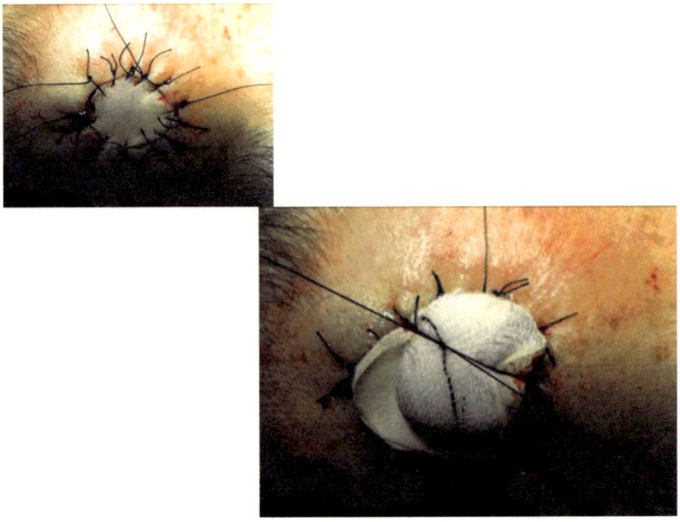

Fig. 9. Graft and tie-on bolsters.

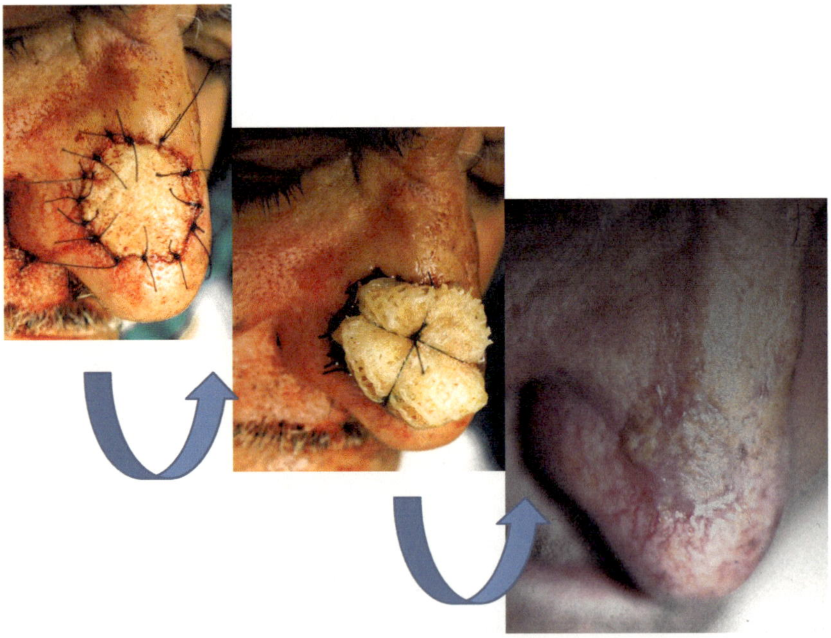

Fig. 10. Nasal graft with a tie-on bolsters. Final results five months later.

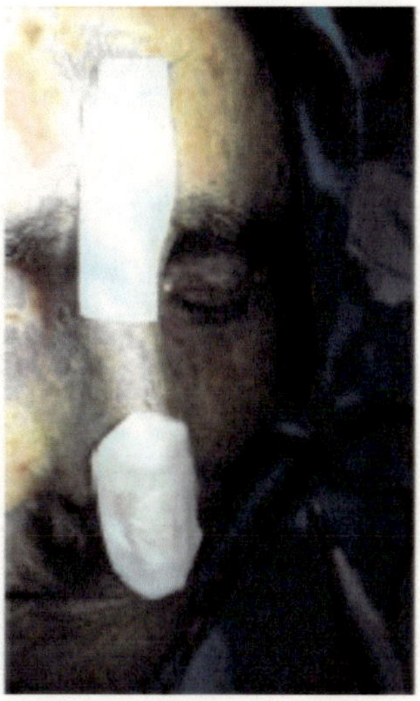

Fig. 11. Hydrocolloid dressings applied directly on the graft and donor area.

We usually use a thin layer of topical antibiotic, fusidic acid mainly on the graft, which is then covered with a hydrocolloid dressing (figure 11). A pressure dressing is then placed and remains in place for 48 hours, repeating the same process again, until the graft has ignited and can be left uncovered.

Finally the closure of the donor area is performed. In the case of nasal grafts, as previously mentioned, the skin will proceed, in most cases, from the glabellar or the preauricular regions, and in some cases from the clavicular region. In the case of the glabellar region, the closure is performed in vertical, perpendicular to the natural lines of the skin, but as it will not alter facial symmetry, aesthetic results tend to be acceptably good. In the other two cases it is easier to guide the scars parallel to the lines of relaxed skin tension, and hide the scars better (figures 12 and 13).

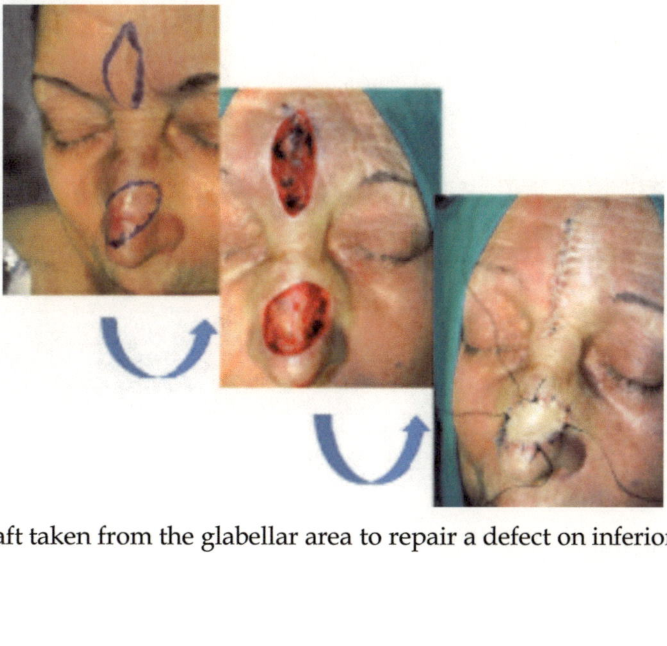

Fig. 12. Nasal graft taken from the glabellar area to repair a defect on inferior nasal dorsum.

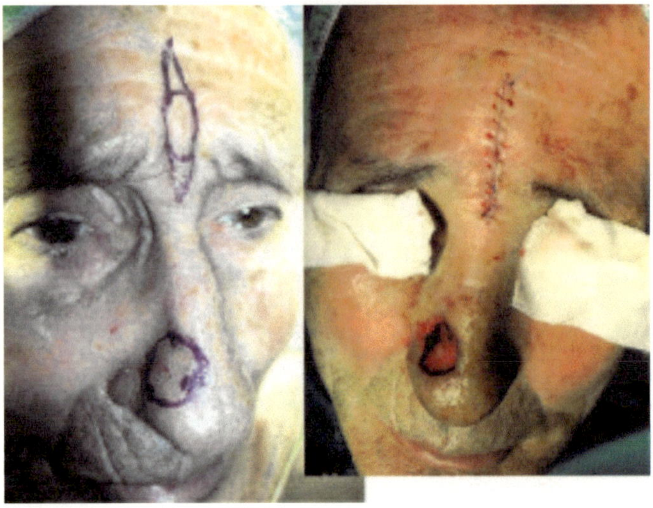

Fig. 13. Nasal graft taken from the glabellar area to repair a defect on alar region.

2.2 Burow's grafts to repair nasal defects

Burow grafting is obtained from the skin adjacent to the defect and allows primary closure of a unit and second unit grafting, using skin with similar cosmetic characteristics.. They are primarily used in the reconstruction of large defects of the nasal dorsum, making the design of Burow's graft in the glabellar region. This will make direct closure of the glabellar region, suturing the graft inferiorly (figures 14-16).

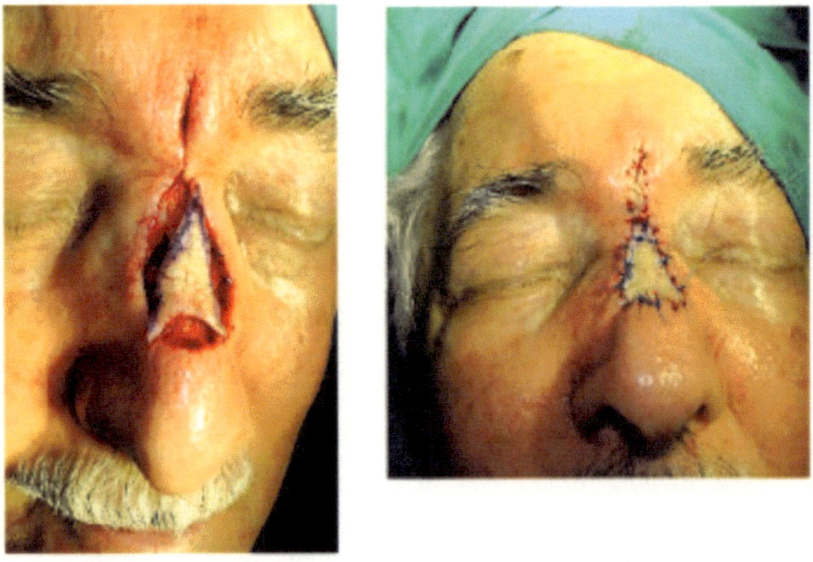

Fig. 14. Burow´s graft from glabellar skin to repair a defect on the upper nasal dorsum.

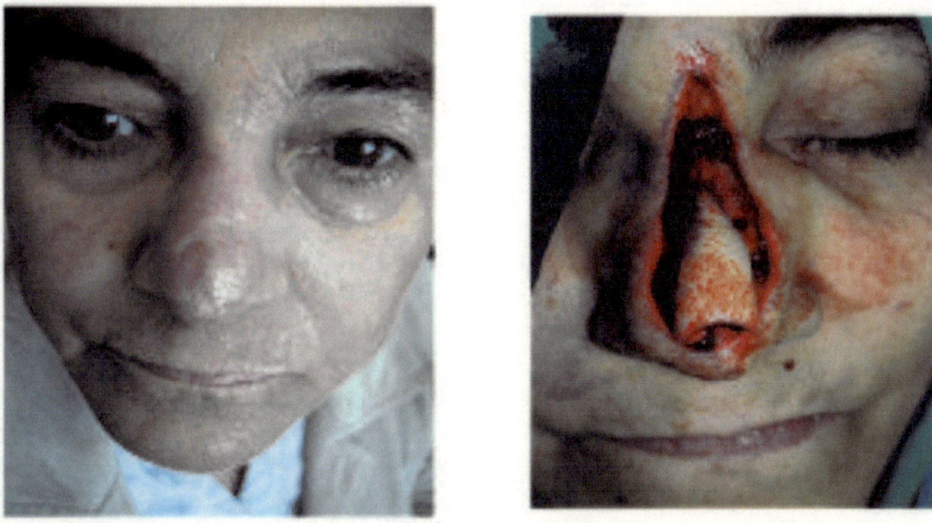

Fig. 15. Burow´s graft from glabellar skin to repair a defect on the nasal dorsum and tip.

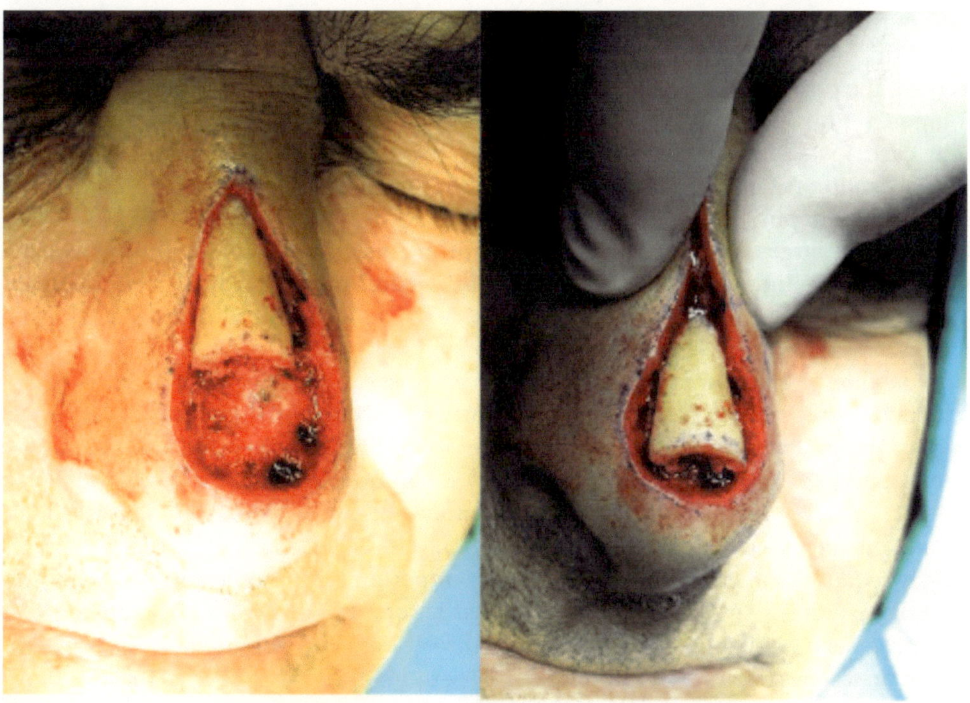

Fig. 16. Burow´s graf from nasal dorsum to repair a defect on the nasal tip.

2.3 Partial thickness skin grafts on the nose

Partial thickness skin grafts contain full thickness epidermis and a variable amount, usually limited of dermis and often lack adnexal structures. Partial thickness skin grafts are further classified by total thickness in millimeters, depending on the amount of dermis included in the graft. The subdivisions are thin (from 0.125 to 0.275 mm), medium (0.275 to 0.4 mm) and thick (0.40 to 0.75 mm). The majority of graft harvest for use in the region of the head and neck are usually 0.3-0.4 mm thick. The main advantages of such grafts include the ability to cover very large defects and the increased likelihood of graft survival, since they need less nutritional intake. In addition, these grafts are thinner and allow earlier detection of tumor recurrence in cutaneous oncology field. The main disadvantages include a less aesthetically desirable colour and texture match with surrounding skin and the need for specialized equipment. The degree of contraction is greater with partial thickness skin grafts than with FTSGs and creates significant granulation that requires more postoperative care.

2.4 Composed and cartilage grafts

The cartilage contributes significantly to the maintenance of the anatomical structure and function of the nose. Sometimes a significant amount of tissue and cartilage support to the nose is removed with oncological surgery, resulting in both structural and functional deficits that require reconstruction. Functional iatrogenic nasal obstruction is a particular risk when working in the wing and supra-alar crease, where the nasal valve is located. In most situations where the loss of cartilage results in a functional deficit, the cartilage must be replaced in order to facilitate the permeability of the nostrils. One method of restoring the lost structure is to use a composite graft or a free cartilage grafts and subsequently cover this with a skin graft, either the same day or several weeks later. If the perichondrium is preserved, the probability of survival of the cartilage will be higher.

A composite graft is a modified graft that contains more than one component of tissue, usually cartilage. However, the survival of composite grafts is dimmer than FTSGs. FTSGs revascularization occurs from vessels throughout the base and edges of the graft, whereas grafts composed only get their new blood supply from the subdermal plexus of the wound and the edges of the graft. Because of problems with vascularization, the size of a composite graft is limited to a maximum graft diameter ranging from 1-2 cm to minimize the risk of necrosis. In the nose, the rich vascular network quite compensates existing problems.

The probability of graft survival can be improved further by improving the basis on which the composite graft will be placed. A hinged flap on the base of the wound may increase the contact of the graft vessel with a suitable base. In addition, the wound can be allowed to heal for a period of several weeks by secondary intention. Particular attention must be paid to this fact, as an excessive contraction may imply functional problems. This is especially important in the nasal valve, so in this location, close monitoring during this phase of healing is required. Patient selection is also very important. We should proceed with caution in elderly patients, smokers, and those with conditions known to cause vascular compromise such as diabetes, vaso-occlusive disease, and prior ioninzing radiation in the receiving area. These conditions can affect the peripheral blood flow and thereby decrease graft survival.

The use of composite grafts is the most commonly used graft in dermatologic surgery to repair defects of the nasal ala, sidewall, and the columella. Alar cartilage loss can lead to nasal valve incompetence and decreased stability of the wing so that during inspiration, nasal tissue is drawn into the nasal septum, resulting in decreased air flow and functional compromise. The cartilage is used as part of the graft to restore the structural integrity of the

wing and maintain the smooth functioning of the prevention of alar collapse during inspiration.
The crus of the helix is most commonly employed, although the helical rim, tragus, antitragus and concha can also be utilized. These areas of the ear has the most of the tissues of the nasal ala, the cartilage is thin and flexible, relatively thin overlying skin and subcutaneous tissue. For areas in the highly sebaceous distal nose are in favor of free cartilage grafts harvested from the ear, but without the skin attached to allow the tissue even better game so superficial, either from another instead of the nose or skin perinasal as a bilobed or nasolabial flap, or in the form of a skin graft melolabial. The shell is most commonly used for reconstruction of lateral nasal wall or nasal columella and large alar defects. The helical crus has the additional advantage of being thicker with a sebaceous texture and a composite graft works well for deeper defects sebaceous, making the nose look more true . (Table1)

NASAL DEFECT LOCATION	FULL-THICKNESS SKIN GRAFT DONOR SITE	CARTILAGE DONOR SITE
Tip, ala/alar rim, alar groove	Preauricular cheek, conchal bowl, melolabial fold, postauricular sulcus, supraclavicular area for larger defects	Conchal bowl, antihelix
Columella	Same locations as other nasal areas	Helical rim, crus, or antihelix

Table 1. Recommended donor sites for full-thickness skin grafts depending on the location of the nasal defect.

3. Conclusion

Nasal defects are a common challenge in daily practice. A multitude of benign and malignant lesions are located in the nasal region. Basal cell carcinoma is the most common skin cancer and is found frequently in this anatomical region. The size of defects secondary to excision of these lesions may not allow primary closure or reconstruction using skin flaps and requires the use of skin grafts. Skin grafts are particularly suitable for large defects occupying almost an entire cosmetic unit and, especially in elderly patients, produce acceptable cosmetic results in many cases.
Full-thickness skin grafts contain the entire epidermis and dermis and preserve adnexal structures, so they are very useful in the reconstruction of these nasal defects. The appropriate choice of donor skin is essential to achieve a cosmetically acceptable result and depends on the nasal cosmetic unit in which the defect is located and on the particular characteristics of the patient's skin. The location of donor skin most commonly used are the glabella and preauricular region, as well as the skin adjacent to the defect that can be obtained by Burow´s technique.

Regarding technical aspects we recommend an adequate fixation of the graft to recipient site with a point made with an absorbable suture. Hydrocolloid dressings placed over the graft are particularly suitable in the first days after surgery as they allow an adequate gas exchange and collaborate in the establishment of the graft to recipient site.
In some cases complex reconstructions are need for big defects affecting the majority of the nasal skin, and skin grafts are always a good option alone or helped by skin flaps (figure 17).

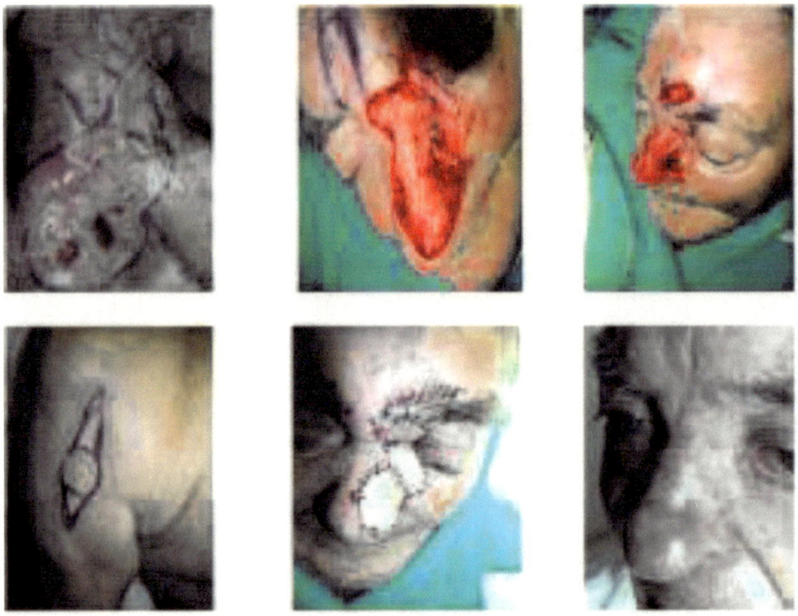

Fig. 17. Basal cell carcinoma affecting the left half of the nose. We repair the defect a rotation flap from glabella and two skin grafts, from the right arm.

4. References

Adams DC, Ramsey ML: Grafts in dermatologic surgery: review and update on full- and split-thickness skin grafts, free cartilage grafts, and composite grafts. Dermatol Surg 2005; 31:1055-1067.
Aden KK, Biel MA: The evaluation of pharmacologic agents on composite graft survival. Arch Otolaryngol Head Neck Surg 1992; 118:175-178.
Adnot J, Salasche SJ: Visualized basting sutures in the application of full-thickness skin grafts. J Dermatol Surg Oncol 1987; 13:1236-1239.
Alcalay J: Cutaneous surgery in patients receiving warfarin therapy. Dermatol Surg 2001; 27:756-758.
Arpey CJ, Whitaker DC, O'Donnell MJ: Skin grafting. New York, McGraw-Hill, 1997.
Arpey CJ, Whitaker DC: Postsurgical wound management. Dermatol Clin 2001; 19:787-797.
Behroozan DS, Goldberg LH: Combined linear closure and Burow's graft for a dorsal nasal defect. Dermatol Surg 2006; 32:107-111.
Bello YM, Falabella AF: Use of skin substitutes in dermatology. Dermatol Clin 2001; 19:555-561.

Bennett JE, Miller SR: Evolution of the electro-dermatome. Plast Reconstr Surg 1970; 45:131-134.

Bumsted RM, Panje WR, Ceilley RI: Delayed skin grafting in facial reconstruction. When to use and how to do. Arch Otolaryngol 1983; 109:178-184.

Burget GC, Menick FJ: The use of composite auricular grafts. Aesthetic reconstruction of the nose. St Louis: Mosby 1994.212-225.

Chester Jr EC: Surgical gem. The use of dog-ears as grafts. J Dermatol Surg Oncol 1981; 7:956-959.

Davenport M, Daly J, Harvey I, et al: The bolus tie-over 'pressure' dressing in the management of full thickness skin grafts. Is it necessary?. Br J Plast Surg 1988; 41:18-32.

Davis DA, Arpey CJ: Porcine heterografts in dermatologic surgery and reconstruction. Dermatol Surg 2000; 26:76-80.

Falabella AF, Valencia IC, Eaglstein WH, et al: Tissue-engineered skin (Apligraf) in the healing of patients with epidermolysis bullosa wounds. Arch Dermatol 2000; 136:1225-1230.

Hirase Y: Postoperative cooling enhances composite graft survival in nasal-alar and fingertip reconstruction. Br J Plast Surg 1993; 46:707-711.

Keck T, Lindemann J, Kühnemann S, et al: Healing of composite chondrocutaneous auricular grafts covered by skin flaps in nasal reconstructive surgery. Laryngoscope 2003; 113:248-253.

Kent DE: Full-thickness skin grafts. New York, McGraw-Hill, 1996.

Kim KH, Gross VL, Jaffe AT, et al: The use of the melolabial Burow's graft in the reconstruction of combination nasal sidewall–cheek defects. Dermatol Surg 2004; 30:205-207.

Kuijpers DI, Smeets MW, Lapière K, et al: Do systemic antibiotics increase the survival of a full thickness graft on the nose?. J Eur Acad Dermatol Venereol 2006; 20:1296-1301.

Kumar P: Classification of skin substitutes. Burns 2008; 34:148-149.

Langtry JA, Kirkham P, Martin IC, et al: Tie-over bolster dressings may not be necessary to secure small full thickness skin grafts. Dermatol Surg 1998; 24:1350-1353.

Lee KK, Mehrany K, Swanson NA: Fusiform elliptical Burow's graft: a simple and practical esthetic approach for nasal tip reconstruction. Dermatol Surg 2006; 32:91-95.

Maves MD, Yessenow RS: The use of composite auricular grafts in nasal reconstruction. J Dermatol Surg Oncol 1988; 14:994-999.

McClane S, Renner G, Bell PL, et al: Pilot study to evaluate the efficacy of hyperbaric oxygen therapy in improving the survival of reattached auricular composite grafts in the New Zealand White rabbit. Otolaryngol Head Neck Surg 2000; 123:539-542.

McLaughlin CR: Composite ear grafts and their blood supply. Br J Plast Surg 1954; 7:274-278.

Papel ID: Facial plastic and reconstructive surgery. 2nd edn. New York, Thieme, 2002.

Park SS: Facial plastic surgery: the essential guide. New York, Thieme, 2005.

Raghavan U, Jones NS: Use of the auricular composite graft in nasal reconstruction. J Laryngol Otol 2001; 115:885-893.

Ratner D, Katz A, Grande DJ: An interlocking auricular composite graft. Dermatol Surg 1995; 21:789-792.

Rigg BM: Importance of donor site selection in skin grafting. Can Med Assoc J 1977; 117:1028-1029.

Rue III LW, Cioffi WG, McManus WF, et al: Wound closure and outcome in extensively burned patients treated with cultured autologous keratinocytes. J Trauma 1993; 34:662-667.

Salasche SJ, Winton GB: Clinical evaluation of a nonadhering wound dressing. J Dermatol Surg Oncol 1986; 12:1220-1222.

Snow SN, Stiff M, Lambert D, et al: Freehand technique to harvest partial-thickness skin to repair superficial facial defects. Dermatol Surg 1995; 21:153-157.

Wright TI, Baddour LM, Berbari EF, et al: Antibiotic prophylaxis in dermatologic surgery: advisory statement 2008. J Am Acad Dermatol 2008; 59:464-473.

10

Surgical Treatment of Post-Burn Trophic Ulcers and Cicatrices of the Foot Calcaneal Area

Babur M. Shakirov
Samarkand State Medical Institute,
Burn department of RSCUMA,
Inter-regional Burn Center, Samarkand
Uzbekistan

1. Introduction

The term 'plantar' ulcer was introduced by Price in 1959 and was defined as a chronic ulceration of the anaesthetic sole of the foot, situated in well-defined areas overlying bony prominences, resistant to local or systemic therapy and characterized by a marked tendency to recurrence.

First time Grabb & Argenta (1981) offered the graft, with blood supply from the artery malleolaris anterior that makes it possible to close the affected zone with limited lesions. Some authors prefer Blair-Brown grafts (Vihriev & Belonogov, 1978).

Initially, Elshahy (1978) had used the local skin and fatty graft, prepared on the lateral or medial surface of ankle joint. According to Amarante et al. (1986), good results were achieved with plasty of defects in the area of the Achilles tendon and with skin-fascial graft on the distal base from medial surface in malleolus.

Shakirov et al., (2009) offered the L-form skin and fatty graft in the case of trophic ulcers in the post-burn wounds of this calcaneal area.

The feature of the clinical course of so - called sandal burns that occurred in the past in some in mountain areas of Middle Asia, where primitive heating devices -sandals, were used, is noteworthy (Shakirov, 2004). Sandal burns are characterized by such severe deep injuries because of a close contact plantar of the foot with ash of coals or woods and include not only skin injuries of various depths but also injuries to underlying tissues: subcutaneous fat, fascia, muscles, and even bones (Shakirov & Tursunov, 2005).

The burn trauma of the posterior surface of talus area and ankle joint with the following formation of cicatrix is often complicated by unhealing trophic ulcer.

Ulcerous cicatrices located in the Achilles tendon zone are constantly traumatised on walking with shoes on, because the area of the tendon adjoining the talus on the surface of the support. As a result, ulcers gradually increase and cicatrices become rough and deep. The wound fundus gets a grey staining and the margins become dense without granulation and with signs of epithelisation. In spite of a large number of methods used, the problem of elimination of extensive defects in a zone of the Achilles tendon is not solved to the end. The study of features of skin structure, blood supply and innervations' of the talus area showed

that soft tissues, located in the area of external talus and lateral surface, are good plastic surgery materials for tendon covering.
The donor area from where the skin and fatty graft had been taken had the following features: first, the skin in the talus area was rather thick and rough, stable to traumatisation with shoes and easily shifted with marked subcutaneous fat layer so it can be taken in a fold; second, it has a good arterial blood supply as there is an artery fubularis behind the donor site and the peripheral ramus of the same artery in front of the donor site that form the vascular network Barsley et. al.,(1983), Holmes et.al. (1984) and third, the area of external talus has axial innervations provided by the sural nerve. The sural nerve passes in the anterior area of the talus. Enumerated anatomical features of blood-supply structure and innervations make the area of lateral talus and foot rather valuable as the donor area for preparation of skin-fatty graft and re-animation of normal-covering tissues above the Achilles tendon and posterior surface of calcaneus.

2. Material and methods

A total of 12 patients (7 men and 5 women, aged 9 to 54 years) have been on under the author's observation at Samarkand Burn Centre, Uzbekistan, for prolonged unhealing ulcers and cicatrices located in the Achilles tendon zone (Table 1). The causes of the trophic ulcers included sandal burns (10 patients), sulphuric acid burns (1 patient), and electro-trauma burns (1 patients). Would assume one since you had 12 total. Ulcers sizes were from 1,0-3,5 to 4-5 sm. in diameter. All patients had undergone operation before (2 - 4 times). The donor area, from where the skin and fatty graft had been taken from, had the following features.

Causes of burns	males		females	
	Quantity	%	Quantity	%
Sandal burns	5	41,7	5	41,7
Sulfuric acid burns	1	8,3	-	-
electro burn	1	8,3	-	-

Table 1.

2.1 The operation technique

After cicatrices dissection, a deep wound measuring 5-11 cm in length was formed. For orientation, we divided the posterior surface of the calcaneal tendon area into three parts: calcaneal, ankle and supramalleolaris areas (Figure 1).
Large wound surfaces can be closed by L-form graft. Posterior crural surface above the Achilles tendon is its base between the distal and middle-third of the leg. The graft is directed lateral and forwards, its posterior border is the margin of cicatrices and its anterior side is about 2 cm farther from the talus apex. Then the graft passes through the lateral surface of the foot at an angle of about 90 along the foot margin. The width of the graft is 5-6 cm and the length is 18-20cm. Of these, the vertical part is 13-14 cm and the horizontal part is 5- 6 sm.

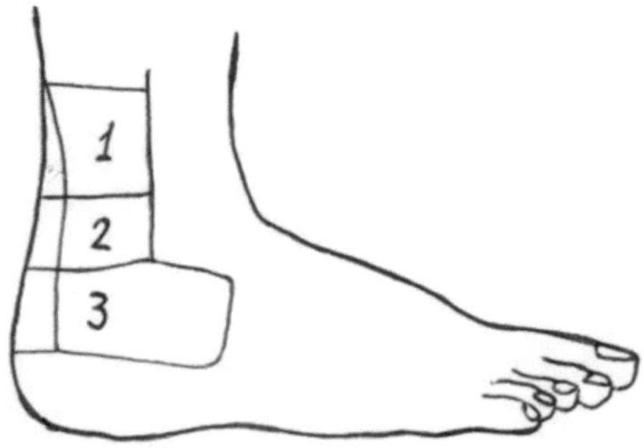

Fig. 1. Division of Achilles tendon into calcaneal, ankle, supramalleolaris areas

The correlation of parts is 3.1, 2.1 and 1.1. Based on the spread of the tissue defect, the graft is planned with a surplus length of 4-5 cm as the graft contracts after mobilisation and when it covers the calcaneal tendon and the calcaneus are fixed on the condition of some extension of width on account of length.

The graft mobilization starts from its apex, penetrating at once to the fascia and covering the muscles by means of the incision and strictly along the fascia from which the graft was raised up to superior distal third of the ankle joint. With this, the terminal branches of artery fibular is intersected and the other branches that penetrated into the graft on the foot from the side of the planta in the zone of the ankle joint, which is higher from the side of the tendon of long fibular muscle, where their number is less than on the foot, the graft was mobilized to be placed above the Achilles tendon. Graft sensitivity is provided by the calf nerve, rete venosum plantare, and arterial blood supply is collateral due to a thick network making up the base of the graft through the long post-fibular muscle, moving away from artery tibialis anterior and also along the anterior border of the pointed muscle, a little more distal to the artery tibialis branch. Depending on the area and localisation of the defects, cicatrices and ulcers, the L-form graft was placed on the wound surface either longitudinally or at an angle when its vertical part, lying across, closed the wound distal zone. The medial margin and the end of the graft were connected with the proper wound margin by one or two rows of sutures, and by means of the lateral margin of the graft, the lateral surface of the Achilles tendon was closed and was fixed by catgut sutures to the fascia through the sub dermal layer. The donor wound was closed with a split thickness skin graft and compression bandage was applied with fixed using stretched sutures.

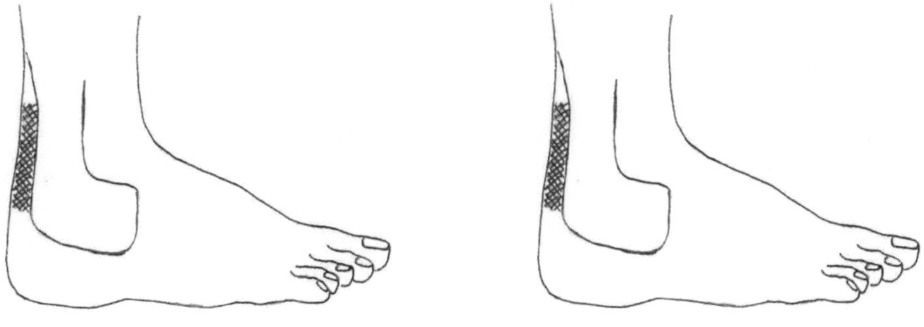

Fig. 2. Ulcerating cicatrix in the area of the Achilles tendon zone. The borders of the L-form skin fascial graft have been pointed out.

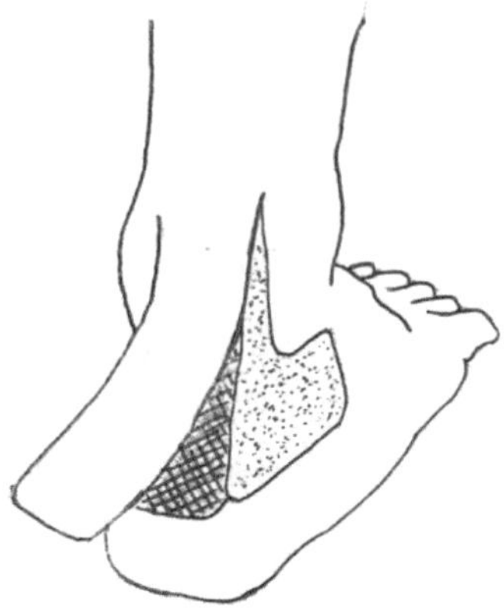

Fig. 3. L-form skin- fascial graft from the inferior third of the crus and foot has been mobilized.

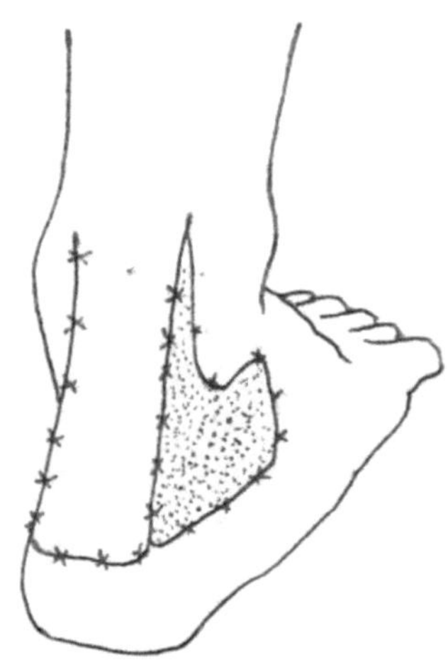

Fig. 4. After ulcerating cicatrices dissection the wound was covered by mobilized skin-fascial graft

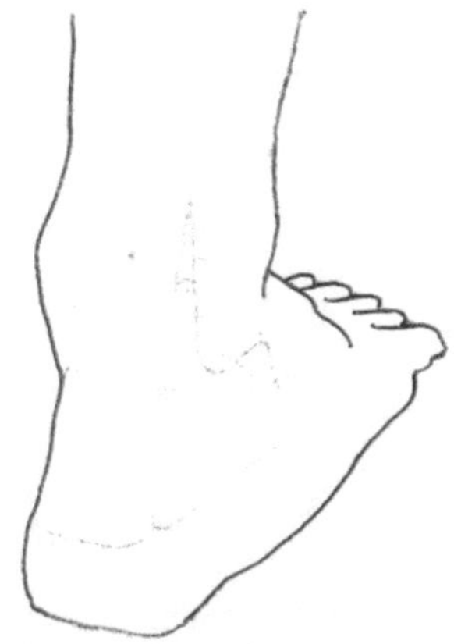

Fig. 5. The result of the Achilles tendon plastics by means of L-form skin-fascial graft.

Patient A., aged 15, was hospitalized with complaints of chronic unhealing wound in the calcaneal area of the left foot. It was determined, from the patient's self-report, that he had received a sandal burn 4 years ago during an epileptic attack. He was treated at Burn Centre. At 3 months after healing, trophic ulcer had developed. The size of the ulcer increased gradually. So the patient was operated on in the Burn Centre for unhealing trophic ulcers, where free-skin transplantation was performed. However, trophic ulcer recurred, and the patient was re-admitted to the Burn Centre. During medical examination of the calcaneal area of the left foot, a post-burn unhealing trophic ulcer (2,0- 2.5 cm in diameter) was revealed.

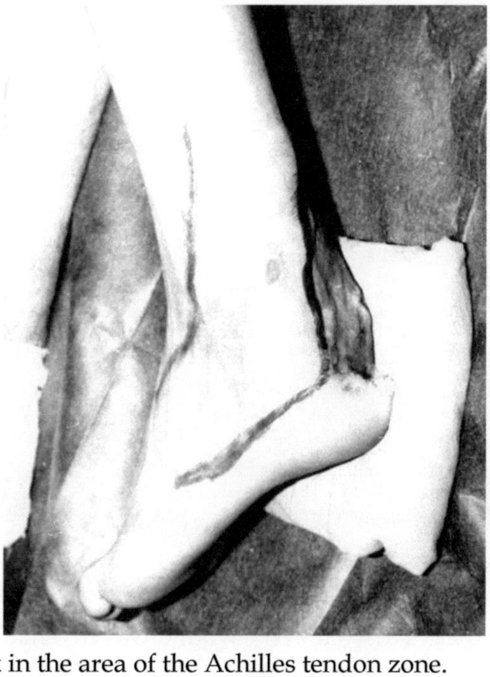

Fig. 6. Ulcerating cicatrix in the area of the Achilles tendon zone.

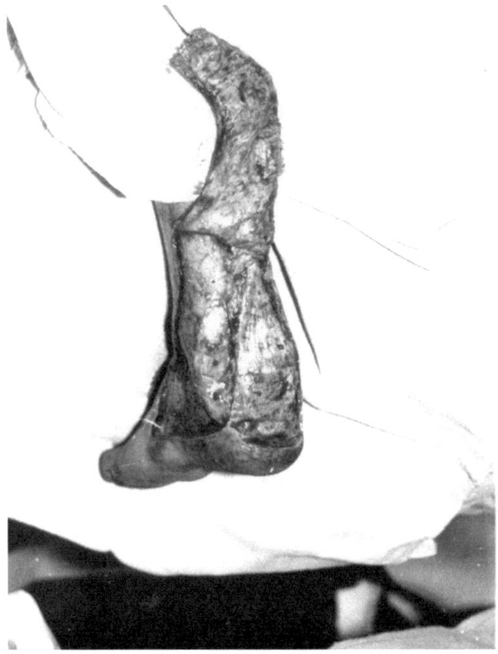

Fig. 7. L-form skin- fascial graft from the inferior third of the crus and foot has been mobilized.

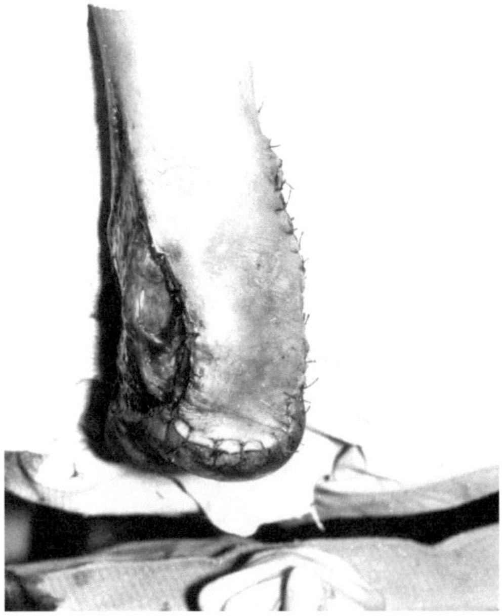

Fig. 8. After ulcerating cicatrices dissection the wound was covered by mobilized skin-fascial graft

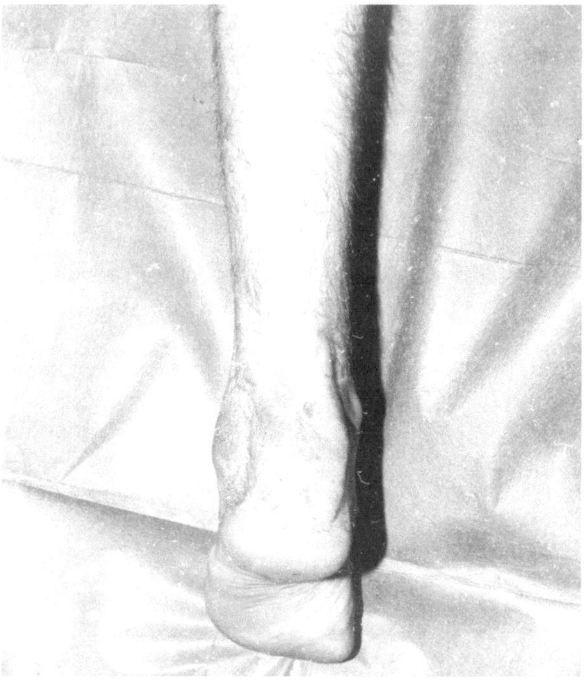

Fig. 9. Result

3. Results

We observed a good result with no complications. The grafts were viable, sensibility was preserved and no marginal necrosis was noticed. Gradually the operation efficacy improved as the cicatrices became softer, and the fossa behind the external talus (donor site) healed. A marginal necrosis was noted on the part of external talus adjoining the ulcer because of the tissue changes only one patient. The necrotized area was removed and the wound was closed by split skin without influencing the good result of the operation.

4. Conclusion

Trophic ulcer is common complication seen in (describe patient population here again) patients and all treatment modalites have significant recurrence rates. In spite of a large number of treatment methods used, the problem of elimination of defects in the area of Achilles tendon has not been solved. As a rule, it is impossible to eliminate them by means of local tissues plasty. Some authors prefer Blair-Brown graft plasty does not ensure good functional and cosmetic results, because the transplanted graft is thin, without tactile or pain sensitivity.

It often undergoes cicatrix formation with trophic ulcer recurrence. Employing plastic surgery in the area of the Achilles tendon, the use of distant-area tissues presents a good effect by means of Italian plastics (crus of the other leg or buttocks) as well as the Filatov's stem; however, these methods are concerned with the inconveniences of the forced position, have many stages and displaced, denervated tissues and have blood supply for the account of traumatic zone.

In L-form skin-fatty graft, produced grafts that were viable and preserved sensibility and saves displacement from mechanical trauma in the natural way. The patients may resume their work in 1.5 months after the operation. However, complete graft adaptation and acclimatization to the place of graft occurs in 2-3 months. During this period, patient must not wear common shoes that press onto the graft.

5. Acknowledgement

We thank K.R. Tagaev for support of this work, Lidia Arkadevna, Nela Ahmedganovna, May Anatollevna and Vladimir Tsibulsky for correcting the English of this manuscript.

6. References

Amarante J, Costa H, Reis J, et al. New distally based fasciocutaneous flap of the leg. Br J Plast Surg 1986; 39:338-40.

Barsley TL, Sharp DT, Chischolm EM. Cross-leg fasciocutaneousm flaps. Plast Reconstruct Surg. 1983; 72:843-52.

Elshahy N.J. The usage of graft on 2 cuttings for the ulcers closing not bearius the load in the area of heel. Acta Chir Plast 1978; 20:30-6.

Grabb W.C, Argenta LC Ibid. 1981. 68. pp. 723-730.

Holmes J, Rauner CR. Lateral calcaneal Artery Island flaps. Br J. Plast Surg 1984; 37:402-5.

Price E.W. 1964. The problem of plantar ulcer. Lepr Rev. 1964; 35:267–72.

Shakirov B.M. Sandal Burns and their Treatment in Children // J. Burn Care Rehabilitation. 2004; 25; 501-505.

Shakirov B.M., K.R Tagaev, B.S. Tursunov, D.A. Achtamov. L- form plastic in the treatment of post-burn trophic ulcers and cicatrices of the foot calcaneal area. J. Plastic, Reconstructive Aesthetic Surgery (2009) 62, e 59-63.

Shakirov B.M., Tursunov B.S. Treatment of severe foot burns in children // J. Burns, 2005; Vol.31, №7: 901-905.

Vihriev B.C, Belonogov LI. Plastic's skin-grafts wound of defects. Herald of surgery; 1984: 89-91.

11

Preputial Skin Grafts

Ahmet Bulent Dogrul[1] and Kaya Yorganci[2]
[1]*Mus State Hospital, Clinic of General Surgery, MUS*
[2]*Hacettepe University Medical School, Department of General Surgery, Ankara*
Turkey

1. Introduction

Although skin grafting originated 2500 to 3000 years ago, it was until the 19 th century that this technique was again introduced as a reconstructive option. While 19th century surgeons used grafts to repair their most difficult cases, skin grafting has since evolved into a modality that is routinely and sometimes preferentially used for the surgical repair of skin defects [1].

In this chapter we will discuss a relatively new type of full thickness skin graft: Preputial skin graft (PSG); regarding its indications, advantages, disadvantages and the valid reasons for the choice of PSG instead of classical full thickness skin graft (FTSG) donor sites for grafting of small defects especially in burned patients.

2. Full thickness skin grafts

A graft is the simplest way to cover superficial skin loss. It consists of the transfer of a section of skin, of variable thickness and size, which is completely detached from its original site and moved to cover the zone to be repaired [2].

Skin grafts can be divided into four types : full thickness grafts, split thickness grafts (STG), composite grafts and cartilage grafts [3]. According to the thickness of the explants, skin grafts are classified as split thickness and full thickness. STGs are further divided into thin (0.15-0.3 mm), intermediate (0.3-0.45 mm and thick (0.45-0.6 mm). FTSGs are usually thicker than 0.6 mm [1, 2].

The outcome of skin grafts can depend on their thickness. An explant usually takes if it is split thickness, that is includes the epidermis and a small portion of the dermis. If the explant is full thickness, that is, consisting of the entire thickness of epidermis and dermis, it only takes if it is relatively small, so that it can be nourished by peripheral, probably lymphatic, imbibitions [2].

Because of poor acceptance of the resulting scars, STGs are usually reserved for deep and full thickness dermal burns, extensive skin losses in areas other than the face, and where the recipient bed is poorly vascularized, full thickness skin grafts, used to cover small areas, provide solid and fairly elastic material, producing satisfactory scarring results not subject to retraction. They are particularly useful for repair of skin losses on the face and fingers, as an alternative to local flaps [1-4].

Full thickness skin grafts are composed of epidermis and the full thickness of dermis, including adnexial structures such as hair follicles and sweat glands. Full thickness skin grafts are most commonly used to repair defects in face and fingers as an alternative to local flaps. FTSGs can provide excellent color, texture and thickness matches for facial defects, and may be especially useful for the repair of defects of the nasal tip, dorsum, ala, and side wall as well as the lower eyelid and ear [1-3].
Selection of a donor site for a FTSG depends on the color, texture, thickness and sebaceous qualities of the skin surrounding the defect [1, 3]. Most FTSGs are taken above the shoulders, whose color, vascular pattern, texture, thickness and density and distribution of adnexial structures best match the tissue surrounding facial defects [1].
The most frequently used grafts, especially for the dermocosmetic purposes, are thick or intermediate split thickness grafts for the repair of areas greater than 3 cm diameter and full thickness grafts for the repair of smaller areas [1].

3. Preputial skin grafts

In last decade, an extraordinary type of FTSG; PSG has been used as an alternative graft source and has promising results. The use of PSG is not a new idea. Its usage is well described in hypospadias surgery till now [5]. In last two decades choice of PSG as a graft source has been reported for many clinical conditions such as burn, release of contractures, syndactly repair, eyelid and anal canal reconstruction, intraoral burn reconstruction, closure of defects after nevus excision and penile skin defect repair [6-12]. Most of these reports are single case reports. Its usage in burned patients is described in literature in relatively larger series of patients [13-15]. But PSG is still not used as a routine full thickness graft side among surgeons [13, 14].
Modern treatment of deep partial-thickness and full-thickness burns are operative debridement with subsequent skin graft coverage. Currently, nearly 95 % success rate is the standard of care for skin grafting. For this success, adequate wound bed preparation, careful selection of donor sites, and appropriate perioperative care are critical. From these factors, careful selection of donor sites is important as donor site problems may occur.
In patients with extensive burns, all unburned areas can be used as donor sites. However, in small burns, selection of donor site can be problematic. Since all donor sites scar to some degree, it is advised to take skin from an area that will be otherwise hidden under most circumstances [16].
Preputial skin graft is a full thickness and expandable graft that can be easily harvested and used [13]. The prepuce is very thin, pliable skin. Its major advantages are its relatively large size and, as a full thickness graft, its very low tendency to contract [14]. Also, like the split thickness graft, it has high viability. A thinning procedure, which is required for the harvest of other donor sites, is not required. Additional advantages of PSG are; they do not need donor site care, do not causes scar, donor site is hidden and can be harvested with simple surgical instruments. In small burns, it has the advantage of not to disrupt any healthy skin area for graft harvesting [13, 14] (Figure 1).
In one series of the patients of which all were burned children, PSG has been used liberally. In this report all of the patients were burned children with an average age of 3,6. Preputial skin graft was the only donor site for 25% of patients and average size of PSG was 6 x 4 cm.

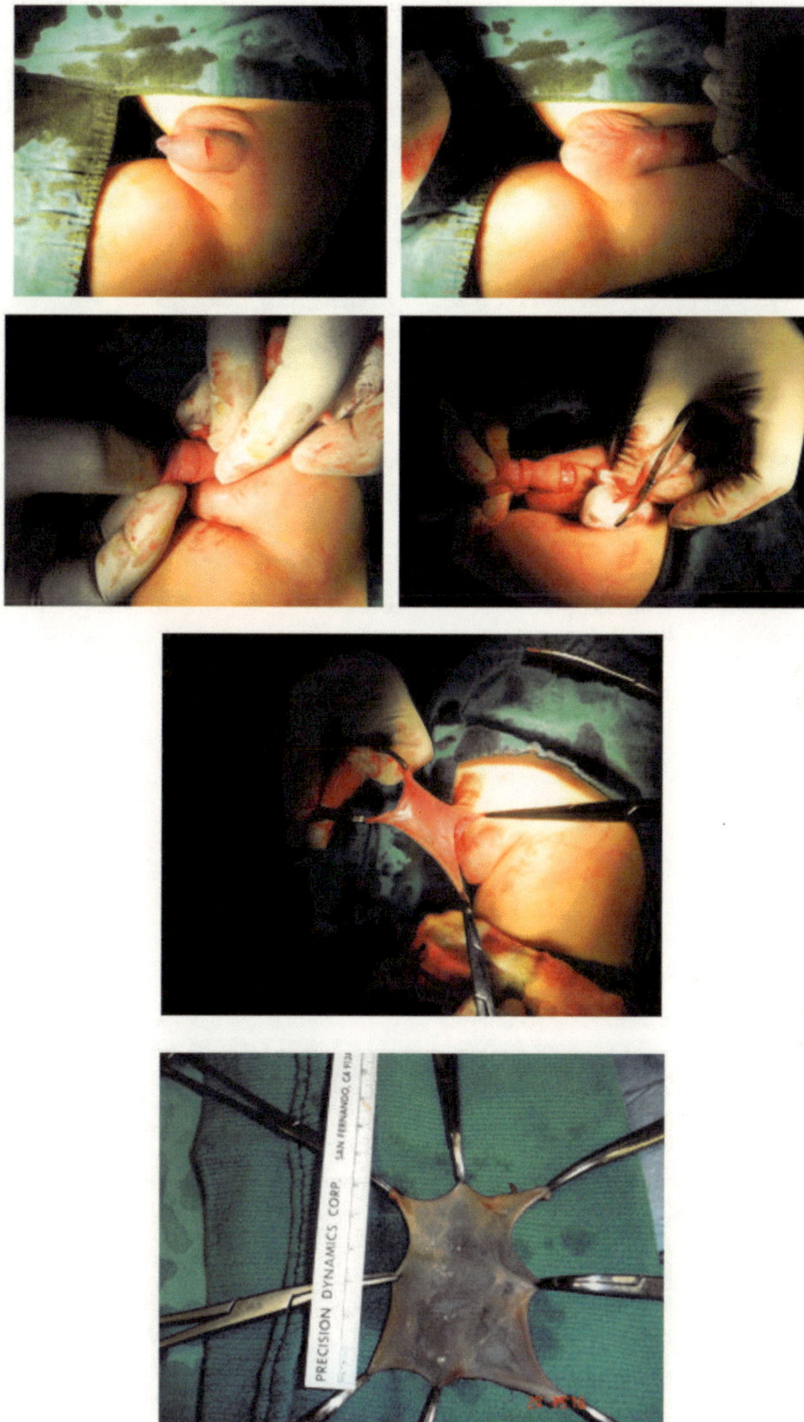

Fig. 1. Circumcision and preparation of skin graft

In 2 patients, PSG was used for periareolar grafting where hyperpigmented healing was preferred (Figure 2). General anesthesia was required in 91% of patients because of need for additional donor sites. Overall graft survival was 100% without any complication of donor site [13] (Table-1).In another series of patients, PSG has been successfully used for burn contracture release, acute burn treatment and for defects in scalp and defects from acute trauma. Mean defect size was 3.5x5.5 cm in this study in which PSG was enough to cover these defects in 90% of the patients. All the recipient area was opened on postoperative day 5. Graft survival was 100 % and no complication on donor site [14] (Table-1).

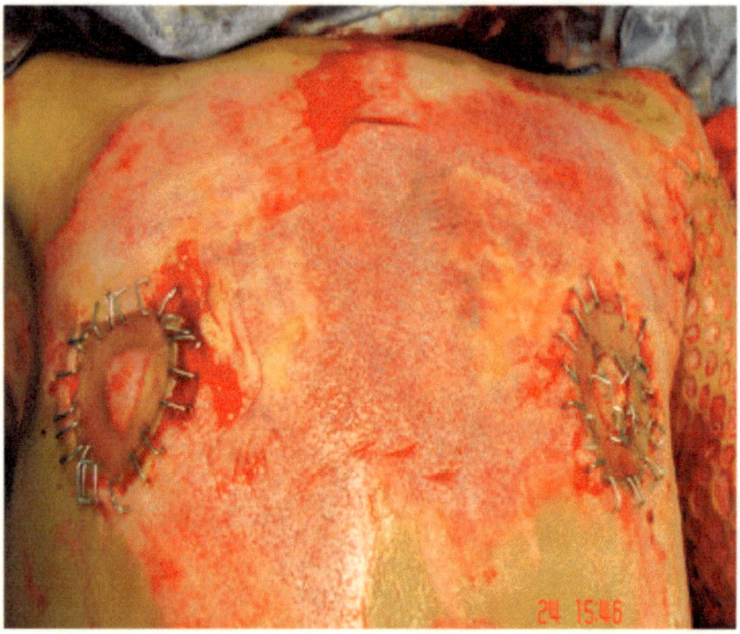

Fig. 2. Periareolar grafting with preputial skin

	Number of Patients	Mean age of Patients	PSG was the only donor Site (%)	Average Defect Size	Mean PSG Size	Graft Survival (%)	Indication for PSG use	Donor site morbidity (%)
Dogrul et al.	12	3.6	25	N/A	6x4 cm	100	Burn	0
Yıldırım et al.	11	7.9	90,9	3.5x5.5 cm	N/A	100	Burn, contracture release, scalp defect and defects from trauma	0

Table 1. Two series of patients in which PSG was liberally used.

Recently in a study performed by Mcheik and et al, keratinocytes isolated from preputial skin after double enzymatic digestion. They cultured keratinocytes and obtained an average of 8.8 million cells per foreskin. And they concluded that keratinocyte resulting from foreskin have a high capacity of division. These cells can divide a long time before differentiation and enabled them to propose with their paitents the keratinocytes from foreskin for wound healing especially for burns in children [17].

Only limitation of PSG is its healing with hyperpigmentation which limits its usage in face and neck region which are the most common recipient side of FTSGs [13, 14]. But it can be used in extremity and scalp defects [14]. But this color mismatch may be an advantage if it is used in special areas like periareolar area [13]. Other limitation of PSG may be potential complications of circumcision.

Circumcision is the surgical procedure for harvesting PSG. As with any surgical procedure, bleeding and infection are probably the most common complications of circumcision [18]. Other complications include hematoma formation, diffuse swelling and pain from inadequate anesthesia and tearing of the sutures due to erection before healing is complete [18]. Urethral injury and penile necrosis are exceptional but reported complications [18]. These complications decrease with experience and can be as low as 0.034 % where circumcision is routinely performed [14] .

In some countries, circumcision is the most common surgical procedure in boys because of religious and cultural reasons. It is routinely performed to all male children with a very low complication rates [13]. There are also some absolute medical indications for circumcision, such as phimosis secondary to balanitis xerotica, obliterans and recurrent balanophosthitis [19, 20]. Relative indications of circumcision are paraphimosis, phimosis, preputial pearls, reduntant foreskin, hypospadias surgery [19]. Besides, it may have some medical benefits such as improved hygiene, reduced risks of urinary and sexually transmitted infections, and of penile and cervical cancer [20]. However, opponents deny or minimize these benefits and put forward complications of circumcision and loss of penile sensation [20]. But we think that; in burn patients, benefits of PSG outweigh from potential complications of circumcision.

Although PSG is still not in routine use in the era of reconstructive surgery, reported series have promising results [13, 14]. Especially in burned children with small sized defects, PSG may be the only graft that adequately used for closure of defects with almost nil donor site complication and 100 % graft survival rate. Only limitation for its usage is hyperpigmentation. Every surgeon must keep PSG in mind as an alternative donor site.

4. References

[1] Ratner, D., *Skin grafting.* Semin Cutan Med Surg, 2003. 22(4): p. 295-305.

[2] Andreassi, A., et al., *Classification and pathophysiology of skin grafts.* Clin Dermatol, 2005. 23(4): p. 332-7.

[3] Ratner, D., *Skin grafting. From here to there.* Dermatol Clin, 1998. 16(1): p. 75-90.

[4] Petruzzelli, G.J. and J.T. Johnson, *Skin grafts.* Otolaryngol Clin North Am, 1994. 27(1): p. 25-37.

[5] Baran, C.N., et al., *What is new in the treatment of hypospadias?* Plast Reconstr Surg, 2004. 114(3): p. 743-52.

[6] Fontenot, C., J. Ortenberg, and D. Faust, *Hypospadiac or intact foreskin graft for syndactyly repair.* J Pediatr Surg, 1999. 34(12): p. 1826-8.

[7] Emory, R.E. and C.H. Chester, *Prepuce pollicization: a reminder of an alternate donor.* Plast Reconstr Surg, 2000. 105(6): p. 2100-1.

[8] D'Alessio, A., et al., *Use of preputial skin as cutaneous graft after nevus excision.* Int J Pediatr. 2010: p. 951270.

[9] Radopoulos, D., I. Vakalopoulos, and P. Thanos, *Preputial graft in penile curvature correction: preliminary results.* Int J Impot Res, 2009. 21(1): p. 82-7.

[10] Silfen, R., D.A. Hudson, and P.J. Skoll, *The use of the prepuce for reconstruction of an intraoral burn.* Ann Plast Surg, 2000. 44(3): p. 317-9.

[11] Oates, S.D. and A.K. Gosain, *Syndactyly repair performed simultaneously with circumcision: use of foreskin as a skin-graft donor site.* J Pediatr Surg, 1997. 32(10): p. 1482-4.

[12] Mak, A.S., A.M. Poon, and M.K. Tung, *Use of preputial skin for the release of burn contractures in children.* Burns, 1995. 21(4): p. 301-2.

[13] Dogrul, A.B., et al., *Preputial skin can be used in all boys with burns requiring grafting.* Ulus Travma Acil Cerrahi Derg, 2009. 15(1): p. 58-61.

[14] Yildirim, S., et al., *The preputium: an overlooked skin graft donor site.* Ann Plast Surg, 2001. 46(6): p. 630-4.

[15] Chlihi, A., et al., *[The use of preputial skin as cutaneous graft after circumcision. Report of 30 clinical cases].* Ann Chir Plast Esthet, 2002. 47(3): p. 214-8.

[16] Helmbach DM, F.L., ed. *Principles of Burn Surgery.* Principles and Practice of Burn Surgery, ed. H.D. Barrett-Nerrin JP. 2005, Mercel Dekker: New York. 135 - 62.

[17] McHeik, J.N., et al., *[Cultured keratinocyte cells from foreskin and future application for burns in children].* Ann Chir Plast Esthet, 2009. 54(6): p. 528-32.

[18] Akoz, T., et al., *Unusual complications of circumcision.* Plast Reconstr Surg, 1998. 101(7): p. 1915-8.

[19] Malone, P. and H. Steinbrecher, *Medical aspects of male circumcision.* BMJ, 2007. 335(7631): p. 1206-90.

[20] Holman, J.R. and K.A. Stuessi, *Adult circumcision.* Am Fam Physician, 1999. 59(6): p. 1514-8.

12

Treatment of Adult-Acquired Buried Penis

W. Britt Zimmerman[1,2] and Richard A. Santucci[1,2]
[1]*Michigan State University – College of Osteopathic Medicine*
[2]*Detroit Receiving Hospital Detroit Medical Center United States of America*

1. Introduction

The first know description of buried penis was by Keyes in 1919. Buried penis was described as the "absence of the penis exists when the penis, lacking its proper sheath of skin, lies buried beneath the integument of the abdomen, thigh or scrotum (Keyes, 1919)." Classically, the entity of buried penis has been primarily discussed in the pediatric population (Boemers & De Jong, 1995, Crawford, 1977, Donatucci & Ritter, 1998, Lim et al., 1995, Maizels et al., 1986, McCahill et al., 1995, Wollin et al., 1990). However, a buried penis afflicts many adults leaving them with the inability to have sexual relations, practice personal hygiene, or stand to void since they are unable to direct their penis during micturition (Cromie et al., 1998). Unlike the pediatric patient population, adults with buried penis have acquired this condition as a result of obesity, over exuberant circumcision, scarring due to lichen sclerosis et atrophicus (previously as known as balanitis xerotica obliterans) or lymphedema (Alici et al., 1998, Chopra et al., 2002, Donatucci & Ritter, 1998, Sivakumar et al., 2004, Tang et al., 2008). This chapter discusses the pathophysiology of a buried penis, patient selection for operative management, and surgical management with associated complications.

2. History of buried penis management

Since the initial description by Keyes and colleagues, various names have been associated with "buried penis" which describes the pathology in both the pediatric and adult population. These names range from buried penis (Keyes, 1919), concealed penis (Wollin et al., 1990) webbed penis (Crawford, 1977), and inconspicuous penis (Maizels et al., 1986). In 1951, Campbell and colleagues described the buried penis as being underneath the perineum, hypogastrium, thigh, or subcutaneous fat of scrotum (Campbell, 1951). Usually, buried penis and concealed penis are used interchangeably (Glanz, 1968).

Two authors have offered classification systems in identifying buried penis. In 1977, Crawford proposed three categories: concealed penis, buried penis (partial or complete) and penoscrotal webs (Crawford, 1977). Later in 1986, Maizels proposed a classification system in four categories: buried penis, webbed penis, trapped penis, and micropenis (Maizels et al., 1986) (Table 1).

Buried Penis Classification		
	Crawford's Classification	Maizel's Classification
1	Concealed penis	Buried penis
2	Buried penis (partial or complete)	Webbed penis
3	Penoscrotal webs	Trapped penis
4		Micropenis

Table 1. Buried penis classification systems

3. Etiology

The underlying pathological process of a buried penis includes an abnormal hypermobility of the ventral skin on dartos fascia and inadequate attachments to the underlying Buck's fascia. The corpora remains stationery and the surrounding tissues (skin and dartos) migrate distally (Alter & Ehrlich, 1999, Casale et al., 1999, Frenkl et al., 2004). Hence, the overlying penile skin acts as a redundant drape, or "tent pole" over which skin is draped. The process may advance because the corporal bodies remain fixed to the pubic bone by the suspensory ligament and because of this fixation, the obese patient's abdomen descends and envelopes the penis. As the penis becomes covered or "buried," excessive moisture begins to develop which then promotes bacterial overgrowth, tissue maceration, and infection. As chronic infections continue and a cycle is established, there is a perpetuation of skin breakdown followed by more inflammation and scarification. In addition, the patient is unable to direct their penis for voiding resulting in urine soilage. Urine is trapped and the cycle continues. Most patients are obese and have associated comorbidities such as diabetes mellitus, which may worsen the patient's prognosis (Donatucci & Ritter, 1998).

4. Patient presentation / selection

Many patients present to their primary care physician or Urologist with in the inability to participate in sexual activity secondary to painful erections or the inability to achieve adequate penile length (Chopra et al., 2002, Cromie et al., 1998) (Figure 1). Additionally, patients may also suffer from social embarrassment, recurrent balanitis, and psychological stress (Chopra et al., 2002, Frenkl et al., 2004).

When selecting patients for surgical correction, many indications exist. Frankl et al (2004) describes; in the pediatric population indications for surgery which include recurrent balanitis, secondary phimosis, difficulty holding the penis during voiding, urinary stream spraying, social embarrassment, and parent's concern for future social embarrassment (Frenkl et al, 2004). These are widely accepted (Adham et al., 2000, Alici et al, 1998, Chuang et al., 2001, Donatucci & Ritter, 1998, Frenkl et al., 2004). However, in dealing with the adult population, the primary indications are related to sexuality. Other indications include complete or partial penile concealment with the inability to stand to void, chronic urinary soilage, dysuria, inability to participate in penetrative intercourse, and erectile pain (Donatucci & Ritter, 1998, Tang et al., 2008).

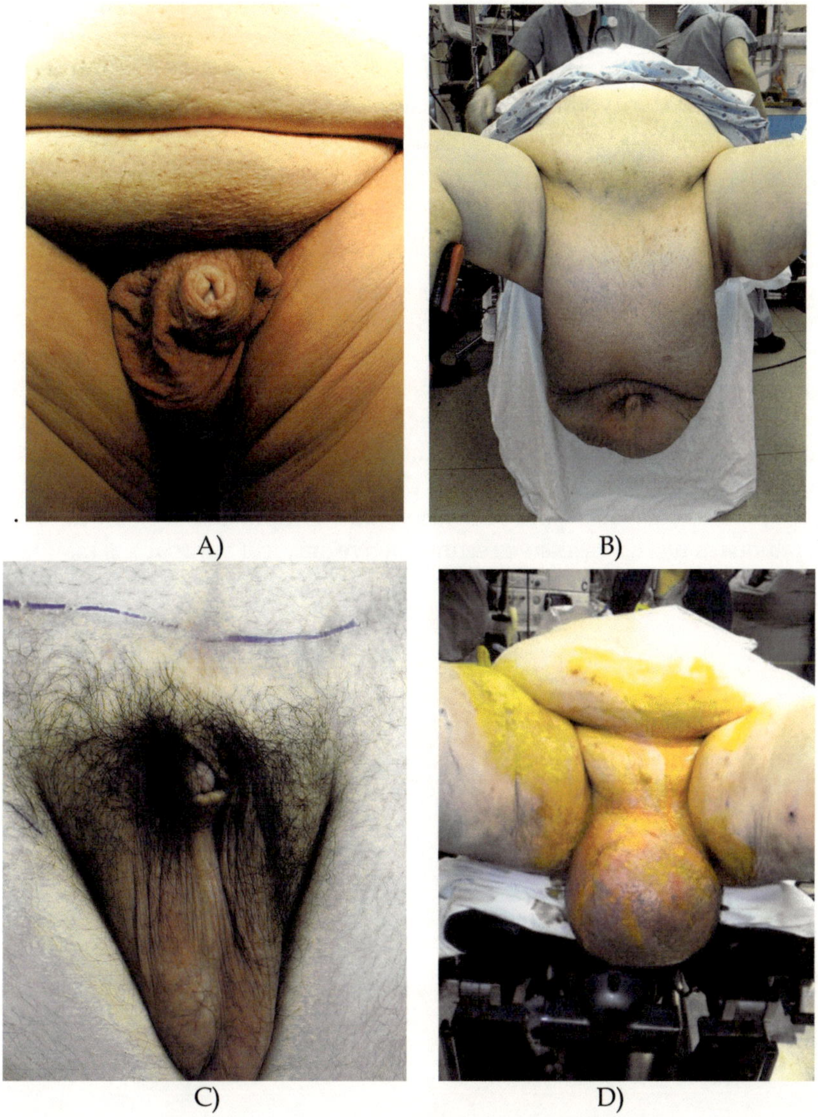

Fig. 1. Buried penis etiologies vary: widely A: Large abdominal pannus, escutcheon and normal size scrotum. B: Large abdominal pannus and severe scrotal lymphedema. C: Buried penis following abdominoplasty, note normal abdomen and scrotum. D: Buried penis as a result of scrotal lymphedema.

The ideal candidates for operative correction of a buried penis are patients who are motivated and prepared for postoperative wound care. Wound complications are reported post-operatively, and these can be significant (Anaya & Dellinger, 2006, Rogliani et al., 2006). Additionally, the patient must be medically and cardiovascular cleared for general anesthesia.

5. Patient preparation

Patient education is paramount during pre-operative management. Many of these patients suffer from depression and some have even considered suicide in the past (Tang et al., 2008). Hence, the patient should be made aware of the extensive postoperative course that will ensue. Obesity and their abdominal girth often have a negative impact on wound healing and may limit their dexterity and ability to care for the groin wounds (Anaya & Dellinger, 2006, Rogliani et al., 2006).

6. Surgical technique

Major reconstructive urologic surgery is required to treat adults with a buried penis. Many techniques have been described. The objectives are all primarily the same: restore the normal anatomy from the underlying pathological process.

Surgical approaches vary and should correlate to the etiology of the buried penis. Some patients present with a normal sized scrotum and abdomen without a pannus (Figure 2). In corollary, many patients suffer from a lack of penile skin as in an over exuberant circumcision. In simple situations like this, the penile skin is released and approximated to the base of the penile shaft, and the defect is covered by split thickness skin grafts. In more complicated scenarios, as in a patient with scrotal lymphedema or an abnormally large abdominal pannus, a more aggressive reconstructive surgical approach is mandated.

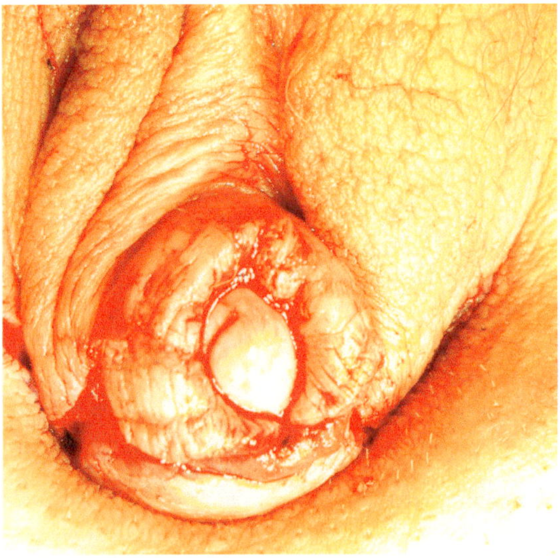

Fig. 2. Buried penis with normal abdomen and scrotal skin and poor penile shaft skin

Various surgical techniques for buried penis have been reported. Maizels et al. (1986) performed a lipectomy of the suprapubic fat pad and suspensory ligament incision. This was accompanied by pubic bone anchoring of the penopubic tissue (Maizels et al, 1986). Similarly, Alter and colleagues (1999) advocated securing the subdermis of the penoscrotal junction to the tunica albugenia ventrally to stabilize the penile and scrotal skin and prevent migration of the penis within the scrotum. Additionally, these authors advocate securing the subdermal penopubic junction to the rectus abdominal fascia (Alter & Ehrlich, 1999).

Wollin et al. (1990) described a complete degloving of penis with lysis of improper ventral dartos attachments. This is followed by an island pedicle flap of preputial skin and transposed to the ventral aspect of the penis (Wollin et al., 1990).

Donatucci et al. (1998) described a treatment algorithm ranging from release of scar contracture and primary closure. If insufficient release of the phallus occurs, then procession to panniculectomy is warranted. Depending on the adequacy of skin or soft tissue in for closure, the next step would be initially to use primary skin closure versus Z-plasty. If native skin is not available and/or of poor quality, then split thickness skin grafts or flaps may be necessary. Skin flaps should only be used when an inadequate graft bed exists (Donatucci & Ritter, 1998).

Chopra et al. (2002) described a technique using a large elliptical panniculectomy with scar excision and penile skin removal. Division of the suspensory ligament of the penis, release of the cicatrix and reattachment of the suspensory ligament of the penis should be undertaken if necessary. Finally, a standard abdominoplasty and full thickness skin grafting to the penis is performed. Skin grafting should be performed in a spiral fashion to diminish any linear scar contraction (Chopra et al., 2002).

Many authors have also addressed the obese patient's overlying suprapubic fat pad by performing dermatolipectomy or suction lipectomy with abdominoplasty (Adham et al., 2000, Alter & Ehrlich, 1999, Horton et al., 1987).

Six principles for success have been summarized in the buried penis patient population by Chopra et al. (2002) (Table 2). First, release of the underlying cicatrix or scar which has anchored the penile tissue preventing it from being mobilized, should occur. Secondly, the majority of the pannus should be removed in the obese patient. Third, with the reduction of the abdominal fat pad, there is a need to reestablish the normal male escutcheon (suprapubic fat pad). The next step, in patients with a normal scrotum, is to reapproximate the median raphe of the scrotum to its' normal anatomic position at the base of the penis. Then, skin resurfacing must be carried out depending on the condition of the penile shaft. This can be achieved with either skin grafts or flaps. However, in the adult patient, non-hair bearing coverage is preferred. Finally, an appropriate dressing needs to be applied as the fragility of the skin graft must be respected (Chopra et al., 2002).

Six Principles for Successful Buried Penis Management	
1	Release/excision of cicatrix
2	Removal of as much pannus as possible
3	Reestablishment of normal male escutcheon
4	Reattachment of median raphe to the base of the penis
5	Resurfacing the denuded penis with a full-thickness skin graft, sutured in spiral fashion to avoid linear contracted scarring
6	Circumferential generic foam dressings applied snugly around the graft for immobilization and splinting

Table 2. Six principle for successful surgical management of buried penis by Chopra et al.

A different surgical approach is described by Tang et al. (2008). This technique in the obese patient includes escutcheonectomy, scrotoplasty, and penile split-thickness grafting with fibrin glue fixation (Tang et al., 2008). This begins with a circumcision incision two to three millimeters proximal to the coronal sulcus. This allows for complete exposure of the glans penis and penile shaft. The penoscrotal webs and aberrant scrotal tissues are released if necessary. If a scrotoplasty is performed, the wound is closed in a two layers and no drain is placed. The escutcheonectomy is made using an elliptical incision and juxtaposition to the base of the penis. We trim any redundant suprapubic fat and secure it as a flap to the superficial suspensory ligaments of the penis using 2-O interrupted polyglactin sutures (Figure 3). We make every effort to close all potential spaces to avoid seroma formation. Closed suction drains are used under the escutcheon flap wherever necessary.

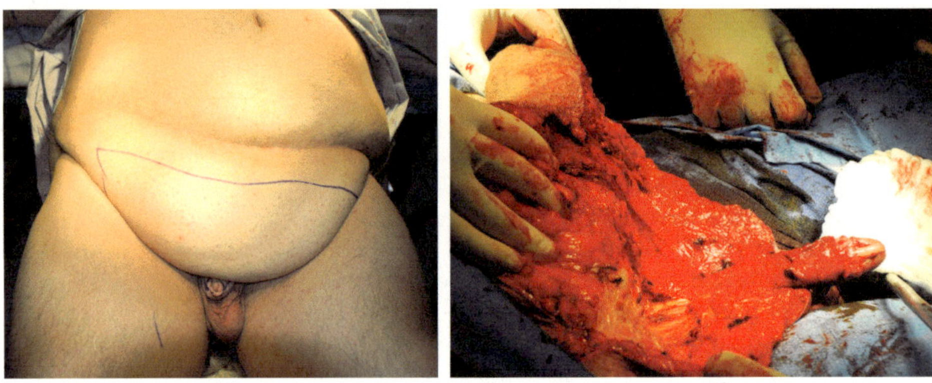

A) B)

Fig. 3. A: An elliptical incision is made on pannus. B: dermatolipectomy is performed.

C. 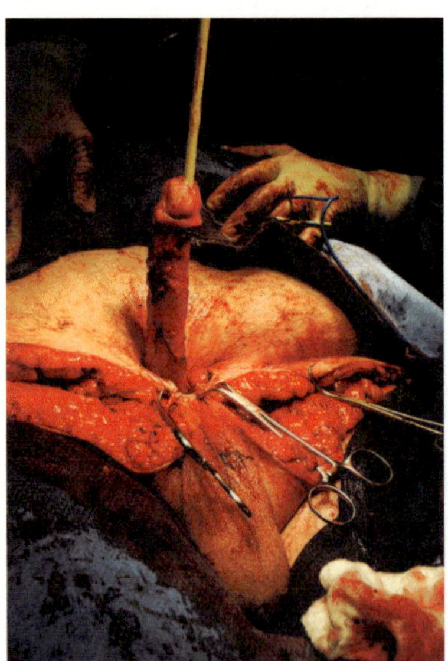

Fig. 3. C: The male escutcheon is reestablished.

In our experience, the remaining penile shaft skin is either non-existent or of poor quality. Hence, we use full thickness skin grafts from the discarded escutcheon or split skin grafts (STSG) from a predetermined location, typically anterior left thigh. The STSG is harvested at a depth of 0.012 to 0.015 inches, using an electric dermatome. The proximal aspect of the skin graft is tacked down using multiple simple interrupted absorbable sutures. To assist in graft success, we use a diluted fibrin sealant (freeze-dried Tissel VH, Baxter, Deerfield, IL) as per manufacturer specifications. We spray the sealant to the entire surface of the penile shaft using the Tissomat fibrin glue spray device (Baxter). By using the dilute fibrin glue concentration (about 10% of the normal calcium concentration of Tissel), we lengthen the time to hardening from seconds to minutes which allows more time for the final graft placement (Figure 4).

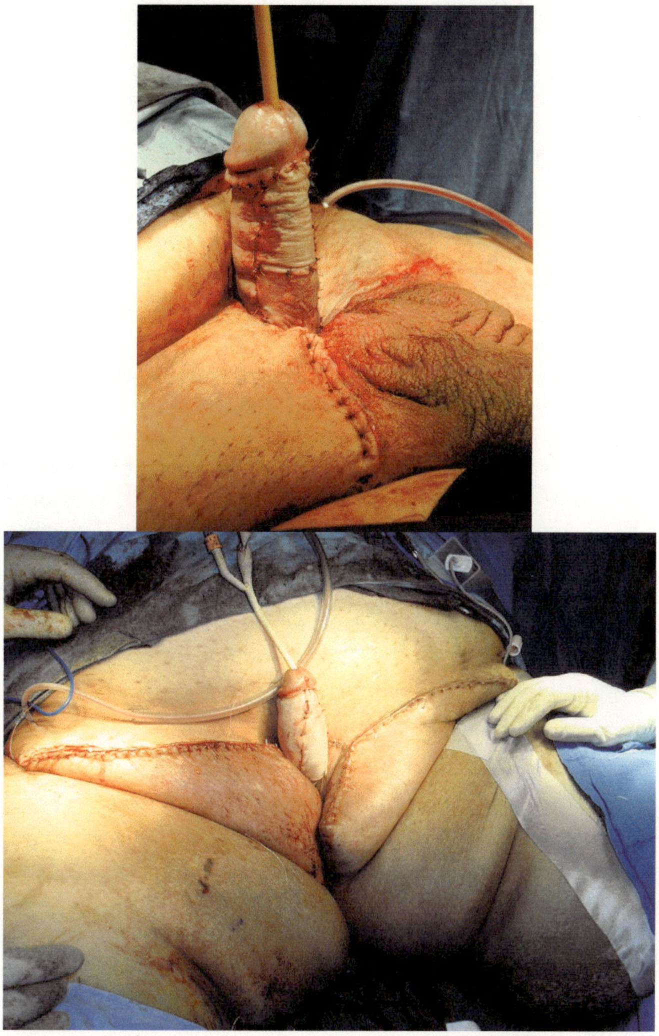

A) B)

Fig. 4. A: Excision of the pannus and skin grafting. B: Pannus excision, scrotoplasty and skin grafting.

The skin graft harvest site is covered with a transparent adhesive dressing (Opsite, Smith & Nephew, London UK) and a small closed suction drain (TLS, Porex Surgical, Newman, GA). This type dressing removes excessive drainage and facilitates the dressing staying longer. The grafted penis is dressed in a 6 inch elastic antimicrobial gauze (Kerlix, Tyco/Kendall, Manfield, MA). Local anesthesia is used with 0.5% bupivacaine containing epinephrine 1:200,000 to lessen any postoperative pain. The skin graft dressing is removed after 24 hours and any seromas (blebs) are incised as necessary.

7. Postoperative care

Immediate postoperative care begins in the hospital. Our patients are admitted to the hospital and are on bed rest for the first three days. On postoperative day four, the patient returns to normal activity and is educated on wound care. Discharge typically takes place on postoperative day five. The patient is continued with oral antibiotics such as amoxicillin/clavulanate for two weeks. The patient is instructed to shower and dress the wounds daily. We recommend 4-inch gauze sponges (eg, Johnson & Johnson "Topper" dressing sponges, or other nonadherent absorbent pads). We recommend against "open weave" gauze sponges as these have a tendency to debride and can result in surgical site breakdown.

8. Complications

In the postoperative period, complications can occur. These can range from surgical site infections to the development of a pulmonary embolism (Tang et al., 2008). In patients suffering from obesity and metabolic syndromes such as diabetes, an increased risk for Surgical Site Infection exists (Anaya & Dellinger, 2006, Rogliani et al., 2006). Patients may also experience erectile dysfunction (ED) postoperatively. The erectile dysfunction may be due to an underlying disease process that initially propagated the buried penis. Hence, ED may only be recognized after the penis is once again revealed. It is also common for the patient to experience decreased sensation over the skin graft site (Donatucci & Ritter, 1998). This will typically improve over time as nerve re-growth occurs.

The most common defense against the aforementioned complications beyond preoperative medical optimization and stringent perioperative care is education. The buried penis patient has often been described as being at the "end of their rope (Tang et al., 2008)." Hence, informed consent and patient expectations need to be framed appropriately.

9. Conclusion

Acquired adult buried penis management is a challenging reconstructive surgery. However, with the proper use of escutcheonectomy, reduction of the suprapubic fat pad, +/- scrotoplasty, and with use of full or split thickness skin grafting, excellent results are possible. With diligent post-operative wound care to manage minor infections and wound dehiscence, the patient can return to sexual activity, have profound improvement in urinary function, and improved self-esteem as a result of improved cosmesis.

10. Acknowledgement

The author would like to acknowledge Dr. Lisa Hall Zimmerman for her dedicated assistance of manuscript editing.

11. References

Adham MN, Teimourian B, Mosca P. (2000). Buried penis release in adults with suction lipectomy and abdominoplasty. Plastic and Reconstructive Surgery, 106, 840-4.

Alici B, Culha M, Ozkara H, Akkus E, Hattat H. (1998). Management of buried penis in adults. Urologia Internationalis, 61, 183-5.

Alter GJ, Ehrlich RM. (1999). A new technique for correction of the hidden penis in children and adults. The Journal of Urology, 161, 455-9.

Anaya DA, Dellinger EP. (2006). The obese surgical patient: a susceptible host for infection. Surgical Infections, 7, 473-80.

Boemers TM, De Jong TP. (1995). The surgical correction of buried penis: a new technique. The Journal of Urology, 154, 550-2.

Campbell M. (1951). Embryology and anomalies of the urogenital tract. In: Clinical Pediatric Urology, pp. 273 W. B. Saunders Co. Philadelphia

Casale AJ, Beck SD, Cain MP, Adams MC, Rink RC. (1999). Concealed penis in childhood: a spectrum of etiology and treatment. The Journal of Urology, 162, 1165-8.

Chopra CW, Ayoub NT, Bromfield C, Witt PD. (2002). Surgical management of acquired (cicatricial) buried penis in an adult patient. Annals of Plastic Surgery, 49, 545-9.

Chuang JH, Chen LY, Shieh CS, Lee SY. (2001). Surgical correction of buried penis: a review of 60 cases. Journal of Pediatric Surgery, 36, 426-9.

Crawford BS. (1977). Buried penis. British Journal of Plastic Surgery, 30, 96-9.

Cromie WJ, Ritchey ML, Smith RC, Zagaja GP. (1998). Anatomical alignment for the correction of buried penis. The Journal of Urology, 160, 1482-4.

Donatucci CF, Ritter EF. (1998). Management of the buried penis in adults. The Journal of Urology, 159, 420-4.

Frenkl TL, Agarwal S, Caldamone AA. (2004). Results of a simplified technique for buried penis repair. The Journal of Urology, 171, 826-8.

Glanz S. (1968). Adult congenital penile deformity. Case report. Plast Reconstr Surg, 41, 579-80.

Horton CE, Vorstman B, Teasley D, Winslow B. (1987). Hidden penis release: adjunctive suprapubic lipectomy. Annals of Plastic Surgery, 19, 131-4.

Keyes EL. (1919). Phimosis-paraphimosis-tumors of the penis. . In: Urology, pp. 649 D. Appleton & Co. New York, NY

Lim DJ, Barraza MA, Stevens PS. (1995). Correction of retractile concealed penis. The Journal of Urology, 153, 1668-70.

Maizels M, Zaontz M, Donovan J, Bushnick PN, Firlit CF. (1986). Surgical correction of the buried penis: description of a classification system and a technique to correct the disorder. The Journal of Urology, 136, 268-71.

McCahill PD, Leonard MP, Jeffs RD. (1995). Epispadias with phimosis: an unusual variant of the concealed penis. Urology, 45, 158-60.

Rogliani M, Silvi E, Labardi L, Maggiulli F, Cervelli V. (2006). Obese and nonobese patients: complications of abdominoplasty. Annals of Plastic Surgery, 57, 336-8.

Sivakumar B, Brown AA, Kangesu L. (2004). Circumcision in 'buried penis'--a cautionary tale. Annals of the Royal College of Surgeons of England, 86, 35-7.

Tang SH, Kamat D, Santucci RA. (2008). Modern management of adult-acquired buried penis. Urology, 72, 124-7.

Wollin M, Duffy PG, Malone PS, Ransley PG. (1990). Buried penis. A novel approach. British Journal of Urology, 65, 97-100.

Part 3

Current Research

13

Skin Graft Preservation

Liangpeng Ge[1], Zhenggen Huang[2] and Hong Wei[3]
[1]*Chongqing Academy of Animal Sciences*
[2]*Northern Hospital*
[3]*Third Military Medical University*
China

1. Introduction

Skin transplants have long been of interest to plastic surgeons for the treatment of burns and other wounds. Skin transplants provide a better micro-enviromental for wound healing and provide physiological barrier which greatly decreases water, electrolyte, protein and heat loss through the wound. However, skin grafts are not always available in adequate quantities for the complete duration of treatment, making skin graft preservation important in meeting the need for skin transplantation.

This chapter highlights progress in the field of skin graft preservation including basic knowledge of skin preservation, harvesting, processing and preservation, and quality control methods and is intended to provide a reference for skin preservation techniques for doctors and researchers.

2. Thermal physics of skin low-temperature preservation

The low-temperature preservation with viable cells and tissues is a complicated procedure, which needs to undergo multiple processes including pretreatment, freezing, preservation under low temperature and thawing in proper order. In these processes, there is unavoidably evident change in the functions and morphology of the tissues. An ideal preservation procedure should be that viable cells and tissues can restore to the original functions and morphology prior to preservation after undergoing all of these processes and then be used for grafting and other purposes like fresh cells and tissue. So far, the effect of low-temperature preservation does not meet the above ideal conditions. Also, doctors and researchers are not fully aware of the change in viable tissue in the preservation processes, especially in the processes of freezing and thawing.

Water occupies a considerable proportion ofviable cells and tissues. The moisture content of skin is about 70%. The quality of skin is closely related to the phase transition of water during low-temperature preservation, which including the solidification in freezing, ebullition in freezing of viable tissue using liquid nitrogen, thawing during freezing and so on.

Water or water vapor can generate more than 10 kinds of solid phase structure, nevertheless, most of them need to be formed under high pressure environment (at least 200 million Pascal（Mpa）), and only hexagonal ice, cube ice or amorphous ice can be generated under low pressure. Water vapor deposits on a cold surface within the temperature range from 0°C slightly below to about -80°C, or forms a hexagonal symmetric ice crystal in a suspended state in the air, snow is a typical case in point, and cubic crystal with diamond structure will be generated under lower temperature (about -80°C~-130°C) and amorphous solid (also called glassy, vitrification) will be formed below -140°C. Liquid water usually only forms a hexagonal symmetric ice crystal upon freezing, however, solutes-bearing water solution more easily realizes vitrification upon freezing compared with pure water. Therefore, some components shall be added before freezing, in order to promote the suspension of cells or tissues to more easily reach vitrification (Zhu et al., 2002).

It is generally believed that there are two kinds of cell damaged in the freezing process: one is intracellular ice crystals damage and the other is solution damage. Ice crystals cause the change of cell wall and ultra-structures in the cells. Even death can occur by intracellular ice crystals growing to a certain degree during freezing. This damage is more serious in the case of quicker freezing. Solution damage causes cell damage by extracellular high-concentration solution because water freezes outside of the cells. The longer cells stay in high-concentration solution, the more serious the solution damage is. For certain types of cells and freezing processes, ice crystals and solution damage exist simultaneously; nevertheless, solution damage dominates in the case of slow cooling and intracellular ice damage dominates in the case of quick cooling. And the solution damage and intracellular ice damage shall be avoided or reduce if ice crystals are avoided (e.g. amorphous or glassy solid are obtained), or ice crystals are formed but fail to grow to change the structure of cells (e.g. partly vitrification) in case of snap freezing.

There are two different protocols used in skin low-temperature preservation: slow freezing and quick freezing/snap frozen. Slow freezing reduces the temperature of the skin treated with antifreeze fluid from about 4 to -60°C at preset rate (e.g. 1-3°C/min) and balanced for 4h using a controlled-rate cooling apparatus, which adopts liquid nitrogen gas to absorb the heat of specimen mainly by convective heat transfer, and then put skin into liquid nitrogen for preservation. It is worthy of note that, the moisture contained in those tissues with greater mass will releases a large amount of latent heat in a cold room at near 0°C, however, liquid nitrogen gas can't rapidly absorb the latent heat of water phase transition due to lower convective heat transfer coefficient, so it makes a probable great difference between the displayed temperature by a controlled-rate cooling apparatus and the actual temperature in the skin tissues, and it is difficult to reduce this temperature difference by increasing cold gas volume. In case of snap frozen, the skin is incubated with antifreeze solution and then transferred directly to liquid nitrogen, and the temperature can be cooled from >0°C to liquid nitrogen temperature within 30s. Being simple, snap frozen eliminates special instrument and reduces cost. However, liquid nitrogen may generate grave ebullition during snap freezing, and the big temperature difference between liquid nitrogen and skin can not be fully utilized at the initial stage of freezing, thus, "thermo-zone platform" (as shown in Fig.1) will be form near zero degree. To avoid this defect, on one hand, antifreeze fluid needs to be optimized, on the other hand, a copper plate pre-cooled with liquid nitrogen shall be used for directly contacting skin graft for snap frozen using heat conduction style, in order to obtain better cooling effect (as shown in Fig.2).

At present, there is inadequate researche on the thawing process of frozen skin. Most standards advocate rapid warming of the skin to optimise viability. This can be achieved by

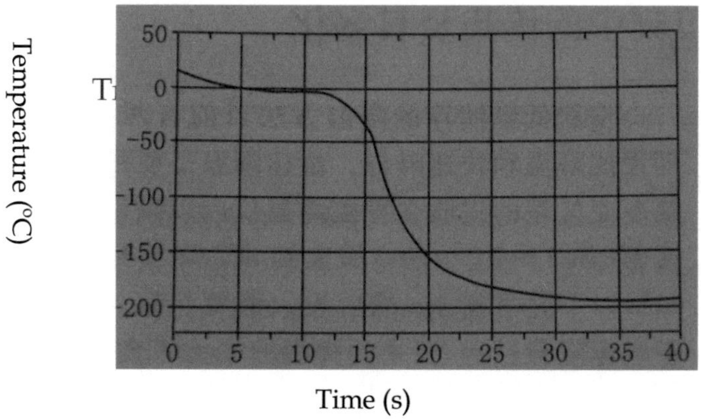

Fig. 1. Temperature (°C) curve of skin immersing in liquid nitrogen (Available from: Basic and application of skin preservation, people's military medical publisher;2002.)

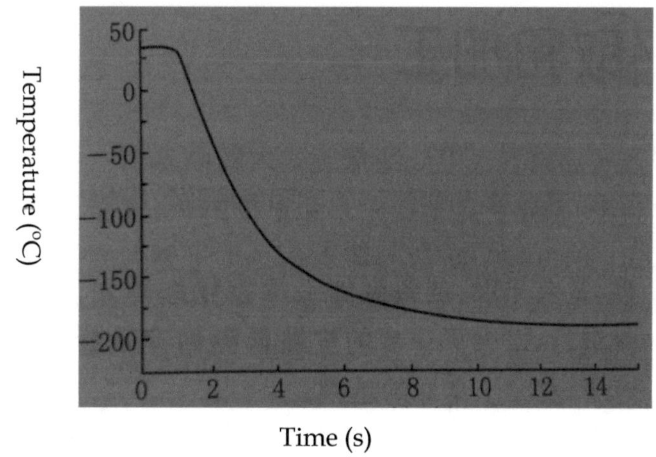

Fig. 2. Temperature (°C) curve of skin in a copper plate pre-cooled with liquid nitrogen (Available from: Basic and application of skin preservation, people's military medical publisher;2002.)

immersion of the packs in a 37°C waterbath. The thawing process of skin is closely related to previous freezing process. In case of snap frozen, glassy solids are formed inside and outside of the cells, and quick rewarming can avoid "devitrification" during temperature rise process. "Devitrification"means glassy water or tiny ice crystals-bearing solid water is recrystallized prior to thawing, or tiny ice crystals are rethawed into large ice crystals, which destroy cell structures and cause cell death(Zieger et al., 1997).

3. Skin harvesting and processing

Processing methods used for banking of skin for subsequent therapeutic use depend on whether the skin is to retain viability or not. For viable skin grafts, sterilisation techniques cannot be applied, however antibiotics and antimycotics may be used to disinfect the tissue with respect to bacteria and fungi (Kearney,2005; Li, 2001; Ninnmam et al,.1978).

3.1 Screening of donor

One of the major concerns with the use of skin grafts from donors is the risk of disease transmission. A case involving the transmission of HIV from a skin donor to a recipient has been reported(Clark, 1987). To reduce the risk of disease transmission, skin donors should be screened before skin harvesting. If skin grafts obtained from cadaveric donors , medical records held by hospitals, family doctors, and others must be screened for conditions that would exclude donation(Delmonico,1998). This may include current systemic infection, diseases of unknown etiology, and previous infections with the possibility of current carrier status (hepatitis, malaria, HIV, syphilis antibodies etc). It may also be prudent to exclude a history of malignant disease particularly if the skin might be used on immunosuppressed patients, for example, those suffering massive burn injuries. Behavioral history may also be grounds for rejection of the donor owing to the high correlations between activities such as intravenous drug abuse and viral infections such as HIV and hepatitis.

3.2 Reducing the population of microorganism

Skin tissue possesses a mixed commensal population of bacteria and fungi that lives primarily in or around the hair and sebaceous follicles (Kearney et al.,1984). Even the commensal bacteria may damage the skin if subsequently allowed to grow during the skin storage period to reach massive population densities. Therefore, it is important to try to eliminate or minimize the microbial population of skin before retrieval.

For viable skin allografts, it is not possible to apply a sterilization technique because sterilization methods tend to inactivate cells at an equal or greater rate than for the bacterial cells. The best that can be achieved is a combination of serology screening for viruses and bacterial disinfection using antibiotic cocktails (Holder et al., 1998). This is generally achieved using skin prepping techniques similar to those used on the skin of patients undergoing operations in hospital. When banking skin in a viable state, it is important to validate that the prepping agents have been adequately removed before harvesting the skin, and that any residuals are not toxic to the skin cells. Although effective in reducing the bioburden, skin prepping is unlikely to totally eliminate bacteria (Lomas et al., 2003). It is therefore essential to prevent proliferation of any residual bacteria after retrieval, during transportation, and during subsequent processing. Maintaining the skin in a refrigerator or at wet ice temperatures prevents the proliferation of most bacteria. To eliminate residual bacteria and fungi in viable skin, an antibiotic/antimycotic cocktail may be used. If used at reduced temperatures (4°C), the skin may be incubated for up to 24 hours in the cocktail; however, only antibiotics that are effective at this temperature should be included. At normothermic temperature (37°C), most antibiotics can be considered; however, the exposure period should be minimized.

For nonviable grafts, a range of sterilization techniques can be considered. Dry heat and autoclaving damage the structure of the skin tissue, including denaturation of collagen, and hence are not suitable. Techniques that have been successfully used include ethylene oxide gas and γ irradiation; however, concerns and limitations of these methods are beginning to appear. Ethylene oxide gas and its reaction product with chloride—ethylene chlorohydrin—are very toxic. Although acceptable levels for these compounds had been proposed, more recent data suggest that there is no safe level of ethylene oxide with respect to genotoxicity. Questions have also been raised about the effectiveness of γ irradiation. Many small viruses and spore-forming bacteria are fairly resistant to γ irradiation. The high doses that would be required to inactivate HIV in a window-period donor (more than 80 kGy) would cause extensive damage to the tissue matrix including collagen denaturation. Therefore, a current consideration is whether "sterilization" can be achieved instead by using combinations of microbial inactivation procedures (Kearney, 1989, 2005; Prolo et al.,1980).

3.3 Time control

Viable skin grafts may be obtained from living donors or, more frequently, from cadaveric donors. In the latter case, the skin becomes ischemic immediately after circulatory arrest. This leads to progressive cell death over a period of days, which is accelerated at higher temperatures. Even if the cadaver is immediately placed into a refrigerator, the body cools at a slow rate, leading to at least some warm ischemia time. Nevertheless, viable skin can still be retrieved up to circa 24 hours after death. If the body is not quickly refrigerated, the skin will be subjected to a much longer warm ischemia period resulting in an accelerated deterioration in viability. Once the skin is removed from the body, it can be cooled rapidly by immersion into a refrigerated solution, thus immediately reducing the rate of cell death. In the other hand, tissue banking standards generally set limits on the maximum warm and cold ischemia times permitted after the death of the donor, because it is known that bacteria from the gut can be released into the vascular system postmortem and migrate to the internal organs and tissues(Kearney, 2005).

3.4 Sample of preparation skin graft from cadaveric donors

3.4.1 Donor selection

Donor skin procurement must comply with local legislation. To ensure skin grafts quality, donors were aged between 8-60 years. The exclusion criteria for harvesting skin are basically the same as for donors of parenchymatous organs. Further exclusion criteria comprise skin diseases, injuries in the areas from which skin may be harvested, and blood samples were tested for HIV, HbA, HbB, HbC and syphilis antibodies.

3.4.2 Skin harvesting

Skin is cleaned with povidone-iodine 10% solution and skin with adipose layer harvested with a knife. Areas from which skin is harvested are limited to the following regions: ventral and dorsal trunk, left and right upper arm, and left and right thigh. Immediately after the removal, grafts were placed in saline, refrigerated and transferred to the processing room. The hair was removed and skin was soaked in 0.1% benzalkonium bromide for 15 min to sterilize. Split skin of 0.2-0.3mm was harvested under sterile conditions by a dermatome. Thereafter split skin was washed extensively and soaked for 10 min 3 times in saline with Penicillin /Streptomycin; then in Neomycin-saline (0.5%) for 10 min, 3 times. All the following procedures are carried out under sterile conditions.

3.5 Sample of preparation skin graft from porcine

Domestic pigs were sacrificed and the skin was washed extensively with soap and water. The hair was removed by razor and the carcass was cleaned with povidone-iodine 10% solution. After cleaning, 0.3 mm to 0.6 mm partial-thickness skin from the pig`s back was harvested with a dermatome. Immediately after the removal, the harvested skins were placed into sterile boxes in normal saline supplemented with penicillin/streptomycin and sent to the laboratory, then soaked in 0.1% benzalkonium bromide for 15 min to sterilise and rinsed thrice in normal saline supplemented with penicillin/streptomycin in a laminar flow hood (Chiu&Burd, 2005).

4. Viable skin grafts preservation

Fresh cadaver allograft is still considered the 'gold standard' biologic dressing for closure of burns. Unfortunately, the use of fresh allografts is severely impeded by their inadequate availability. Skin graft preservation for the purpose of delayed application is still a basic tool in burn treatment and plastic and reconstructive surgery. Even if the skin is placed into an oxygenated nutrientrich medium, ischemic necrosis of the tissue still occurs because the diffusion path from the tissue periphery to the central cells is extensive, oxygen and nutrients cannot diffuse fast enough to supply the cells, and toxic metabolites cannot be removed quickly enough. Therefore, method for the viable storage of skin is to reduce the temperature hence reduces the metabolic rate of the cells and the nutritional demands and metabolite production (Bravo et al,. 2000; Ge et al., 2010; Robb et al., 2001; Sterne et al., 2000).

4.1 Storage in 4°C

As early as 1903, Wentscher reported the successful storage and grafting of skin autografts at temperatures near 0°C for 14 days (Wentscher, 1903). Further studies by Carrel using normothermic and hypothermic storage conditions confirmed the utility of the latter (Carrel, 1912). Eventually, refrigerator storage for skin autografts became the norm in burn units. The simplest technique was to fold the skin so that the cut surfaces were in apposition and then wrap the skin sandwich in tulle gras and/or saline gauze to prevent desiccation. Using this method, autologous skin can be used after around 2 weeks of storage, although cell viability is very low at this point. Unlike autograft, allograft has already lost some viability by the time it is retrieved; therefore, maximum storage times using this method are reduced to 7 or 8 days. Many attempts have been made to extend the refrigerator storage period for skin. The addition of homologous serum at 10% to 33% was found to be beneficial because it provided nutrients and diluted and buffered acids produced as byproducts of metabolism (Allgower & Blocker, 1952). Alternatively, tissue culture media as a source of nutrients and various buffering systems have been evaluated. The buffering systems, however, only extend slightly the period of useful storage. Different methods for storing skin grafts around 4°C are shown in Table 1 and show a large variance in storage time although the storage methods are similar. The main reason for this variance may be criteria incompatible and the absence of reliable detection methods of early research especially before 1970. The storage of skin grafts in a 4°C refrigerator is a simple and practicable technique; however, the skin showed a very slow viability decrease with time stored at 4°C (Chang et al., 1998; DeBono et al., 1998; DeLW, 1980; Matsuka et al., 1993; May & Wainwright, 1985). The preservation time of fresh skin should not exceed 3 days when stored in normal saline and must be used within two weeks even when stored in tissue culture media with 10% serum.

4.2 Storage in -20°C

Wang has success develop non-freeze complex cryoprotectants(10% DMSO, 10% propylene glycol, 10% PEG, 10% glycerin) to avoid ice crystal formation when skin stored in -20°C, the skin remain 76% activity in 14th day, higher than that of stored at liquid nitrogen（60-70%）, then skin activity lower than that of stored at liquid nitrogen in the following time, but still remain 50% viability(the ultimate rate to survival post-transplantation) in 60 days, so skin grafts stored at -20°C should be first consider if skin will be used within 2 weeks.(Wang et al., 2002).

Year	Author	Category	Stored method	Stored time
1903	Wentsch	Human	Exsiccatus ice-box	3-14d
1912	Carrel	chicken	0°C, normal saline with serum, paraffin oil	Several weeks
1912	Carrel	Dog	0°C, normal saline，blood	Several months
1922	Filatov	Human	0°C	Several days
1945	Matthews	Human	3-6°C，normal saline，oxygen deficiency	3-8 weeks
1949	Hanks，Wallace	Rabbit	0-8°C，10% serum	2 weeks
1952	Allgower，Blocker	Human	5°C,10% serum	14 days
1952	Hyatt	Human	4°C,10% serum	185 days
1954	Skoog	Rat	3°C	3 weeks
1957	Perry	Human	4°C，Earle medium，10% serum	84 days
1963	Grasham	Human	4°C，10% serum	6-8 weeks
1971	Bondoc，Burke	Human	4°C，serum	14 days
1972	Lawrene	Human	4°C，normal saline	1 week
1985	May，Wainwright	Pig	4°C，Earle medium	1 week
2002	Alotto	Human	4°C，RPMI 1640, 1% human serum albumin	72 hours
2003	Castagnoli	Human	4°C，RPMI 1640, 1% human serum albumin	4 days
2010	Ge	Pig	4°C，normal saline or DMEM	72/96hours

Table 1. Effect of skin stored around 4°C

4.3 Deep freezing

Deep freezing is preservation of skin grafts in ultra-low temperature refrigerator, which generally maintain temperature under -80°C, and now -150°C ultra-low temperature refrigerator has been made in China. The advantage of this method is simplicity of operator, low maintain cost and relative long preservation time (not exceed 1 year) (May et al., 1985, 1988).

To achieve high viability of skin grafts, cryoprotective agents (CPAs) should be added before freezing. The general properties of cryoprotectants are that the molecules can pass through the cell membrane into the cell and be relatively nontoxic at very high multimolar concentrations. Several cryoprotective chemicals have been identified. CPAs are glycerol and dimethyl sulfoxide. Cryoprotective agents are able to prevent solution effect injury. CPAs mode of action is probably 2-fold. First, they act as solvents for the salt, thus reducing the salt concentration that the cells are subjected to at the high subzero temperatures (where solution effects are most damaging). Secondly, the presence of CPAs within the cells prevent excessive shrinkage of the cells during this cooling phase. Therefore, in the presence of CPAs, it is possible to use very slow cooling rates that minimize intracellular ice formation while protecting the cells against solution effects. High viabilities of all cell types can thus be achieved using this slow cooling rate.

Although CPAs are relatively nontoxic at low temperatures, the toxicity can become significant at higher temperatures. In addition, the rate at which CPAs enter the cells is temperature and CPA dependent, being faster at higher temperatures. Therefore, the optimum temperature and the exposure time need to be validated. The basal medium into which the CPA is dissolved for incubation of the skin tissue should be a balanced salt solution, in which the zwitterionic buffers hydroxyethyl piperazine ethanesulfonic acid (HEPES) and trimethylamino-ethanesulfonic acid (TES) have been shown to work well (Basaran et al., 2006). To avoid osmotic lysis of the cells, either the saline can be added gradually or an impermeant solute such as sucrose can be added to the saline to reduce the difference in osmolarity.

4.4 Cryopreservation

A better method for the long-term preservation of skin grafts is cryopreservation. The cryopreservation technique facilitates the cooling of the tissues to ultralow temperatures while protecting the viability of the cells (Aggarwal et al., 1985; Bondox & Burke, 1971; Cui et al., 2007; Fujita et al., 2000; Marrel et al., 1986). Once the skin is at a temperature lower than -130°C, no further loss of cell viability is incurred. The boiling point of nitrogen gas is -196°C, so skins immersed into liquid nitrogen should be able to keep viabily indefinitely in abstracto.

There are two different cryopreservation protocols used in skin preservation: slow freezing and quick freezing/snap frozen. Slow freezing can be achieved using a controlled-rate cooling apparatus (Blondet et al., 1982). There is an optimum cooling rate for any cell type that produces maximum cell survival. On either side of this optimum, the survival rate falls. In the presence of CPA, a cooling rate of -1 °C per minute will ensure survival of most of the cells within skin tissue. As the cooling rate is increased, cell populations are sequentially and adversely affected. Many cells in the body derived from leukocytes or closely related lineages are known to be exquisitely sensitive to cryogenic injury. The depletion of immunostimulatory "passenger leukocytes" was demonstrated by increasing the cooling rate for pancreatic islets of Langerhans while maintaining the viability of the insulin-producing islet cells (Ingham et al., 1993). This concept of cooling rate–dependent immunomodulation was evaluated for skin tissue. A cooling rate of -30°C/min was shown to maintain the viability of keratinocytes and fibroblasts while reducing the immunogenicity (as assessed by the mixed epidermal cell/lymphocyte response assay) of murine allografts by 95%. This was assumed to be due to an effect of the faster cooling rate on the major immunostimulatory cell in the skin—the Langerhans cell.

Quick freezing/snap frozen is skin vitrification technique. Vitrification is defined as "the instant solidification of a solution brought about by an extreme elevation in viscosity during cooling, without ice crystal formation". In other words, vitrification is faster and lacks some of the typical disadvantages seen in traditional slow freezing (Mukaida, 2003). It bypasses the ice-crystal formation phase and instantaneously solidifies into a glass-like structure, moves the water directly into a glass-like phase. In a glass, the molecules do not rearrange themselves into grainy ice crystals as the solution cools, but instead become locked together while still randomly arranged as in a fluid, forming a "solid liquid" as the temperature falls below the glass transition temperature (Silvestre et al., 2002). This technique was simple, and no expensive equipment was needed. Initially, this method needed a 2-step procedure because the cryoprotective agent was toxic. Kasai et al., (1990) modified this impractical to a 1-step method and incubated the skin with vitrification solution at room temperature and was transferred directly into liquid nitrogen.

Ben-Bassat et al., (1996, 2001) evaluation graft performance of cryopreserved cadaveric skin by programmed freezing (1°C/min). The results demonstrate that graft performance of cryopreserved skin decreased with time as seen in the lower percent of samples with high scores of separate histologic criteria after prolonged storage (Ben-Bassat et al., 1996). Nevertheless, paired comparison analysis between cryopreserved and fresh skin indicated that this decrease was not significant for storage of 5 years; however, it was highly significant for 6 years of storage (Ben-Bassat et al., 2001).
Table 2 shows the distinction of different preservation and the viability of skin frozen at -20°C attenuated to 50% (the ultimate rate to survival post-transplantation) in 60 days. Skin grafts stored at -20°C should be used within two months. To be similar, the skins should be transplanted in one year of freezing in -80°C and 5 years in liquid nitrogen. Viability declines rapidly after thawing of the skin and further storage before use cannot be recommended.

	Commom refrigerator	Freezer	ultra-low temperature refrigerator	Liquid nitrogen
Temperature(°C)	4	-18～-20	-80	-196
Equipment cost	Cheap	Cheap	Costly	moderately
Sustain cost	Cheap	Cheap	Cheap	Costly
Electricity effect	Great	Great	Great	None
Storage time	3～7days	60days	1 year	5 years
Viability（%）	30～80	50～60	50～60	60～70

Table 2. Comparison of different preservation methods

5. Nonviable skin grafts preservation

With non-viable skin (or dermis) there is no requirement to maintain the viability of tlhe skin cells. Nevertheless, it is still important that degradative changes do not adversely affect the tissue matrix and bacteria are not allowed to proliferate; therefore, many of the practices discussed earlier will still apply. A major difference from viable skin, however, is that much more effective disinfection or sterilisation methods can be applied to the skin, including virucidal treatments.

5.1 Freeze drying

In the early 1950s, the US Navy Tissue Bank was the first to commence large-scale freeze drying of human tissues for implantation. In 1955, the use of freeze-dried skin was first reported (Brown et al., 1955). It was subsequently shown that freeze drying reduced the immunogenicity of skin without interfering with its beneficial properties（Abbott & Hembree , 1970）.This process involves the removal of water from skin in the frozen state by sublimation, which is achieved by applying a vacuum to the tissue and condensing the removed water molecules downstream. Sublimation from the frozen state helps to protect molecules that would otherwise be adversely affected by high salt concentrations at higher temperatures, for example, denaturation of proteins. Drying must continue until enough water has been removed to prevent degradation reactions, which equates to less than 5% residual water as measured gravimetrically. Although accepted in most tissue banking standards, "residual water" is not identical to "water activity", which is the most appropriate measure.

5.2 Glycerolization preservation

In 1980s, glycerin was applied in clinical practice as skin graft preservation fluid, and had very good effect (Hermans, 1989; Huang et al., 2004; Richter et al., 1997; Van Baare et al., 1994,1998; Vuola & Pipping, 2002). EuroSkin Bank has done considerable fruitful work in the area and developed a solute preservation method using glycerol (De Backere & Mackie, 1997; Mackie, 1997). The skin was incubated in successively more concentrated glycerol solutions (50%, 70%, and 85%) and maintained long term in 85% glycerol. More recently, the glycerol and water flux kinetics have been characterized and a more efficient validated protocol was proposed. Study demonstrated that the 85% concentration originally chosen by the Euroskin Bank is optimal for minimizing degradative reactions (Ross & Kearney, 2004). It is very important that the glycerol is removed from the skin before clinical use. Failure to remove glycerol may lead to high systemic concentrations when used on open wounds. This is achieved by repeatedly washing the skin in physiological saline, and at least 30 to 60 minutes are required to remove most of the glycerol.

5.3 Glutaraldehyde preservation

As early as 1975, Schetnter reported the successful grafting of glutaraldehyde- preserved skin in clinical (Schetnter, 1975). The morphology of skin grafts has not evident change after treated with glutaraldehyde, and skin antigenicity was greatly reduced because antigen determinant site was closed by cross-linking of protein in the skin grafts. Glutaraldehyde-treated skin grafts can be used for escharectomy and tangential excision wounds and granulation wound covering, and has been shown to promote the formation of granulation tissues. However, such skin grafts have least elasticity, that is, with the extension of preservation duration, the skin becomes harder. Fresh allograft skin or lyophilized skin shall be immersed in 0.5% glutaraldehyde solution for 7-20min and be washed with normal saline for three times prior to use. There is no evident change in the elasticity and softeness of such skin, but its antignicity is decreased, which helps to extend the adhesion duration of grafted skin.

5.4 Irradiation preservation

Irradiated porcine skin is the most commonly used burn wound covering in China. Fresh porcine skin graft is sealed in a plastic bag and is irradiated with 60Co or an accelerator, then put into an ordinary refrigerator for preservation. After being irradiated, porcine skin can achieve integral asepsis, and its antignicity can be decreased. For gamma irradiation, the most resistant microorganisms are viruses, D10-values as high as 13 KGy have been reported for certain small viruses. Application of the commonest used dosage (25 KGy) to these viruses would only reduce the bioburden by 2 logs10. The high doses that would be required to inactivate HIV in a window-period donor (more than 80 kGy) would cause extensive damage to the tissue matrix including collagen denaturation. There are two possible effects on the macromolecular structure of skin matrix resulting from ionising irradiation. The first is scission which results in the breaking of bonds thus weakening the matrix. In the presence of water a second process involves crosslinking by new bond formation resulting from the generation of free radicals which may lead to stiffening of the matrix.

6. Quality control

A variety of national/international organisations have issued standards or guidelines for tissue banking, including the National Blood Service, British Association for Tissue Banking, and European Association of Tissue Banks, etc (Baxter, 1985; Ben-Bassat et al., 2000; British Association for Tissue Banking, 2011; Chua et al., 2004; European Association of Tissue Banks, 2011; Freedlander et al., 1998; Janezic, 1999; Kalter, 1997; Kearney, 1998; May, 1990; Pillipp et al., 2004; Pianigiani et al., 2005). The core principle of skin banking quality control is to avoid the risk of cross infection and provide high-quality skin grafts for clinical. Therefore, donor selection, microbial/viral tests, skin viability detection and transplantation performance will be discussed in this paper.

6.1 Donor selection

With respect to medical/behavioural history screening, the regulatory and standards documents are once again very specific with a good deal of international consensus. Sources of medical/behavioural information include the next of kin (or partner/close friend) of the deceased who must be interviewed regarding medical history and any factors, practices or behaviour that may have increased the risk of exposure to HIV/Hepatitis. In addition, the family doctor, hospital records, and autopsy report should be consulted as additional sources of medical and behavioural history. Evaluation of the risk of virus exposure must be explored in detail with other aspects of medical and behavioural history. The exclusion criteria for harvesting skin are basically the same as for donors of parenchymatous organs including cancer, diseases of unknown aetiology and various viral, bacterial and parasitic diseases. Further exclusion criteria comprise other skin diseases and injuries in the areas from which skin may be harvested.

6.2 Microbial/viral tests

There is a widespread consensus on the testing of donors to preclude certain virological diseases, including HIV, Hepatitis B, Hepatitis C, syphilis antibodies ,and in general these follow the National Blood Service testing regimens for each country. Screening for CMV is important when recipients are CMV negative and will receive immunosuppressive drugs following organ transplantation. However, the natural immunosuppression associated with burns does not appear to lead to CMV related problems in skin allograft recipients. Many tissue banks do not screen for CMV. The microbial tests are generally done on allograft samples and the viral tests on blood samples.Skin samples for microbial tests are incubated in Thioglycollate and Roswell Park Memorial Institute (RPMI) 1640 without antibiotics, in a 37°C incubator for 10 days.

6.3 Skin viability

The viability of graft skin is fundamental for surgical procedures involving graft taking, and the American Association of Tissue Banks indicates that the viability of skin is an essential prerequisite for good-quality grafts (American Association of Tissue Banks, 2011). It is a necessity that a skin bank should certify, not only the sterility, but also the viability of the skin allografts used and that routine quality controls be carried out to certify that grafts are viable before transplantation. The of viability assays is two-fold: one is that of supplying an "experimental assay": used to optimize the various parts of a preservation procedure during experimental development. The other offers a "predictive assay": used to predict the "quality" of an individual sample that has been stored by an established tested technique. Various methods, both qualitative and quantitative, are currently used to determine skin grafts viability such as cell culture, succinate dehydrogenase, trypan blue dye, skin oxygen consumption, Tetrazolium salts (MTT/WST-1), SYTO/EB dyes and so on (Alotto et al., 2002). The MTT method is most widely used because it is simple, quick and precise (Castagnoli et al., 2003; Klein, 1996; Pegg, 1989; Yang et al., 2000; Zieger et al., 1993).

6.4 Transplantation performance

Skin transplantation experiment is a straightforward and reliable skin graft quality evaluation method. For any skin graft and preservation method, the final result is to identify that the skin graft can survive in the living body. For evaluation of transplantation performance of preserved skin, samples of skin were often grafted onto mice and rats and the experiment animals were sacrificed after 4 or 7 days. The grafts were then assessed by gross inspection including adherence to wound bed, color and pliability and by histologic evaluation including epidermis integrity, epidermal–dermal junction, collagen organization, the presence of fibroblasts and graft adherence (Cinamon et al., 1993).

7. Conclusions

Skin graft preservation for the purpose of delayed application is still a basic tool in burn treatment and plastic and reconstructive surgery. It is therefore important to provide a framework for selecting optimal guidelines for procurement, processing, preservation, and quality control of skin grafts for doctors and researchers, thus ensuring high levels of safety and efficacy of skin grafts.

8. References

Abbot, W.M. & Hembree, J.S. (1970). Absence of antigenicity in freeze-dried skin allografts. *Cryobiology*, Vol.6, No.5,(Mar-Apr),pp. 416-418, 0011-2240

Aggarwal, S.J.; Baxter, C.R. & Diller, KR. (1985). Cryopreservation of skin: an assessment of current clinical applicability. *J Burn Care Rehabil*, Vol.6,No.6,(Nov-Dec),pp.469-476, 0273-8481

Allgower, M. & Blocker, T.G. (1952). Viability of skin in relation to various methods of storage. *Tex Rep Biol Med*, Vol.10, No.1, (Jan), pp.3-21, 0040-4675

Alotto, D.; Ariotti, S.; Graziano, S.; Verrua, R.; Stella, M. & Magliacani, G., et al. (2002). The role of quality control in a skin bank: tissue viability determination. *Cell Tissue Bank,* Vol.3, No.1, (Nov),pp.3–10. 1389-9333

American Association of Tissue Banks. Standards. Available from: www.aatb.org

Basaran, O.; Ozdemir, H.; Kut, A.; Sahin, F.I.; Deniz, M.. & Sakallioglu, E.A., et al. (2006). Effects of different preservation solutions on skin graft epidermal cell viability and graft performance in a rat model. *Burns,*Vol.32,No.4, (Jun),pp.423–429, 0305-4179

Baxter, C.R. (1985). Skin banking in the USA. *J Burn Care Rehabil,* Vol.6, No.4, (Jun-Aug), pp.322,0273-8481

Ben-Bassat, H.; Chaouat, M.; Segal, N.; Zumai, E.; Wexler, M.R. & Eldad, A. (2001).How long can cryopreserved skin be stored to maintain adequate graft performance? *Burns,* Vol.27,No.5,(Aug),pp.425-431. 0305-4179

Ben-Bassat, H.; Chaouat, M. ; Zumai, E. ; Segal, N. ; Cinamon, U. & Ron, M., et al.(2000). The Israel National Bank: quality assurance and graft performance of stored tissues. *Cell Tissue Bank,* Vol.1, No.4, pp.303–312, 1389-9333

Ben-Bassat, H.; Strauss, N.; Ron, M.; Chaouat, M.; Breiterman, S. & Israeli, A., et al. (1996). Transplantation performance of human skin cryopreserved by programmed or stepwise freezing and stored at −80°C or −180°C. *J Burn Care Rehabil,* Vol.17, No.5, (Sep-Oct),pp.17:421-428, 0273-8481

Blome-Eberwein, S.; Jester, A.; Kuentscher, M.; Raff, T.; Germann, G. & Pelzer, M., et al. (2002). Clinical practice of glycerol preserved allograft skin coverage. *Burns,* Vol.28, No.Suppl.1, (Oct),pp.S10-12. 0305-4179

Blondet, R.; Gibert-Thevenin, M.A.; Pierre, C. & Ehrsam, A. (1982). Skin preservation by programmed freezing. *Br J Plast Surg,*Vol.35, No.4, (Oct), pp.530-536. 0007-1226

Bondox, C.C. & Burke, H.F. (1971). Clinical experience with viable frozen human skin and frozen skin bank. *Ann Surg,*Vol.174, No.3, (Sep), pp.371–382. 0003-4932

Bravo, D.; Rigley, T.H.; Gibran, N.; Strong, D.M. & Newman-Gage, H. (2000).Effect of storage and preservation methods on viability in transplantable human skin allografts. *Burns,*Vol.26, No.4, (Jun), pp.367-378, 0305-4179

British Association for Tissue Banking. General standards and technical guidelines. Available from: www.batb.org.uk/standards.htm

Brown, J.B.; Fryer, M.P. & Zaydon T.J. (1955). A skin bank for postmortem homografts. *Surg Gynecol Obstet,* Vol.101, No.4, (Oct), pp. 401-412, 0039-6087

Carrel A. (1912). The preservation of tissues and its application in surgery. *J Am Med Assoc,* Vol.59, No.7, (Jun); 523-527.0002-9955

Castagnoli, C.; Alotto, D. ; Cambieri, I. ; Casimiri, R. ; Aluffi, M. & Stella, M., et al. (2003). Evaluation of donor skin viability: fresh and cryopreserved skin using tetrazolioum salt assay. *Burns,*Vol.29, No.8, (Dec), pp.759–767, 0305-4179

Chiu, T. & Burd, A. (2005). "Xenograft" dressing in the treatment of burns. *Clin Dermatol,* Vol.23, No.4,(Oct), pp. 419–423, 1175-0561

Chang, P.; Rosenquist, M.D.; Lewis, R.W. & Kealey, G.P. (1998). A study of functional viability and metabolic degeneration of human skin stored at 4°C. *J Burn Care Rehabil,* Vol.19, No.1 Pt 1,(Jan-Feb),pp.25-28, 0273-8481

Chua, A.; Song, C. ; Chai, A. ; Chan, L. & Tan, K.C. (2004). The impact of banking and the use of its cadaveric skin allografts for severe burn victims in Singapore. *Burns,* Vol.30, No.7, (Nov), pp.696–700, 0305-4179

Cinamon, U.; Eldad, A.; Chaouat, M.; Wexler, R.M.; Israeli, A. & Zanger, U., et al. (1993). A simplified testing system to evaluate performance after transplantation of human skin preserved in glycerol or in liquid nitrogen. *J Burn Care Rehabil,*Vol.14, No.4, (Jul-Aug), pp.435–439, 0273-8481

Clark, J. (1987). HIV transmission and skin grafts. *Lancet,* Vol.329, No.8539, (Apr),pp.983. 0140-6736

Cui, X.; Gao, D.Y.; Fink, B.F.; Vasconez, H.C. & Rinker, B. (2007). Cryopreservation of composite tissues and transplantation: Preliminary studies. *Cryobiology,* Vol.55, No.3, (Dec), pp.295-304, 0011-2240.

DeBackere, A.C.J. & Mackie, D. (1997). The Euro Skin Bank: development and application of glycerol-preserved allografts. *J Burn Care Rehabil,* Vol.18, No.1 Pt 2,(Jan-Feb),pp.7-9, 0273-8481

DeBono, R.; Rao, G.S. & Berry, R.B. (1998). The survival of human skin stored by refrigeration at 4°C in MacCoy's 5A medium: does oxygenation of the medium improve storage time? *Plast Reconstr Surg,*Vol.102,No.1,(Jul),pp.78-83, 0032-1052

De, L.W.; De, W.F. & Penninckx, F. (1980). Metabolic changes in human skin preserved at −3°C and at −196°C. *Cryobiology,* Vol.17, No.1,(Feb),pp.46-53,0011-2240

Delmonico, F. (1998). Organ donor screening for infectious diseases. *Transplantation,* Vol.65, No.5, (Mar),pp.603-610, 2090-0015

European Association of Tissue Banks. Standards. Available from: www.eatb.de/html/standards.htm.

Freedlander, E.; Boyce, S.; Ghosh, M.; Ralston, D.R. & MacNeil, S. (1998). Skin banking in the UK: the need for proper organization. *Burns,*Vol.24, No.1,(Feb),pp.19–24, 0305-4179

Fujita, T.; Takami, Y.; Ezoe, K.; Saito, T.; Sato, A.K. & Takeda, N., et al. (2000). Successful preservation of human skin by vitrification. *J Burn Care Rehabil,* Vol.21, No.4, (Jul-Aug), pp.304-309, 0273-8481

Ge, L.; Sun, L.; Chen, J.; Mao, X.; Kong, Y. & Xiong, F., et al. (2010). The viability change of pigskin in vitro. Burns,Vol.36, No.4,(Jun),pp.533-538, 0305-4179

Hermans, M.H.E. (1989). Clinical experience with glycerol-preserved donor skin treatment in partial thickness burns. *Burns* ,Vol.15, No.1,(Feb),pp.57-59, 0305-4179

Holder, I.A.; Robb, E. & Kagan, R. (1998). Antimicrobial mixtures used by tissue banks for harvested skin: comperative in vitro activity. *Burns,* Vol.24, No.7, (Nov), pp.604-608, 0305-4179

Huang, Q.; Pegg, D.E. & Kearney, J.N. (2004). Banking of non-viable skin allografts using high concentrations of glycerol or propylene glycol. *Cell Tissue Bank,* Vol.5,No.1, pp.3-21, 1389-9333

Ingham, E.; Matthews, B.; Kearney, J.N. & Gowland, G. (1993). The effects of variation of cryopreservation protocols on the immunogenicity of allogeneic skin grafts. *Cryobiology,* Vol.30, No.5,(Oct), pp.443-458, 0011-2240

Janezic, T.F. (1999). Then and now: 25 years at the Ljubljana burns unit skin bank. *Burns,*Vol.25, No.7,(Nov),pp.599–602, 0305-4179

Kalter, E.S.; de By, T.M. (1997). Tissue banking programmes in Europe. *Br Med Bull,* Vol.53, No.4, pp.798-816, 0007-1420

Kasai, M.; Komi, J. H.; Takakamo, A.; Tsudera, H.; Sakurai, T. & Machida, T. (1990). A simple method for mouse embryo cryopreservation in a low toxicity vitrification solution, without appreciable loss of viability. *J Reprod Fertil,* Vol.89,No.1, (May), pp. 91-97, 0022-4251

Kearney, J.N. (1998). Quality issues in skin banking: a review. *Burns,*Vol.24, No.4, (Jun), pp.299-305. 0305-4179

Kearney, J.N. (2005). Guidelines on processing and clinical use of skin allografts. *Clin Dermatol* , Vol.23,No.4,(Jul-Aug),pp.357-364,1507-5516

Kearney, J.N.; Harnby, D.; Gowland, G. & Holland K.T. (1984). The follicular distribution and abundance of resident bacteria on human skin. *J Gen Microbiol.* Vol.130, No.4, (Apr), 130:797- 801.

Kearney, J.N.; Franklin, U.C.; Aguirregoicoa, V. & Holland, K.T. (1989). Evaluation of ethylene oxide sterilisation of tissue implants. *J Hosp Infect,* Vol.13, No.1, (Jan), pp.71-80, 0195-6701

Klein, M.B.; Shaw, D.; Barese, S.; Chapo, G.A. & Cuono, C.B. (1996). Reliable and cost-effective in vitro assay of skin viability for skin banks and burn centers. *J Burn Care Rehabil,* Vol.17, No.6 Pt 1, (Nov-Dec),pp.565–570, 0273-8481

Li, A. (2001).*LI AO Burns,* 1st ed., Shanghai Science & Technique Press, ISBN:7-5323-5910-7, Shanghai, China

Lomas, R.J.; Cruse-Sawyer, J.E.; Simpson, C.; Ingham, E.; Bojar, R. & Kearney, J.N. (2003). Assessment of the biological properties of human split skin allografts disinfected with peracetic acid and preserved in glycerol. *Burns,*Vol.29, No.6,(Sep),pp.515-525, 0305-4179

Mackie, D.P. (1997). The Euro skin bank: development and application of glycerol-preserved allografts. *J Burn Care Rehabil,* Vol.18, No.1 Pt 2,(Jan-Feb),pp.S7-9, 0273-8481

Marrel, S.W.; Shelby, J.; Saflle, J.R.; Krueger, G.G. & Navar, P.D. (1986). An invivo test of viability for cryopreserved human skin. *Curr Surg,*Vol.43, No.4, (Jul-Aug), pp.296–300, 0149-7944

Matsuka, K.; Hata, Y.; Yano, K.; Ito, O. & Matsuda, H. (1993). Epidermal cell viability in rat skin preserved at 4 degrees C. *Ann Plast Surg,* Vol.31, No.4,(Oct),pp.358–363, 1536-3708

May, S.R. (1990). The future of skin banking. *J Burn Care Rehabil,* Vol.11, No.5, (Sep-Oct), pp.484-486, 0273-8481

May, S.R.; Guttman, R.M. & Wainwright, J.F. (1985). Cryopreservation of skin using an insulated heat sink box stored at -70°C. *Cryobiology,*Vol.22,No.3,(Jun),pp.205-214, 0011-2240

May, S.R. & Roberts, D.P. (1988). Development of a passive device for freezing large amounts of transplantable skin at one time in a -70°C mechanical refrigerator. *Cryobiology,* Vol.25, No.3,(Jun),pp.186-196, 0011-2240

May, S.R. & Wainwright, J.F. (1985). Integrated study of the structural and metabolic degeneration of skin during 4°C storage in nutrient medium. *Cryobiology,* Vol.22, No.1, (Feb), pp.18-34, 0011-2240

Mukaida, T.; Nakamura, S.; Tomiyama, T.; Wada, S.; Oka, C.; Kasai, M. & Takahashi, K. (2003). Vitrification of human blastocysts using cryoloops: clinical outcome of 223 cycles. *Hum Reprod.* Vol.18,No.2, (Feb), pp.384-391, 0268-1161

Ninnmann, J.L.; Fisher, J.C. & Frank, H.A. (1978). Clinical skin banking: a simplified system for processing, storage and retrieval of human allografts. *J Trauma,* Vol.18, No.10, (Oct), pp.723–725. 0022-5282

Pegg, D.E. (1989). Viability assays for preserved cells, tissues, and organs. *Cryobiology,* Vol.26, No.3,(Jun),pp.212–231, 0011-2240

Philipp, S.; Hans, L. & Hans-Ulrich, L. (2004). Five Years of Experience with the Dortmund Skin Bank. *Euro J Trauma,*Vol.30,No.2,(Mar),pp.116-119, 1439-0590

Pianigiani, E.; Ierardi, F.; Cherubini, D.S.F. & Andreassi, A. (2005). Skin bank organization. *Clin Dermatol,* Vol.23,No.4,(Jul-Aug),pp.353-356, 1175-0561

Prolo, D.J.; Pedrotti, P.W. & White DH. (1980). Ethylene oxide sterilisation of bone, dura mater and fascia lata for human transplantation. *Neurosurgery,* Vol.6, No.5, (May), pp.529-539, 1524-4040

Richter, C.D.; Hoekstra, M.J.; van Baare, J.; du Pont, J.S. & Kamperdijk, E.W.A. (1997). Immunogenicity of glycerol-preserved human cadaveric skin in vitro. *J Burn Care Rehabil,* Vol.18,No.3,(May-Jun),pp.228-233, 0273-8481

Robb, E.C.; Bechmann, N.; Plessinger, R.T.; Boyce, S.T.; Warden, G.D. & Kagan, R.J. (2001). Storage media and temperature maintain normal anatomy of cadaveric human skin for transplantation to full-thickness skin wounds. *J Burn Care Rehabil,* Vol.22, No.6, (Nov-Dec),pp.393-396, 0273-8481

Ross, A. & Kearney, J.N. (2004). The measurement of water activity in allogeneic skin grafts preserved using high concentration glycerol or propylene glycol. *Cell Tissue Bank,* Vol.5, No.1, pp.37- 44, 1389-9333

Schechter, I. (1975). Prolonged retention of glutaraldehyde-treated skin allografts and xenografts: immunological and histological studies. *Ann Surg,* Vol.182, No.6, (Dec), pp.699-704, 0003-4932

Silvestre, M.A.; Saeed, A.M.; Escribá, M.J. & García-Ximénez, F. (2002). Vitrification and rapid freezing of rabbit fetal tissues and skin samples from rabbits and pigs. *Theriogenology,* Vol.58, No.1,(Jul),pp.69-76, 0093-691X

Sterne, G.D.; Titley, O.G. & Christie, J.L. (2000) A qualitative histological assessment of various storage conditions on short term preservation of human split skin grafts.Br *J Plast Surg,* Vol.53,No.4,(Jun),pp.331-336, 0007-1226

Van Baare, J.; Buitenwerf, J.; Hoekstra, M.J. & du Pont, J.S. (1994). Virucidal effect of glycerol as used in donor skin preservation. *Burns,* Vol.20, suppl. 1,pp.S77-S80,0305-4179

Van, Baare. J.; Cameron, P.U.; Vardaxis, N.; Pagnon, J.; Reece, J. & Middelkoop, E., et al. (1998). Comparison of glycerol preservation with cryopreservation methods on HIV-1 inactivation. *J Burn Care Rehabil,* Vol.19,No.6,(Nov-Dec),pp.494-500, 0273-8481

Vuola, J. & Pipping, D. (2002). Maintaining a glycerolized skin bank—a practical approach. *Burns,* Vol.28, Suppl. 1, (Oct), pp.S31-33,0305-4179

Wang X.H.; Wu J.; Zhang N.; Chen X.W.; Zhou L.X. & Xiao G.X. An experimental study on preservation of human split thickness skin samples with -20°C non-freezing composite cryoprotective solution. *ACTA Academiae Medicinae Militaris Tertiae* . Vol.24, No.2, (Feb), pp.225-226, 1000-5404

Wentscher, J. (1903). A further contribution about the survivability of human epidermal cells. *Dtsch Z Chir,* Vol..70, pp.21-44, 0367-0023

Yang, H.; Jia, X.M.; Acker, J.P.; Lung, G. & McGann, L.E. (2000). Routine assessment of viability in split-thickness skin. *J Burn Care Rahabil,* Vol.21,No.2,(Mar-Apr), pp.99–104, 0273-8481

Zhu, Z.M.; Chai, J.K. & Jia, X.M. (2002). *Basic and application of skin preservation,* 1st ed., People's military medical publisher, ISBN: 7-80157-604-7, Beijing, China

Zieger, M.A.J.; Tredget, E.E. & McGann, L.E. (1993). A simple, effective system for assessing viability in split-thickness skin with the use of oxygen consumption. *J Burn Care Rehabil,* Vol.14,No.3,(May-Jun),pp.310-318, 0273-8481

Zieger, M.A.J.; Tredget, E.E.; Sykes, E.D. & McGann, L.E. (1997). Injury and protection in split-thickness skin after very rapid cooling and warming. *Cryobiology,*Vol.35,No.1, (Aug), pp.53-69, 0011-2240

14

Comparative Study of Skin Graft Tolerance and Rejection in the Frog *Xenopus Laevis*

Hristina Nedelkovska and Jacques Robert
Department of Microbiology and Immunology, University of Rochester Medical Center, Rochester USA

1. Introduction

Over the last few decades, the amphibian *Xenopus laevis*[1] has been used as a unique comparative model to study the developmental and immunological aspects of tissue transplantation as well as self tolerance (Du Pasquier, Schwager et al. 1989; Robert and Ohta 2009). The immune system of *X. laevis*, one of the best defined outside mammals and chickens, is fundamentally similar to that of mammals. Notably, the evolutionary distance of *X. laevis* from mammals permits distinguishing species-specific adaptations from more conserved features of the immune system. In addition, advanced genetic resources including the full genome sequence of the *X. leavis* sister species *X. tropicalis*, a large collection of EST, cDNA and genomic (BAC, Fosmid) libraries for both species, efficient transgenesis and genome wide mutagenesis has markedly empowered *X. laevis* as a biomedical model. Furthermore, several different major histocompatability complex (MHC) defined inbred strains of *X. laevis*, as well as clones sharing identical MHC haplotypes but differing at multiple minor histocompatibility (H) loci, provide a unique opportunity to study T cell regulation *in vivo* by skin graft. More information about these resources can be found on the Xenbase website (http://www.xenbase.org/common/) (Bowes, Snyder et al. 2009) and the *X. laevis* research resource for immunobiology (http://www.urmc.rochester.edu/mbi/resources/Xenopus/) (Robert 2006).

The objectives of this review are first to provide short background information on the immune system and skin graft biology in *X. laevis*, and then to examine the use of the minor H-Antigen (Ag)-disparate skin grafting model system in *X. laevis* isogenic clones and to investigate *in vivo* the immunostimulatory properties of certain heat shock proteins (hsps) such as gp96 and hsp70 with particular emphasis on minor H-Ag specific T cell responses. We will also consider the possible role of nonclassical MHC class Ib molecules in this context. Furthermore, we will re-evaluate old data on induction of long term immunological memory and immune tolerance in *X. laevis* larvae to skin graft Ags in the context of immune regulation. Finally, we will discuss the possibility to use hsps and new genetic tools

[1] All animals were handled under strict laboratory and UCAR regulations (Approval number 100577 / 2003-151), minimizing discomfort at all times.

(genomic and transgenic technology) to revisit this immune regulation to skin Ags during development of *X. laevis*. It is our conviction that by integrating the unique biological features of *X. laevis* with the recently advanced genetic resources of this comparative model, it will be possible to answer critical questions about the development of self-tolerance as well as autoimmunity.

2. The immune system of *Xenopus laevis*

The frog *X. laevis* has been used to study skin graft rejection as well as tolerance for the last few decades. The immune system of *X. laevis*, a genus whose common ancestors with mammals diverged 350 million years ago (Kobel and Du Pasquier 1975; Evans 2008), is fundamentally similar to that of mammals. Importantly, this extensive evolutionary distance allows one to distinguish species-specific adaptation from conserved features of the immune system. The *X. laevis* immune system is characterized by T and B lymphocytes with RAG-mediated rearranging TCR and Ig genes, MHC class I- and class II-restricted T cell recognition (Du Pasquier, Schwager et al. 1989; Robert and Ohta 2009), as well as innate immune cells such as macrophages and NK cell (Horton, Horton et al. 1998; Horton, Minter et al. 2000; Robert, Ramanayake et al. 2008; Morales, Abramowitz et al. 2010). Interestingly, *X. laevis* lacks lymph nodes but it does have both a thymus and a spleen similarly to mammals.

The additional developmental transition occurring during metamorphosis in *X. laevis* results in two different life stages, the larvae and the adult, which provides a unique opportunity of working with two distinct immune systems. Unlike mammals, larvae have external development; therefore, they are amenable to experimental manipulation and there is easy accessibility of early developmental stages free of maternal influences. For example, since large areas of the larvae are transparent, the thymus is easily distinguishable and it is also relatively simple to perform thymectomy on these animals which will render them free of T cells in their larval as well as adult life. During metamorphosis the immune system undergoes a remarkable developmental transformation during which surface major histocompatability complex (MHC) class Ia (class Ia) expression becomes detectible for the first time on erythrocytes and splenic leukocytes (Flajnik, Kaufman et al. 1986; Flajnik and Du Pasquier 1988; Rollins-Smith, Flajnik et al. 1994). Interestingly, NK cells that are not detected during larval life emerge concurrently with class Ia expression (Horton, Stewart et al. 2003). *X. laevis* larvae are different from adults since they are naturally class Ia deficient, but importantly these animals are immunocompetent and they have thymus-dependent CD8 T cells (Flajnik, Kaufman et al. 1986). In addition, certain nonclassical MHC class Ib (class Ib) genes have been found to be expressed in the thymic anlage very early in ontogeny and preferentially by thymocytes (Goyos, Ohta et al. 2009; Goyos, Sowa et al. 2011). The implication of this on the T cell repertoire of early larval stages is under investigation. MHC class II antigen expression during larval life is restricted to the thymic epithelium centrally, and to B lymphocytes and accessory cells in the periphery: whereas, it is constitutively expressed on virtually all thymocytes and mature peripheral T as well as B cells in adults (Flajnik, Kaufman et al. 1986; Du Pasquier and Flajnik 1990; Flajnik, Ferrone et al. 1990).

Thus, the larval and adult *X. laevis* immune systems have critical differences as well as similarities. As such, comparisons between these two developmental stages afford unique opportunities to investigate *in vivo* developmental and immunological aspects of tissue transplantation. Also the differential expression of class Ia together with the ease of larval experimental manipulation allows us to explore questions regarding MHC-restriction, autoimmunity, and the development of self-tolerance that can not be easily studied in other animal models.

A major attribute of the *X. laevis* model is the availability of different MHC-defined strains and clones. In addition to the MHC homozygous inbred strains, the J and F strains (Du Pasquier and Chardonnens 1975; Tochinai and Katagiri 1975), the *X. laevis* model also includes MHC-defined isogenic clones of frogs, such as the LG-15 and LG-6 that share the same heterozygous MHC haplotypes (a/c) but differ at multiple minor histocompatability (H) loci (Kobel and Du Pasquier 1975; Kobel and Du Pasquier 1977). These clones are generated by gynogenesis, a procedure where diploid eggs from *X. laevis/X. gilli* hybrids are only activated by UV irradiated sperm, and thus the spermatozoid DNA does not contribute any genetic material to the offspring. This system allows us to easily pool cells from different frogs and perform adoptive cell transfers since the clones share identical genetic make up (Maniero and Robert 2004). In addition, we also have available a transplantable thymic lymphoid tumor named 15/0 (originally a spontaneously growing tumor derived from a LG-15 clone) that is tumorigenic in both LG-15 and LG-6 clones (Robert, Guiet et al. 1994; Robert, Guiet et al. 1995; Robert and Cohen 1998). Interestingly this tumor does not have class Ia protein expression however it does express several class Ib molecules (Robert, Guiet et al. 1994; Salter-Cid, Nonaka et al. 1998; Rau, Cohen et al. 2001). As a result, the accessibility of different animals and reagents has provided us the unique opportunity to study T cell regulation *in vivo* by skin transplantation.

3. Skin graft rejection in adult *Xenopus laevis*

Skin graft rejection is a well-established technique in *X. laevis* that has been used for determining the segregation of both major and minor H-Ag loci (Chardonnens and Du Pasquier 1973; Du Pasquier and Bernard 1980; Ramanayake, Simon et al. 2007).

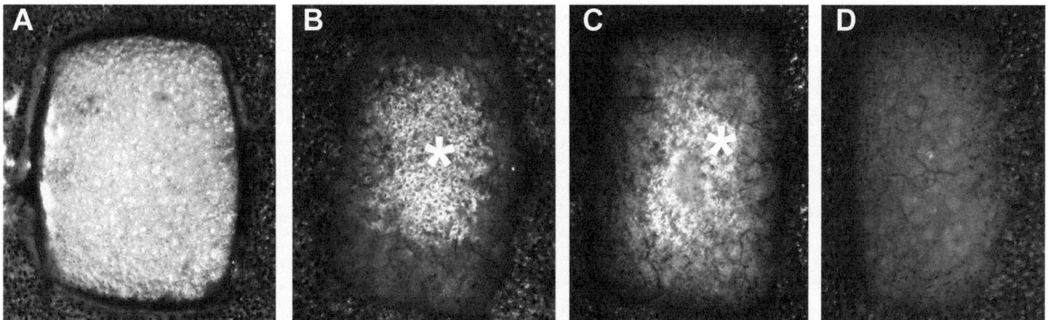

Fig. 1. Skin graft rejection in *Xenopus laevis*. (A) Allograft one day post transplantation, 0% rejection. The entire graft appears silvery due to the presence of irridophores. In (B) and (C) the grafts are undergoing rejection 50 and 90% respectively. (*) indicates areas of the graft that are still surviving. The rejected areas of the grafts are highly vascularized. (D) Representative image of a fully (100%) rejected skin graft. This graft is "dull" and does not have any more surviving irridophores.

We have recently described this technique in details (Nedelkovska, Cruz-Luna et al. 2010). Succinctly, *X. laevis* adults are skin grafted by cutting a 5mm^2 piece of donor ventral skin (abdominal skin which appears silvery due to the presence of irridophores) and inserting it under the dorsal skin of the recipient (Chardonnens and Du Pasquier 1973; Nedelkovska, Cruz-Luna et al. 2010). It is critical to handle the graft gently and avoid damage with the forceps, which would obscure the results. Also care must be taken to avoid introducing large air bubbles under the skin because that can cause displacement or loss of the graft. After 24 hours, a window of overlaying host skin covering the graft is removed and then the graft can be easily visualized using a dissecting microscope. Skin graft rejection is then monitored by determining the percent of irridophore destruction over time. Rejection is considered complete when the entire exposed graft has become "dull" and all the irridophores have been entirely destroyed (Figure 1).

3.1 Conserved role of T cells in skin graft rejection

In adult *X. laevis,* as in mammals, the kinetics of skin graft rejection are dependent on the number of MHC mismatches as well as minor H-Ags between the donor and the recipient frogs. If the graft is either an autograft, syngenic or an isograft, it will never be rejected by the host. However, if the donor skin displays one or two MHC haplotype mismatches, then there will be an acute skin graft rejection that will take 18 to 22 days at 21°C to complete (Table 1). Furthermore, if the frogs share the same MHC haplotype but only differ by minor H-Ags then the graft will undergo chronic rejection, which will take between 30 to more than 100 days at 21°C for full rejection depending of the genetic combinations (Table 1). With *X. laevis* being ectothermic, temperature has a profound effect on skin graft rejection. For instance, at 27°C minor H-Ag-disparate grafts between individuals of the partially inbred F strain are rejected in 23-37 days, which is significantly faster than the rejection at 21°C that takes 60-100 days (Robert, Guiet et al. 1995). *In vitro, X. laevis* immune functions are also affected by temperature (Hsu 1998). For example, *in vitro* T-cell proliferation in MLR (Mixed Lymphocyte Reaction) or induced by mitogen (Meier 2003) and proliferation of lymphoid thymic tumor cell lines (Robert, Guiet et al. 1994), occurs faster at 27°C (optimum) than at lower temperature (18–25°C). Therefore, temperature has to be taken in account when comparing *in vivo* and *in vitro* responses against alloantigens.

The strict T cell dependency of skin rejection has been clearly established in *X. laevis* by thymectomy at early developmental stages before the full differentiation of T cell precursors (5-6 days post-fertilization; st. 47/48 (Horton, Horton et al. 1998) stages based on (Nieuwkoop and Faber 1967)). Adult frogs that have been thymectomized at early developmental stage fail to reject both MHC as well as minor H-Ag-disparate allografts (Barlow and Cohen 1983; Arnall and Horton 1987; Robert, Guiet et al. 1997). In contrast, adults that have been thymectomized either during mid larval (st. 53-55) or late larval (st. 56-58) development remain capable to reject MHC-disparate grafts. This most likely is due to the fact that mature T cells are able to migrate out of the thymus before it is removed; therefore, they can have effector functions in the periphery. These data demonstrated that skin graft rejection in adult *X. laevis* is thymus dependent and suggested that like in mammals allograft rejection is mediated by CD8 as well as CD4 T cells. Additionally, there is immunological memory against minor H-Ag because second set skin grafts are rejected in an accelerated fashion while third party grafts are not, suggesting that these responses are specific to the immunizing alloantigens (Table 1) (Nagata and Cohen 1983).

In order to assess more directly the role that CD8 T cells play in these responses *in vivo,* depletion by antibody treatment was used. CD8 T cells were depleted using the AM22 mouse anti-*X. laevis* CD8 monoclonal antibody (Flajnik, Ferrone et al. 1990). AM22 is specific for CD8 T cells because cells stained with this antibody express a pan-T cell marker (XT-1) as well as high levels of CD5 and CD45 (Gravenor, Horton et al. 1995; Robert, Sung et al. 2001). Moreover, cells stained by AM22 are not detected in frogs that are thymectomized during early larval life and lack T cells (Gravenor, Horton et al. 1995; Robert, Guiet et al. 1997). AM22 depletion experiments showed that in the absence of CD8 T cells MHC-disparate allografts did not undergo the typical acute rejection pattern but underwent slower rejection that took 7 days longer to complete (Rau, Cohen et al. 2001). Interestingly, these grafts were indeed completely rejected even if more mAb AM22 injections were used to prolong the CD8 T cell depletion effect. This suggests that other cells like CD4 T cells may also be involved in the response against skin Ags. To date this possibility has not been investigated due to the unavailability of antibodies against *X. laevis* CD4. However, recently our lab has generated and is currently characterizing a single chain CD4 antibody which will allow exploration of the importance of CD4 T cells in allograft rejection.

To further characterize the CD8 T cells involved in graft rejection, our lab adapted a whole-mount immunohistology technique. This procedure allows us to visualize lymphocytic infiltration into unfixed transplanted skin tissues using fluorescent antibodies (Ramanayake, Simon et al. 2007). Additionally, this method preserves the tissue structure and we can use several antibodies conjugated to different fluoropores to see exactly where cells are located and distinguish what kind of cells are present in the grafts. Therefore, this technique is a powerful tool which we can use to characterize and monitor immune effector cells mediating the immune responses of *X. laevis* against skin rejection Ags.

Using whole-mount immunohistology we found that, unlike isograft controls, MHC-disparate grafts that were undergoing rejection were infiltrated with a large number of CD8 T cells. These CD8 T cells were mainly distributed in areas where the graft was not yet rejected and the silvery irridophores were still persisting. Moreover, there was an inverse correlation between the percent rejection and number of infiltrating cells. For example the most prominent CD8 T cell infiltration occurred at day 7 when there was only 50% rejection. Additionally, these grafts also had significant infiltration of class II positive cells which were more numerous than the CD8 T cells. As mentioned before all adult leukocytes have class II expression in adult *X. laevis,* therefore, the majority of the class II positive cells in MHC-disparate grafts were actually CD8 T cells (~80%). This was also seen by cell morphology since most of the cells were small round lymphocytes although this does not exclude CD4 T cells. Besides lymphocytes, other cells morphologically similar to macrophages and dendritic cells (such as Langerhan cells) were seen in both allografts and isografts. These cells were already present in the grafts before transplantation, which suggests that they could potentially serve as antigen presenting cells (APCs). However, more of these cells from the recipient animal can infiltrate the graft and then migrate out to the spleen to prime more CD8 T cells.

As previously discussed, the main difference between MHC-disparate and minor H-Ag-disparate grafts is the time it takes for complete graft rejection, which is either acute or chronic, respectively. Therefore, one might assume that this is due to the lesser number of infiltrating effector T cells since only minor H-Ags are involved in these responses. On the contrary, however, we found that minor H-Ag-disparate grafts were infiltrated by similar numbers of both CD8 and class II positive cells, but with delayed kinetics (Ramanayake, Simon et al. 2007). In these minor H-Ag-disparate allografts the peak of immune cell infiltration was also observed when the graft was about 50% rejected which in this case occurred 15 days after transplantation, rather than 7 days as in the case of MHC mismatched grafts (Table 1).

Whole-mount immunohistology is a very powerful technique to study infiltration of immune cells; therefore, we are currently using different antibodies such as *X. laevis* CD4 and HAM56 (a human macrophage marker which cross-reacts with *X. laevis* macrophages) which will allow us to visualize both effector cells as well as APCs, respectively.

3.2 Characterization of the immunological properties of heat shock proteins (HSPs) using skin graft rejection

Our *X. laevis* skin grafting model has been instrumental to get better insight into the immunological properties of certain hsps such as gp96 and hsp70. Hsps are evolutionarily ancient and highly conserved intracellular molecular chaperones that help with intracellular transport, folding of newly synthesized proteins, and prevent protein aggregation. In addition, hsps have been implicated in a variety of innate as well as adaptive immune responses. Notably, hsps have the intrinsic property to carry exogenous antigenic peptides from the tissues which are purified from and interact with endocytic receptors expressed by APCs. Once the hsp-Ags complexes enter the APCs the peptides are shuttled into the MHC class Ia cross-presentation pathway where they are processed and presented by class Ia molecules to CD8 T cells. Therefore, hsps have the ability to elicit potent CD8 T cell responses against the chaperoned Ags. Gp96 and hsp70 bind Ags differently. While the peptide binding of gp96 is unclear, hsp70 has defined peptide binding which is ATP dependent (Blachere, Li et al. 1997). Peptides can be loaded *in vitro* onto hsp70 by simply adding ADP to the reaction, whereas ATP addition results in peptide disassociation. Hsp70 preferentially binds peptides that contain 4-5 hydrophobic residues flanked by two basic residues (Castellino, Boucher et al. 2000), but it has been shown that 30 amino acid long synthetic peptides can also be complexed (Calderwood, Theriault et al. 2005).

As mentioned, the LG-6 and LG-15 clones share the same MHC haplotypes but differ by minor H-Ags, and frogs primed with a first set of minor H-Ag-disparate skin graft reject a second set skin significantly faster. Furthermore, this accelerated rejection is thymus-dependent and Ag specific (e.g., a third party skin graft rejection is not accelerated). This system has revealed to be ideal in investigating whether the ability of hsps to generate CD8 T cell responses is conserved between mammals and amphibians.

We found that if we first immunize LG-6 clones with either gp96 or hsp70 purified from LG-15 liver (meaning that those hsps would carry LG-15 minor H-Ags) and then graft them with an LG-15 allograft, the graft undergoes accelerated rejection in comparison to control unimmunized animals or animals that were immunized with LG-6 derived hsps (carrying self-Ags) (Robert, Gantress et al. 2002). Additionally, syngenic grafts were never rejected regardless of the immunization status of the animal, which rules out possible Ag-independent pro-inflammatory effect induced by the hsps. Furthermore, these *in vivo* responses are specific to the Ags chaperoned by the hsps because if an LG-6 animal is immunized with LG-46 derived hsp and is grafted with both LG-15 as well as LG-46 skin (these three LG clones share the same MHC haplotype (a/c) but differ in multiple minor H-Ags) only the LG-46 graft will have accelerated rejection, while the LG-15 graft will undergo a typical chronic rejection (Table 1). Moreover, immunization with hsp70-peptide complexes results in accelerated skin graft rejection, while immunization with hsp70 free of Ags (i.e.,

Ags eluted by ATP-agarose chromatography) does not change the rejection kinetics in comparison to unimmunized animals. These data indeed show that both gp96 and hsp70 are able to generate potent specific T cell responses *in vivo* against minor H-alloantigens.

Type of skin grafts¶	**Minor H-Ag disparate**	**1 MHC haplotype disparate**	**2 MHC haplotype disparate**
Rejection at 21°C	30 - 100	18 - 22	18 - 22
Peak CD8 T cell infiltration	15	7	7
Rejection after priming with same first set graft	16 – 30	ND	ND
Rejection after gp96 or hsp70 immunization	20 - 30	ND	ND

Table 1. Summary of allograft rejection and immunological memory in adult *X. laevis*. Data is represented in days. ND, Not done or data not found in literature.

In mammals it is known that immune responses generated by hsps are mediated by CD8 cytotoxic T lymphocytes (CTLs). Using an *in vitro* killing assay, our lab confirmed that as in mammals, immunization with gp96 and hsp70 results in the generation of anti-minor H-Ag CTLs. Specifically, CD8 T cells purified from LG-6 animals primed with LG-15 tissue-derived hsp70 were able to kill class Ia positive LG-15 lymphoblast but not class Ia positive LG-6 blast targets nor class Ia negative 15/0 tumor targets. In contrast, CD8 T cells from animals immunized with Ag free hsp70 or unimmunized animals did not kill any of the blast targets. The same results were obtained using gp96 and different combinations of cloned frogs. Besides showing that the ability of hsps to generate CTL responses is conserved in amphibians, this study has provided definitive evidence of MHC class Ia restriction and Ag specificity of cytotoxic CD8 T cell effectors in *X. laevis*.
To explore *in vivo* the anti-minor H-Ag CD8 T cell effector capacity generated by gp96, our lab adapted a carboxyfluorescein diacetate succinimidly ester (CFSE) proliferation assay for *X. laevis* (Robert, Gantress et al. 2004). CFSE is a fluorescent dye that is incorporated into viable cells and upon cell division the CFSE content gets diluted in half, meaning that each daughter cell will have half the CFSE fluorescent intensity in comparison to undivided cells. This technique allows us to label, follow and calculate the percent of dividing cells as well as to determine the number of divisions that occurred. Using this approach, splenocytes from LG-6 frogs immunized with LG-15 gp96 were first labeled with CFSE and then were adoptively transferred into naïve LG-6 recipients that were previously grafted with a LG-15 skin allograft or a LG-6 syngenic graft. These experiments showed that the transferred CFSE labeled splenocytes accumulated in the spleens of animals that carried minor H-Ag-disparate skin grafts, while no such accumulation was detected in animals with syngenic grafts (Maniero and Robert 2004). Furthermore, by flow cytometry staining it was shown that the majority of CFSE+ dividing cells in these animals were CD8 T cells, which underwent several rounds of proliferation (3-4 cycles). This proliferation is not as robust as the one seen in mammals where up to 8 divisions can be seen. This can be due to several reasons including the difference in temperature as mentioned earlier or the strength of the TCR signal. Currently we do not know the status of other subsets of gp96 primed T cells to

minor H-Ags; however, since we know that CD8 depletion alone is not enough to completely abrogate skin graft rejection, this would suggest that other immune effector cells are also involved.
To test the effector function of adoptively transferred CFSE+ cells we monitored skin graft rejection. We found that unimmunized frogs carrying a minor H-Ag-disparate graft had accelerated skin graft rejection which reached 45-90% by day 10 after adoptive transfer of splenocytes (Maniero and Robert 2004). On the other hand, animals that carried isogenic grafts did not show signs of rejection. These rejection kinetics are reminiscent of a secondary T cell mediated rejection that occurs with animals primed with gp96 carrying minor H-Ag complexes. This means that gp96 is able to prime CD8 effector T cells that when adoptively transferred can recognize minor H-Ags presented *in vivo* by an allograft and kill the transplanted skin.

3.3 Possible role of nonclassical MHC class Ib genes in skin transplantation

As discussed above, CD8 T cells are critically involved in skin graft rejection in *X. laevis* and these responses are MHC class Ia restricted. However, the involvement of nonclassical MHC class Ib (class Ib) molecules in allorecognition has not been addressed. Class Ib genes in comparison to class Ia are heterogeneous genes with a limited tissue distribution and low polymorphism (Hofstetter, Sullivan et al. 2011). Both class Ia and most class Ib molecules have similar structure and need to associate with β2-m in order to be presented at the cells surface (Goyos, Guselnikov et al. 2007). Class Ib molecules, unlike class Ia, usually present Ags of a more limited variability or PAMPs including peptides as well as lipids and glycolipids. In *X. laevis* there are as many as 20 *X. laevis* class Ib (XNC) genes divided into 11 subfamilies (Flajnik, Kasahara et al. 1993; Goyos, Ohta et al. 2009). We have demonstrated that *X. laevis* has the ability to generate unconventional class Ib restricted anti-15/0 CTLs after hsp immunization (Goyos, Cohen et al. 2004). There is a possibility that after allograft or hsp immunization a population of class Ib mediated T cell effectors can arise. These effector cells can be both CD8 positive as well as CD8 negative as in the case in human and mice. Interestingly, we recently found expression of the XNC11 gene, in the skin of adult frogs. The XNC11 gene has a very unique expression pattern; it is almost exclusively expressed at low levels in the thymus, and at high levels by several thymic lymphoid tumors including 15/0 (Goyos, Ohta et al. 2009). We now have evidence of faint but consistent expression of XNC11 in the skin. So far attempts to modify the expression pattern of XNC11 by any inflammatory stimuli such as LPS and heat killed bacteria or by viral infection has been unsuccessful. Currently, we are working under the hypothesis that XNC11 is mainly found in the skin macrophages, Langerhan cells or unconventional T cells. If this hypothesis is correct, it is possible that XNC11 can present Ags to effector cells during allograft recognition or is involved in the regulation of specialized or unconventional skin resident T cells. Our lab is in the process of generating monoclonal antibodies against several different class Ib molecules including XNC11. These tools will allow us to directly address if XNC11 or other class Ib genes are involved in immune responses against skin minor H-Ags.

4. Immune responses and tolerance to skin antigens during larval and metamorphic stages

Of particular relevance for the immunological aspects of tissue transplantation, is the fact that unlike mammals, the *X. laevis* immune system undergoes striking developmental remodeling twice during its life: first during embryogenesis, and then again during the transition from larva to adult. The thymus, first colonized by embryonic stem cells a few days after fertilization, undergoes a second wave of stem cell immigration after losing most of its lymphocytes during metamorphosis. The embryonic and larval periods of thymocyte differentiation take place in different environments since during metamorphosis the whole organism is remodeled and many new proteins are expressed that could be considered antigenic by the larval immune system. The emerging adult lymphocytes, therefore, are likely to be subjected to a new wave of negative selection by the adult "self," resulting in a new balance of self-tolerance. In addition, MHC class I and class II genes are differentially regulated during metamorphosis. Although, larvae like adults have CD8 T cells, there is no consistent expression of MHC class Ia until metamorphosis, especially in the thymus.

In this section we will discuss the ability of *X. laevis* larvae to become tolerant to skin alloantigens. The induction of allotolerance is a very complex process governed by several different variables; therefore some conflicting data have been reported concerning its ontogeny as will be discussed later in detail. One of the differences that may affect tolerance induction is technical variability. Skin grafting in larvae is similar to grafting in adults but with several important differences. A first notable difference is that due to its fragility larval skin does not support transplantation onto a larval hosts and immune rejection is difficult to distinguish from tissue degeneration (Horton, Horton et al. 1993). For this reason, the use of ventral adult, instead of larval skin, graft onto larval recipients has been and is still favored. The adult skin is introduced under the larval skin on the head between the ears of the recipient (Chardonnens and Du Pasquier 1973). Another difference is that compared to adults, larvae are transparent. The adult skin is usually firmly fixed one day after transplantation and the transparent host skin retracts from the graft therefore removing the overlaying skin is unnecessary (Figure 2). Graft rejection is scored similarly to adults where the percent of irridophore destruction is determined. Several factors have been shown to affect the outcome of adult skin transplantation in tadpoles, including the size of the transplanted skin, as well as the genetic background and the developmental stage. Changes in temperature do not affect the percent of skin graft rejection; however they do influence the kinetics of rejection at all developmental stages. At 21°C grafts differing by 1 MHC haplotype are rejected in 40-55 days in comparison to 25-35 days at 24°C (Cohen, DiMarzo et al. 1985). Furthermore, size of the graft is very important for tolerance induction and in general larger grafts have an increased chance to be tolerized. Experiments that use outbred animals, which are genetically heterogeneous, should be considered with caution when compared to those that use MHC defined frogs differing by minor H-Ag loci only or by minor H-Ag loci plus one or two MHC haplotypes.

Another possible source of conflicting results concerns development, especially metamorphosis, which may play the most important role in generating tolerance. Metamorphosis in frogs, both initiation and completion, is under the control of the thyroid hormone (Furlow and Neff 2006; Tata 2006). The thyroid hormone starts being produced around stage 50, peaks at stage 60, and the levels are back to normal at the end of metamorphosis (Figure 3). Also there are two different thyroid receptors- α and β. Thyroid receptor-α is expressed early on after hatching while β comes up concomitantly with the thyroid hormone (Figure 3). In addition, the action of the thyroid hormone during metamorphosis is local and not systemic. This means that in certain tissues the changes associated with metamorphosis may start earlier than in other tissues and this may directly impact the ontogeny of tolerance. The complexity of the metamorphic transition is likely to result in marked individual variation even in clonal animals, including the differences in

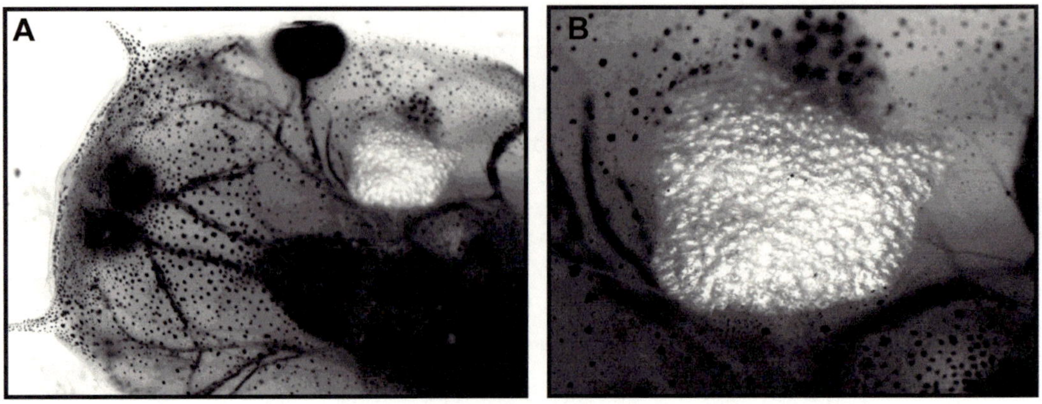

Fig. 2. Larval skin graft. A. Minor H-Ag-disparate adult skin graft inserted on the head region of a tadpole. B. Enlarged image of the graft shows the presence of silvery irridophores, 0% rejection.

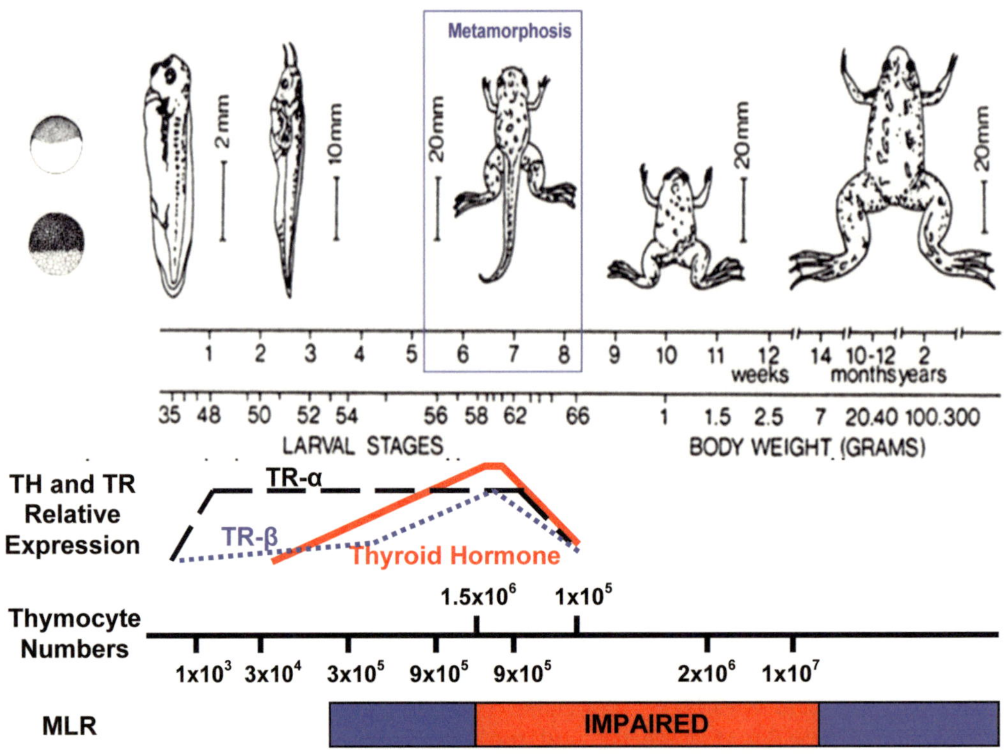

*Figure adapted from (Du Pasquier, Schwager et al. 1989) and (Furlow and Neff 2006)

Fig. 3. Overview of the changes occurring during metamorphosis. The different developmental stages of *X. laevis* are illustrated including the period of metamorphosis along with the morphological criteria used. Additionally, the relative expression of the thyroid hormone as well as the thyroid hormone receptors TR-α and TR-β is depicted. Also, total thymocyte number, which significantly decreases during metamorphosis, is shown to correlate with impaired T cell function (MLR activity).

the immune system. This is indeed observed by the individual variation in morphological changes (e.g. there are easily several day differences in the time of complete tails loss in cloned progeny).

In order to address some discrepancies in the literature we will first discuss the induction of tolerance to minor H-Ag followed by MHC-disparate grafts. The mechanism(s) as well as possible effector cells involved in allotolerance will also be considered. Finally, we will provide some perspective on using new tools and methodologies to more conclusively answer questions associated with tolerance.

4.1 Immune response and allotolerance in *X. laevis* larvae to minor H skin antigens

X. laevis tadpoles develop allorecognition at stage 49 (12 days post fertilization) which is accompanied by lymphocytic infiltration of the grafts (Horton 1969). In *X. laevis* there are three distinct periods throughout development during which there is a difference in the immune responses against skin allografts (Chardonnens and Du Pasquier 1973). Those include the periods before, during and after metamorphosis. Sibling studies showed that at stage 53 (period before metamorphosis or premetamorphosis) allografts from siblings were completely rejected (Table 2). Furthermore, larvae at the same stage were also grafted with allografts from unrelated donors and again the majority of grafts underwent complete rejection. Moreover, these tadpoles primed by a first skin graft, rejected a second set skin grafted from the same donor at stage 58 (beginning of metamorphosis period) with accelerated kinetics suggesting immunological memory similar to second set adult grafts. Therefore, *X. laevis* larvae are immunocompetent and can indeed be sensitized against the grafts. Also young adults (2 months post metamorphosis, postmetamorphic animals) similarly to larvae were able to completely and acutely reject sibling allografts in 100% of the cases with mean rejection time of 20 days (Table 2).

In contrast, during metamorphosis (which actually includes the time spanning 15 days before (st. 58) and about a month after metamorphosis, perimetamorphic animals) up to 50% of the sibling grafts were actually tolerized (i.e., not rejected), and those that were rejected followed a very slow rejection kinetics (20 - 80 days for complete rejection) in comparison to grafts on young larvae or adults (10 - 20 days). This suggests that metamorphosis is a special developmental time during which immune tolerance can be induced. This could be due to the fact that the immune system is undergoing complete remodeling and there is reduced number of lymphocytes. For example, more than 50% thymocytes die during metamorphosis (Du Pasquier and Weiss 1973). However, several pieces of evidence do not support the hypothesis that tolerance induction at metamorphosis is due to an insufficient number of lymphocytes. For instance, regardless whether the grafts are rejected or tolerized they are infiltrated by lymphocytes (Horton 1969; Bernardini, Chardonnens et al. 1970), while autografts are not. This implies that the grafts are recognized as non-self although they are not rejected. Also if tolerance is induced due to the lack of lymphocytes one would assume that once metamorphosis is completed and the number of lymphocytes is recovered, these grafts would be rejected. However, that is not the case since these grafts survive for more than two years. Interestingly, this tolerance can be broken by a third party graft (Bernardini, Chardonnens et al. 1970), which suggests that some H-Ags may be shared between the two different grafts. Therefore, once a T cell response is initiated against the third party graft that response can also be cross-reactive to the tolerized graft. Thus, it appears that during metamorphosis *X. laevis* larvae are capable of inducing active allotolerance against certain H loci shared by the different outbred *X. laevis* used (Chardonnens and Du Pasquier 1973; Chardonnens 1975).

On the other hand, allograft tolerance capacity was found to occur also at premetamorphic stages (Table 2) when more genetically defined and homogeneous animals were used (DiMarzo 1980; DiMarzo and Cohen 1982a; DiMarzo and Cohen 1982b). Remarkably, both pre and perimetamorphic larvae of inbred strains were able to induce tolerance against allografts that were either minor H locus or even MHC-disparate, whereas all postmetamorphic froglets rejected 100% of the grafts (Table 2). In addition, differences in rejection depending on the developmental stage were noted; in general younger larvae (st. 47/48) had a higher propensity for becoming tolerant while older larvae (st. 57/58) had the ability to reject more grafts. In either case, the grafts were rejected with delayed kinetics in comparison to postmetamorphic animals. Despite the discrepancy on the ontogeny of allotolerance in *X. laevis*, it is clear that perimetamorphic larvae are indeed able to become tolerant to allografts in all cases. The inconsistency may be in part due to individual variation of thyroid hormone levels and the impact it has on initiation of metamorphosis. It is also possible that different tolerance mechanisms or regulatory cells are involved in premetamorphic and metamorphic stages.

4.2 Immune response and allotolerance in *X. laevis* larvae to MHC-disparate grafts

Although early experiments have indicated that during metamorphosis allotolerance is induced to minor H-Ags (Chardonnens and Du Pasquier 1973; Chardonnens 1975; DiMarzo 1980; DiMarzo and Cohen 1982a; DiMarzo and Cohen 1982b), other work has revealed that the immunogenetics of tolerance are complex. Family studies using field-collected outbred adult *X. laevis* showed that when grafted during metamorphosis skin that differed by one-MHC haplotype had prolonged survival (more than 75 days) and the majority of those grafts were never rejected suggesting long lasting tolerance (Barlow, DiMarzo et al. 1981). In contrast, all post metamorphic frogs rejected their grafts. Notably, grafts that were rejected by animals grafted during metamorphosis took at least twice as long for complete rejection. When two-MHC haplotype-disparate grafts were transplanted during metamorphosis the majority of grafts were rejected. However, even in this case, grafts did enjoy prolonged survival (more than 42 days for complete rejection in comparison to 18 days in postmetamorphic hosts, Table 2). In this study even though similar results were obtained using six different families, there was also variability from one family to another which suggests that genetics play a large role in the induction of tolerance (Barlow, DiMarzo et al. 1981).

In order to bypass undefined genetic variation, Barlow et al. (1981) used MHC defined inbred strains of *X. laevis*. In two different MHC combination when the donor and the recipient differed by one-MHC haplotype there was 93% graft survival in perimetamorphic hosts, while 100% grafts were rejected by postmetamorphic recipients (Table 2). When the graft differed by two-MHC haplotypes only 30% of grafts on perimetamorphic hosts survived more than 50 days. These data clearly show that during metamorphosis allotolerance can easily be induced to minor H-Ags as well as one-MHC haplotype-disparate grafts but rarely to grafts differing by two MHC haplotypes.

In addition to the genetic background of the grafts, as mentioned before, graft size plays an important role which can tip the balance between rejection and tolerance (Bernardini, Chardonnens et al. 1970; Chardonnens and Du Pasquier 1973; Barlow and Cohen 1983). In general smaller grafts (1-2 mm^2) are more readily rejected (can reach up to 90% rejection) in perimetamorphic animals when there is a one MHC haplotype difference between donor and host. On the other hand, larger grafts (4-9 mm^2) almost always induce tolerance. The same trend holds true for grafts differing by two MHC haplotypes except the capacity for rejection is greater since tolerance is not easily induced in this case.

4.3 Mechanisms of allotolerance

Cell transfer approaches were developed to investigate the cellular mechanism responsible for tolerance induction and maintenance of skin Ags in *X. laevis*. In a set of experiments, isogenic frogs carrying minor H-Ag-disparate grafts were injected with thymocytes and splenocytes from isogenic metamorphosing larvae. This cell transfer induced significantly delayed skin graft rejection in comparison to control animals that received either adult cells or were not adoptively transferred with any cells (Du Pasquier and Bernard 1980). Importantly, multiple injections of metamorphosing immune cells were necessary to achieve suppression of graft rejection since a single injection did not result in the specific delay. Additionally, this effect was not permanent; once the injections stopped the grafts were rejected. Similarly, splenocytes from larvally tolerant frogs that were adoptively transferred into normal frogs drastically suppressed the rejection of semi-allogeneic grafts (Nakamura, Maeno et al. 1987). This indicates that the thymus and spleen of metamorphosing animals contain cells, presumably lymphocytes that have tolerogenic or suppressive activity against skin minor H-Ags. The need for repeated transfers of these cells to delay graft rejection may be due to their low frequency and/or short life span in the spleen and thymus of the metamorphic donor or as a result of the cell transfer. Additionally, the fact that the effect does not last suggests that tolerance induction to skin grafts during metamorphosis is regulatory (requiring the presence of regulatory cells) rather than deletional (absence or deletion of potentially reactive T cells). This possibility is further supported by experiments showing that maintenance of tolerance to minor H-Ag-disparate skin grafts can be broken by cyclosphosphamide treatment (Horton, Horton et al. 1989).

In a complementary set of experiments, adoptive cell transfer was used to determine if tolerance to skin minor H-Ags can be broken (Du Pasquier and Bernard 1980). Splenocytes from isogenic adults primed by minor H-Ag-disparate skin grafts were adoptively transferred into isogenic metamorphic recipients with tolerized skin graft genetically identical to the one used to prime the adults. This adoptive transfer of primed anti-minor H-Ag lymphocytes was not able to break tolerance in animals that tolerated the grafts for at least six months. However, if a second graft, identical to the tolerized graft, was placed at the time of the adoptive transfer, an acute rejection of this graft was initiated but stopped within 10 days. The result was a graft that was half rejected and half healthy. This suggests that even though the animal is tolerant to the allograft, the primed transferred cells are able to cause graft destruction although the number and/or survival of these reactive cells is not sufficient to complete the rejection. Presumably, if another transfer was done the graft may be fully rejected. Another possibility is that a subset of regulatory cells home to the skin at the time of transplantation to induce and maintain tolerance or suppression, and that the presence of adoptively transferred anti-minor H-Ag lymphocytes prevent or delay the migration of these regulatory cell in the transplanted skin. Taken together, these data strongly suggest that tolerance in larvae does not depend upon deletion of alloreactive cells but rather is maintained by suppressor or regulatory cells that can be adoptively transferred.

The preponderant role of T cells in larvally-induced allotolerance has been established by thymectomy. When larvae were thymectomized during early larval life before the migration of T cell precursors into the thymic anlage, graft rejection of premetamorphic larvae as well as postmetamorphic froglets was severely impaired (Table 2) demonstrating that without the thymus alloreactive cells can not develop (Horton and Manning 1972; Barlow and Cohen 1983; Kaye and Tompkins 1983; Nagata and Cohen 1983). Furthermore, the impaired rejection capacity of premetamorphic larvae that were thymectomized at early developmental stage can be rescued by implantation of an intact larval or adult thymus (Arnall and Horton 1986). When these T cell deficient thymectomized larvae are implanted with an isogenic thymus their capacity to reject both minor H-Ags and MHC-disparate skin grafts was fully restored. However, when thymectomized larvae were reconstituted with a thymus that was either MHC-disparate or differed even by minor H-Ags from the host, rejection was restored only to grafts that were MHC incompatible both to the host and the thymus donor. Interestingly, these reconstituted animals had an impaired ability to reject minor H-Ag-disparate grafts. Notably, when MHC incompatible thymi were transplanted, skin grafts from the same donor were tolerated even though they were able to elicit proliferative responses against the thymus donor cells in an *in vitro* MLR (Arnall and Horton 1986). This split tolerance was further substantiated *in vivo* by injecting irradiated splenocytes from the thymus donor into reconstituted animals (Arnall and Horton 1987). Again there was an *in vivo* response against the transferred splenocytes, although the grafts were still not rejected. In addition, if live MHC-disparate splenocytes from the thymus donor were injected, animals developed graft versus host disease and died. Based on these results it has been concluded that the cytotoxic rather than the proliferative alloresponse is suppressed in thymus reconstituted thymectomized animals.

In contrast to early thymectomy, late larval thymectomy did not have an effect on rejection (Table 2). Interestingly, however, thymectomy performed during mid-larval stages significantly impaired the ability of animals to become tolerant to allografts (Table 2) (Barlow and Cohen 1983). Moreover, this impairment was dependent on the number of different MHC haplotypes as well the size of the grafts.

In conclusion, it is clear that *X. laevis* larvae can become tolerant to allografts although the developmental stage at which this tolerance can be established, the types and amount of skin Ags that can be tolerized, and the cellular mechanisms involved still remain unclear. During metamorphosis the larval immune system is drastically remodeled and larvae develop tolerance against newly expressed adult self-antigens; therefore, allotolerance may be a consequence of this period. This does not mean that there are not enough effector cells or CTLs to reject the grafts since it was clearly demonstrated that MLR in these animals was positive meaning that T cells can proliferate in the presence of alloantigens. A most likely scenario is that during metamorphosis there is a general suppressive state where putative T regulatory cells suppress immune responses against adult tissues in order to avoid auto-immunity. The thyroid hormone signaling which initiates metamorphosis may be one plausible factor of individual variability for premetamorphic larvae to become tolerant to allografts. As explained earlier, thyroid hormone acts locally and it is possible that in some cases animals start producing larger quantities of this hormone in certain tissues such as the skin, which would mean that even if the animal is not showing general changes associated with metamorphosis certain organs or tissues may be. It is possible that particular organs or tissues will be associated with a more suppressive environment suited for induction of tolerance. Although, the tolerance ability of premetamorphic stages may result from the establishment of this regulatory process that would peak during the metamorphic climax, it is also possible that it results from a different mechanism such as insufficient or immature T cell response. This can especially be the case at earlier larval stages (eg. st. 53) when peripheral T cells are still few (~10,000 to 100,000).

	Premetamorphic	Perimetamorphic	Postmetamorphic
Developmental Stage	47 - 58	58 – 1 month post metamorphosis	2 months post metamorphosis
Minor-H-Ag disparate grafts	Tolerance induction +*	Tolerance induction +++	Rejection 100%
1 MHC haplotype disparatre grafts	Tolerance induction +*	Tolerance induction +++	Rejection 100%
2 MHC haplotypes disparate grafts	Rejection	Rejection MST 42	Rejection MST 18
Early larval life thymectomy	Impaired graft rejection	No effect	Impaired graft rejection
Mid larval life thymectomy	No effect	Impaired tolerance	No effect
Late larval life thymectomy	No effect	No effect	No effect

Table 2. Summary of tolerance induction in *X. laevis* larvae and the effects of thymectomy.

*Discrepancy between different studies. Chardonnens and Du Pasquier (1973) reported that premetamorphic larvae were capable of rejecting grafts similary to postmetamophic froglets while several reports from the Cohen lab reported that premetamoprhic larvae (as early as stage 47) had the capacity to induce tolerance.

+, low incidence of tolerance induction

+++, high incidence of tolerance induction

MST: Mean Survival Time (in days)

4.4 New tools to study tolerance

During metamorphosis, as described before, *X. laevis* larvae have to become tolerant to newly emerging adult self-antigens, which can be recognized as foreign by the larval immune system, and lead to autoimmunity. It is highly plausible that the same mechanisms that are involved in allotolerance are also involved in tolerance to self; therefore, *X. laevis* provides a unique model to study autoimmunity. This is illustrated by the observation that certain animals that are thymectomized at stage 56 and than transplanted with MHC-disparate graft have a high incidence of death due to "red disease" (Barlow and Cohen 1983). This is a disease that is autoimmune in nature and is characterized by cutaneous hemorrhaging around the eyes and legs and by internal hemorrhaging in the liver and kidneys.

There is still much unknown regarding the mechanism(s) associated with suppression during allotolerance. For instance, we still don't know which effector cells are involved, even though we speculate that they might be T regulatory cells. The mode and site of action of these regulatory cells is also not defined. Using some newly generated tools and techniques we can start to answer some of these questions. Initially, it will be of great interest to immunize perimetamorphic larvae with hsps carrying either MHC or minor H-Ags and then look for immunological memory toward skin grafts (same genetic background as the Ags carried by the hsp) transplanted post metamorphosis. These experiments will show if the Ags alone are capable of generating tolerance by possibly negatively selecting reactive thymocytes in the thymus or by generating specific T regulatory cells toward those particular Ags.

To further investigate the effector cells involved in these responses, we will be able to use transgenic animals. Transgenesis in *X. laevis* has been widely used over the last several years and the most common technique used is REMI (Restriction Enzyme Mediated Integration) which requires integration of the transgene into the sperm nuclei which are than transplanted into unfertilized eggs (Kroll and Amaya 1996). However, for generating transgenics with our isogenic clones this technique is not useful since they are maintained by gynogenesis. Therefore, our laboratory adapted a new transgenic approach using the I-SceI Meganuclease (Ogino, McConnell et al. 2006; Pan, Chen et al. 2006). This method requires a plasmid that carries the transgene of interested flanked by I-SceI recognition sites which is digested by the meganuclease and the entire digest is injected into activated eggs. This causes stable integration of the transgene into one to two different sites in the genome. An added advantage of working with the clones is that all of the progeny of a given founder will be transgenic which will give us enough larvae for experimentation.

As mentioned in the introduction the genome of the *X. laevis* sister species, *X. tropicalis* has been fully sequenced and annotated. This has provided new possibilities to identify immune genes using, for example, gene synteny (Robert and Ohta 2009). Furthermore, the full sequencing of the *X. laevis* genome using the homozygous inbred strain J from our resource center is now ongoing and the first assembly is already available (R. Harland, personal communication). With these new available resources, it will become possible to identify and isolate regulatory regions of immunologically relevant genes and produce transgenic reporter animals expressing fluorescent reporter genes (such as GFP) under the control of these regulatory regions as in mouse and zebra fish (Smith, Ataliotis et al. 2005; Doherty, Johnson Hamlet et al. 2007; Hall, Flores et al. 2009). *X. laevis* transgenic lines expressing, for example, GFP under the transcriptional control of the CD4 (CD4 T cells) or the Foxp3 (T regulatory cells) promoter regions (i.e., homologs of these genes have already been identified in the *X. tropicalis* genome), would permit to localize and follow the fate of these cells in transplanted skin tissues during rejection and tolerance induction. Since tadpoles are transparent this will allow us to easily visualize the trafficking pattern of these cells and see if those are the effector cells that are found infiltrating tolerated grafts. Also we can sort these cells based on their GFP expression and than adoptively transfer them into postmetamorphic frogs to check if indeed these cells are involved in the induction of tolerance. Additionally, by using cloned animals we will be able to pool enough larval cells to perform the adoptive transfers as well as to use multiple transfers to see if the number of transferred cells will have an effect on allotolerance.

Another area of investigation where *X. laevis* may reveal useful involves the possible role of certain class Ib molecules in tolerance induction. In mice and humans certain NKT cells that are educated onto class Ib molecules seem to be involved in autoimmunity. The partial characterization of skin γδ T cells as well as dendritic cells has recently been reported in adult *X. laevis* (Mescher, Wolf et al. 2007). It would be interesting to determine the similarity and potential difference in the larval skin, since old data suggest that in contrast to adult, larval skin does not have Langerhan cells (Du Pasquier and Flajnik 1990). Furthermore, since *X. laevis* tadpoles do not have consistent class Ia expression until metamorphosis their T cells may be educated on class Ib molecules that are expressed in the thymus during early development. We can test if certain class Ib molecules are involved in tolerance induction by down regulating these genes *in vivo* by transgenesis. We have already established a protocol to silence *X. laevis* genes, including class Ibs, using RNA interference (Goyos, Guselnikov et al. 2007; Nedelkovska and Robert unpublished). We can also generate specific shRNAs targeting genes critical for T regulatory cell function to determine if impairment of this cell type will lead to loss of tolerance and induction of autoimmunity.

5. Conclusion

The studies reviewed here highlight the versatility and attractiveness of *X. laevis* to study skin graft rejection as well as immune tolerance. Due to the dual nature of its immune system, larval and adult, *X. laevis* can be used as a useful model for investigating T cell regulation as well as long term immunological memory. Furthermore, this system already demonstrated and will further explore the conserved ability of heat shock proteins to elicit Ag specific CD8 T cell responses. Finally, *X. laevis* provides a powerful model to study self-tolerance by dissecting the mechanisms involved in induction of allotolerance. The advent of new genetic and genomic tools and technologies will allow better insight into the complex regulation and development of allotolerance which is of general relevance for generating self-tolerance, as well as autoimmunity.

6. Acknowledgment

We would like to thank Nikesha Haynes and Juan Oves for critically reading the manuscript. Also we would like to acknowledge the *X. laevis* research resource for immunobiology (http://www.urmc.rochester.edu/mbi/resources/Xenopus/) for providing animals used in experiments performed in the authors' lab. Research support: NIH *AI-07285* (H. N.), *1R03-HD061671-01, R24-AI-059830-06* and NSF *IOS-0923772* (J. R.).

7. References

Arnall, J. C. and J. D. Horton (1986). "Impaired rejection of minor-histocompatibility-antigen-disparate skin grafts and acquisition of tolerance to thymus donor antigens in allothymus-implanted, thymectomized Xenopus." Transplantation 41(6): 766-776.

Arnall, J. C. and J. D. Horton (1987). "In vivo studies on allotolerance perimetamorphically induced in control and thymectomized Xenopus." Immunology 62(2): 315-319.

Barlow, E. H. and N. Cohen (1983). "The thymus dependency of transplantation allotolerance in the metamorphosing frog Xenopus laevis." Transplantation 35(6): 612-619.

Barlow, E. H., S. J. DiMarzo, et al. (1981). "Prolonged survival of major histocompatibility complex-disparate skin allografts transplanted to the metamorphosing frog, xenopus laevis." Transplantation 32(1): 51-57.

Bernardini, N., X. Chardonnens, et al. (1970). "[Tolerance of cutaneous allografts in Xenopus laevis. Influence of the size and age of the graft]." C R Acad Sci Hebd Seances Acad Sci D 270(19): 2351-2354.

Blachere, N. E., Z. Li, et al. (1997). "Heat shock protein-peptide complexes, reconstituted in vitro, elicit peptide-specific cytotoxic T lymphocyte response and tumor immunity." J Exp Med 186(8): 1315-1322.

Bowes, J. B., K. A. Snyder, et al. (2009). "Xenbase: gene expression and improved integration." from http://www.xenbase.org/common/.

Calderwood, S. K., J. R. Theriault, et al. (2005). "Message in a bottle: role of the 70-kDa heat shock protein family in anti-tumor immunity." Eur J Immunol 35(9): 2518-2527.

Castellino, F., P. E. Boucher, et al. (2000). "Receptor-mediated uptake of antigen/heat shock protein complexes results in major histocompatibility complex class I antigen presentation via two distinct processing pathways." J Exp Med 191(11): 1957-1964.

Chardonnens, X. (1975). "Tissue typing by skin grafting during metamorphosis of the toad Xenopus laevis (Daudin)." Experientia 31(2): 237.

Chardonnens, X. and L. Du Pasquier (1973). "Induction of skin allograft tolerance during metamorphosis of the toad Xenopus laevis: a possible model for studying generation of self tolerance to histocompatibility antigens." Eur J Immunol 3(9): 569-573.

Cohen, N., S. J. DiMarzo, et al. (1985). The ontogeny of allo-tolerance and self-tolerance in larval *Xenopus laevis*. Metamorphosis. M. Balls and M. Bownes. Oxford, Clarendon Press.

DiMarzo, S. J. (1980). Ontogeny of alloreactivity in the toad, *Xenopus laevis*, University of Rochester. PhD.

DiMarzo, S. J. and N. Cohen (1982a). "Immunogenetic aspects of in vivo allotolerance induction during the ontogeny of Xenopus laevis." Immunogenetics 16(2): 103-116.

DiMarzo, S. J. and N. Cohen (1982b). "An in vivo study of the ontogeny of alloreactivity in the frog, Xenopus laevis." Immunology 45(1): 39-48.

Doherty, J. R., M. R. Johnson Hamlet, et al. (2007). "A flk-1 promoter/enhancer reporter transgenic Xenopus laevis generated using the Sleeping Beauty transposon system: an in vivo model for vascular studies." Dev Dyn 236(10): 2808-2817.

Du Pasquier, D. and X. Chardonnens (1975). "Genetic aspects of the tolerance to allografts induced at metamorphosis in the toad *Xenopus laevis*." Immunogenetics 2: 431-440.

Du Pasquier, L. and C. C. Bernard (1980). "Active suppression of the allogeneic histocompatibility reactions during the metamorphosis of the clawed toad Xenopus." Differentiation 16(1): 1-7.

Du Pasquier, L. and M. F. Flajnik (1990). "Expression of MHC class II antigens during Xenopus development." Dev Immunol 1(2): 85-95.

Du Pasquier, L., J. Schwager, et al. (1989). "The immune system of Xenopus." Annu Rev Immunol 7: 251-275.

Du Pasquier, L. and N. Weiss (1973). "The thymus during the ontogeny of the toad Xenopus laevis: growth, membrane-bound immunoglobulins and mixed lymphocyte reaction." Eur J Immunol 3(12): 773-777.

Evans, B. J. (2008). "Genome evolution and speciation genetics of clawed frogs (Xenopus and Silurana)." Front Biosci 13: 4687-4706.

Flajnik, M. F. and L. Du Pasquier (1988). "MHC class I antigens as surface markers of adult erythrocytes during the metamorphosis of Xenopus." Dev Biol 128(1): 198-206.

Flajnik, M. F., S. Ferrone, et al. (1990). "Evolution of the MHC: antigenicity and unusual tissue distribution of Xenopus (frog) class II molecules." Mol Immunol 27(5): 451-462.

Flajnik, M. F., M. Kasahara, et al. (1993). "A novel type of class I gene organization in vertebrates: a large family of non-MHC-linked class I genes is expressed at the RNA level in the amphibian Xenopus." EMBO J 12(11): 4385-4396.

Flajnik, M. F., J. F. Kaufman, et al. (1986). "Major histocompatibility complex-encoded class I molecules are absent in immunologically competent Xenopus before metamorphosis." J Immunol 137(12): 3891-3899.

Furlow, J. D. and E. S. Neff (2006). "A developmental switch induced by thyroid hormone: Xenopus laevis metamorphosis." Trends Endocrinol Metab 17(2): 40-47.

Goyos, A., N. Cohen, et al. (2004). "Anti-tumor MHC class Ia-unrestricted CD8 T cell cytotoxicity elicited by the heat shock protein gp96." Eur J Immunol 34(9): 2449-2458.

Goyos, A., S. Guselnikov, et al. (2007). "Involvement of nonclassical MHC class Ib molecules in heat shock protein-mediated anti-tumor responses." Eur J Immunol 37(6): 1494-1501.

Goyos, A., Y. Ohta, et al. (2009). "Novel nonclassical MHC class Ib genes associated with CD8 T cell development and thymic tumors." Mol Immunol 46(8-9): 1775-1786.

Goyos, A., J. Sowa, et al. (2011). "Remarkable conservation of distinct nonclassical MHC class I lineages in divergent amphibian species." J Immunol 186(1): 372-381.

Gravenor, I., T. L. Horton, et al. (1995). "Ontogeny and thymus-dependence of T cell surface antigens in Xenopus: flow cytometric studies on monoclonal antibody-stained thymus and spleen." Dev Comp Immunol 19(6): 507-523.

Hall, C., M. V. Flores, et al. (2009). "Transgenic zebrafish reporter lines reveal conserved Toll-like receptor signaling potential in embryonic myeloid leukocytes and adult immune cell lineages." J Leukoc Biol 85(5): 751-765.

Hofstetter, A. R., L. C. Sullivan, et al. (2011). "Diverse roles of non-diverse molecules: MHC class Ib molecules in host defense and control of autoimmunity." Curr Opin Immunol 23(1): 104-110.

Horton, J. D. (1969). "Ontogeny of the immune response to skin allografts in relation to lymphoid organ development in the amphibian Xenopus laevis Daudin." J Exp Zool 170(4): 449-465.

Horton, J. D., T. L. Horton, et al. (1998). "T-cell and natural killer cell development in thymectomized Xenopus." Immunol Rev 166: 245-258.

Horton, J. D., T. L. Horton, et al. (1993). "Incomplete tolerance induced in Xenopus by larval tissue allografting: evidence from immunohistology and mixed leucocyte culture." Dev Comp Immunol 17(3): 249-262.

Horton, J. D., T. L. Horton, et al. (1989). "Attempts to break perimetamorphically induced skin graft tolerance by treatment of Xenopus with cyclophosphamide and interleukin-2." Transplantation 47(5): 883-887.

Horton, J. D. and M. J. Manning (1972). "Response to skin allografts in Xenopus laevis following thymectomy at early stages of lymphoid organ maturation." Transplantation 14(2): 141-154.

Horton, T. L., R. Minter, et al. (2000). "Xenopus NK cells identified by novel monoclonal antibodies." Eur J Immunol 30(2): 604-613.

Horton, T. L., R. Stewart, et al. (2003). "Ontogeny of Xenopus NK cells in the absence of MHC class I antigens." Dev Comp Immunol 27(8): 715-726.

Hsu, E. (1998). "Mutation, selection, and memory in B lymphocytes of exothermic vertebrates." Immunol Rev 162: 25-36.

Kaye, C. and R. Tompkins (1983). "Allograft rejection in Xenopus laevis following larval thymectomy." Dev Comp Immunol 7(2): 287-294.

Kobel, H. R. and L. Du Pasquier (1975). "Production of Large Clones of Histocompatible, Fully Identical Clawed Toads (Xenopus)." Immunogenetics(2): 87-91.

Kobel, H. R. and L. Du Pasquier, Eds. (1977). Strains and species of *Xenopus* for immunological research. Developmental Immunobiology. Amsterdam, Elsevier/North Holland Publishing Co.

Kroll, K. L. and E. Amaya (1996). "Transgenic Xenopus embryos from sperm nuclear transplantations reveal FGF signaling requirements during gastrulation." Development 122(10): 3173-3183.

Maniero, G. D. and J. Robert (2004). "Phylogenetic conservation of gp96-mediated antigen-specific cellular immunity: new evidence from adoptive cell transfer in xenopus." Transplantation 78(10): 1415-1421.

Meier (2003). T cell development and the diversification and selection of the *Xenopus* T cell recpetor beta chain repertoire, University of Alberta.

Mescher, A. L., W. L. Wolf, et al. (2007). "Cells of cutaneous immunity in Xenopus: studies during larval development and limb regeneration." Dev Comp Immunol 31(4): 383-393.

Morales, H. D., L. Abramowitz, et al. (2010). "Innate immune responses and permissiveness to ranavirus infection of peritoneal leukocytes in the frog Xenopus laevis." J Virol 84(10): 4912-4922.

Nagata, S. and N. Cohen (1983). "Specific in vivo and nonspecific in vitro alloreactivities of adult frogs (Xenopus laevis) that were thymectomized during early larval life." Eur J Immunol 13(7): 541-545.

Nakamura, T., M. Maeno, et al. (1987). "Tolerance induced by grafting semi-allogeneic adult skin to larval Xenopus laevis: possible involvement of specific suppressor cell activity." Differentiation 35(2): 108-114.

Nedelkovska, H., T. Cruz-Luna, et al. (2010). "Comparative in vivo study of gp96 adjuvanticity in the frog Xenopus laevis." J Vis Exp(43).

Nieuwkoop, P. D. and J. Faber (1967). Normal table of Xenopus laevis (Daudin). Amsterdam, Elsevier.

Ogino, H., W. B. McConnell, et al. (2006). "High-throughput transgenesis in Xenopus using I-SceI meganuclease." Nat Protoc 1(4): 1703-1710.

Pan, F. C., Y. Chen, et al. (2006). "I-SceI meganuclease-mediated transgenesis in Xenopus." Dev Dyn 235(1): 247-252.

Ramanayake, T., D. A. Simon, et al. (2007). "In vivo study of T-cell responses to skin alloantigens in Xenopus using a novel whole-mount immunohistology method." Transplantation 83(2): 159-166.

Rau, L., N. Cohen, et al. (2001). "MHC-restricted and -unrestricted CD8 T cells: an evolutionary perspective." Transplantation 72(11): 1830-1835.

Robert, J. (2006). "*Xenopus laevis* research resource for immunobiology." from http://www.urmc.rochester.edu/mbi/resources/Xenopus/.

Robert, J. and N. Cohen (1998). "Evolution of immune surveillance and tumor immunity: studies in Xenopus." Immunol Rev 166: 231-243.

Robert, J., J. Gantress, et al. (2004). "Xenopus as an experimental model for studying evolution of hsp--immune system interactions." Methods 32(1): 42-53.

Robert, J., J. Gantress, et al. (2002). "Minor histocompatibility antigen-specific MHC-restricted CD8 T cell responses elicited by heat shock proteins." J Immunol 168(4): 1697-1703.

Robert, J., C. Guiet, et al. (1997). "Effects of thymectomy and tolerance induction on tumor immunity in adult Xenopus laevis." Int J Cancer 70(3): 330-334.

Robert, J., C. Guiet, et al. (1994). "Lymphoid tumors of Xenopus laevis with different capacities for growth in larvae and adults." Dev Immunol 3(4): 297-307.

Robert, J., C. Guiet, et al. (1995). "Ontogeny of the alloimmune response against a transplanted tumor in Xenopus laevis." Differentiation 59(3): 135-144.

Robert, J. and Y. Ohta (2009). "Comparative and developmental study of the immune system in Xenopus." Dev Dyn 238(6): 1249-1270.

Robert, J., T. Ramanayake, et al. (2008). "Phylogenetic conservation of glycoprotein 96 ability to interact with CD91 and facilitate antigen cross-presentation." J Immunol 180(5): 3176-3182.

Robert, J., M. Sung, et al. (2001). "In vitro thymocyte differentiation in MHC class I-negative Xenopus larvae." Dev Comp Immunol 25(4): 323-336.

Rollins-Smith, L., M. Flajnik, et al. (1994). "Expression of MHC class I antigens during ontogeny in *Xenopus* is metamorphosis independent." Dev Comp Immunol(18): S95.

Salter-Cid, L., M. Nonaka, et al. (1998). "Expression of MHC class Ia and class Ib during ontogeny: high expression in epithelia and coregulation of class Ia and lmp7 genes." J Immunol 160(6): 2853-2861.

Smith, S. J., P. Ataliotis, et al. (2005). "The MLC1v gene provides a transgenic marker of myocardium formation within developing chambers of the Xenopus heart." Dev Dyn 232(4): 1003-1012.

Tata, J. R. (2006). "Amphibian metamorphosis as a model for the developmental actions of thyroid hormone." Mol Cell Endocrinol 246(1-2): 10-20.

Tochinai, A. and C. Katagiri (1975). "Complete abrogation of immune responses to skin allografts and rabbit erythrocytes in the early thymectomized *Xenopus*." Dev Growth Differ (17): 283-294.

15

The Effect of Human Recombinant Erythropoietin (rHuEPO) and Tacrolimus (FK506) in Autologous and Homologous Full Thickness Skin Graft (FTSG) Take and Viability in a Rat Model

Dimitrios Karypidis, Despina Perrea,
Othon Papadopoulos and Alkiviadis Kostakis
2nd Propedeutic Surgical Department and Department of Experimental Surgery Athens University School of Medicine
Greece

1. Introduction

The use of autologous skin grafts comprises a well established method of reconstruction in large areas involving partial thickness defects. Additionally, when skin availability is limited due to associated trauma or injury (e.g. burns) the use of homologous skin grafts from a compatible donor appears to be a valid alternative. The effort to maximize effectiveness of skin grafting in terms of increasing graft take, protecting viability, reducing full healing time and achieving improved postoperative outcomes without impairing function has also been constant especially in cases of impaired general condition.

Human recombinant erythropoietin (rHuEPO) is a glycoprotein with primarily a hemopoietic role due to the inhibition of precursor erythrocytes and the promotion of their proliferation. Its genetic expression is being regulated by hypoxia. It is primarily synthesized by the fetal kidneys and liver and by the adult kidneys (Paschos et al. 2008).

The biological activity of rHuEPO is promoted by its interaction with the cell surface erythropoietin receptor (EPOR) (Brines and Ceramic 2008) which is a type I cytokine expressed by precursor erythrocytes as well as in other non hemopoietic systems such as the central and the peripheral nervous system in response to trauma (Galeano et al. 2004), in cardiac muscle cells, vascular endothelial smooth muscle cells and in subcutaneous mast cells with potent anti-ischaemic action (Brines and Ceramic, 2008; Galeano et al. , 2004).

Current research has focused on its non-hemopoietic role. Many studies report the local production of erythropoietin (EPO) in response to trauma prior to the local concentration of pre-inflammatory cytokines and EPO acting antagonistically to them by reducing edema, inhibiting cellular apoptosis, promoting neovascularization by enhancing endothelial cell mitosis and promoting wound healing (Paschos et al. 2008).

Since endogenous local EPO production is inadequate, it has been shown that the exogenous administration of rHuEPO enhanced wound healing and revascularization in experimental studies on healthy rats, rats with genetically induced diabetes mellitus and rats with burn injuries (Galeano 2006). In clinical studies including human subjects, the wound healing promoting properties of rHuEPO have been reported following γ-knife for brain surgery and recently in patients who underwent destruction osteogenesis (Mihmanli et al. 2009)

Vascular endothelial growth factor (VEGF) comprises a heparin-binding, dimeric glycoprotein which initiates the proliferation and migration of endothelial cells to participate in the development of new vascular lumens, and increases the penetration and extravasation of plasma macromolecules (Hom et al., 2005; Paschos et al., 2008). VEGF receptors are found in endothelial cells and are expressed under conditions of hypoxia and following endothelial damage. Two high-affinity endothelial cell receptors, KDR/Flk-1 and flt-1 mediate VEGF effects on tissue physiology (Lantieri et al. 1998)

VEGF has been shown to participate in wound healing enhancement, embryo development, growth of certain solid tumors, and ascites formation (Isogai et al., 2006; Schultze-Mosgau et al., 2003). In this study, the immunohistochemical detection of VEGF expression is used as a method of skin graft take evaluation.

Tacrolimus (FK-506), has recently been established as a valid immunosuppressant and comprises a well-known calcineurin (a serine/threonine phosphatise) inhibitor. It has been shown that FK-506 inhibits TGF-β induced VEGF production by antagonizing calcineurin which leads to the attenuation of the activation and translocation of the nuclear factor that activates T-cells (nft) (Mori et al 1997). FK-506 also inhibits: a) interleukin-2 induced interleukin-5 production by CD4+ T cells and b) T-cells proliferation stimulated by interleukin-2 and interleukin-7 (Mori et al 1997). Confirmation was provided by similar studies which showed that rapamycin, another immunosuppressant which does not inhibit calcineurin, did not have any effect on TGF-β induced VEGF production while cyclosporine A, which is also a calcineurin inhibitor, resulted in reduction of VEGF production (Marumo et al. 1995). The action of FK-506 is mediated by immunophilins, a class of proteins which bind to immunosuppressive drugs, giving to FK-506 the ability to interact with calcineurin and to interfere with its access and dephosphorylation of various substrates. The primary immunophilin was shown to be FKBP 13 which is localized to the endoplasmic reticulum lumen, where processing and presentation of antigen in the immune system are thought to take place (Nigam et al. 1993). The liver and the intestinal mucosa are the main sites of FK-506 metabolism by the cytochrome P4503A4 enzyme. Subsequently, FK-506 is eliminated through biliary excretion. (Lampen et al., 1995; Nakazawa et al., 1998; Plosker & Foster, 2000). FK-506 has been widely used systemically, maintaining a profile of safety during the long-term experience with the drug. Most side effects appear to be related to whole-blood concentrations and refer to nephrotoxicity, cardiovascular toxicity, metabolic and neurotoxicity. However, almost all of the reports of FK-506 toxicity are derived from its use in solid-organ transplantation, in which much higher doses are used compared to those for skin transplantation (Mayer et al., 1997; Pirsch et al. 1997). The aim of this animal study is to investigate the effect of human recombinant erythropoietin (rHuEPO) and tacrolimus (FK-506) on autologous and homologous full thickness skin grafts in an experimental research design including Wistar rats.

2. Methods and material

Thirty adult inbred female Wistar rats (n=30), with weights ranging from 220 to 300 gr, were selected for this study. Two control and 3 experimental groups were formed, each consisting of 6 subjects. This experimental study followed the National Research Council's Guide for the Care and Use of Laboratory Animals and was approved by the National Bioethics Committee. This study used the minimum number of animals needed in order to establish a valid conclusion and statement regarding the specific subject. All necessary refinements and design methods have been performed and planned according to accredited established protocols. All surgical procedures were performed under general anesthesia with the use of ketamine hydrochloride (80 mg/kg intramuscularly) and xylazine (2 mg/kg intramuscularly).

After induction of general anesthesia the surgical site was shaved and prepped with povidone iodine and chlorhexidine solution. The animals were covered with sterile surgical drapes with only the operative site exposed.

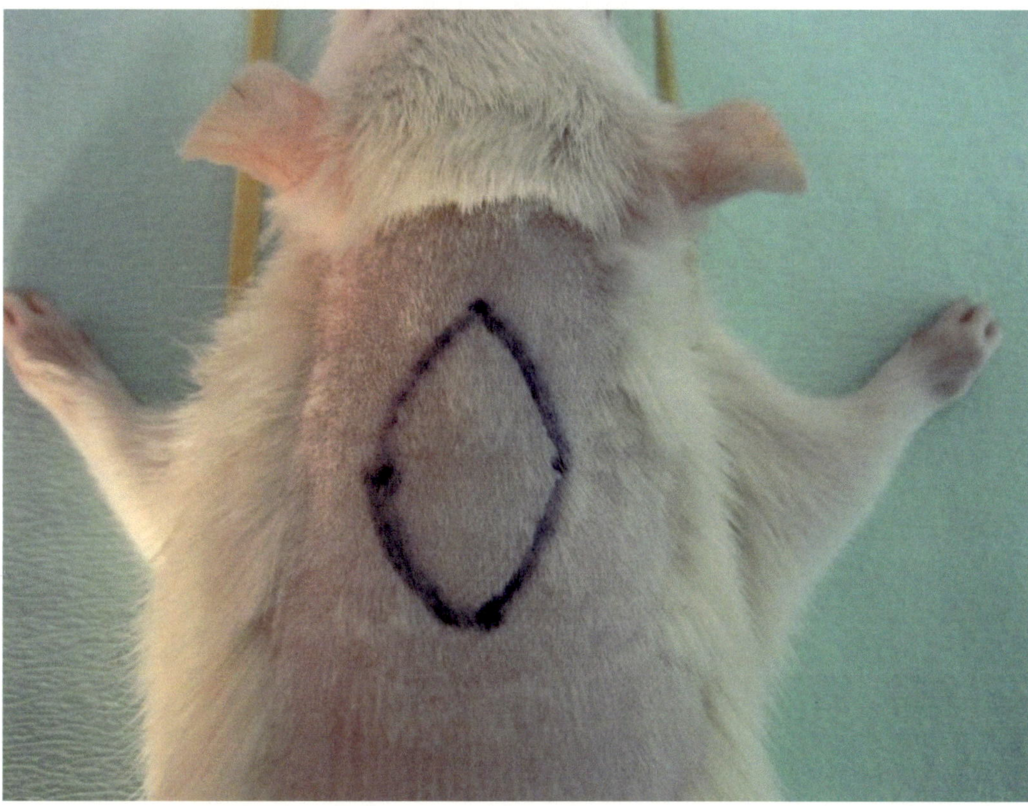

Fig. 1. Preoperative design of the FTSG on the back of the subject

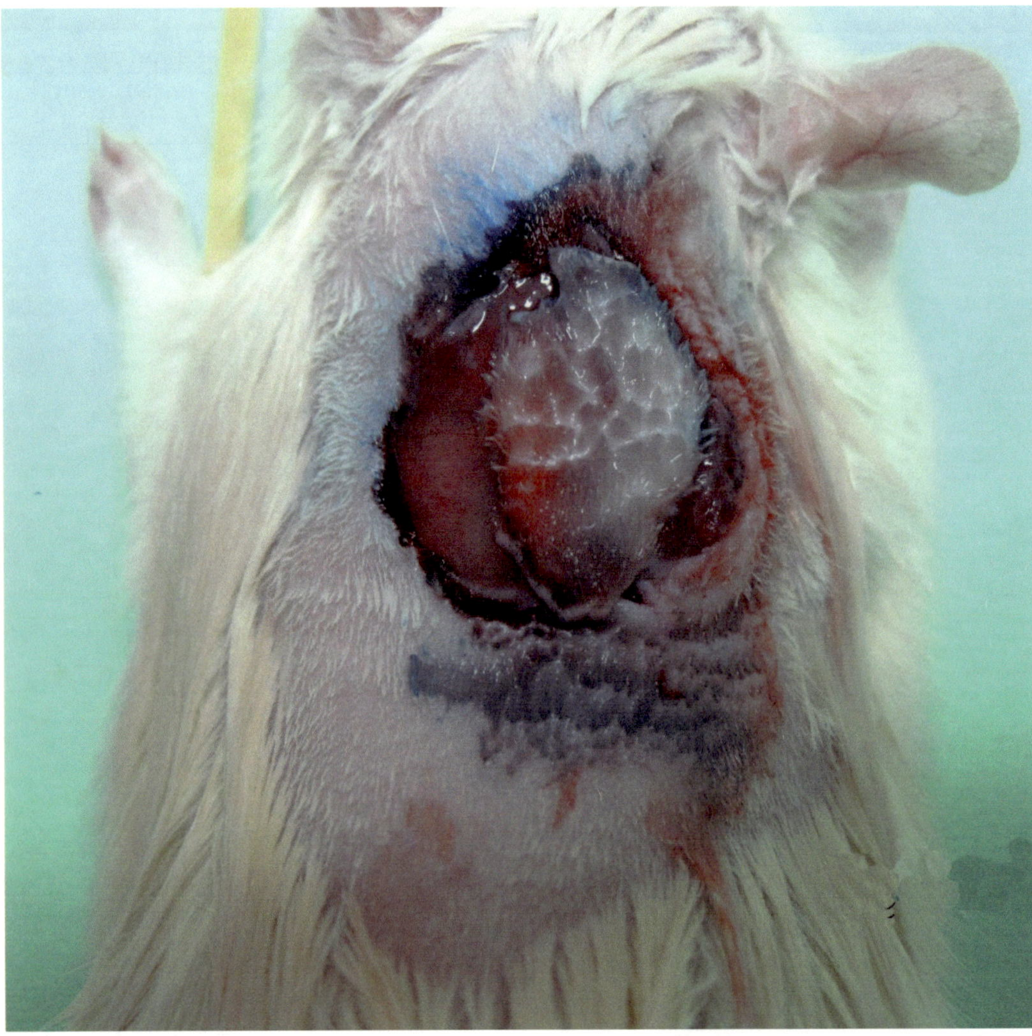

Fig. 2. Dissection and harvesting of the FTSG and then rotation of the FTSG on the wound bed by 180° so as the previously caudal edge becomes rostral and the donor site can be used as the recipient site

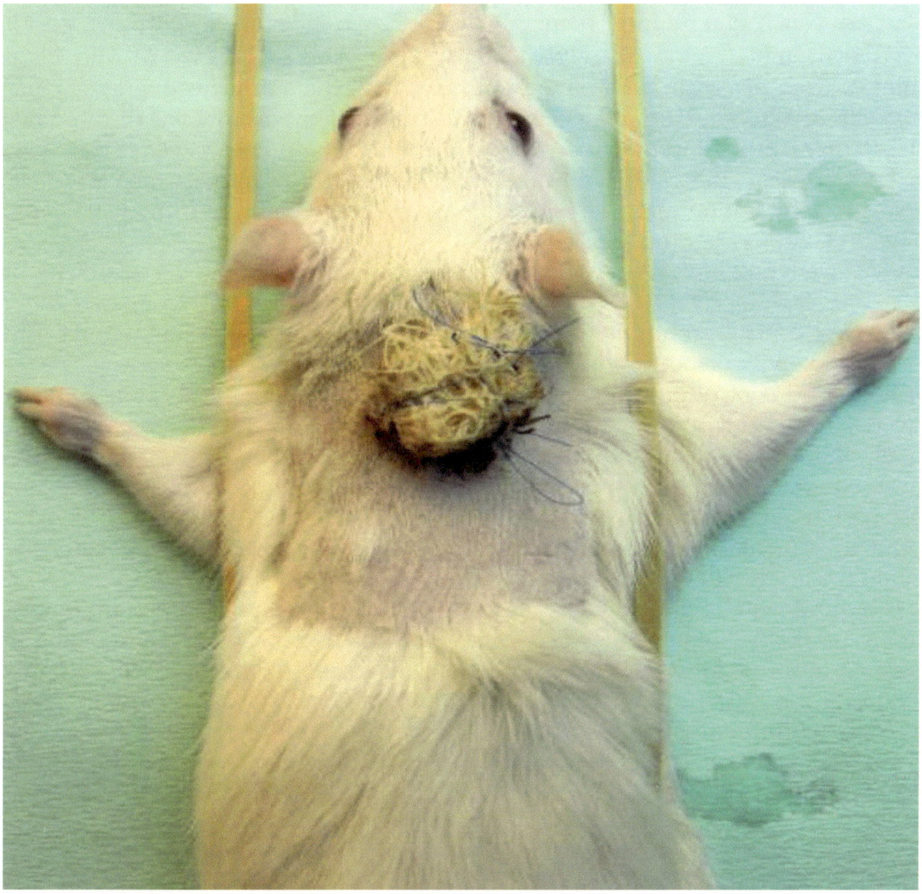

Fig. 3. Cleaned wound area and dressing application on the FTSG

A full thickness skin graft was harvested from the area between the two scapula bones on the dorsum of each rat. The skin graft was elliptical in shape, with a long diameter of 2 cm and a small diameter of 1 cm (Figure 1). During harvesting, the panniculus layer was carefully removed from the bed of the skin graft and recipient site. The skin graft was kept in phosphate-buffered saline before being transferred to the recipient site. In this experimental model, each skin graft was repositioned in the same area from which it was harvested after being rotated by 180 degrees in the vertical axis, so as the severed vascular axons in the skin graft remain misaligned to the vascular axons of the recipient bed. In this way each donor site also serves as a recipient site since revascularization and new vascular connections between skin graft and recipient bed are still required due to the preserved vascular misalignment in the new graft position. When a homologous FTSG was required, animals underwent surgery in pairs and a FTSG was harvested in the aforementioned way from each animal and it was then transplanted into the donor site of the other after being similarly rotated by 180 degrees (see subject groups below).

The location of the recipient bed is conveniently situated between the scapular bones, unreachable by the rats and well fixated on a minimally mobile area causing negligible irritation to the rats. No animal involved in this project was subjected to discomfort, pain, or

distress. Any such discomfort, pain, or distress was alleviated with the appropriate approved medication (Figure 1-3). Nylon 5-0 non-absorbable sutures were invariably used.
The animals were placed in a warm environment with the aid of heating lamps and were continuously monitored. Pain management was carried out with the use of Buprenorphine at 0.05-0.10 mg/Kg, SC, and then twice daily. The animals were observed for their pattern of breathing, alertness, ability for food and drink uptake. After surgery rats were carefully observed for dehydration and diarrhea. Rats were kept separately in their housing cages which were standard filter top secured cages.
The animals were randomized into the following groups according to the treatment that was used:
Group A (First control group, n=6): An autologous FTSG was harvested and repositioned. Local infiltration with water for injection was also performed as a control.
Group B (Second control group, n=6): Animals underwent surgery in pairs. Consequently there were 3 pairs in this group. A homologous FTSG was harvested from each animal of each pair and transplanted into the donor site of the other. FK506 (tacrolimus) was administered systematically to prevent rejection. Local infiltration with water for injection was also performed as a control.
Group a (experimental, n=6): An autologous FTSG was harvested and repositioned. Local infiltration with rHuEPO was performed.
Group b (experimental, n=6): Animals underwent surgery in pairs as in group B, forming a total of 3 pairs. A homologous FTSG was harvested from each animal and it was transplanted into the donor site of the other while FK506 (tacrolimus) was administered systematically (local infiltration) to prevent immunologic response. Local infiltration with rHuEPO was performed.
Group c (experimental, n=6): An autologous FTSG was harvested and repositioned and local infiltration with FK506 was performed. Table 1 summarizes the details regarding each animal group.

Group	Type	Number of subjects	FTSG	FK506	rHuEPO	wfi
A	control	6	autologous	no	no	yes
B	control	6	homologous	for immunosuppression	no	yes
a	experimental	6	autologous	no	factor	no
b	experimental	6	homologous	for immunosuppression	factor	no
c	experimental	6	autologous	factor	no	no

Table 1. The animal groups in the study. FTSG: full thickness skin graft, for immunosuppression: FK506 is used in order to prevent rejection, not as tested factor, factor: FK506 or rHuEPO are used as local infusion around the recipient bed and their effect on graft viability and healing is tested, wfi: water for injection used for local infiltration as a placebo, when one of the previously mentioned factors were not used

FK-506 (Fujisawa USA, Inc.) was dissolved in 80% ethanol and 20% cremaphor to create a stock solution with a concentration of 10 mg/ml. This stock was then diluted with 75%

propylene glycol and 25% water to a final concentration of 0.5 mg/ml. The diluted solution was replaced every 3 days.

In groups B and b, FK-506 was subcutaneously administered daily at a dose of 2mg/Kg. The use of FK-506 either as a systematic immunosuppressant (groups B and b) or as a local agent (group c) always involved local, subcutaneous infiltration. In groups a and b, 400UI/kg in a 100μL solution of rHuEPO were subcutaneously administered, daily. Local infiltration of agents was invariably performed around and under the recipient bed.

The effect of FK-506 and rHuEPO administration in the aforementioned experimental groups was investigated. The investigation consisted of the clinical, histological and immunohistochemical evaluation of the grafts and their viability-take on the 10th post grafting day. All subjects were euthanized on the 10th post grafting day by prolonged inhalation in a closed diethyl-ether inhalation chamber.

Skin graft take area and viability were assessed using digital photographs and manual measurements. The photographs were processed by digital image surface area analysis software (Pixcavator Image Analysis Software 2.3). Specimens of autologous and homologous skin grafts were then harvested together with a marginal recipient bed skin, along the perimeter of the graft for histological examination and immunohistochemistry. The formalin fixed, paraffin embedded tissue sections were treated with hematoxylin-eosin stain as well as by two antibodies. Standard procedures as recommended by the manufacturer were performed.

The antibodies used in our study were:

Monoclonal Mouse Anti-Human Vascular Endothelial Growth Factor, Clone VG1, isotype: IgG1, kappa antibody was used to label the VEGF-121, VEGF-165, and VEGF-189 isoforms of vascular endothelial growth factor (VEGF) Clone VG1.

Monoclonal Mouse Anti-Human CD31, Endothelial Cell, Clone JC70A, isotype: IgG1, kappa, (Dako A/S, Glostrup

Denmark Autostainer/Autostainer Plus) antibody was used to label endothelial cells of newly formed vessels to determine angiogenesis.

Histology findings were evaluated for vascular presence and endothelial condition, lymphocytic infiltration, dermal/epidermal interphase reaction (spongiosis, incomplete, complete epidermal separation) and necrosis. More specifically, due to the relatively variable macroscopic presentation of homologous graft rejection, histology findings and criteria were solely used to describe and categorize potential rejection according to the established method of Tatsuya et al (1997) which includes the following three grades:

Grade 1: intraepidermal blister formation,

Grade 2: incomplete epidermal separation from the dermis;

Grade 3: complete epidermal separation from the dermis.

Immunochemistry analysis aimed at demonstrating the degree of angiogenesis in the skin grafts as a direct sign of vascular network rearrangement and development, viability and effective graft take.

Manual measurement and clinical assessment of graft take was performed using light microscopy and corresponded adequately with the digital image analysis.

Spleens were harvested and subjected to the mixed lymphocyte reaction, to assess the degree of immunosuppression. Liver and kidneys were also harvested and examined for signs of potential hepato- and nephrotoxicity.

3. Statistical analysis

Areas of graft take comprise numeric data which are presented with approximation of two decimal digits. Means are presented ±SD where applicable, and the *t* test for independent samples has been used for statistical analysis of the results. SPSS 17.0 (IBM Corporation Somers, NY 10589) was used. Statistical significance was considered for $p<0.05$.

4. Results

Clinical results were classified according to the mean area of inadequate graft take - graft necrosis (N). In control group A N=40.98 mm^2, in control group B N=71.2 ± 4.67mm^2, in experimental group a N= 15.22 ± 4.76 mm^2 in experimental group b N= 29.2± 4.70 mm^2, in experimental group c N=46.52 ± 4.60 mm^2. Manual measurements corresponded well with the aforementioned digital image analysis measurements. The corresponding percentages (over the total area of each graft which was 20 x 10 mm^2= 200 mm^2) of mean graft necrotic areas were: group A: 20.49%, group B: 35.6%, group a: 7.6%, group b: 14.6%, group c: 23.26% ($p<0.001$ in all group comparisons: A-a, B-b and A-c) (Figures 4-9).

Histological findings using hematoxylin-eosin stain showed the differences in graft revascularization and take among groups (10th post-grafting day) (Figures 10-19)

Immunohistochemistry resulted in significant observations regarding graft revascularization in the each group (Figures 20-27).

Clinical, histological and immunohistochemical findings consistently show the resulting quality of graft take and degree of revascularization among the various groups: graft take in group a>group b> group A> group c> group B.

No signs of hepato- and nephro-toxicity were found.

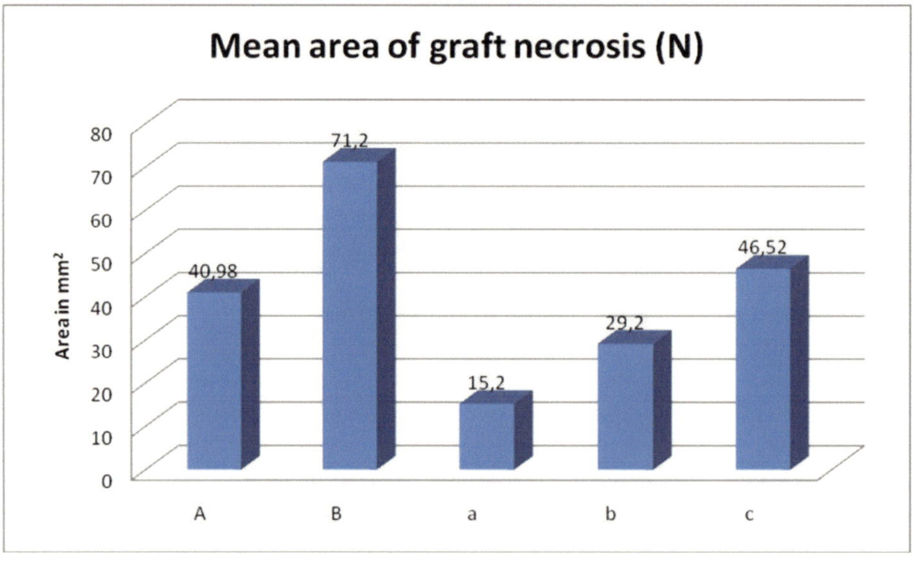

Fig. 4. Mean inadequate graft take-necrosis percentage per group. A, B, a, b and c correspond to animal groups

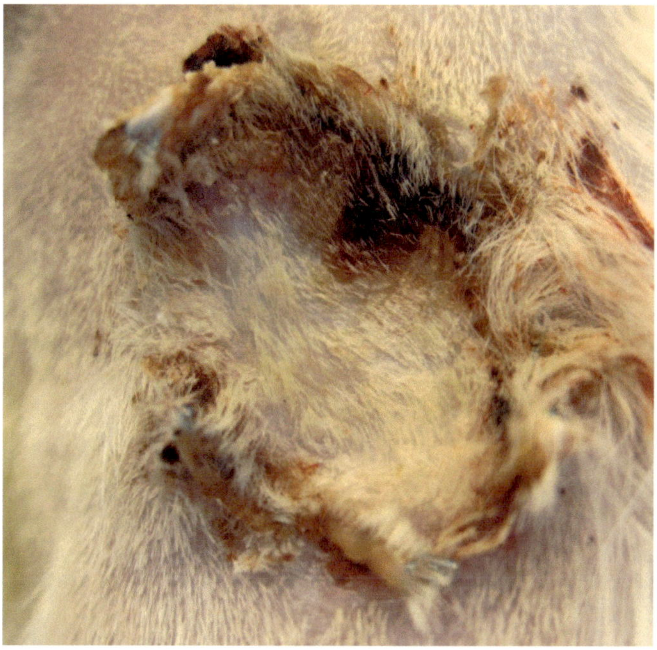

Fig. 5. Group A macroscopic presentation. Mild peripheral necrosis, good overall take

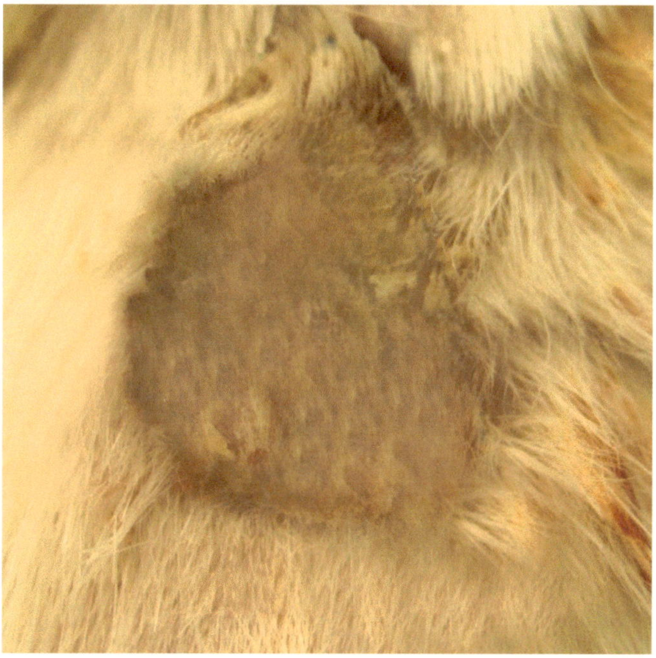

Fig. 6. Group a macroscopic presentation. Full graft take, no signs of necrosis, excellent graft viability

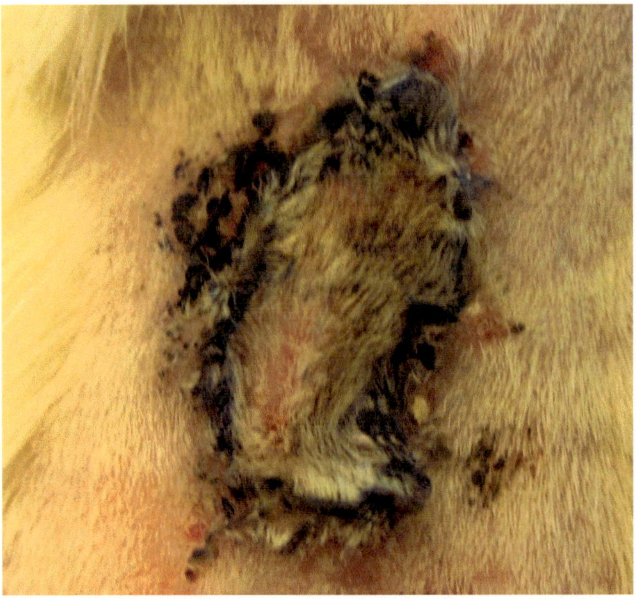

Fig. 7. Group B macroscopic presentation. Considerable peripheral graft rejection. Central graft take and viability

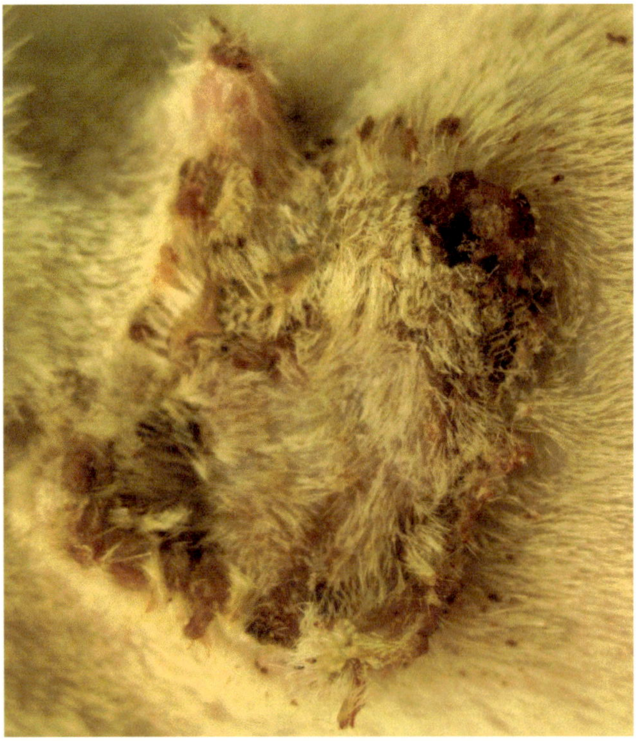

Fig. 8. Group b macroscopic presentation. Minimal peripheral rejection and nearly complete graft take.

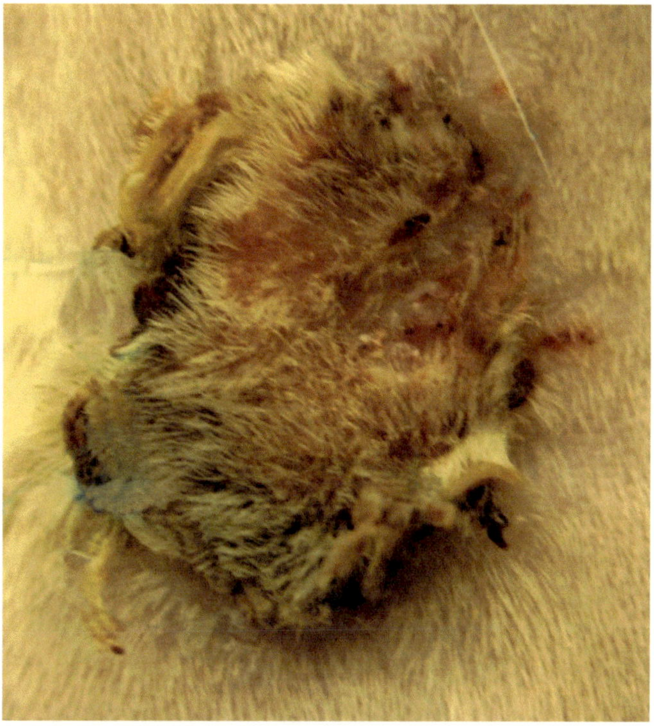

Fig. 9. Group c macroscopic presentation. Partial graft necrosis, not uniform graft take compared to control group A.

Groups A-a

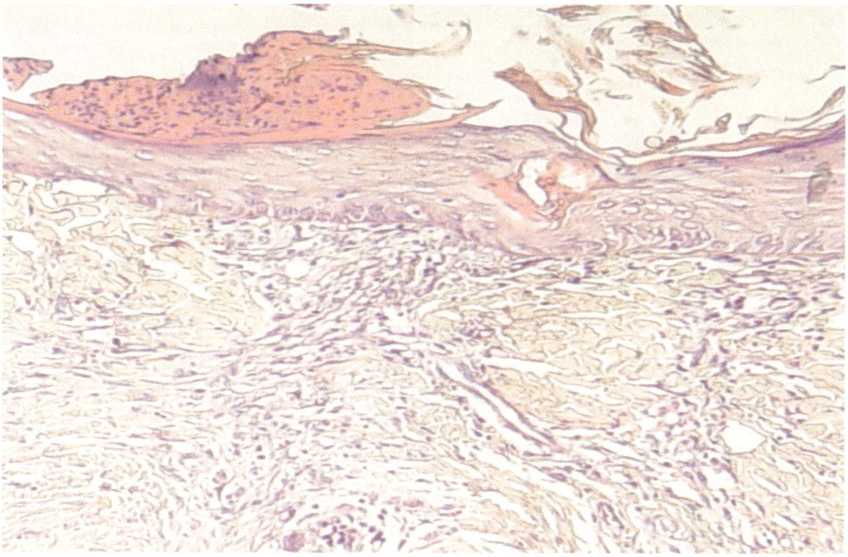

Fig. 10. Formalin fixed, paraffin embedded FTSG x50 in group A. Normal graft take with intermediate inflammatory inflammation demonstrating FTSG take without the use of exogenous active factors.

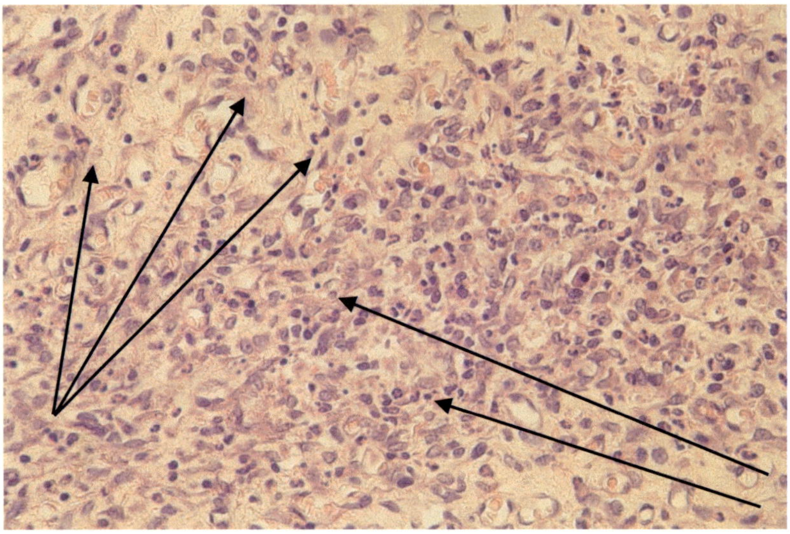

Fig. 11. Formalin fixed, paraffin embedded autologous FTSG x200 in group A. Vascular lumens with erythrocytes (v), polymorphonuclear cells(p), lymphocytes (l) and other inflammatory cell intermediate concentrations are also shown. The number of vessels is indicative of the quality of graft take and viability

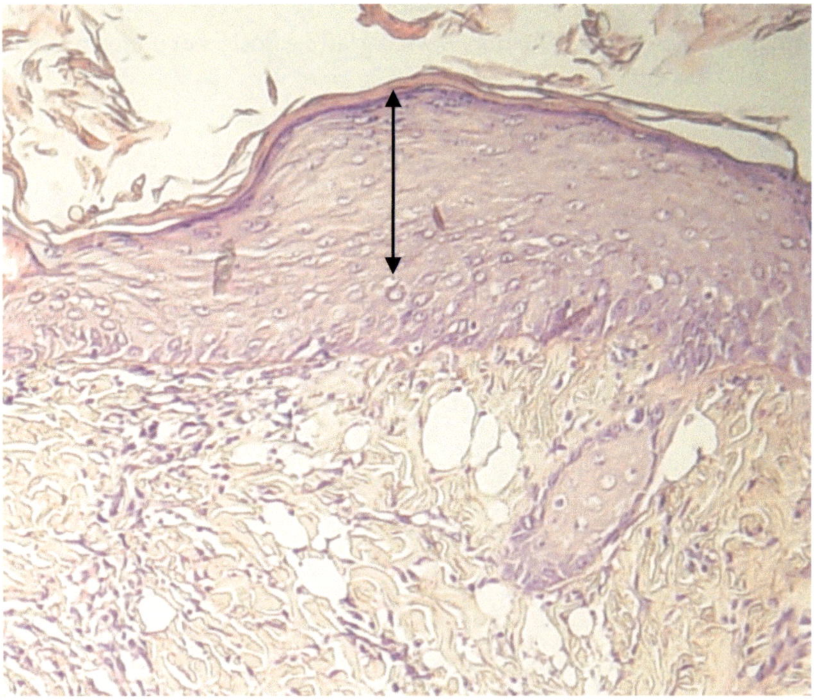

Fig. 12. Formalin fixed paraffin embedded autologous FTSG x50 in group a. Higher vessel concentration, more uniform and higher epidermal layer (double arrow line), less inflammatory infiltration than in control group A

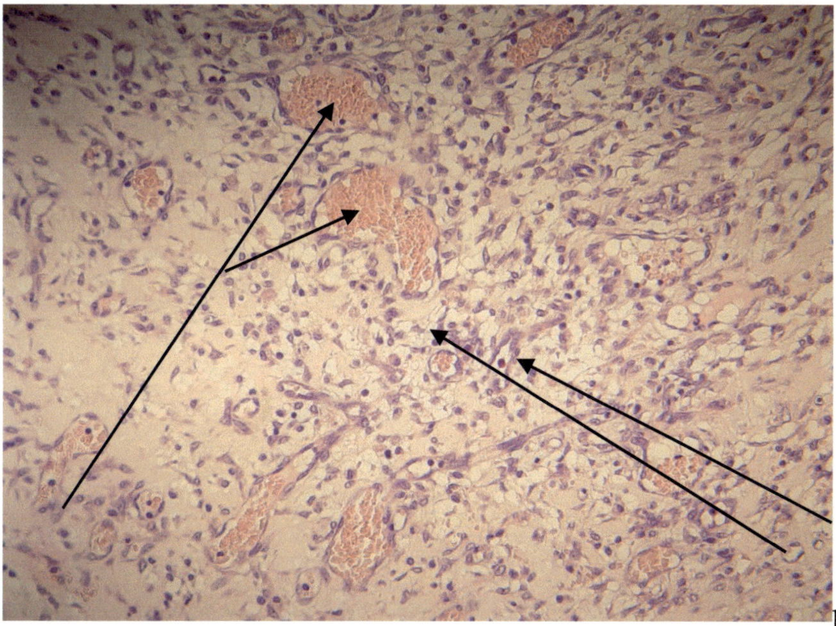

v p l

Fig. 13. Formalin fixed, paraffin embedded autologous FTSG x200 in group a. Vascular lumens with erythrocytes (v), polymorphonuclear cells(p), lymphocytes (l) and other inflammatory cell concentrations are also shown. Note the increased number of vessels and the milder inflammatory response which are indicative of better quality of graft take and viability than in the control group

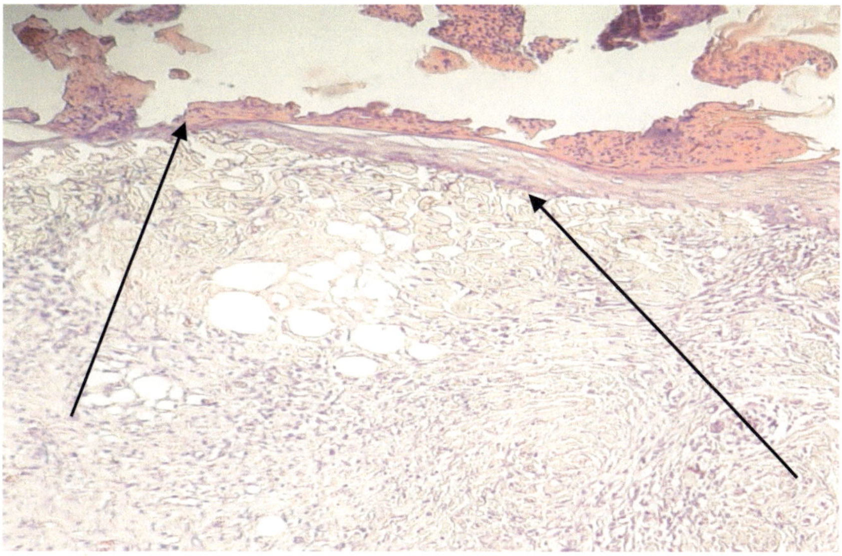

s b

Fig. 14. Homologous FTSG x50 in group B. Increased intraepidermal blisters (b), dermoepidermal lack of cohesion (s) and increased inflammatory infiltration compatible with grade 2-3 of rejection according to Tatsuya et al (1997).

Groups B-b

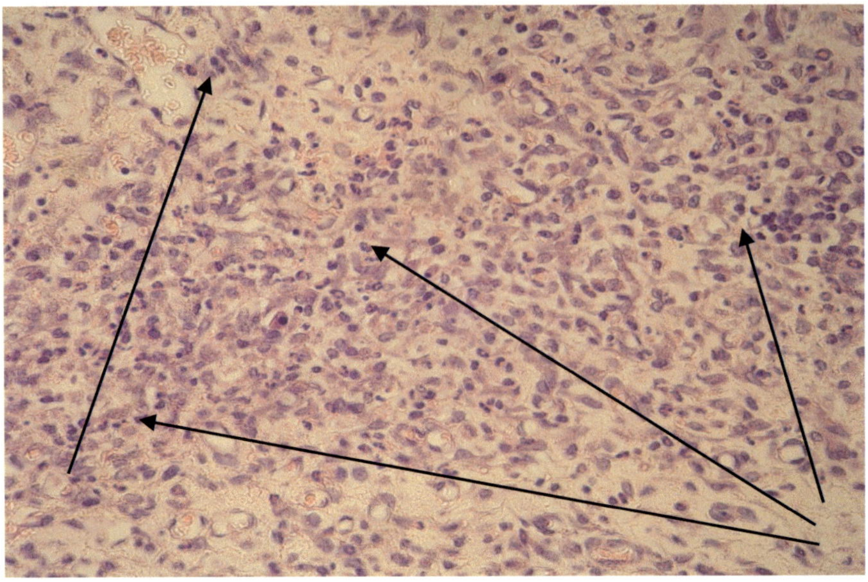

v e

Fig. 15. Formalin fixed, paraffin embedded homologous FTSG x200 in group B. Inflammatory response and mild revascularization compatible with the initial stages of rejection, impairing the ongoing course of graft revascularization (v) and take. Inflammatory cells include large eosinophils concentrations (e) characteristic of the aforementioned response type.

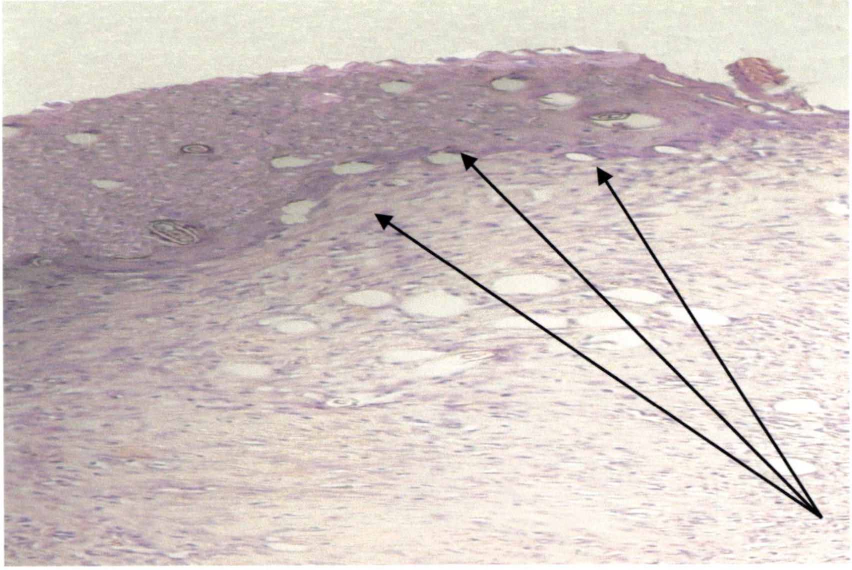

b

Fig. 16. Formalin fixed, paraffin embedded homologous FTSG x50 in group b. Intraepidermal blisters (b) but lack of partial dermoepidermal separation. Better quality of graft take and minimal rejection response than in control group B.

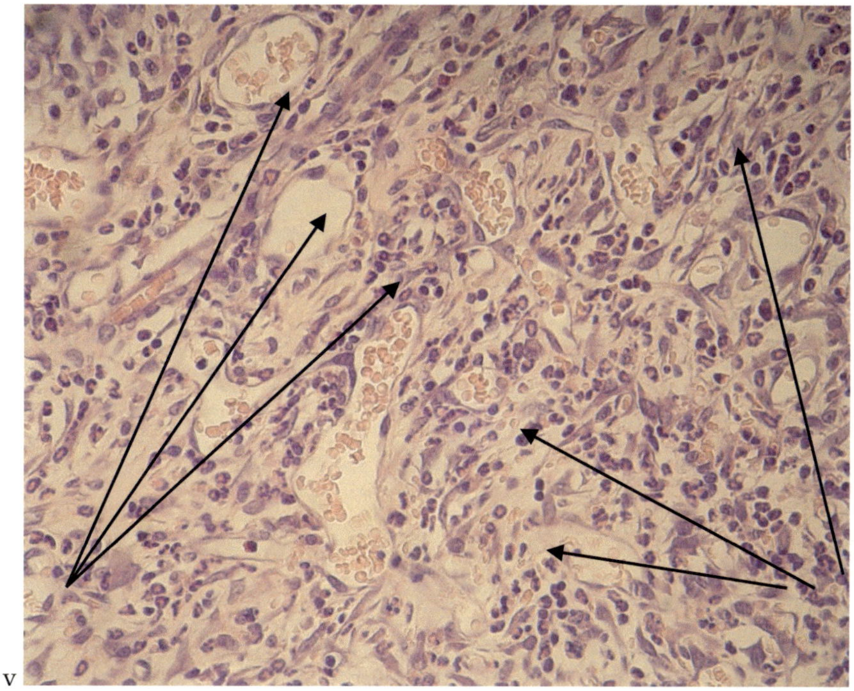

Fig. 17. Formalin fixed, paraffin embedded homologous FTSG x200 in group b. Inflammatory response with concentrations of eosinophils (e), lymphocytes (l) and polymorphonuclear cells (p) but also nearly unimpaired revascularization (v) demonstrating a considerably better quality of graft take and milder rejection response than in control group B.

Group c

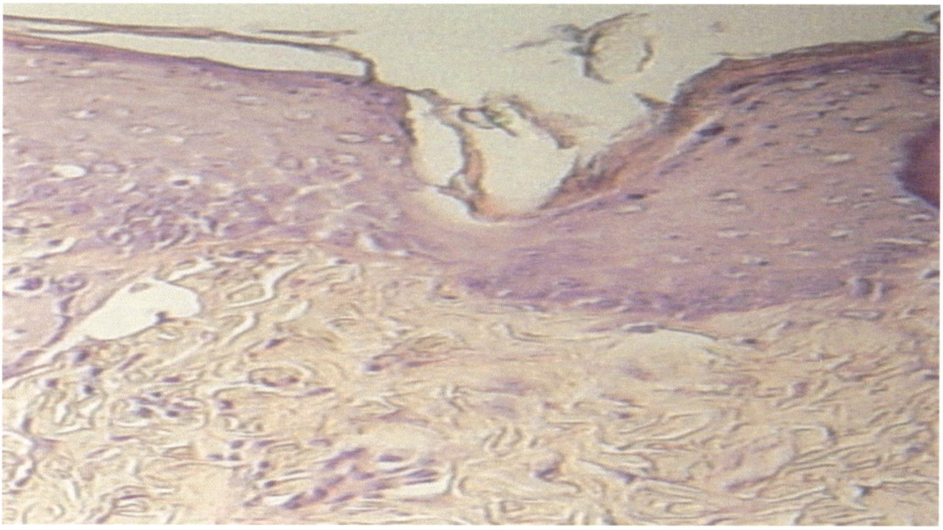

Fig. 18. Formalin fixed, paraffin embedded autologous FTSG x50 in group c. Nearly normal graft take with minimal inflammatory response, firm dermoepidermal cohesion but marginally decreased new vessels development than in control group A.

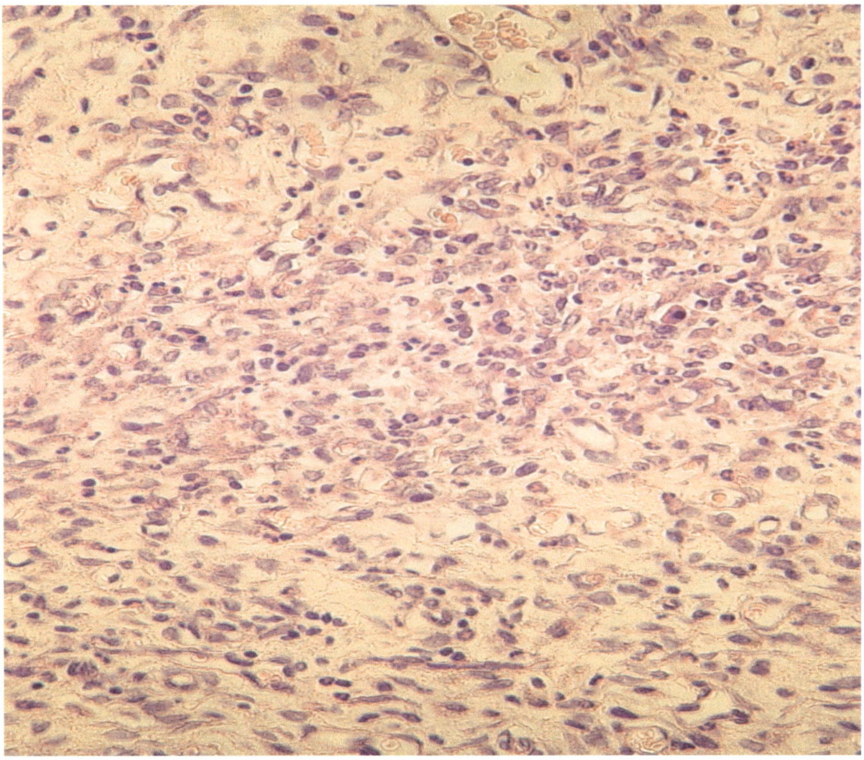

Fig. 19. Formalin fixed, paraffin embedded autologous FTSG x200 in group c. Nearly normal graft take with minimal inflammatory response and decreased revascularization compared to group A.

Groups A-a

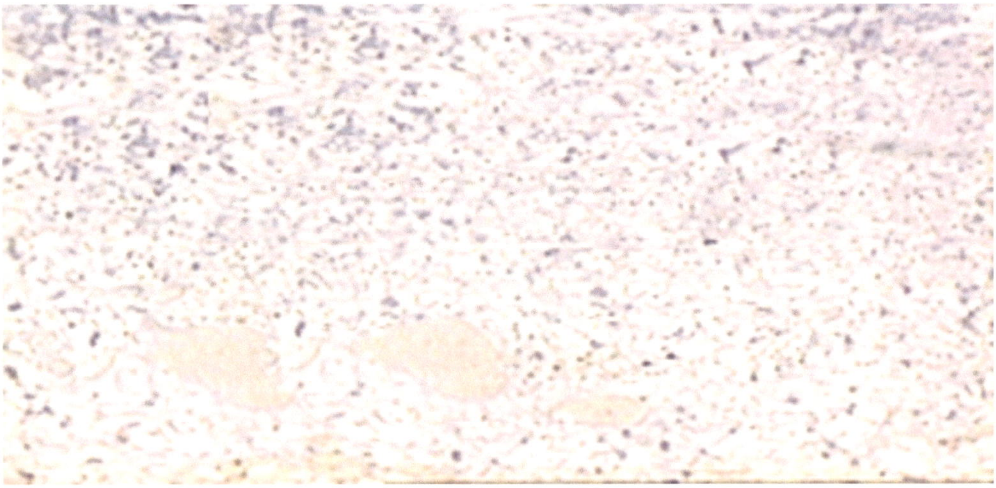

Fig. 20. VEGF expression in group A, as detected by treating tissues with human VEGF monoclonal antibody. Low or absent stain in the normal autologous grafting group.

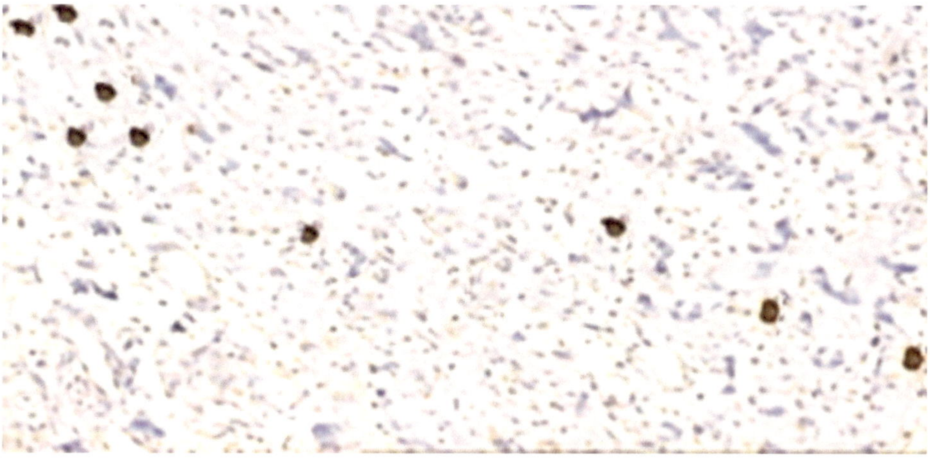

Fig. 21. VEGF expression in group a, as detected by treating tissues with human VEGF monoclonal antibody. Stained-activated macrophages (brown) are noted indicating an increase in revascularization process compared to the control group A

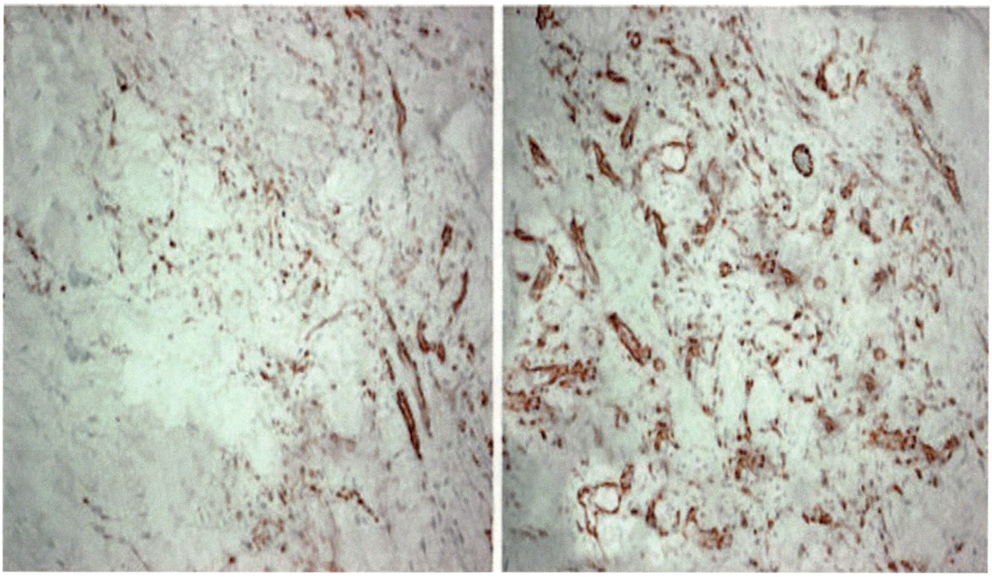

Fig. 22. CD31 stained endothelial cells of newly formed vessels (copper color) in control group A (left) and group a (right). Notably increased angiogenesis is shown in group a

Groups B-b

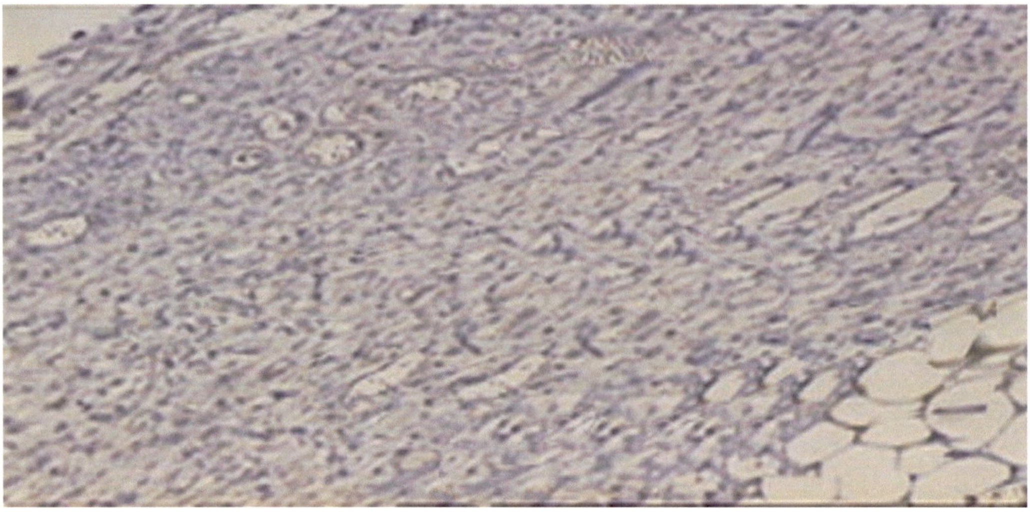

Fig. 23. VEGF expression in group B, following tissue treatment with human VEGF monoclonal antibody. Low or absent stain in the homologous grafting group. Blisters are also noted, indicative of early rejection response signs.

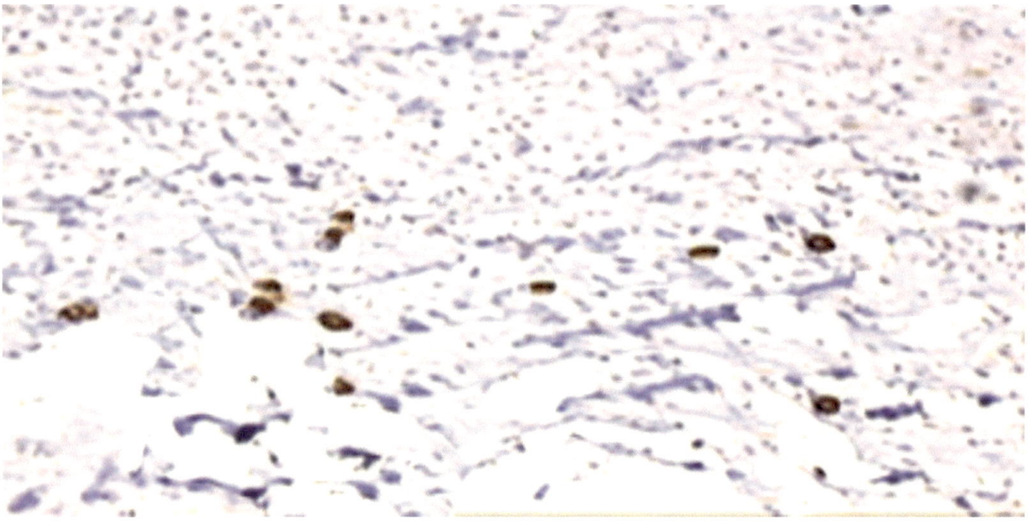

Fig. 24. VEGF expression in group b after the use of VEGF monoclonal antibody. Stained-activated macrophages (brown) are noted compared to their absence in group B tissues, indicative of increased angiogenesis.

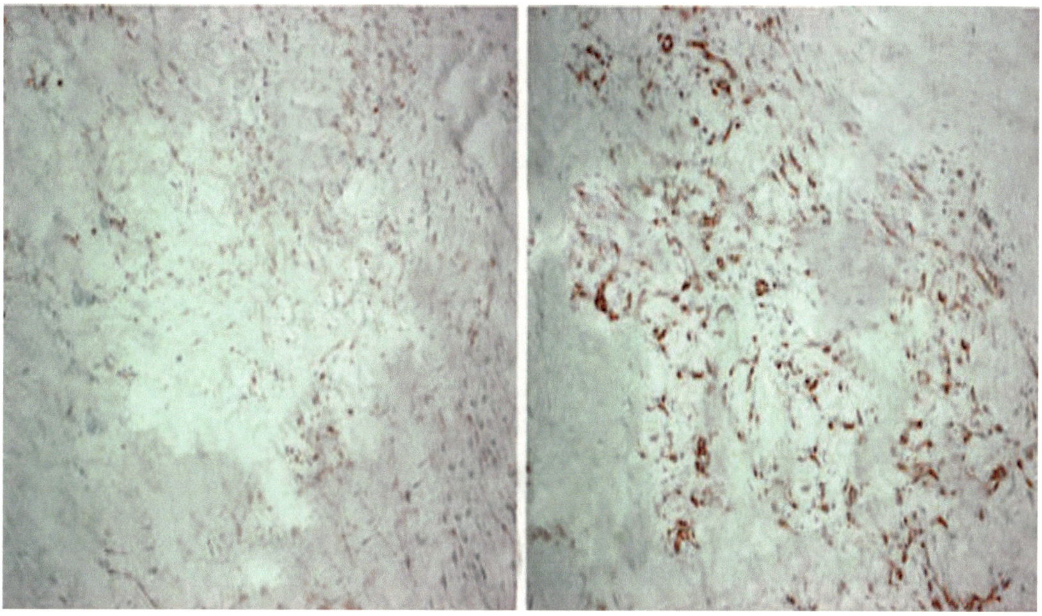

Fig. 25. CD31 stained endothelial cells of newly formed vessels (copper color) in control group B (left) and group b (right). Note the absence of endothelial concentrations in group B and the increased angiogenesis in group b

Groups c

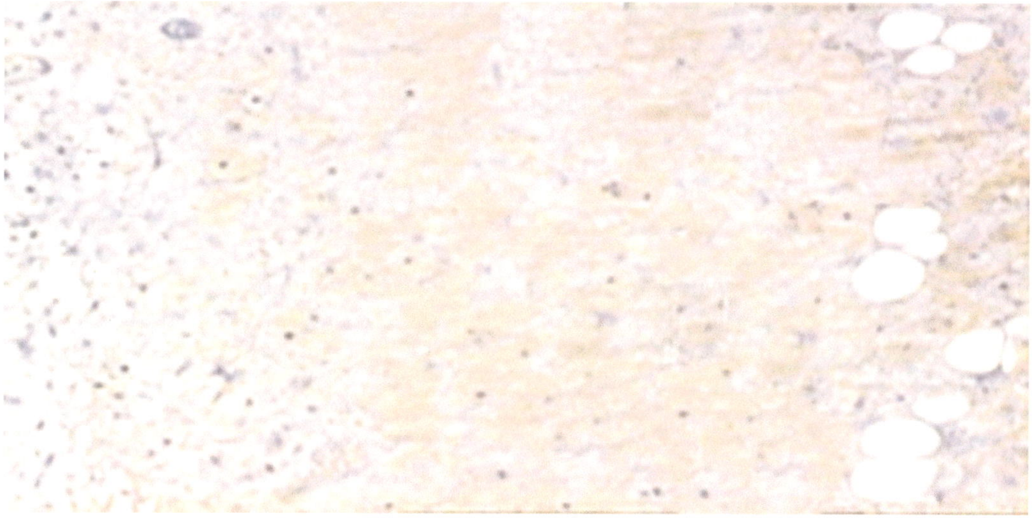

Fig. 26. VEGF expression in group c, after treating tissues with human VEGF monoclonal antibody. Minimal stain in the autologous grafts included in group c.

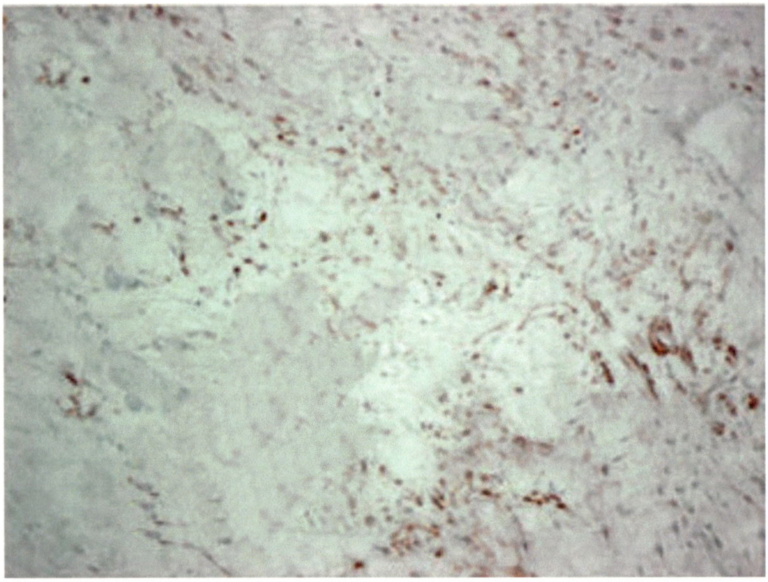

Fig. 27. CD31 stained endothelial cells of newly formed vessels in group c. Considerable decrease in angiogenesis compared to control group A

5. Discussion

Between days 3 and 8 after grafting, the transient formation of spherical protrusions in the graft capillaries resembling angiogenic buds is taking place in what appears to be an angiogenic response of the autochthonous graft capillaries (Lindenblatt et al 2010). Proangiogenic molecules in the recipient bed and the graft tissue were revealed by immunohistochemical analysis which showed that the wall of the aforementioned buds expressed CD31 and desmin, indicating the presence of both endothelial cells and pericytes (Gerhardt & Betsholtz 2003). A docking of sprouting vascular formation takes place from the recipient bed which connects to the aforementioned spherical protrusions of the pre-existing graft vessels unlike the previously suggested neovascularization theory which requires weeks to complete. Additionally, there is rather no vessel inosculation from the recipient bed to the graft as it was previously accepted but there is what appears to be a gradual angiogenic response leading to newly formed vascular buds (Goretsky et al., 1995; Okada ,1986; Young et al., 1996).

The traditional vessel inosculation theory implies vessel re-formation and lumen restoration of already existing vessels via direct approximation of vessels of the recipient bed and the ones in the graft. Since it is nearly impossible to assume that simple graft positioning leads to an effective number of successful graft-bed vessel couplings, the aforementioned angiogenetic process has been recently described. Conversely, it has also been suggested that pre-existing channels in the graft allow vessels from the recipient bed to invade the graft from the periphery replacing a considerable number of graft vessels (Capla et al. 2006)

In order to provide the physiologic mechanism of graft take process it could be suggested that during the initial stages (hours) following transplantation, blood, nutrients and angiogenic factors cover the graft area and bed. Hypoxia along with the substrate of available factors creates the signal for the angiogenic response which commences at 2-3 postgrafting days. According to our findings it was noted that the center of the graft contains a higher density of vascular buds and vessels suggesting that angiogenesis begins there and continuous outwardly towards the periphery of the graft. It is controversial whether angiogenesis takes place before the 2-3td postgrafting day since there are authors who claim that the graft on its own has the physiologic potential to perform angiogenesis much earlier (Laschke et al., 2008; Shepherd et al., 2004). However, it is generally accepted that revascularization is a process that involves the presence of both the recipient bed and the graft itself since it is their interaction which leads to effective angiogenesis. Additionally, after the initial angiogenic response, vessels from the recipient bed gradually take over and invade-merge with the existing vascular infrastructure of the graft and with the newly formed vascular buds. Following that, endothelial cells initially migrate into the perivascular space creating gradually enlarging vascular lumens which in turn are covered by a migrating pericytes from the inner side of the vascular wall. Pericytes control and further organize the formation of effective vascular structure by producing VEGF and by signalling the end of aberrant angiogenesis where it takes place.

Wang et al (1996) in their study including 22 Sprague-Dawley rats, used human platelet derived wound healing factor (HPDWF) from burn patients and porcine pituitary extract on the recipient bed of 6 pieces of FTSG placed 1 cm apart on the back of each rat and investigated their effect on wound healing. The recipient site was actually the bed of a previously raised dermocutaneous local flap which was subsequently re-positioned on top of the grafts after interposing a completely occlusive sheet between the flap and the grafts. They found approximately 14.4% for the HPDWF and 13.16% for the PPE group improvement in terms of the time needed to bridge the gaps between the FTSGs. However, limitations in their study are the fact that there was no account of the role of the overlying flap in graft wound healing despite its suggested occlusive nature by adding for example a control group without the flap covering technique as well as the lack of evidence regarding the histochemical compatibility of the used factors with the subjects and the potential adverse effects of their use. Additionally the study refers to autologous skin grafts only.

Tatsuya et al (1997) found that the topical application of FK-506 on rat skin allografts may prolong their viability and prevent the rejection cascade phenomena. Nevertheless there was no attempt to further improve graft take results like in our study where the additional use of rHuEPO provided additional graft healing improvement in terms of lowering the percentage of post-grafting necrosis by 21% compared to the control group where only FK-506 was used (35.6% vs 14.6). In our study, rHuEPO had a considerably favorable effect on graft take and viability by achieving 12.89% less graft necrotic area (20.49%-7.6%). According to Kaemmer et al. (2010) the formation of granulation tissue in soft tissue wounds is promoted by rHuEPO primarily under tissue hypoxia. More specifically, rHuEPO promotes cell migration, proliferation, myo-fibroblasts and VEGF production, solely under hypoxia but not under normoxia. Consequently, hypoxia in the graft tissue comprises the signal for the initiation of rHuEPO promoting effect on the graft healing process.

In group b, the additional administration of rHuEPO achieved 21% smaller area of graft necrosis. The favorable effect of rHuEPO was shown in homologous skin grafting. New drugs have been developed in order to achieve prevention of the rejection process without causing toxicity is a goal in transplantation with calcineurin inhibitors (CNIs) comprising one o them. Rejection was prevented by the use of FK-506, which is a CNI, while rHuEPO promoted gradual healing of the graft area due to its effect on cell migration and new vessel formation. It could be suggested that preventing excessive inflammatory response and tissue rejection 'bought' the necessary time for rHuEPO to have its favorable effect in graft and wound healing. Additionally, it has been demonstrated that rHuEPO inhibits the production of pro-inflammatory cytokines by inflammatory cells, antagonizing the

activation of local mechanisms which trigger potential innate injury response (Strunk et al. 2008). Thus it could be suggested that the tissue protective action of rHuEPO complemented indirectly the rejection preventing role of FK-506.
Graft take and revascularization were lower in group c where FK-506 was administered in subjects with autologous skin grafts than in the control group A. According to Mori et al (1997) the explanation could be suggested to be the multiple inhibitory action of FK-506 to many wound healing mediator molecules, primarily to TGF-β induced VEGF, leading to angiogenesis impairment and consequently to graft take interference. However, it was shown that graft take obstruction by FK-506 is neither irreversible nor detrimental since the process of graft take appears to progress achieving optimum or nearly optimum levels. It could therefore be suggested that FK-506 creates a new equilibrium, unfavorable to graft revascularization, prolonging the required time for complete graft take and increasing the risk of impaired viability for a part of the graft tissue. Nevertheless, more studies are required to clarify the exact FK-506 mechanism of action in graft take and healing.
The potential clinical investigations that the finding of this study could include are the use of rHuEPO in immunologically challenged patients (such as patients with extensive trauma, burn injuries, transplanted organs, cancer, immunocompromising infectious disease, special medication treatments, radioactivity injuries, hematological diseases etc) in order to promote or/and sustain good quality skin graft take during the course of their hospitalization or even permanently, as a definitive treatment. In our knowledge this is the first time rHuEPO has been used in conjunction with FK-506 in homologous skin grafting with favorable results.
When it comes to the potential use of skin graft promoting factors to patients, considerations regarding adverse effects also concern the use of rHuEPO as its systemic administration has been associated with strong pro-coagulant and hemodynamic effects which are likely to lead to thrombotic complications especially in patients with cancer, infection, or trauma. Exacerbating the abnormal retinal angiogenesis in patients presenting with retinopathy and the tumor growth supporting effect of rHuEPO have also been reported (Bennett et al., 2008; Corwin et al., 2007). Nevertheless, there is not enough evidence to support any of the aforementioned adverse effects. Cautious use in patients with history of diabetes, heart disease, cancer and extensive trauma is always required.

6. Conclusion

Human recombinant erythropoietin promotes autologous FTSG take and viability in rats. It also appeared to have a favorable effect on homologous FTSG in rats, with the use of FK-506 as an immunosuppressant. When used alone in rats with autologous skin grafts, FK-506 was shown to have a moderately unfavorable effect on graft take. Overall, rHuEPO was shown to promote graft take and viability in rats. Clinical considerations regarding both the favorable and the adverse effects of special factors when used in patients, require future studies which could provide additional insight and feedback.

7. References

Bennett, CL., Silver, SM., Djulbegovic, B., Samaras, AT., Blau, CA., Gleason, KJ., Barnato, SE., Elverman, KM., Courtney, DM., McKoy, JM., Edwards, BJ., Tigue, CC., Raisch, DW., Yarnold, PR., Dorr, DA., Kuzel, TM., Tallman, MS., Trifilio, SM., West, DP., Lai, SY., Henke, M. (2008). Venous thromboembolism and mortality associated with recombinant erythropoietin and darbepoetin administration for the treatment of cancer-associated anemia. *Journal of American Medical Association*, 299, pp. 914 24.

Brines, M., Ceramic, A., (2008). Erythropoietin-mediated tissue protection: reducing collateral damage from the primary injury response. Journal of International, *Medicine*, 264(5), pp.405-32.

Capla, JM., Ceradini, DJ., Tepper, OM. (2006). Skin graft vascularization involves precisely regulated regression and replacement of endothelial cells through both angiogenesis and vasculogenesis. *Plastic and Reconstructive Surgery*, 117, pp. 836–844

Corwin, HL., Gettinger, A., Fabian, TC., May, A., Pearl, RG., Heard, S., An, R., Bowers, PJ., Burton, P., Klausner, MA., Corwin, MJ., EPO Critical Care Trials Group. (2007). Efficacy and safety of epoetin alfa in critically ill patients, *New England Journal of Medicine*. 357(10), pp.965-76.

Galeano, M., Altavilla, D., Cucinotta, D., Russo, GT., Calò, M,, Bitto, A., Marini, H., Marini, R., Adamo, EB., Seminara, P., Minutoli, L., Torre, V., Squadrito, F. (2004). Recombinant human erythropoietin stimulates angiogenesis and wound healing in the genetically diabetic mouse, *Diabetes*, 53(9), pp. 2509-17.

Galeano, M., Altavilla, D., Bitto, A., Minutoli, L., Calò, M., Lo, Cascio. P, Polito, F., Giugliano, G., Squadrito, G., Mioni, C., Giuliani, D., Venuti, FS., Squadrito, F. Recombinant human erythropoietin improves angiogenesis and wound healing in experimental burn wounds (2006) *Critical Care Medicine* , 34(4), pp.1139-46.

Gerhardt, H., Betsholtz, C. (2003), Endothelial-pericyte interactions in angiogenesis. *Cell Tissue Research*, 314, pp.15–23.

Goretsky, MJ.,Breeden,M., Pisarski G, Harriger, MD., Boyce,, ST,Greenhalgh DG. (1995) Capillary morphogenesis during healing of full-thickness skin grafts: An ultrastructural study. *Wound Repair and Regeneration*, 3, pp. 213–220.

Hom, DB., Unger, GM., Pernell, KJ., Manivel, JC. (2005). Improving surgical wound healing with basic fibroblast growth factor after radiation. *Laryngoscope*, 115(3), pp.412-22.

Isogai, R., Takahashi, M., Aisu, K., Horiuti, Y., Aragane, Y., Kawada, A., Tezuka, T. The receptor for erythropoietin is present on cutaneous mast cells (2006). *Archives of Dermatologic Research*, 297(9), pp.389-94

Kaemmer, DA., Otto, J., Binneboesel, M., Klink, C., Krones, C., Jansen, M., Cloer, C., Oettinger, A., Schumpelick, V., Klinge, U. (2010). Erythropoietin (EPO) influences colonic anastomotic healing in a rat model by modulating collagen metabolism. *Journal of Surgical Research* 163(2), pp.e67-72

Lampen, A., Christians, U., Guengerich, FP., Watkins, PB., Kolars, JC., Bader, A., Gonschior, A-K., Dralle, H., Hackbarth, I., Sewing, K-F. (1995). Metabolism of the immunosuppressant tacrolimus in the small intestine: Cytochrome P450, drug interactions, and interindividual variability. *Drug Metabolism and Disposal* 23, pp.1315–1324.

Lantieri, LA., Martin-Garcia, N., Wechsler, J., Mitrofanoff, M., Raulo, Y., Baruch, JP. (1998). Vascular endothelial growth factor expression in expanded tissue: A possible mechanism of angiogenesis in tissue expansion. *Plastic and Reconstructive Surgery*, 101, pp.392

Laschke, MW., Rucker, M., Jensen, G. (2008). Improvement of vascularization of PLGA scaffolds by inosculation of in situ- preformed functional blood vessels with the host microvasculature, *Annals of Surgery* 248, pp. 939–948.

Lindenblatt, N., Platz, U., Althaus, M., Hegland, N., Schmidt, CA., Contaldo, C., Vollmar, B., Giovanoli, P., Calcagni, M., (2010). Temporary Angiogenic Transformation of the Skin Graft Vasculature after Reperfusion, *Plastic and Reconstructive Surgery*, 126, pp. 61-60

Marumo, T., Nakaki, T., Hishikawa, K., Suzuki, H., Kato, R., Saruta, T. (1995). Cyclosporin A inhibits nitric oxide synthase induction in vascular smooth muscle cells, *Hypertension* 25, pp.764–8.

Mayer, AD., Dmitrewski, J., Squifflet, JP. (1997). Multicenter randomized trial comparing tacrolimus (FK506) and cyclosporine in the prevention of renal allograft rejection: A report of the European Tacrolimus Multicenter Renal Study Group, *Transplantation,* 64, pp.436-443

Mihmanli,A., Dolanmaz, D., Avunduk, MC., Erdemli, E. (2009). Effects of recombinant human erythropoietin on mandibular distraction osteogenesis, *Journal of Oral and Maxillofacial Surgery,* 67(11), pp.2337-43.

Mori, A., Suko, M., Kamimuma, O. (1997). IL-2-induced IL5 synthesis but not proliferation of human CD+ T cells is suppressed by FK506, *Journal of Immunology,* 158, pp.3659-3665

Nakazawa, Y., Chisuwa, H., Ikegami, T., Hashikura, Y., Terada, M., Katsuyama, Y., Iwasaki, K., Kawasaki, S. (1998). Relationship between in vivo FK506 clearance and in vitro 13-demethylation activity in living-related liver transplantation. *Transplantation ,* pp.1089–1093.

Nigam, S., Jin, YJ., Jin, MJ., Bush, KT., Bierer, B., Burakoff, SJ. (1993). Localization of the FK506-binding protein, FKBP 13, to the lumen of the endoplasmic reticulum, *Journal of Biochemistry,* 294, pp. 511-514

Okada, T. (1986). Revascularization of free full thickness skin grafts in rabbits: A scanning electron microscope study of microvascular casts. *British Journal of Plastic Surgery,* 39, pp. 183–189.

Paschos, N., Lykissas, MG., Beris, AE., (2008). The role of erythropoietin as an inhibitor of tissue ischemia. *International Journal of Biologic Science* 10; 4(3), pp. 161-8.

Pirsch, JD., Miller, J., Deierhoi, MH., (1997). A comparison of tacrolimus (FK506) and cyclosporine for immunosuppression after cadaveric renal transplantation. FK506 Kidney Transplant Study Group. *Transplantation* 63, pp.977-983

Plosker, GL., Foster, RH. (2000). Tacrolimus: A further update of its pharmacology and therapeutic use in the management of organ transplantation. *Drugs* 59, pp. 323–389.

Schultze-Mosgau, S., Wehrhan, F., Rödel, F., Amann, K., Radespiel-Tröger, M., Grabenbauer, GG. (2003). Improved free vascular graft survival in an irradiated surgical site following topical application of rVEGF. *International Journal of Radiation Oncology and Biologic Physicjs* 57(3), pp.803-12.

Shepherd,BR., Chen,HY., Smith,CM., Gruionu,G., Williams,SK., Hoying,JB. (2004). Rapid perfusion and network remodeling in a microvascular construct after implantation. *Arteriosclerosis T V Biology,* 24, pp. 898–904

Strunk, T., Hartel, C., Temming, P., Matzke, N., Zimmer, J., Schultz, C. (2008). Erythropoietin inhibits cytokine production of neonatal and adult leukocytes. *Acta Paediatrica,* 97, pp. 16–20.

Tatsuya, F., Shuji, T., Atsuhito, Y., Kowichi, J., Noriyuki, S. (1997). Prolonged survival of rat skin allograft by treatment with FK506 ointment *Transplantation,* 27; 64(6), pp.922-5.

Wang, HJ., Wan, HL., Yang, T.S., Wang, DS., Chen, TM., Chang, DM. (1996). Acceleration of skin graft healing by growth factors, *Burns,* 22(1), pp. 10-14

Young, DM., Greulich, KM., Weier, HG. (1996). Species-specific in situ hybridization with fluorochrome-labeled DNA probes to study vascularization of human skin grafts on athymic mice. *Journal of Burn Care and Rehabilitation,* 17, pp. 305–310

16

Recent Innovation in Pretreatment for Skin Grafts Using Regenerative Medicine in the East

Hitomi Sano[1] and Shigeru Ichioka[2]
[1]*Department of Surgical Science, Graduate School of Medicine, the University of Tokyo*
[2]*Department of Plastic and Reconstructive Surgery Saitama medical university hospital Japan*

1. Introduction

Chronic ulcers remain a significant health care concern today, especially in the elderly and immobile population. Pedicled or free flap transfers are usually applied to deep wounds in which bone and/or tendon are exposed. Despite improvements in reconstructive surgery techniques, operative invasion and complications, including flap necrosis and infection, are serious problems in patients whose general condition is unfavorable. For these patients, skin graft provides less invasive coverage of wounds as compared to the flap procedures. However, skin graft cannot survive on deep and poorly vascularized defects. Conversion of such defects to applicable beds to simple skin graft requires technologies to induce high-quality granulation tissue on compromised wounds. Stimulating the repair process after surgical debridement may achieve granulation tissue formation and shorten the period for skin grafts. For this purpose, regenerative medicine has attracted our attention. The characteristics of the methodology include the use of the three main tools of regenerative medicine; biomaterials, cytokines, and cells. This section introduces the technologies of regenerative medicine for wound bed preparation with particular focus on their progress in Asia.

All the patients illustrated in this chapter consented to the treatment. Clinical trials were approved by the Institutional Review Board (IRB) of Saitama Medical University.

2. Regenerative medicine for wound bed preparation

As already mentioned, the methodology includes the use of biomaterials, cytokines and cells, regenerative medicine's three main tools.

2.1 Biomaterials

Collagen is a natural substratum for various types of animal cells and is contained in tissues in large amounts as compared to other proteins (Linsenmayer, 1985). Advanced purification techniques can feasibly extract biocompatible and biodegenerative collagen matrix from animal tissues. These properties support the collagen matrix as one of the most suitable components of artificial tissue substitutes for reconstruction of damaged tissues and organs (Chvapil et al., 1973; Doillon & Silver, 1986). Several types of collagen-based artificial skin have been reported since the initial description by Yannas and Burke (1980) (Leipziger et al., 1985; Doillon et al., 1986; Boyce et al., 1988; Bel et al, 1981).

In the West, Integra ® (Siad Healthcare, Milano, Italy) has been generally used, and recently approved in Japan, but only for the treatment of burns. On the other hand, clinicians in Japan have widely used two types of artificial collagen matrix substitute dermis composed of an atelocollagen matrix (collagen matrix) with a silicone layer, namely TERUDERMIS (Terumo Corp, Tokyo, Japan) and Pelnac (Smith and Nephew Co., Ltd, Tokyo, Japan). These have been officially approved for the treatment of various skin defects caused by acute wounds as well as chronic wounds (Dantzer et al., 2001; Ichioka et al., 2003).

When these matrix substitutes are applied to a tissue defect, sprouting capillaries and fibroblasts migrate into the collagen, which acts as a scaffold for regeneration, resulting in induction of angiogenesis and fibroplasia. The autogenous regenerating tissue then gradually replaces the atelocollagen, and poorly vascularized deep defects are resurfaced by high-quality granulation tissue that can be easily covered with a simple skin graft (Ichioka et al., 2003). Collagen matrices have been reported to achieve less invasive reconstruction of severe defects with bone and/or tendon exposure that formerly required invasive tissue transfer (Braden & Bergstrom, 1989; Dantzer & Braye, 2001).

2.2 Cytokines

Cohen (1962) noticed that the purification of submaxillary gland extracts led to earlier eyelid separation and eruption of the incisor in mice, which eventually led to the isolation of the first growth factor as epidermal growth factor (EGF) as part of his Nobel Prize winning work. Since Cohen's discovery, it has been revealed that many growth factors are implicated in the processes of angiogenesis and wound healing (Greenhalgh, 1996; Stadelmann et al., 1998). In the chronic wound, the balance between stimulation and inhibition is destroyed (Stadelmann et al., 1998; Doughty & Sparks-Defriese, 2007) and fibroblasts have been reported to be less responsive to growth factors (Harding et al., 2002). The analysis of the supernatant from chronic pressure ulcers has shown decreased levels of growth factors, compared with the values in acute wound supernatant (Cooper et al., 1994). Deficiencies of growth factors in chronic ulcers suggest that the supplement of these factors might accelerate tissue repair processes. Therefore, growth factors have been proposed as therapeutic agents.

2.2.1 Cytokines for critical limb ischemia

Peripheral artery disease (PAD) is a major cause of the most difficult chronic limb ulcers. The occlusion of large limb arteries leads to ischemia, and can progress to critical limb ischemia (CLI). The treatment for ischemia is given priority in wound care. The main treatment strategy for severe, limb-threatening ischemia is either surgical or endovascular revascularization. If revascularization has failed or is not possible, major amputation is often inevitable. This relates to about 30% of all cases of severe limb ischemia (Adam et al., 2005). Regenerative medicine has been spotted as a new therapeutic option to induce angiogenesis. Recently gene therapies using cytokines have been developed as novel treatment strategies. The first in-human studies of gene therapy for the treatment of PAD and coronary artery

disease(CAD) were reported in the late 1990s (Isner et al., 1996; Schumacher et al., 1998; Laitinen et al., 1998). Since these initial reports, several gene therapies have been reported using growth factors, including vascular endothelial growth factor (VEGF) (Isner et al., 1996), fibroblast growth factor (FGF) (Nikol et al., 2008), hypoxia-inducible factor (HIF) (Rajagopalan et al., 2007), developmentally regulated endothelial locus (Del-1) (Grossman et al., 2007), and hepatocyte growth factor (HGF) (Powell et al., 2008). Among these studies, VEGF has been the most commonly employed approach. The beneficial effects of therapeutic angiogenesis using VEGF gene transfer have been reported in human patients with CLI and CAD (Isner et al., 1998; Baumgartner et al., 1998; Baumgartner et al., 2000; Losordo et al., 1998; Vale et al., 1999; Vale et al., 2000; Rosengart et al., 1999).
On the other hand, in Japan, Morishita et al (1999, 2002) have focused on HGF. HGF is also a potent angiogenic growth factor (Belle et al. 1998; Hayashi et al., 1999; Taniyama et al., 2001; Aoki et al., 2000), is a potent mitogen for a wide variety of cells and has angiogenic, antiapoptotic, and antifibrotic properties (Azuma et al., 2006; Matsumoto et al., 1996; Bussolino et al., 1992; Morishita et al., 2004). It is suggested that even in high-risk conditions for atherosclerosis, over expression of HGF is enough to stimulate collateral formation to treat ischemic symptoms (Taniyama e al., 2001). Furthermore, the mitogenic activity of HGF has been reported to be more potent than that of VEGF (Belle et al., 1998; Nakamura et al., 1996). Serum levels of HGF, but not VEGF, are elevated in CAD patients with collaterals, and elevated HGF levels are associated with better prognoses in patients with acute coronary syndromes (Lenihan et al., 2003; Heeschen et al., 2003). Morishita et al. (1999; 2004) conducted preclinical investigations and initial human safety studies of HGF gene therapy, which subsequently led to the phase II HGF-STAT trial. Patients with CLI were randomized to treatment with placebo or 1 of 3 doses of HGF plasmid (Powell et al., 2008). $TcPO_2$ was significantly more improved in patients who received the highest dose of HGF plasmid than in patients in whom a placebo or the lower HGF plasmid doses were administered. The authors concluded that intramuscular injection of HGF plasmid has an acceptable safety profile for the treatment of patients with CLI. Intramuscular injection of HGF plasmid may have a favorable effect on limb perfusion as measured by $TcPO_2$ in patients with CLI. Based on these findings, the phase III trial is now underway to determine whether HGF has a clinically meaningful effect on wound healing, limb salvage, and survival.

2.2.2 Cytokine products for topical application

Topical application of cytokines might be effective for wound healing. In the West, the growth factor product generally used is recombinant human platelet-derived growth factor (PDGF) (Regranex®). In South Korea, products based on PDGF, epidermal growth factor (EGF) (Easyef®) and basic fibroblast growth factor (bFGF) (Fibrast®) are available. In Japan, a bFGF product has been licensed since 2001 for use on various skin defects such as diabetic foot wounds, pressure ulcers, venous ulcers and trauma. The following subsections introduce EGF and bFGF for wound bed preparation.

2.2.2.1 Epidermal growth factor (EGF)

Epidermal growth factor (EGF) is a polypeptide of 53 amino acids that was first isolated from the mouse submaxillary gland by Cohen (1962) as previously mentioned. EGF acts by binding with the high affinity to epidermal growth factor receptor (EGFR) which is expressed in almost all types of tissue, triggering an increase in the expression of certain genes that ultimately lead to DNA synthesis and cell proliferation (Herbst, 2004). EGF has been observed to stimulate the differentiation of epithelial cells, endothelial chemotaxis and angiogenesis, and fibroblast migration and proliferation, and to regulate extracellular matrix turnover (Deasy et al., 2002). Enhanced wound healing has been noted in dermal wounds treated with topical or subcutaneous EGF (Starkey et al., 1975). Franklin & Lynch (1979) recorded quicker epithelial regeneration and less scar contracture in EGF-treated wounds in rabbits.

With the introduction of recombinant human EGF in the 1980s, the range of studies increased to include burn wounds and chronic ulcers (Brown et al., 1989; Falanga et al., 1992). Studies with partial thickness human burn wounds and topical EGF confirmed a decrease in wound healing time (Brown et al., 1989). Although the use of EGF in human impaired wound healing by Falanga et al. (1992) showed a modest improvement in wound healing times and rate of epithelialization, the results were not statistically significant. Some other reports also suggested that the efficacy of EGF in chronic wounds is limited (Franklin & Lynch 1979; Brown et al., 1989). Therefore, no conclusions about the efficacy of EGF for chronic wounds can be made at present.

2.2.2.2 Basic fibroblast growth factor (bFGF)

In 1974, Gospodarowicz isolated a protein that accelerated the proliferation of fibroblasts from bovine pituitary glands and termed it the fibroblast growth factor (FGF) (Gospodarowicz et al., 1987; Gospodarowicz et al., 1988; Greenhalgh et al., 1990). One of the best-known FGF activities includes the stimulation of fibroblast proliferation leading to granulation tissue formation (Floss et al., 1997). FGF also plays a key role in proliferation of endothelial cells and keratinocytes and the mitogenesis of mesenchymal cells (Floss et al., 1997; Menetrey et al., 2000). Experimental studies have demonstrated that bFGF accelerates angiogenesis, granulation, and epithelialization (Gospodarowicz et al., 1988). Some clinical studies have shown the efficacy and safety of bFGF for the treatment of various wounds including diabetic ulcers, pressure ulcers and burns (Ishibashi et al., 1996; Ichioka et al., 2005).

2.3 Cell therapies

Stimulation of the microcirculation and enhancement of angiogenesis may promote granulation tissue formation on compromised wounds. For this purpose, several technologies using autologous cells have been developed. Bone marrow firstly attracted our attention as a possible beneficial material for wound healing, because it contains multipotential progenitor cells that can differentiate into endothelial cells and secrete several growth factors. Several reports have illustrated the potential of bone marrow to induce angiogenesis and also that it might contain early stem cells that can differentiate into non-hematopoietic tissues such as the skin (Ichioka et al., 2004; Yamaguchi et al., 2005). Asahara and colleagues (1999; 1997). have shown that vascular endothelial progenitor cells (EPCs), the population of mononuclear cells, from the bone marrow passed through the peripheral circulation and migrated locally to tumors, injured or ischemic regions. Furthermore, it has been suggested experimentally that bone marrow cells contribute to the formation of a matrix (Fathke et al., 2004; Badiavas et al., 2003), vascular formation (Asahara t al., 1999), secretion of angiogenic cytokines (Kamihata et al., 2001; Sanchez-Guijo et al., 2010), and stimulation of muscle cells. (Tateno et al., 2006.)

2.3.1 Cell therapies for critical limb ischemia

Several experiments have demonstrated therapeutic relevance of cell therapy for the ischemic limb. *Ex vivo*-expanded human EPCs transplanted into limb ischemia mice models showed a recovery of blood flow, an enhanced collateral density, and a 60% limb salvage (7% in controls) (Kalka et al., 2000). Iba et al. (2002) demonstrated that implantation of Peripheral blood mononuclear cells and platelets into ischemic limbs effectively induced collateral vessel formation using rat models, suggesting that this cell therapy is useful for therapeutic angiogenesis.

Some reports indicated the efficacy and feasibility of the clinical use of cell therapy (Tateishi-Yuyama et al., 2002; Kajiguchi et al., 2007; Matoba et al., 2008; Miyamoto et al., 2004). Therapeutic angiogenesis using cell transplantation (TACT) is a treatment strategy for no-option patients with CLI in Japan. Tateishi-Yuyama et al. (2002) reported the first large clinical study on the use of bone marrow derived mononuclear cells in the treatment of limb ischemia. According to this report, injection of bone marrow derived mononuclear cells into the muscle of the ischemic limb apparently improved the ankle-brachial index (ABI), transcutaneous oxygen pressure ($TcPO_2$), rest pain, and the pain free walking distance. The Japanese Ministry of Health, Labour and Welfare has approved this technology, namely "Therapeutic angiogenesis using bone marrow cell transplantation", as advanced medicine for critical limb ischemia. In addition, two other technologies using autologous cells, "Therapeutic angiogenesis using peripheral mononuclear cells" and "Therapeutic angiogenesis using peripheral blood stem cells", have been also approved (Matoba et al., 2008; Kajiguchi et al., 2007; Miyamoto et al., 2004).

2.3.2 Topical application of autologous cells

Topical application of bone marrow cells and platelet rich plasma (PRP) have been experimentally and clinically well-reported for their efficacy in the promotion of angiogenesis and wound healing (Wu et al., 2010; Lacci & Dardik, 2010).

2.3.2.1 Bone marrow

Bone marrow has long been known to participate in wound healing by providing inflammatory cells which produce cytokines and orchestrate a cascade of events (Gillitzer & Goebeler, 2001). Recent bodies of evidence suggest that bone marrow might also serve as a resource to provide skin progenitor cells (Krause et al., 2001; Liang & Bickenbach, 2002). Several reports have experimentally illustrated that topically applied bone marrow cells might promote wound healing (Badiavas et al., 2003; Sivan-Loukianova et al., 2003; McFarlin et al., 2006).

Badiavas et al. (2003) indicated that wounding stimulated the engraftment of bone marrow cells to the skin and induced bone marrow-derived cells to be incorporated and differentiate into non-hematopoietic skin structures using mice models. The authors concluded that bone marrow might be a valuable source of stem cells for the skin and possibly other organs. The application of peripheral blood mononuclear cells accelerated the neovascularization and epidermal healing in a model of chronic full-thickness skin wounds in diabetic mice (Sivan-Loukianova et al., 2003). McFarlin et al. (2006) found that local injection of mesenchymal stem cells significantly improved wound healing in an animal wound model. Bone marrow-derived cells have been reported as transit-amplifying cells in injured tissue where they differentiate into keratinocytes, using a mouse wound model (Borue et al., 2004).

Based on the results of the experimental studies, bone marrow-derived stem cells have been clinically used in the treatment of chronic wounds (Badiavas & Falanga, 2003; Ramsey et al.,

1999; Metcalfe & Ferguson, 2007). Badiavas & Falanga (2003) showed that topically applied autologous bone marrow-derived cells can bring about closure of long-standing and hard-to-heal wounds. These authors reported that bone marrow-derived cultured mesenchymal stem cells accelerated the healing of cutaneous wounds (Falanga et al., 2007). A similar clinical approach has been performed by Rogers et al (2008) and reported that topical application and injection into the wound periphery of bone marrow can be a useful and a potentially safe adjunct to wound simplification and ultimate closure (Rogers et al., 2008). It was reported that locally applied mononuclear bone marrow cells restored angiogenesis and promoted wound healing of an ulcer of the lower leg in a type 2 diabetic patient (Humpert et al., 2005).

In Japan, several methods of applying bone marrow derived cells for wound have also been tried. Mizuno et al. (2010) employed the combination of mononuclear bone marrow cells and allogeneic cultured dermal substitute for the treatment of intractable ulcers in critical limb ischemia. The authors injected mononuclear cells intramuscularly into the lower leg and around the wound area and applied allogeneic cultured dermal substitute on the wound surface (Mizuno et al., 2010). In our strategy, we impregnated autologous bone marrow cells into a collagen matrix (Terdermis): bone marrow-impregnated collagen matrix, (Fig.1) that has been utilized for the treatment of chronic wounds.

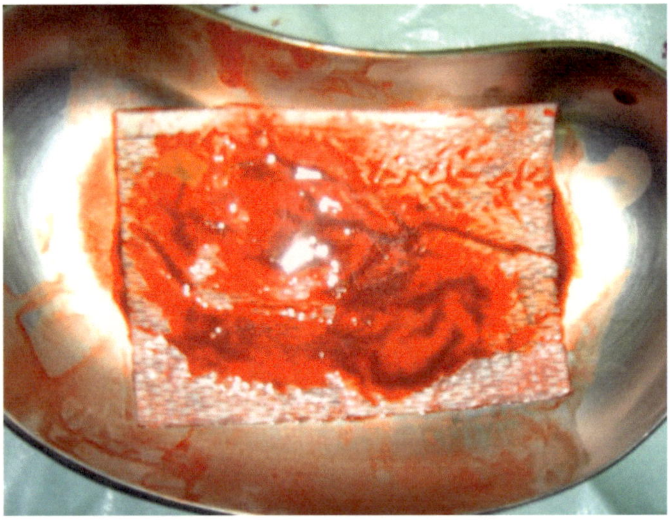

Fig. 1. The macroscopic finding of a bone marrow-impregnated collagen matrix

We have experimentally and clinically suggested the efficacy of this procedure for chronic ulcer treatment (Ichioka et al., 2005, 2009). One typical case is presented to illustrate the outcomes.

[patient 1] A-48-year-old woman suffered from a venous leg ulcer that had not healed despite seven years of standard conventional wound therapy (Fig. 2. A). Surgical debridement followed by bone marrow-impregnated collagen matrix application was undertaken under lumbar anesthesia (Fig. 2. B, C). Twenty-two days later, well-vascularized healthy granulation tissue had developed (Fig. 2. D), split-thickness skin graft was performed. The patient has remained free of complications for 29 months since treatment (Fig. 2. E).

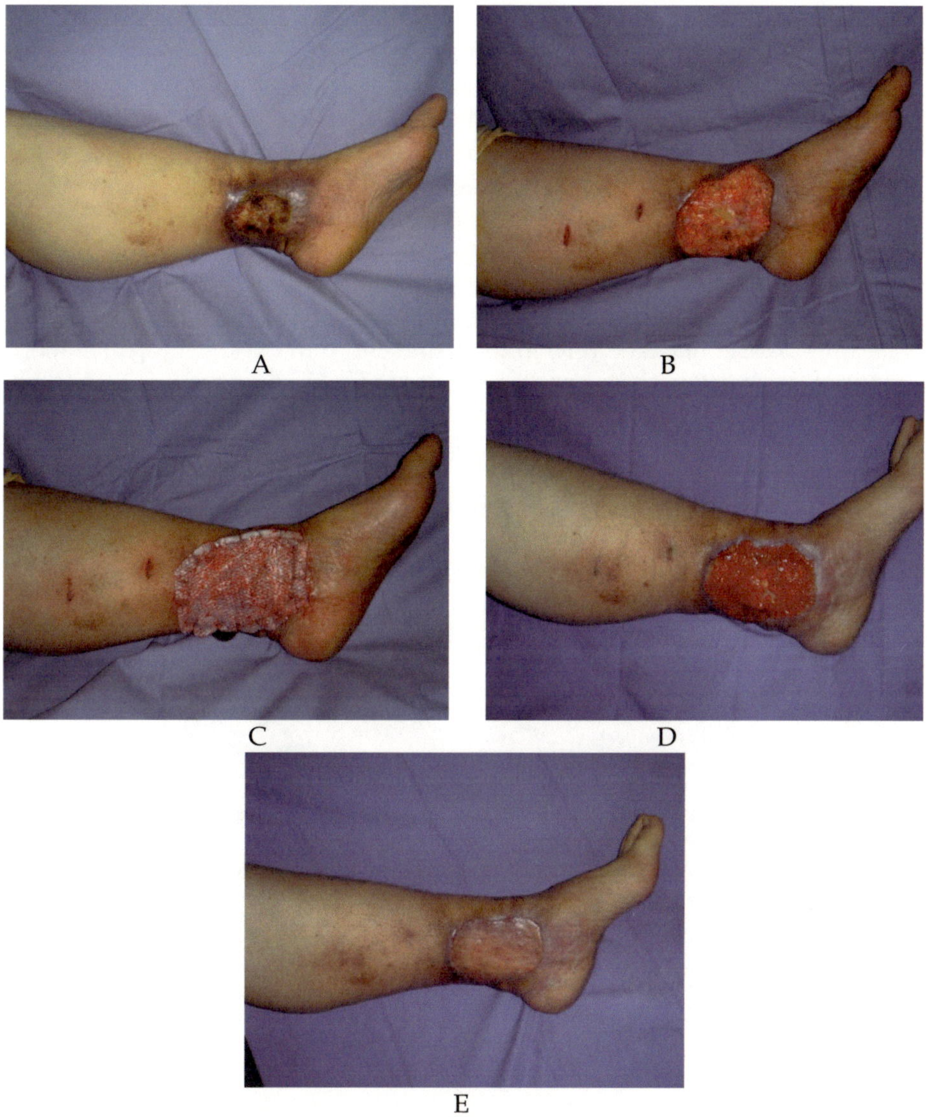

Fig. 2. (A) Nonhealing ulcer on the left lower limb before wound debridement. (B) Application of the bone marrow-impregnated collagen matrix after debridement. (C) Robust granulation tissue 3 weeks after PRP collagen application. (D) Split-thickness mesh skin grafting was performed. (E) Healed wound.

2.3.2.2 Platelet-rich plasma (PRP)

Besides the fundamental role in hemostatsis at the injured site, platelets initiate and enhance wound healing by releasing numerous plasma proteins and various growth factors (Everts et al., 2006; Knighton et al., 1986; Knighton et al., 1988). Platelets stimulate angiogenesis, proliferation and migration, and collagen synthesis. The main growth factors produced by platelets include platelet-derived growth factor (PDGF) (Bennett et al., 2003), transforming growth factor beta (TGF-β) (Assoian & Sporn., 1986), insulin-like growth factor (IGF-I)

(Hock et al., 1988), endothelial growth factor (EGF), vascular endothelial growth factor (VEGF) (Mohle et al., 1997), fibroblast growth factor (FGF) (Brunner et al., 1993). Platelet-rich plasma (PRP) is defined as a portion of the plasma fraction of autologous blood having a platelet concentration above baseline (Mehta &Watson, 2008; Marx, 2001). PRP can be supplied with a simple centrifugation procedure using solely autologous blood, suggesting that it is a minimally invasive method (Shashikiran et al., 2006; Bhanot & Alex, 2002). Roberts and Sporn (1993) and Marx (1998; 2001) have contributed a wealth of knowledge for the topical application of PRP in dentistry. In wound treatments, several investigations have reported the beneficial effects of PRP since its first report in 1985 (Driver et al., 2006). Margolis et al. (2001) reported a retrospective cohort study devised to estimate the effectiveness of platelet releasate (PR) in the treatment of diabetic neuropathic foot ulcers. The wounds of the 26,599 patients enrolled in this study, 43.1% of patients healed within 32 weeks, including 50% of patients treated with PRP and 41% of patients not treated with PR treatment. The investigators concluded that PRP was more effective than the standard care (Margolis et al., 2001). Driver et al. (2006) carried out the first prospective, randomized, controlled multicenter trial in the United States regarding the use of autologous PRP for the treatment of diabetic foot ulcers. The authors found the PRP treatment group attained significantly better outcomes as compared with the control group. (Driver et al., 2006). In our strategy, PRP is adapted with a collagen matrix to prepare the wound bed for skin graft or spontaneous closure (Fig. 3), and is applied to the debrided wound.

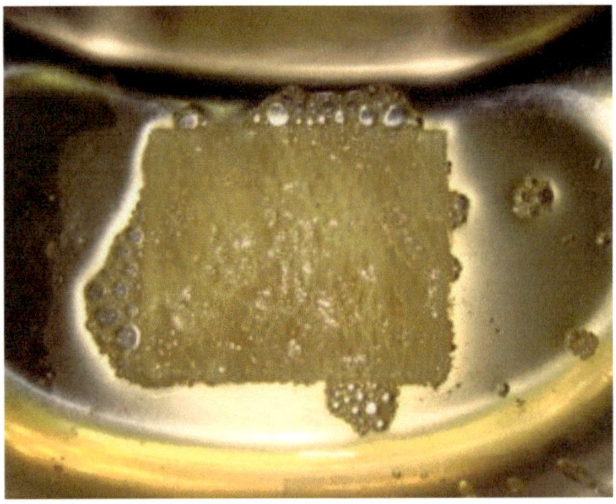

Fig. 3. Collagen matrix impregnated with PRP

Some recent studies have examined the clinical application of PRP using a drug delivery system (DDS). O'Connell et al. (2008) reported that a newly developed material containing PRP, which they named platelet-rich fibrin matrix membrane (PRFM), exhibited a gradual steady-state release of platelet-derived growth factors for as long as 7 days and potentially provided a fibrin scaffold to further facilitate the tissue repair process (O'Connell, et al. 2008). In Japan, Yazawa et al. (2003) reported that when a platelet concentrate was used in conjunction with fibrin glue as a carrier, the contents were released over a period of about 1 week. We have also reported that platelet-protein film (PPF) as an autologous fibrin clot which PRP and plasma proteins, might continuously release growth factors to the wound bed (Fig. 4) (Tanaka et al., 2007).

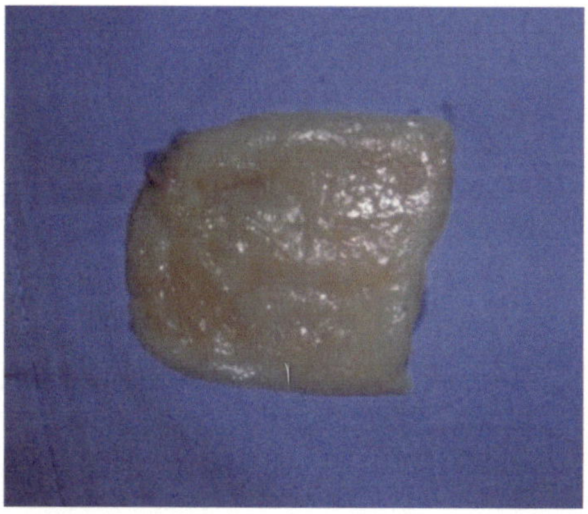

Fig. 4. The macroscopic finding of PPF

One successful case is presented to illustrate the possible outcome of treatment using PRP.
[Patient 1]
A 89-year-old female developed a pressure ulcer over the left lower limb; the ulcer had not healed despite three months of standard conventional wound therapy (Fig. 5 A). Surgical debridement followed by PRP collagen application was performed under general anesthesia (Fig. 5 B). Three weeks later, well-vascularized, healthy granulation tissue had developed (Fig. 5 C), and a split-thickness skin graft was performed to completely close the wound (Fig. 5 D). The patient has remained free of complications for 4 months since treatment (Fig. 5 E).

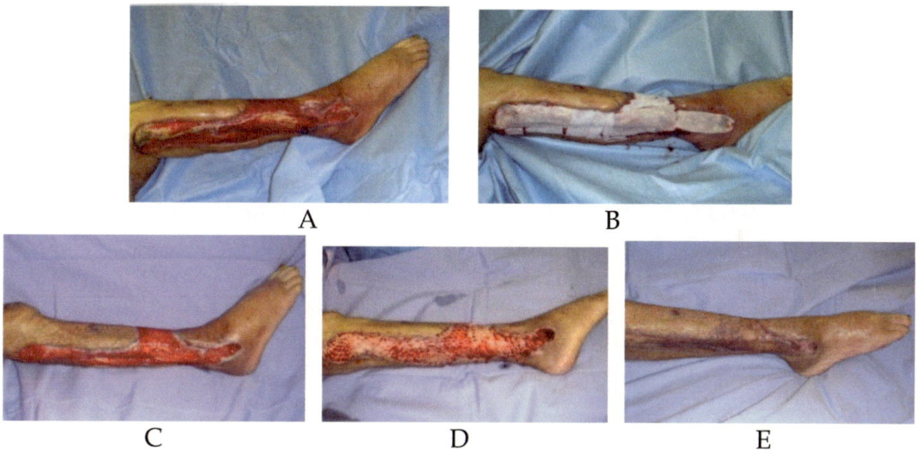

Fig. 5. (A) Nonhealing ulcer on the left lower limb before wound debridement.(B) Application of PRP collagen after debridement.(C) Good granulation tissue 3 weeks after PRP collagen application.(D) Split-thickness mesh skin graft was performed.(E) Healed wound.

3. Conclusion

Advanced regenerative medicine-based technologies currently provide successful and less invasive wound closure with spontaneous healing or can be used in combination with skin grafting instead of invasive surgical tissue transfer. Recent developments in physical therapies including negative pressure wound therapy (NPWT) reinforce the efficacy of conservative wound treatment. However, we should always bear in mind that topical therapeutic management strategies work effectively only on adequately perfused wound beds under a moist environment without devitalized tissue or a critical bacterial burden.

4. References

Adam, DJ., Beard, JD., Cleveland, T et al. (2005). Bypass versus angioplasty in severe ischemia of the leg (BASIL): multicentre, randomized controlled trial. *Lancet,* 366, pp. 1925–1934, ISSN 0140-6736.

Aoki, M., Morishita, R. Taniyama, Y et al. (2000). Angiogenesis induced by hepatocyte growth factor in non-infarcted myocardium and infracted myocardium: up-regulation of essential transcription factor for angiogenesis, ets. *Gene Ther.* 7, pp. 417–427, ISSN 0969-7128

Asahara, T., Masuda, H., Takahashi, T et al. (1999). Bone marrow origin of endothelial progenitor cells responsible for postnatal vasculogenesis in physiological and pathological neovascularization. *Circ Res* 85, pp. 221-228, ISSN 0009-7330

Asahara, T., Murohara, T., Sullivan, A et al. (1997). Isolation of putative progenitor endothelial cells for angiogenesis. Science 275, pp. 964-967, ISSN 0036-8075

Assoian, RK. & Sporn, MB. (1986). Type beta transforming growth factor in human platelets: release during platelet degranulation and action on vascular smooth muscle cells. *J Cell Biol,* 102, pp. 1217–1223, ISSN 0021-9525

Azuma, J., Taniyama, Y., Takeya, Y et al. (2006). Angiogenic and antifibrotic actions of hepatocyte growth factor improve cardiac dysfunction in porcine ischemic cardiomyopathy. *Gene Ther,* 13, pp. 1206–1213, ISSN 0969-7128

Baumgartner, I., Pieczek, A., Manor, O et al. (1998). Constitutive expression of phVEGF165 after intramuscular gene transfer promotes collateral vessel development in patients with critical limb ischemia. *Circulation,* 97, pp. 1114–1123, ISSN 0009-7322

Baumgartner, I., Rauh, G., Pieczek, A et al. (2000). Lower-extremity edema associated with gene transfer of naked DNA encoding vascular endothelial growth factor. *Ann Intern Med,* 132, pp.880–884, ISSN 0003-4819

Badiavas, EV., & Falanga, V. (2003). Treatment of chronic wounds with bone marrow-derived cells. *Arch Dermatol,* 139, pp. 510–516. ISSN 0003-987X

Badiavas, EV., Abedi, M., Butmarc, J et al. (2003). Participation of bone marrow derived cells in cutaneous wound healing. *J Cell Physiol,* 196(2), pp. 245-50, ISSN 0021-9541

Bel, E., Ehrlich, HP., Buttle, DJ et al. (1981). A living tissue formed in vitro and accepted as a full thickness skin equivalent. *Science,* 211, pp. 1042-1054, ISSN 0036-8075

Belle, EV., Witzenbichler, B., Chen, D et al. (1998). Potentiated angiogenic effect of scatter factor/hepatocyte growth factor via induction of vascular endothelial growth factor: the case for paracrine amplification of angiogenesis. *Circulation,* 97, pp. 381–390, ISSN 0009-7322

Bennett, SP., Griffiths, GD., Schor, AM et al. (2003). Growth factors in the treatment of diabetic foot ulcers. *Br J Surg,* 90, pp. 133–146, ISSN 0007-1323

Bhanot, S. & Alex, JC. (2002). Current applications of platelet gels in facial plastic surgery. *Facial Plast Surg.* 18(1), pp. 27-33, ISSN 1521-2491

Borue, X., Lee, S., Grove, J et al. (2004). Bone marrow-derived cells contribute to epithelial engraftment during wound healing. *Am J Pathol,* 165, pp. 1767-1772, ISSN 0002-9440

Boyce, ST., Christian, DJ. & Hansbrough, JF. (1988). Structure of collagen-GAG dermal skin substitute optimized for cultured human epidermal keratinocyte. *J Biomed Master Res,* 22, pp. 939-957, ISSN 1552-4973

Braden, BJ. & Bergstrom, N. (1989). Clinical utility of the Braden scale for predicting pressure sore risk. *Decubitus,* 2, pp. 44–46, 50–51, ISSN 0898-1655

Brown, G., Nanney, L., Griffen. J et al. (1989). Enhancement of wound healing by topical treatment with epidermal growth factor. *N Eng J Med,* 321, pp. 76-89, ISSN 0028-4793

Brunner, G., Nguyen, H., Gabrilove, J et al. (1993). Basic fibroblast growth factor expression in human bone marrow and peripheral blood cells. *Blood,* 81, pp.631–638, ISSN 0006-4971

Bussolino, F., DiRenzo, MF., Ziche, M et al. (1992). Hepatocyte growth factor is a potent angiogenic factor which stimulates endothelial cell mobility and growth. *J Cell Biol,* 119, pp. 629–641, ISSN 0021-9525

Chvapil, M., Kronenthal, RL. & Winkle, WV. Jr. (1973). *Medical and surgical applications of collagen. International Review of Connective Tissue Research,* vol. 6, Hall D.A.and Jackson D. S. (eds), Academic Press, New York, pp. 1-61, ISBN 9780123637109

Cooper, DM., Yu, EZ., Hennessey, P et al. (1994). Determination of endogenous cytokines in chronic wounds. *Ann Surg,* 219, pp. 688-692, ISSN 0003-4932

Cohen, S. (1962). Isolation of a mouse submaxillary gland protein accelerating incisor eruption and eyelid opening in the new-born animal. *J Biol Chem,* 237, pp. 1555–1562. ISSN 0021-9258

Dantzer, E. & Braye, FM. (2001). Reconstructive surgery using an artificial dermis (Integra): results with 39 grafts.*Br J plast Surg,* 54, pp.659-664, ISSN 0007-1226.

Deasy, BM., Qu-Peterson, Z., Greenberger, JS et al. (2002). Mechanisms of muscle stem cell expansion with cytokines. *Stem Cells,* 20, pp. 50–60, ISSN 1066-5099

Doillon, CJ. & Silver, FH. (1986). Collagen-based wound dressing: Effects of hyaluonic acid and fibronectin on wound healing. Biomaterials, 7, pp. 3-8,.ISSN 0142-9612

Doillon, CJ., Whyne, CF., Brandwein, S. et al. (1986). Collagen-based wound dressing: Control of the pore structure and morphology. J Biomed Mater Res, 20, pp. 1219-1228, ISSN 1552-4973

Doughty, D. &Sparks-Defriese, B. (2007). Wound healing physiology. In: Bryant RA, Nix DP, eds. *Acute&Chronic Wounds: Current Management Concepts.* 3rd ed. St. Louis: Mosby/Elsevier, 56–81, ISBN 9780323030748

Driver, VR., Hanft, J., Fylling, CP et al. (2006). Autologel Diabetic Foot Ulcer Study Group. A prospective, randomized, controlled trial of autologous platelet-rich plasma gel for the treatment of diabetic foot ulcers. *Ostomy Wound Manage.* 52(6), pp. 68-70, 72, 74 passim, ISSN 0889-5899

Everts, PA., BrownMahoney, C., Hoffmann, JJ et al. (2006). Platelet-rich plasma preparation using three devices: implications for platelet activation and platelet growth factor release. *Growth Factors.* 24(3), pp. 165-71, ISSN 0897-7194

Falanga, V., Iwamoto, S. & Chartier M. (2007). Autologous bone marrow-derived cultured mesenchymal stem cells delivered in a fibrin spray accelerate healing in murine and human cutaneous wounds. *Tissue Eng,* 13, pp. 1299-1312, ISSN 1076-3279

Fathke, C., Wilson, L., Hutter, J et al. (2004). Contribution of bone marrow-derived cells to skin: collagen deposition and wound repair. *Stem Cells,* 22(5), pp. 812-22, ISSN 1066-5099

Franklin, J. & Lynch, J. (1979). Effects of topical applications of epidermal growth factor on wound healing. *Plast Reconstr Surg,* 64. pp. 766-70, ISSN 0032-1052

Floss, T., Arnold, HH. & Braun, T. (1997). A role for FGF-6 in skeletal muscle regeneration. *Genes Dev,* 11, pp. 2040–5, ISSN 0969-7128

Gillitzer, R. & Goebeler, M. (2001). Chemokines in cutaneous wound healing. J *Leukoc Biol,* 69, pp. 513–521, ISSN 0741-5400

Greenhalgh, DG., Sprugel, KH., Murray, MJ et al. (1990). PDGF and FGF stimulate wound healing in the genetically diabetic mouse. *Am J Pathol.* 136, pp. 1235–46, ISSN 0002-9440

Greenhalgh, D. (1996). The role of growth factors in wound healing. *J Trauma,* 41, pp. 159-67, ISSN 0022-5282.

Gospodarowicz, D. (1988). Molecular and developmental biology aspects of fibroblast growth factor. *Adv Exp Med Biol,* 234, pp. 23–39, ISSN 0065-2598

Gospodarowicz, D., Ferrara, N., Schweigerer, L et al. (1987). Structural characterization and biological functions of fibroblast growth factor. *Endocr Rev,* 8, pp. 95–114, ISSN 0163-769X

Grossman, PM., Mendelsohn, F., Henry TD et al. (2007). Results from a phase II multicenter, double-blind placebo-controlled study of Del-1 (VLTS-589) for intermittent claudication in subjects with peripheral arterial disease. *Am Heart J,* 153, pp. 874–880, ISSN 0002-8703

Humpert, PM., Bartsch, U., Konrade, I et al. (2005). Locally applied mononuclear bone marrow cells restore angiogenesis and promote wound healing in a type 2 diabetic patient. *Exp Clin Endocrinol Diabetes,* 113, pp. 538-540, ISSN 0947-7349

Harding, KG., Morris, HL. & Patel GK. (2002). Science, medicine and the future: Healing chronic wounds. *BMJ,* 324, 160–163

Hayashi, S., Morishita, R. & Nakamura, S. (1999). Potential role of hepatocyte growth factor, a novel angiogenic growth factor, in peripheral arterial disease: down-regulation of HGF in response to hypoxia in vascular cells. *Circulation.* 100, pp. II301–II308, ISSN 0009-7322

Heeschen, C., Dimmeler, S. & Hamm, CW. (2003). Prognostic significance of angiogenic growth factor serum levels in patients with acute coronary syndromes. *Circulation,* 107, pp. 524–530, ISSN 0009-7322

Herbst, RS. (2004). Review of epidermal growth factor receptor biology. *Int J Radiat Oncol Bio Phys,* 59(Suppl 2), pp.21-6, ISSN 0360-3016

Hock, JM., Gentrella, M. & Canalis, E. (1988). Insulin-like growth factor I has independent effects on bone matrix formation and cell replication. *Endocrinology,* 122, pp. 254-60, ISSN 0013-7227

Iba, O., Matsubara, H. & Nozawa, Y. (2002). Angiogenesis by Implantation of Peripheral Blood Mononuclear Cells and Platelets Into Ischemic Limbs. *Circulation.* 106, 2019-2025, ISSN 0009-7322

Ichioka, S., Ohura, N., Sekiya, N et al. (2003). Regenerative surgery for sacral pressure ulcers using collagen matrix substitute dermis (artificial dermis). *Ann Plast Surg,* 51(4), pp. 383–9, ISSN 0148-7043

Ichioka, S., Kudo, S., Shibata, M et al. (2004) Bone marrow cell implantation improves flap viability after ischemia-reperfusion injury. Ann Plast Surg, 52(4), pp. 414-8, ISSN 0148-7043

Ichioka, S., Ohura, N., Nakatsuka, T et al. (2005). The positive experience using a growth factor product on deep wounds with bone exposure. *Journal of Wound Care.* 14(3), pp. 105-109. ISSN 0969-0700

Ichioka, S., Kouraba, S., Sekiya, N et al. (2005). Bone marrow-impregnated collagen matrix for wound healing: experimental evaluation in a microcirculatory model of angiogenesis, and clinical experience. *Br J Plast Surg,* 58, pp. 1124-30. ISSN 0007-1226

Ichioka, S., Yokogawa, H., Sekiya, N et al. (2009). Determinants of Wound Healing in Bone Marrow impregnated Collagen Matrix Treatment: Impact of Microcirculatory Response to Surgical Debridement. *Wound Repair Regen,* 17(4), pp. 492-7, ISSN 1067-1927

Ishibashi, Y., Harada, S., Takemura, T et al. (1996). Clinical effectiveness of KCB-1(bFGF) on patients with skin ulcerations clinical trial for 12 weeks. *J Clin Therapeut Med,* 12, pp. 2117–29, ISSN 0910-8211

Isner, JM., Pieczek, A., Schainfeld, R et al. (1996). Clinical evidence of angiogenesis after arterial gene transfer of phVEGF165 in patient with ischaemic limb. *Lancet.* 348, pp. 370 –374, ISSN 0140-6736

Isner, JM., Baumgartner, I., Rauh, G et.al. (1998). Treatment of thromboangiitis obliterans (Buerger's disease) by intramuscular gene transfer of vascular endothelial growth factor: preliminary clinical results. *J Vasc Surg,* 28, pp. 964–973, ISSN 0741-5214

Kajiguchi, M., Kondo, T., Izawa H et.al. (2007). Safety and Efficacy of Autologous Progenitor Cell Transplantation for Therapeutic Angiogenesis in Patients With Critical Limb Ischemia, *Circ J,* 71, pp. 196 –201, ISSN 1346-9843

Kalka, C., Masuda, H., Takahashi, T et al. (2000). Transplantation of ex vivo expanded endothelial progenitor cells for therapeutic neovascularization. *Proc Natl Acad Sci USA,* 97, pp. 3422–3427, ISSN 0027-8424

Kamihata, H., Matsubara, H., Nishiue, T et al. (2001). Implantation of bone marrow mononuclear cells into ischemic myocardium enhances collateral perfusion and regional function via side supply of angioblasts, angiogenic ligands, and cytokines. *Circulation,* 104(9), pp. 1046-1052, ISSN 0009-7322

Knighton, DR., Ciresi, KF., Fiegel, VD et al. (1986). Classification and treatment of chronic nonhealing wounds. Successful treatment with autologous platelet-derived wound healing factors (PDWHF). *Ann Surg,* 204(3), pp. 322-30, ISSN 0148-7043

Knighton, DR., Doucette, M., Fiegel, VD et al. (1988). The use of platelet derived wound healing formula in human clinical trials. *Prog Clin Biol Res,* 266, pp. 319-29, ISSN 0361-7742

Krause, DS., Theise, ND., Collector, MI et al. (2001). Multi-organ, multilineage engraftment by a single bone marrow-derived stem cell. *Cell,* 105, pp. 369–377, ISSN 0092-8674

Lacci, KM. & Dardik A. (2010) Platelet-rich plasma: support for its use in wound healing. *Yale J Biol Med.* 83(1), pp 1-9, ISSN 0044-0086

Laitinen, M., Makinen, K., Mannienen, H et al. (1998). Adenovirus-mediated gene transfer to lower limb artery of patients with chronic critical leg ischaemia. *Hum Gene Ther,* 9, pp. 1481–1486, ISSN 1043-0342

Leipziger, LY., Gllushko, V., Dibernardo, B et al. (1985). Dermal wound repair: Role of collagen matrix implants and synthetic polymer dressing, *J Am Acad Dermatol*, 12, pp. 409-419, ISSN 0190-9622

Lenihan, DJ., Osman, A., Sriram, V et al. (2003). Evidence for association of coronary sinus levels of hepatocyte growth factor and collateralization in human coronary disease. *Am J Physiol Heart Circ Physiol*, 284, pp. H1507–H1512, ISSN 0363-6135

Liang, L., & Bickenbach, JR. (2002). Somatic epidermal stem cells can produce multiple cell lineages during development. *Stem Cells*, 20, pp. 21–31, ISSN 1066-5099

Linsenmayer, TF. (1985). collagen," in *Cell biology of extracellular matrix*, E.D. Hay(ed.), Plenum Press, New York, pp.5-37, ISBN 9780306439513

Losordo, DW., Vale, PR., Symes, JF et.al. (1998). Gene therapy for myocardial angiogenesis: initial clinical results with direct myocardial injection of phVEGF165 as sole therapy for myocardial ischemia. *Circulation*, 98, pp. 2800–2804, ISSN 0009-7322

Margolis, DJ., Kantor, J., Santanna, J et al. (2001). Effectiveness of platelet releasate for the treatment of diabetic neuropathic foot ulcers. *Diabetes Care*, 24(3), pp. 483-488, ISSN 0149-5992

Marx, RE. (2001). Platelet-rich plasma (PRP): what is PRP and what is not PRP? *Implant Dent*, 10(4), pp. 225-228, ISSN 1056-6163

Marx, RE., Carlson, ER., Eichstaedt, RM et al. (1998). Platelet-rich plasma: Growth factor enhancement for bone grafts. *Oral Surg Oral Med Oral Pathol Oral Radiol Endod*, 85, pp. 638-646, ISSN 1079-2104

Matsumoto, K. & Nakamura, T. (1996). Emerging multipotent aspects of hepatocyte growth factor. *J Biochem*, 119, pp. 591- 600, ISSN 0021—924X

Matoba, S., Tatsumi, T., Murohara, T et al. (2008) Long-term clinical outcome after intramuscular implantation of bone marrow mononuclear cells (Therapeutic Angiogenesis by Cell Transplantation [TACT] trial) in patients with chronic limb ischemia. *Am. Heart J*, 156(5), pp. 1010-1018, ISSN 0002-8703

McFarlin, K., Gao, X., Liu, YB et al. (2006). Bone marrowderived mesenchymal stromal cells accelerate wound healing in the rat. *Wound Repair Regen*, 14, pp. 471–478, ISSN 1067-1927

Menetrey, J., Kasemkijwattana, C., Day, CS et al. (2000). Growth factors improve muscle healing in vivo. *J Bone Joint Surg Br*, 82, pp. 131–137 ISNN 0301-620X

Metcalfe, AD. & Ferguson, MW. (2007). Tissue engineering of replacement skin: the crossroads of biomaterials, wound healing, embryonic development, stem cells and regeneration. *J R Soc Interface*, 4, pp. 413–437, ISSN 1742-5689

Mehta, S. & Watson, JT. (2008). Platelet rich concentrate: basic science and current clinical applications. *J Orthop Trauma*, 22(6), pp.432-438, ISSN 0890-5339

Miyamoto, M., Yasutake, M., Takano, H et al. (2004). Therapeutic angiogenesis by autologous bone marrow cell implantation for refractory chronic peripheral arterial disease using assessment of neovascularization by 99mTc-tetrofosmin (TF) perfusion scintigraphy. Cell Transplant, 13(4), pp. 429-437, ISSN 0963-6897

Mizuno, H., Miyamoto, M., Shimamoto, M et al. (2010). Therapeutic angiogenesis by autologous bone marrow cell implantation together with allogeneic cultured dermal substitute for intractable ulcers in critical limb ischaemia. J Plast Reconstr Aesthet Surg, 63(11), pp. 1875-1882, ISSN 1748-6815

Mohle, R., Green, D., Moore, MA et al. (1997). Constitutive production and thrombin-induced release of vascular endothelial growth factor by human megakaryocytes and platelets. *Proc Natl Acad Sci USA*, 94, pp. 663–668, ISSN 0027-8424

Morishita, R., Nakamura, S,; Hayashi, S et al. (1999). Therapeutic angiogenesis induced by human recombinant hepatocyte growth factor in rabbit hind limb ischemia model as cytokine supplement therapy. *Hypertension*, 33, pp. 1379–1384, ISSN 0194-099X

Morishita, R., Sakaki, M., Yamamoto, K et al. (2002). Impairment of collateral formation in Lp(a) transgenic mice: therapeutic angiogenesis induced by human hepatocyte growth factor gene. *Circulation*, 105, pp. 1491–1496, ISSN 0009-7322

Morishita, R., Aoki, M., Hashiya, N., (2004). Therapeutic angiogenesis using hepatocyte growth factor (HGF). *Curr Gene Ther*. 4, pp. 199–206, ISSN 1566-5232

Morishita, R., Aoki, M., Hashiya, N., (2004). Safety evaluation of clinical gene therapy using hepatocyte growth factor to treat peripheral arterial disease. *Hypertension*, 44, pp. 203–209, ISSN 0194-911X

Nakamura, Y., Morishita, R., Higaki, J et al. (1996). Hepatocyte growth factor is a novel member of the endothelium- specific growth factors: additive stimulatory effect of hepatocyte growth factor with basic fibroblast growth factor but not with vascular endothelial growth factor. *J Hypertens*, 14, pp. 1067–1072, ISSN 0263-6352

Nikol, S., Baumgartner, I., Van Belle E et al. (2008). Therapeutic angiogenesis with intramuscular NV1FGF improves amputation-free survival in patients with critical limb ischemia. *Mol Ther*, 16, pp. 972–978, ISSN 1525-0016

O'Connell, SM., Impeduglia, T., Hessler, K et al. (2008). Autologous platelet-rich fibrin matrix as cell therapy in the healing of chronic lower-extremity ulcers. *Wound Repair Regen*, 16(6), pp. 749-56, ISSN 1067-1927

Powell, RJ., Simons, M., Mendelsohn, FO et al. (2008). Results of a double-blind, placebo-controlled study to assess the safety of intramuscular injection of hepatocyte growth factor plasmid to improve limb perfusion in patients with critical limb ischemia. *Circulation*, 118, pp. 58–65, ISSN 0009-7322

Ramsey, SD., Newton, K., Blough, D et al. (1999). Incidence, outcomes, and cost of foot ulcers in patients with diabetes. *Diabetes Care*, 22, pp. 382–387, ISSN 0149-5992

Rajagopalan, S., Olin, J., Deitcher, S et al. (2007). Use of a constitutively active hypoxia-inducible factor-1alpha transgene as a therapeutic strategy in no-option critical limb ischemia patients: phase I doseescalation experience. *Circulation*, 115, pp. 1234 –1243, ISSN 0009-7322

Roberts, AB. & Sporn, MB. (1993). Physiological actions and clinical applications of transforming growth factor-beta (TGFbeta). *Growth Factors*, 8, pp. 1-9, ISSN 0897-7194

Rogers, LC., Bevilacqua, NJ. & Armstrong, DG. (2008). The use of marrow-derived stem cells to accelerate healing in chronic wounds. *Int Wound J*, 5(1), pp.20-5, ISSN 1742-4801

Rosengart, TK., Lee, LY., Patel, SR et al. (1999). Six-month assessment of a phase I trial of angiogenic gene therapy for the treatment of coronary artery disease using direct intramyocardial administration of an adenovirus vector expressing the VEGF121 cDNA. *Ann Surg*, 230, pp. 466–470, ISSN 0003-4932.

Rosengart, TK., Lee, LY., Patel, SR et al. (1999). Angiogenesis gene therapy: phase I assessment of direct intramyocardial administration of an adenovirus vector expressing VEGF121 cDNA to individuals with clinically significant severe coronary artery disease. *Circulation*, 100, pp. 468–474, ISSN 0009-7322

Sanchez-Guijo, FM., Oterino, E., Barbado, MV et al. (2010). Both CD133(+) cells and monocytes provide significant improvement for hindlimb ischemia, although they do not transdifferentiate into endothelial cells. *Cell Transplant*, 19(1), pp. 103-112, ISSN 0963-6897

Schumacher, B., Pecher, P., von Specht, BU et al. (1998). Induction of neoangiogenesis in ischemic myocardium by human growth factors: first clinical results of a new treatment of coronary heart disease. *Circulation*, 97, pp. 645- 650. ISSN 0009-7322

Shashikiran, ND., Reddy, VV., Yavagal, CM et al. (2006). Applications of platelet-rich plasma (PRP) in contemporary pediatric dentistry. *J Clin Pediatr Dent*, 30(4), pp. 283-286, ISSN 1053-4628

Sivan-Loukianova, E., Awad, O., Stepanovic, V et al. (2003). CD34_ blood cells accelerate vascularization and healing of diabetic mouse skin wounds. *J Vasc Res*, 40, pp. 368–377, ISSN 1018-1172

Stadelmann, WK., Digenis, AG. & Tobin GR. (1998). Physiology and healing dynamics of chronic cutaneous wounds. *Am J Surg*, 176, pp. 26S–38S, ISSN 0002-9610

Starkey, R., Cohen, S. & Orth D. (1975). Epidermal growth fator: identification of a new hormone in human urine. *Science*, 189, pp. 800-802, ISSN 0036-8075

Tanaka, R., Ichioka, S., Sekiya, N et al. (2007). Elastic plasma protein film blended with platelet releasate accelerates healing of diabetic mouse skin wounds. *Vox Sang*, 93(1), pp. 49-56, ISSN 0042-9007

Taniyama, Y., Morishita, R., Aoki, M et al. (2001). Therapeutic angiogenesis induced by human hepatocyte growth factor gene in rat and rabbit hind limb ischemia models: preclinical study for treatment of peripheral arterial disease. *Gene Ther*, 8, pp. 181–189, ISSN 0969-7128

Taniyama, Y., Morishita, R., Hiraoka, K et al. (2001). Therapeutic angiogenesis induced by human hepatocyte growth factor gene in rat diabetic hind limb ischemia model: molecular mechanisms of delayed angiogenesis in diabetes. *Circulation*, 104, pp. 2344–2350, ISSN 0009-7322

Tateishi-Yuyama, E., Matsubara, H., Murohara, T et al. (2002). Therapeutic angiogenesis for patients with limb ischaemia by autologous transplantation of bone-marrow cells: a pilot study and a randomised controlled trial. *Lancet*, 360, pp. 427–435, ISSN 0140-6736

Tateno, K., Minamino, T., Toko, H et al. (2006). Critical roles of muscle-secreted angiogenic factors in therapeutic neovascularization. *Circ Res*, 98(9), pp. 1194-1202, ISSN 0009-7330

Vale, PR., Losordo, DW., Milliken, CE et al. (1999). Images in cardiovascular medicine: Percutaneous myocardial gene transfer of phVEGF-2. *Circulation*, 100, pp. 2462–2463, ISSN 0009-7322

Vale, PR., Losordo, DW., Milliken, CE et al. (2000). Left ventricular electromechanical mapping to assess efficacy of phVEGF165 gene transfer for therapeutic angiogenesis in chronic myocardial ischemia. *Circulation*, 102, pp. 965–974, ISSN 0009-7322

Wu, Y., Zhao RC. & Tredget, EE. (2010). Concise review: bone marrow-derived stem/progenitor cells in cutaneous repair and regeneration. *Stem cells*, 28(5), pp. 905-915, ISSN 1066-5099

Yamaguchi, Y., Kubo, T., Murakami, T et al. (2005). Bone marrow cells differentiate into wound myofibroblasts and accelerate the healing of wounds with exposed bones when combined with an occlusive dressing. *Br J dermatol*, 152, pp. 616-622, ISSN 0007-0963

Yannas, IV. & Burke, JF. (1980). Design of an artificial skin Ⅰ. Basic design principles. *J Biomed Mater Res*, 14, pp. 65-81, ISSN 1552-4973

Yazawa, M., Ogata, H., Nakajima, T et al. (2003). Basic studies on the clinical applications of platelet-rich plasma. *Cell Transplant*, 12, pp. 509-518, ISSN 0963-6897

17

Application of the Nanocrystalline Silver in Treatment of Burn Wounds in Children

Maya Argirova and Ognian Hadjiiski
N.I. Pirogov, Centre of Burns and Plastic Surgery, Sofia
Bulgaria

1. Introduction

Infection is one of the most frequent and major complications in patients with burn injuries and is the main cause for prolonged in-hospital stay and death in cases of wide-spread burns despite marked progress in the development of treatments methods for these patients. Burn infections get complicated by the development of multi-resistant organisms. The colonization and infection of these wounds are a dual clinical problem. On one hand, a slowing of the healing process is possible based on a damaged immune system and inadequate perfusion to the wound. On the other hand, the infected wound may be a potential source of spreading of antibiotic-resistant microorganisms. The infected wound is a cause for pain and discomfort for patients, as well as life-threatening septic conditions. Thus, the treatment cost and the medical care increase, respectively.

The topical treatment of the wound is an integral part of the general treatment of the burns. The topical treatment agents should posses some important characteristics such as a broad spectrum of antibacterial activity, low resistance level, decreased vapour loss, dehydration prevention, limited adverse effects, pain control, ease of use and limited toxic risk. Due to the wide variety of suitable agents, the choice of the agent depends on the assessment of the wound. The most important considerations for the choice of a burn wound dressing are the level of its antiseptic effect, the influence of its bioactive abilities on the epithelization and its abilities for management of the wound infection. The perfect dressing for children should provide optimal protection, reparation and minimization of pain and burn sequelae. Over the last 30 years, the knowledge of the mechanism of wound healing has made incredible progress as a result of intensive technological and clinical research. The new technologies have focused on the development of antiseptic products releasing the antiseptic agent slowly and steadily, which allows a lower and more efficient concentration. The wide-spread antiseptic agents containing silver have a long history of usage and a wide spectrum of activity (Klasen, 2000; Landsdown, 2006; Fong & Wood, 2006). Silver dressings are the most commonly and frequently used in burn wound treatment.

The perfect silver dressing should contain such silver concentration which creates a free (or limited) side antibacterial effect. The silver nitrate solution is not applied any more due to its toxic effect, change of ionic balance and low penetration in depth. The silver sulphadiazine SSD (Flammazine, Dermazin, Silvadene, Silverdin®, etc.) is the most frequently used agent for topical treatment of children with burns. SSD has a powerful antibacterial effect against a broad spectrum of Gram-positive and Gram-negative bacteria, and especially MRSA and

Candida spp. The antibacterial effect can be achieved two hours after application and its maximum activity lasts approximately six hours. The majority of the comparative clinical studies, utilizing biological and non-biological dressings, involves silver sulphadiazine, which shows that it is used as a standard agent for treatment in most burn centres (Huang et al., 2007; Cuttle et al., 2007).

Creams and solutions containing silver have been used as main agents in burn wound treatment for a long time. Attempts to utilize the excellent antiseptic properties of silver and keep the principles of maintaining the moisture environment in the wound on the one hand, and avoid the disadvantages of SSD and silver nitrate on the other, have led to the development of a new generation of silver dressings. New technologies allowing impregnating substances with "antimicrobial" effect in materials or medical equipment have been exploited. Silver dressings have preventive and healing effect on the wound surface (Burrell, 2003; Orvington, 2001).

The new silver-impregnated dressings, developed over the last 20 years, have overcome to a great extent the disadvantages and limitations of the older silver dressings and especially the fast silver inactivation. In these new dressings, when silver is consumed by interaction with target cells or inactivated by protein and anion complexes in wound exudate, additional silver is released in the wound. Thus, a sustained and steady supply of active silver is achieved on the wound surface (Leaper, 2006). The innovation in these dressings is not the properties of silver, which are well-known, but the amount of silver incorporated in the dressings themselves. Since the properties of silver are beyond doubt, the choice of dressing is determined by the characteristics of the silver-carrying material and by the way of silver delivery to the wound. The dressing components vary as well including mesh, nylon, hydrocolloid or methylcellulose. In order to be biologically active, the structure of silver should have dissolution properties, e.g., Ag^+ or Ag^0. Ag^+ is a known ionic form present in silver nitrate, silver sulfadiazine and other ionic silver compounds. Ag^0 is the metallic or uncharged form of silver occurring in crystalline and nanocrystalline silver structures (Demling & De Santi, 2001; Orvington, 2001).

In the treatment practice, various silver-impregnated dressings are used. Dressings of this type differ mostly in their silver "reservoirs". Some examples are Acticoat (Smith & Nephew), Actisorb Silver 220 (Johnson & Johnson), Aquacel - Ag (Convatec), Arglaes (Medline, Mundelein), Contreet - H (Coloplast, Marietta), SilvaSorb (Medline) and Silverlon® (Argentum LLC). The comparison of the silver dressings is usually based on the bacteriology (Cavanagh et al., 2010). Thus, differences are noticed in the field of inhibition, with Minimum Inhibitory Concentration (MIC) and Minimum Bactericidal Concentration (MBC) as a result of the antimicrobial activity of the agent. The results of the in-vitro studies of these products with respect to their antimicrobial effect are comparatively identical, and most of them demonstrate that Acticoat has a more powerful and broader-spectrum antibacterial effect (Yin, 2003; Yin, Langford & Burrell, 1999). For example, MIC is reached in concentration of Ag at the range of 5-50 ppm for the most bacteria of clinical interest and 60.5 ppm for MRSA. Ag concentration for Acticoat is 70 ppm. Acticoat and Aquacel-Ag are shown to be most efficient among the silver-impregnated dressings. It has to be pointed out that only few prospective clinical studies on the use of these products in patients with burns have been published. The nanocrystalline silver dressing was produced using nanotechnology and was introduced by R.E. Burrell in 1998 (Wright et al., 1998; Burrell et al., 1999).

Acticoat has biological, clinical and practical advantages. The biological advantages are: i) excellent antimicrobial activity; ii) decrease in the inflammatory reaction of the wound by diminishing exudation and control of wound contamination; and iii) creation of optimal environment for the healing process of the wound by maintaining moisture, stimulating epithelization and controlling wound contamination (Gravante et al., 2009).
The antimicrobial activity of silver ions has been studied in detail. It has been found that this activity is due to: i) interruption of the cell respiratory chain; ii) intervention in the electronic and ionic transport of the bacterial cell; iii) attaching to bacterial DNA and influence on cell replication; and iv) interaction with the cell membrane and damaging of its structure and receptor function.
The aim of our study was to assess the quality and efficacy of the nanocrystalline silver dressing in treatment of burn wounds and to determine the potential advantages over the older silver dressings.

2. Materials and methods

2.1 Prospective clinical study involving children treated with Acticoat

A prospective clinical study involving a clinical contingent of 112 children treated with Acticoat has been carried out. The protocol was approved by the local ethics committee and written informed consent was provided by the children's parents prior the commencement of the study. The approval of reporting the results of the study has been obtained. The nanocrystalline silver dressing has been applied on children of both genders, stationary treated for a period of one and a half year in 2009 and 2010. **Acticoat**™ and **Acticoat Flex** with 3- and 7-day-wear time have been used. **Acticoat**™ consists of three layers – two outer and one inner. The inner layer is an absorbent core of rayon and polyester, which controls the silver release. The two outer layers are a silver-coated, high-density polyethylene mesh. The silver dressing coating has a specific physical structure consisting of silver nanocrystalline, organised in a coarse columnar structure. The thickness of the silver layer is approximately one micrometer and contains 0.24±0.4 mg silver per mg polyethylene mesh. Acticoat-7 dressing consists of three layers of polyethylene mesh coated with nanocrystalline silver and two layers of rayon polyester.
Acticoat Flex is a new, modern formula of the unique silver nanotechnology. Acticoat Flex has an open-weave structure. The open weave structure allows good contact with the wound and easy exudate migration, thus reducing the risk of maceration and does not require constant moistening. The dressing can be perfectly combined with vacuum negative pressure therapy in cases of soft tissue defects.
The monitored children were in the group age of 9 months to 18 years (mean age – 5.26 years) and had burn area of 0.5% to 95% (mean – 7.89%). The burn wounds had various depth and localization. Among them predominated the second-degree superficial burns (IIAB. The studied contingent was grouped into five groups:

- The first and largest group comprised 78 children with second-degree superficial burns (IIAB) having mean burn area of 6.82%;
- The second group involved 19 children with deep burn wounds – mean area of the deep burn wounds of 15.76%.
- The third group comprised 5 children on whom the Acticoat dressing was applied on excised wounds with mean area of 6.75%.
- The fourth group comprised 5 children with application of the dressing on autografts.

- The fifth group comprised 5 children with application of the dressing on fresh donor sites.

The assessment methods used included clinical, microbiological, statistical and photo documentation.

2.2 Comparative analysis

A comparative clinical and cost analysis between **Acticoat™** and **SSD** (**Dermazin**) has been carried out, since the latter agent has proven antiseptic properties and is widely used for the treatment of burns in children in comparison with the other epithelotonic and less antiseptic agents such as iodic and chlorine-hexidine (Tonkin & Wood, 2005). The clinical contingent for this comparative analysis is different from the previous one and involved 111 children. The patients were randomized into two groups. The comparative assessment has been performed for 68 children with **Acticoat™** and 43 children with **Dermazin** and the following parameters have been monitored:

- Clinical – wound type (initial and post dressing change), wound clearing time, epithelization time and hospital stay;
- Microbiological – dynamically monitoring the microbial flora, prior and post each dressing change;
- Pharmacological and cost parameters.

2.3 Method of use

The way of application depends on the type **of Acticoat**. The application is easy and identical regardless of the age, area, localization and the depth of the burn, excised area, area covered with autograft or donor site. The wound areas are mechanically cleaned by hydro-procedure using Hibiscrub. Prior to use, **Acticoat**™ is moistened with sterile water and applied on the burn wound, excised area, autograft or donor site. The dressing is trimmed according to the shape of the treated area. **Acticoat**™ is covered with a four-layer moistened gauze followed by four layers of dry gauze whose purpose is to drain the surplus amount of fluid. The dressing is held in place with a bandage or mesh. The moisture maintenance is an important condition for the dressing efficacy and can be done by means of the following two ways:

- Moistening the dressing by irrigation or watering once or twice daily. The outer gauze layer is changed.
- Covering the dressing with polyethylene foil which helps maintain moisture.

An alternative but a more expensive way to maintain the moisture is to use Intrasite gel or Allevyn foam.

In case of heavy exudate wounds, additional moistening of the wounds is not necessary. The dressing is changed 3 or 7 days after application, but this period may differ depending on the estimation. **Acticoat Flex** is used after an identical preparatory wound treatment and is moistened with sterile water prior to application. It is cut to the desired shape and size, and exploiting its elasticity applied to the wound area. The dressing is covered with a four-layer moistened gauze followed by four layers of dry gauze. It is not additionally moistened until the next dressing. In wide spread burns, the dressing change is performed by using a general anaesthesia (Tancheva, 2008). In cases of limited and small burn areas, a general anaesthesia is not necessary due to the painless dressing change.

Microbiological quantitative (tissue biopsy samples) and qualitative (wound surface swab) analysis of the flora in the treated areas were carried out before initial application and at

every dressing change. The studied contingent was monitored for presence of pain or discomfort after the dressing as well as for side effects - general and local.
The treatment of 62 children from the first group started within 24 hours after the burn and for the remaining 16 children –24 hours after the burn. The treatment of 7 children from the second group began within 24 hours after the burn and for the remaining 12 children - within 42 hours.
In all burn centres **SSD** is changed every 12 hours. In this study the **Dermazin** dressings were changed every 24 hours. The microbiological analysis was performed at the beginning of the treatment and at every dressing change. The closed method of application was used. After a hydro-procedure with Hibiscrub and cleansing using disinfection solution, the agent of 2-3 mm layer was applied directly on the wound and covered with dry, sterile and dense bandage-gauze dressing (Atiyeh, 2009).

3. Clinical observations

3.1 Clinical observation of the wounds treated with Acticoat

The treatment with Acticoat of the first group of children (78) with superficial burns was conducted according to the described method. Decreasing of the exudation and demarcation of devitalized tissue was observed as early as in the first dressing. In wounds and areas of second degree (IIA), the dermis was deeply red with beginning epithelization. In cases of abundant exudation and of deep dermal burns, a bright and jelly-like coating was observed on the wound surface and the Acticoat bed, which was caused by protein coagulation. Attempting to remove this coating led to heavy wound bleeding. The wound resembled the "infected" one, but bacterial growth was absent. There was no inflammation area around the wound. A dark brown or grey pigmentation of the wound and intact skin was observed, which was transient and disappeared within 2 to 14 days. The intact skin was changed by the hydration but not macerated. The hydrated skin appeared white or lighter than the surrounding skin with a wrinkled or prune-like look, while the macerated skin was soft and tissue became bright red, progressing to blistering and breakdown. When Acticoat Flex was applied on this type of burns, a good fixation of the agent on the wound and hardly any exudation was observed. In most cases, the dressing could be removed only after a prolonged moistening. The dressing structure allows good control of the wound and a new dressing was not applied, regardless of the Acticoat Flex wear time (3 or 7 days), providing the dressing was properly fixed. When the dressing was applied on a heavily exudating wound, the exudation decreased after one or two dressings (6 children). The exudation level was subjectively assessed by the type and size of the coating on the wound surface and on the dressing. In burns above 10%, where wound infection was not present, smell appeared after the removal of the dressing. The patients did not feel pain immediately after the dressing application and between the dressing changes.
A discomfort after the dressing application was observed in 8 children, which disappeared within 3-4 hours. In the deep dermal burn wounds, a very rapid demarcation and removal of the necrotic tissue was observed (in the 2nd or 3rd dressing). The mean wound clearing time is 8.92 days and the mean epithelization time is 12.98 days, shorter in comparison with the agents used thus far. The second (IIA) degree burn wounds epithelialized within 5-6 days. In the case of cleared wound and beginning epithelization, the dressing could be replaced by another type of epithelotonic dressing such as Bactigras. (Bactigras is a sterile gauze dressing made of cotton impregnated with soft paraffin containing 0.5%

chlorhexidine acetate). When the Acticoat dressing was applied on infected wounds, the clinical type of the wound remained the same, but the coating on the dressing bottom was more mucous and thick, and a 4-5-day delay in the wound clearing was observed. Wound sites in which a pathogenic flora was isolated during the treatment did not clinically change the wound type. In these rare cases the only clinical sign was the delay of the wound clearing and epithelization, respectively.
The application of Acticoat™ and Acticoat Flex for treatment of superficial burns is demonstrated (Figures 1-15).

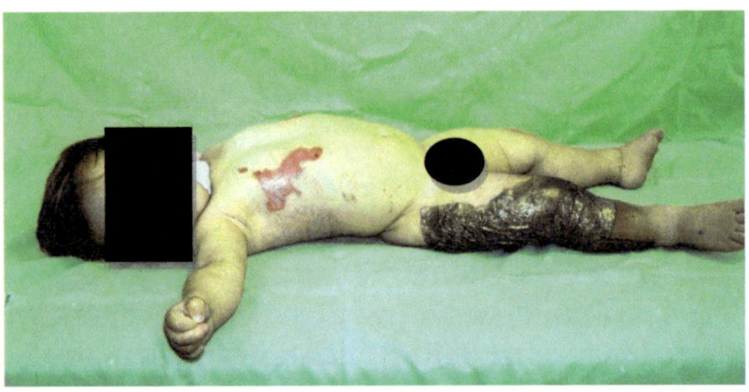

Fig. 1. The beginning of treatment

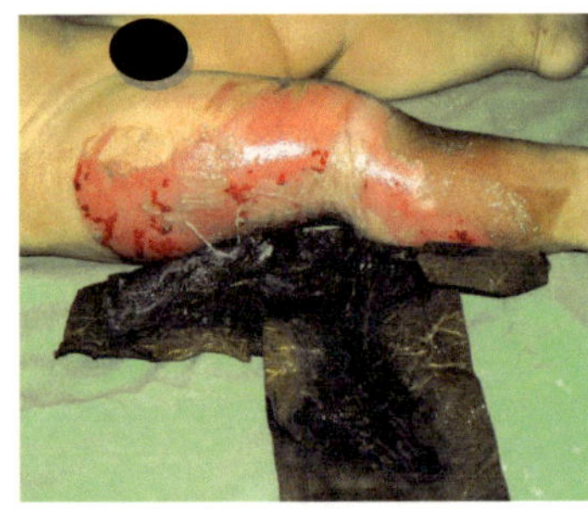

Fig. 2. Result after the 1st dressing

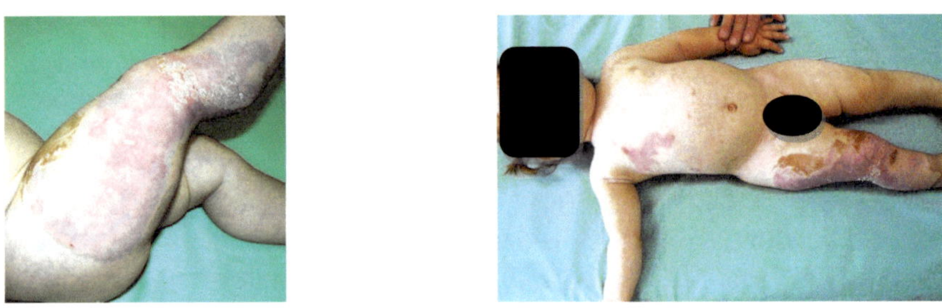

Fig. 3. Result after the 2st dressing - complete epithelization

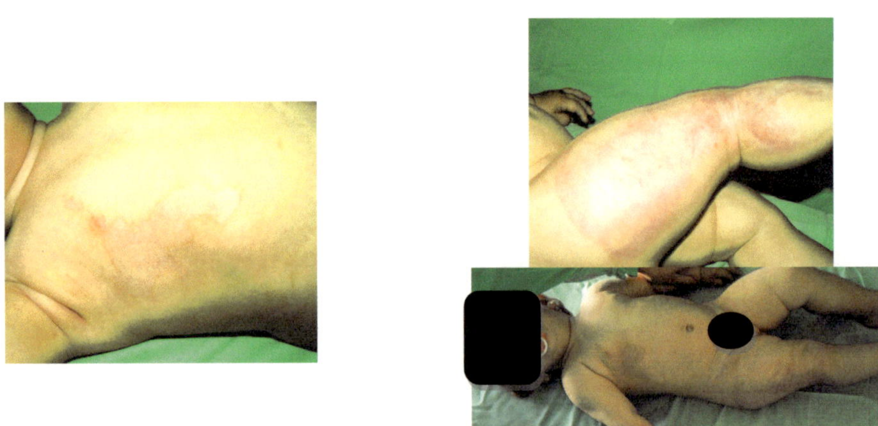

Fig. 4. Final result - 30th day after the burn

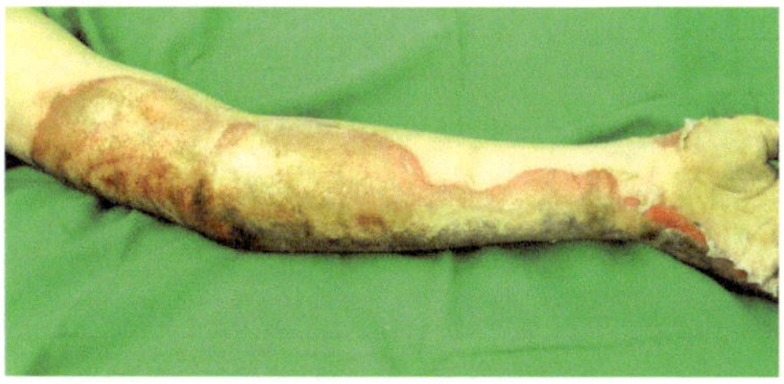

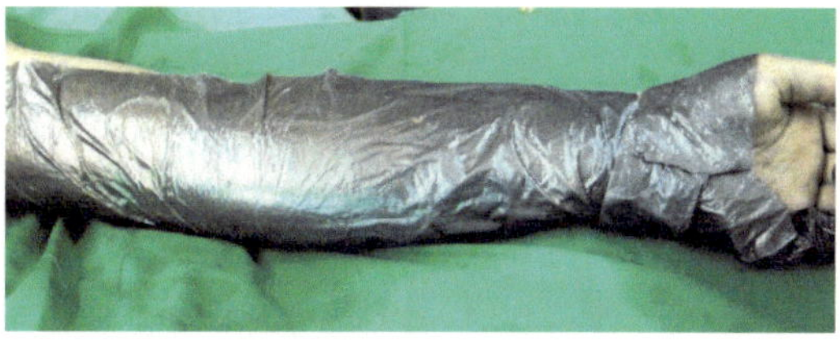

Fig. 5. The beginning of the treatment with Acticoat™ of a left arm with deep dermal flame burn –

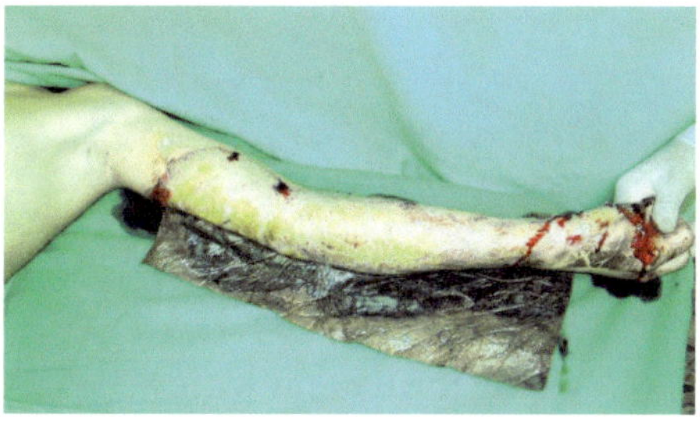

Fig. 6. Wound condition after the 1st dressing

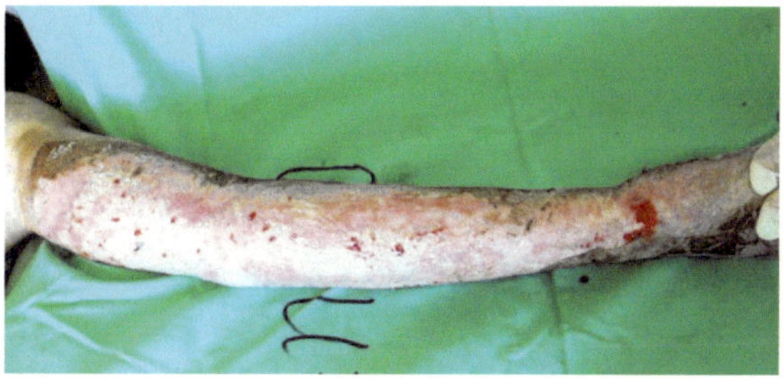

Fig. 7. Wound condition after the 2nd dressing

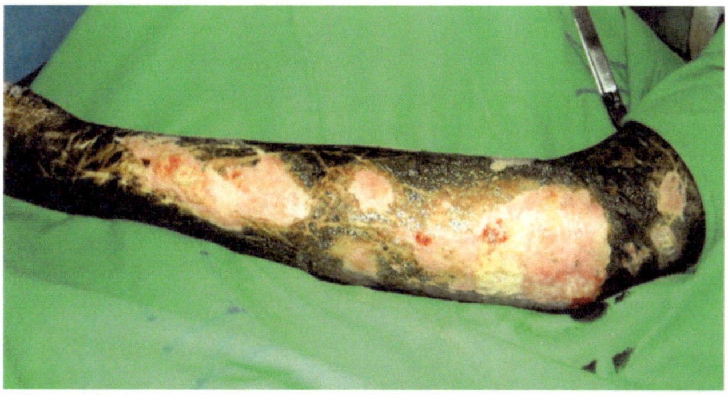

Fig. 8. Wound condition after the 3rd dressing – epithelialized surface with scattered small wounds and distinguished hyperpigmentation resulted from the application of the silver dressing

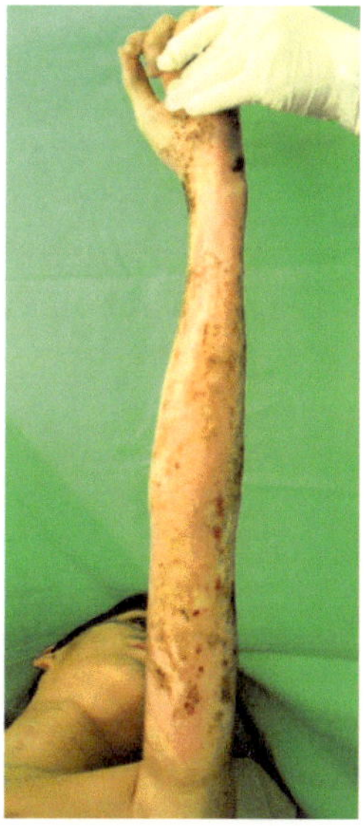

Fig. 9. The 16th day after burn. Full epithelization with disappearing hyperpigmentation

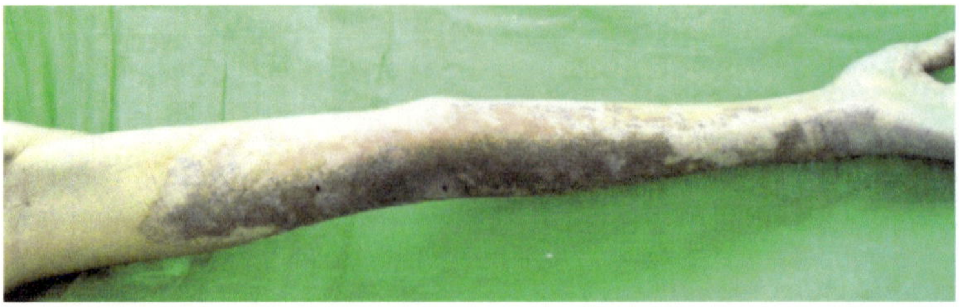

Fig. 10. Final outcome

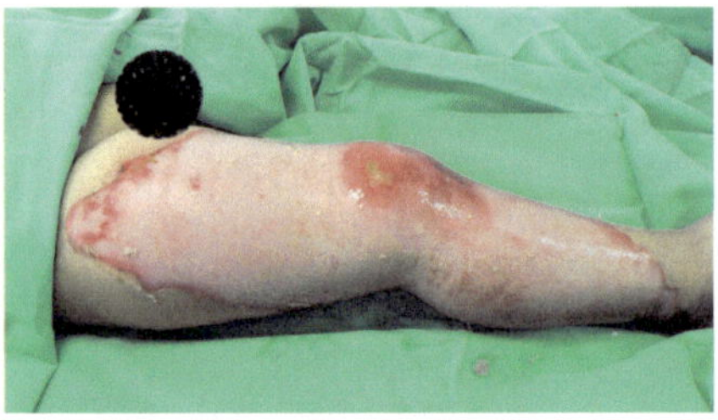

Fig. 11. Scalding of the right leg

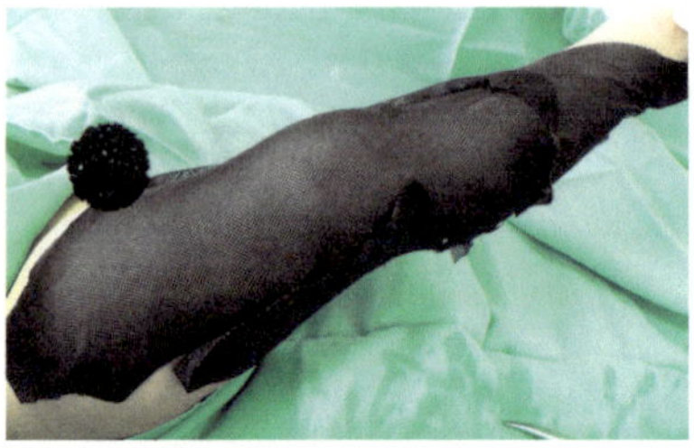

Fig. 12. Covering the wound with Acticoat Flex 7

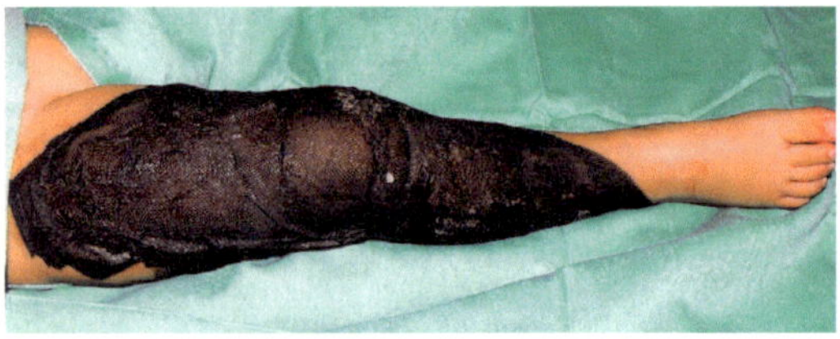

Fig. 13. The result after the 1st dressing on the 7th day of the treatment

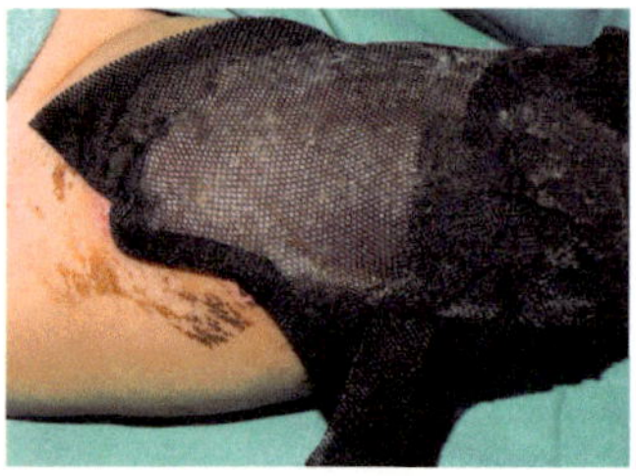

Fig. 14. Epithelializing wound covered with Acticoat Flex

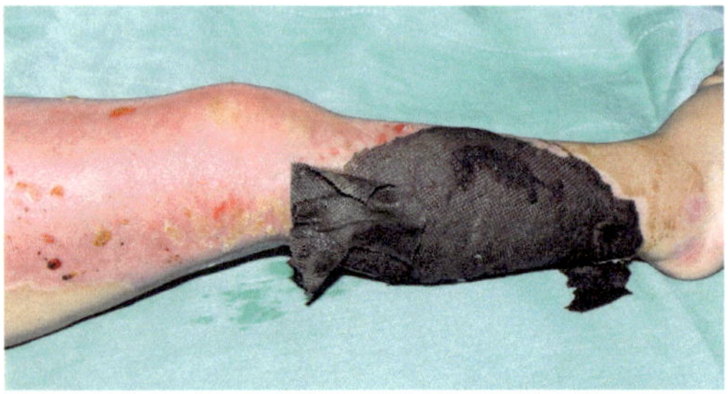

Fig. 15. The 12th day of the treatment - fully epithelialized wound of the thigh and progressing wound epithelization of the lower leg

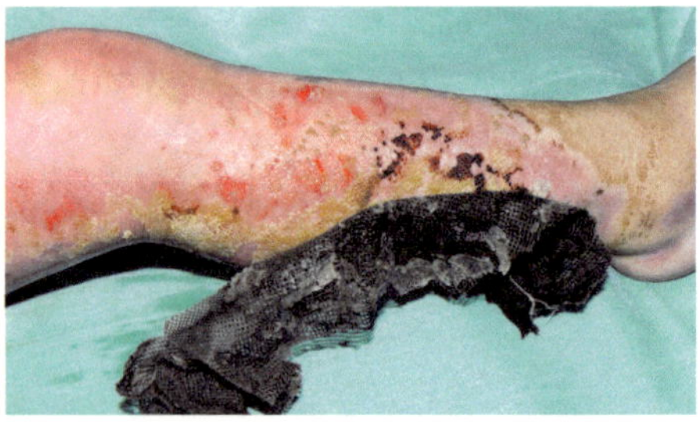

Fig. 16. Early result (15th day) - removing of the dressing after moistening. The wound is almost fully epithelialized

The dressing was applied on 19 children from the second group with deep burns with various area (from 0.5% to 95%, mean - 15.76%) and various localization. All children underwent operation. An early surgical excision at one, two or three stages was performed on 16 children between the 2nd and the 6th day after the burn. Three children were operated on after the 10th day of the burn. The dressing changes for this group conformed to the times of surgical treatment. On those patients operated on after the 10th day, the dressing was applied according to the described standard method. The demarcation and separation of the devitalized tissue in these patients occurred after the second or third dressing. The burns were clear and without exudation. The formed necroses were greenish and not dry for Acticoat™, while those for Acticoat Flex were greenish-brown and drier. Dressing removal was easy and without bleeding, and a clear wound with a short and fresh granulation was formed, ready for autografting.

In 5 children from the third group, Acticoat was applied on fresh excised sites of burn wounds (mean area of 6.75%), where multistage excision was carried out. After the dressing removal, the excised site was covered with bright yellow coating without smell and exudation. This coating could be easily removed and the wound area was fresh and ready for autografting without any additional surgical treatment. Hyperpigmentation of the wound was not observed.

The dressing was applied on autografts in 5 of the clinically monitored children, who had above 15% burn and deep burn area ranging from 6% to 72%. Using the standard method, Acticoat was applied directly on the autografts, which had various areas (300 cm^2 to 800 cm^2) and was meshed at 1:2 ratio using mesh-graft dermatome (1:4 ratio for one patient only). The dressing was removed on the 4th day after the operation (in two children on the 5th day) and well-healed autografts with hyperpigmentation, scant smell and without exudation was observed. The epithelization of the mesh splits was 95%.

In 5 children, the dressing was applied on fresh donor sites situated on the thighs. The autografts with thickness of 0.2 - 0.5 mm were harvested from these areas with electric dermatome. The standard way of dressing application was used. After the removal of the dressing on the 4th day, the donor site had pink colour and was covered with silver scattered particles. This site did not have any smell, exudate or coating. Epithelization of 95% occurred in one child on the 4th day. The complete epithelization occurred in the remaining patients within 8 days after the dressing application. Hyperpigmintation of the intact skin was observed in all patients. The donor sites were monitored up to six months after the epithelization and there were no signs of hypertrophic scarring according to the Vancouver Scar Scale (VSS).

The following figures demonstrate a clinical case with Acticoat™ application (Figures 17-28): i) treatment of deep burns localized on the legs; ii) application on excised area; iii) application on auto- and allograft; iv) application on donor sites.

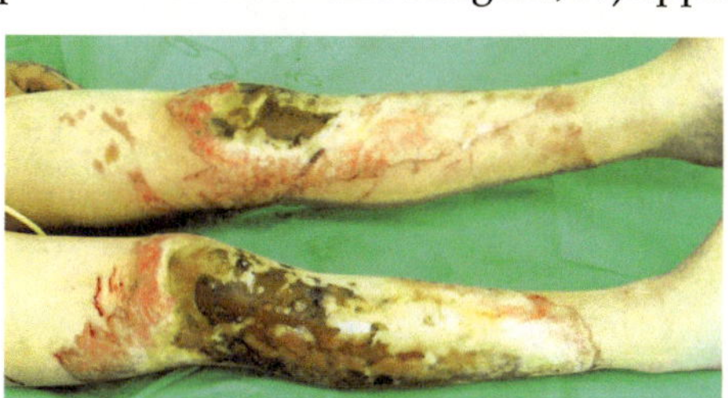

Fig. 17. Deep burn

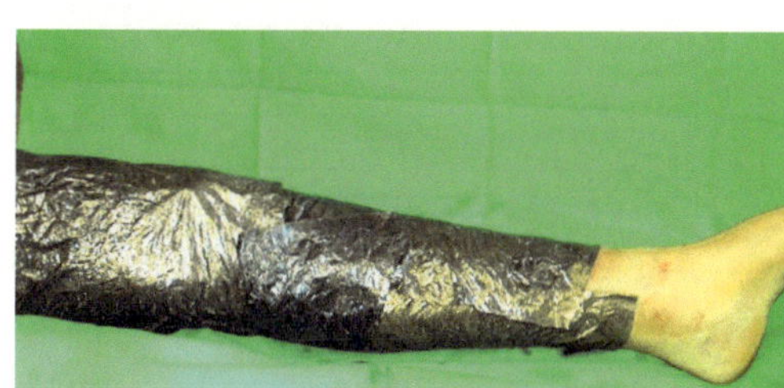

Fig. 18. Application of Acticoat™ as a pre-operative preparation

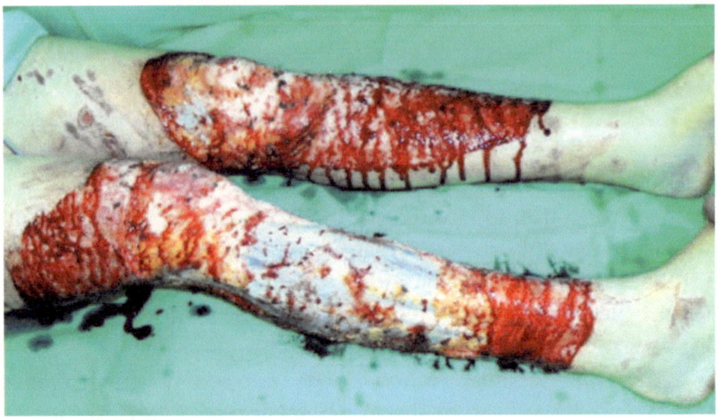

Fig. 19. Total surgical excision

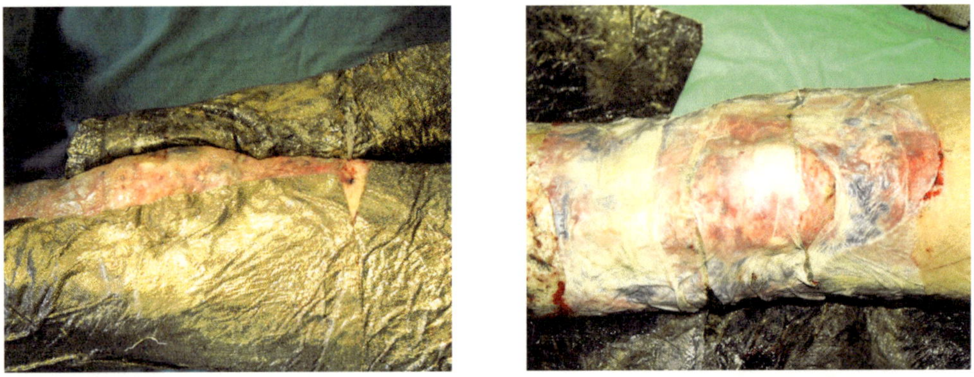

Fig. 20. Application of Acticoat™ on fresh autograft

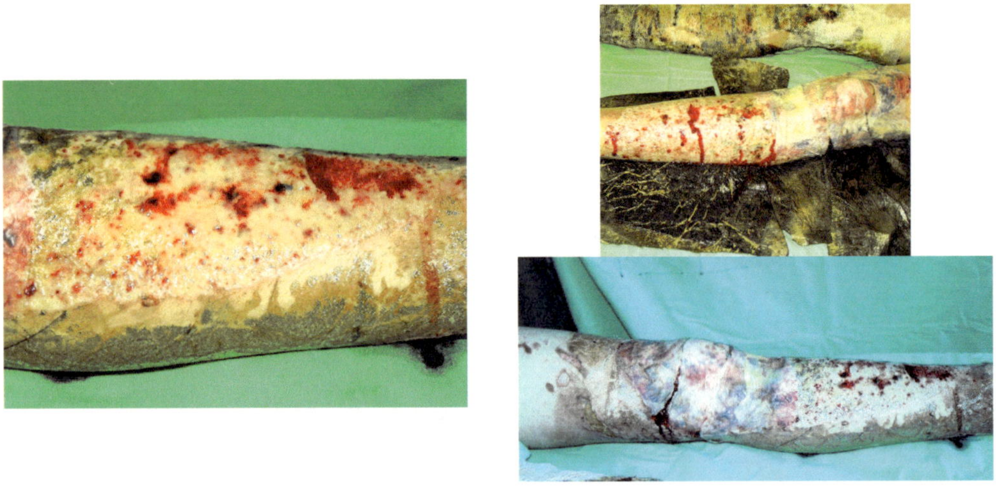

Fig. 21. A stable whole autograft on knee and condition of the excised site on the lower leg after Acticoat™ removal

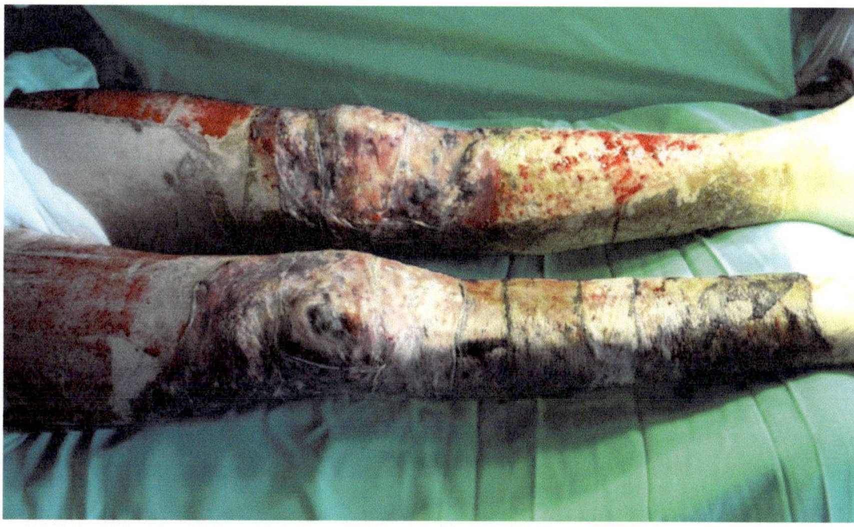

Fig. 22. A stage of the treatment – healed autografts in the knee area, healed autografts in the right lower leg; and clinical condition of the excised site on the left lower leg after Acticoat™ application

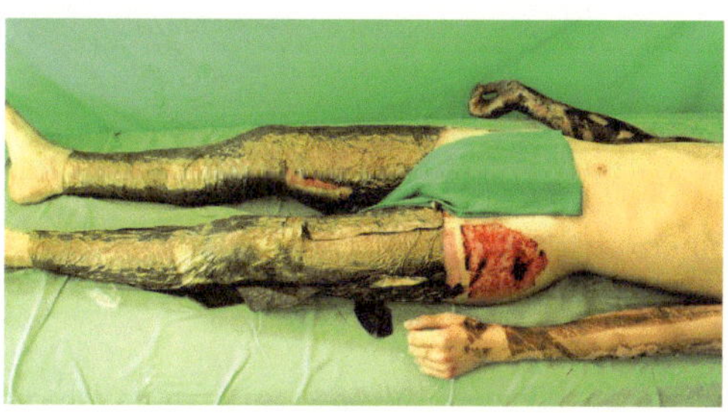

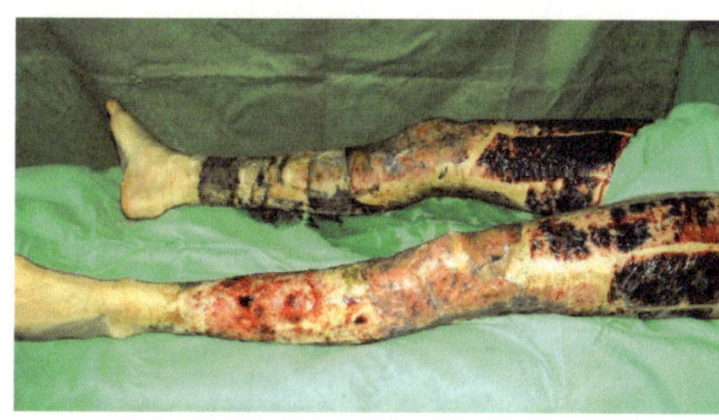

Fig. 23. Autografts covered with Acticoat and donor sites on both legs

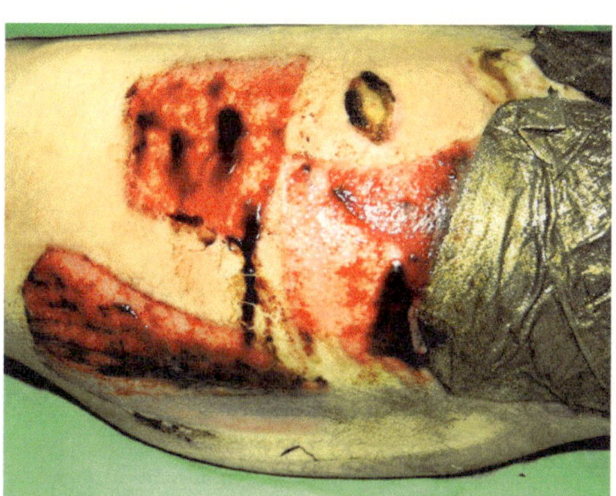

Fig. 24. Donor sites after the 1st Acticoat™ dressing

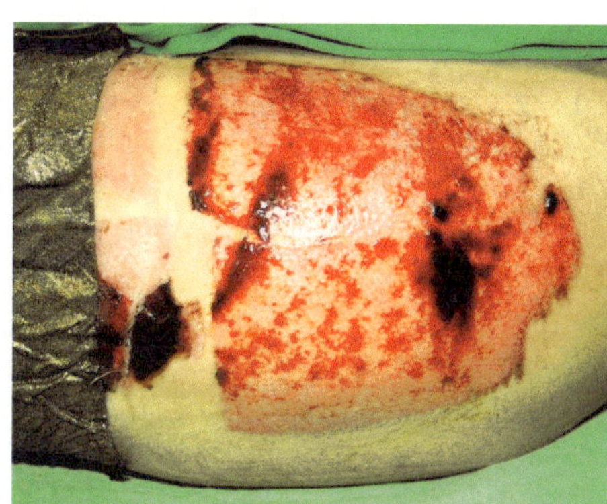

Fig. 25. Epithelialized donor site at the 2nd dressing and neighbouring donor site after the 1st dressing

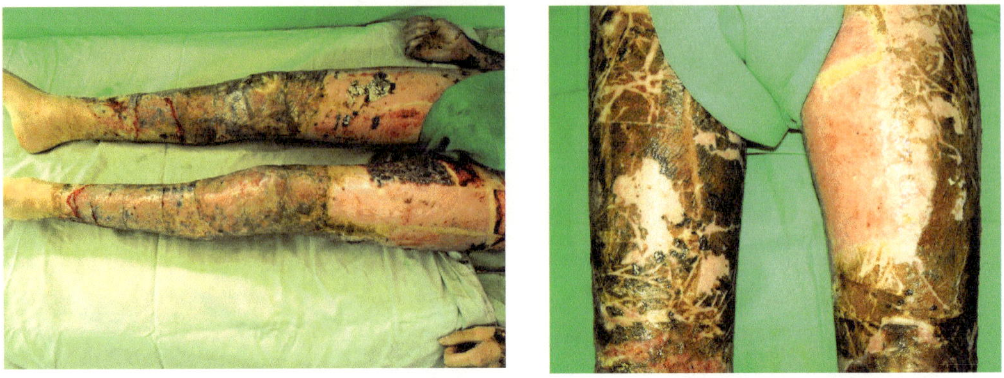

Fig. 26. Wounds covered with stable autografts and fully epithelialized donor sites. Persistent hyperpigmentation on operated and donor sites due the Acticoat™ use

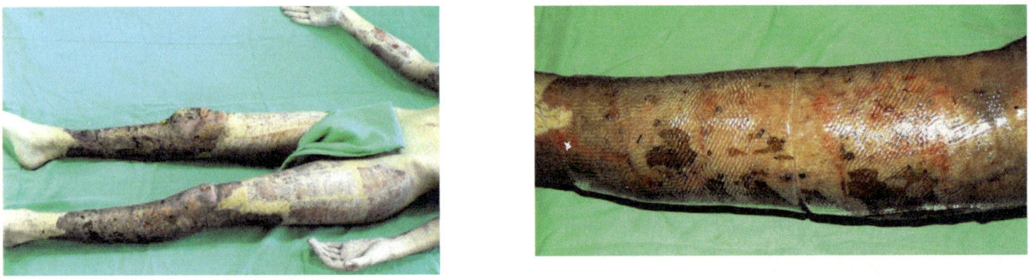

Fig. 27. Outcome at the end of the treatment and beginning of the prophylaxis of the scars with silicone sheets

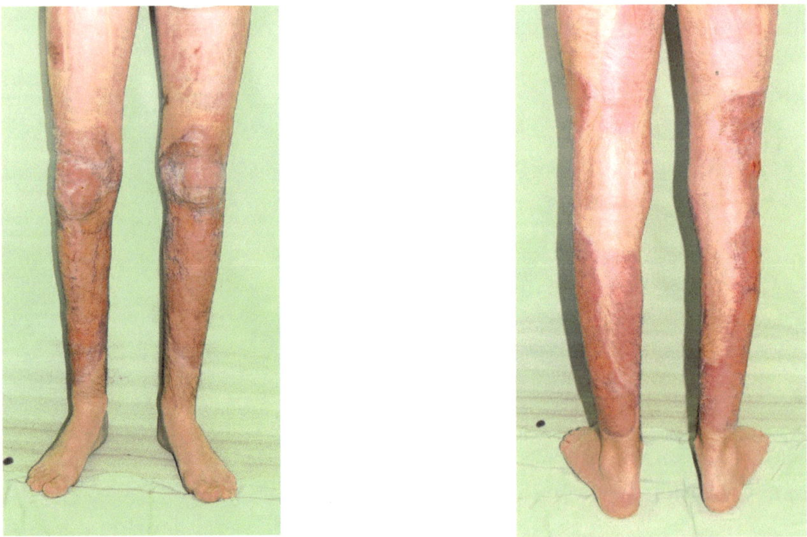

Fig. 28. The patients after the end of the treatment

3.2 Clinical observation of the wounds treated with Dermazin

The application time of the agent was registered until the beginning of stable epithelization of the wound in the patients with superficial burns. In the deep burns, this period included the time until the wound clears or the surgical treatment begins. The local treatment continued further with other agents for both groups of patients, depending on the wound type. In 32 patients with superficial burns, on which Dermazin was applied, the wounds were covered with "an abundant amount of fester-like exudate", which created an impression of worsened local status (Figure 29). The bacteriological analysis showed that in most of the cases this exudate was sterile and was caused by the mixing of the wound exudate and the agent. Forming of "pseudonecrosis", which was difficult and painful to remove, was observed (Figure 30). For this reason, the dressing change required general anaesthesia even in burns with small area. Moist and soft necroses with grey metallic colour, which were irremovable, were observed in deep-dermal and deep burn wounds (Tonkin & Wood, 2005). In patients who did not undergo operations, these necroses were slowly and tangentially detached in due course. In case of local infection, the dressings were wet at the time of dressing change due to the abundant amount of exudates, while swelling, reddening, firm wound edges and smell were observed.

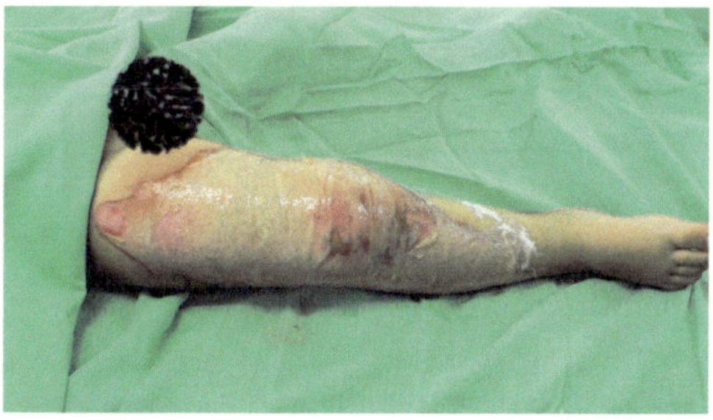

Fig. 29. Clinical state of a wound treated with Dermazin

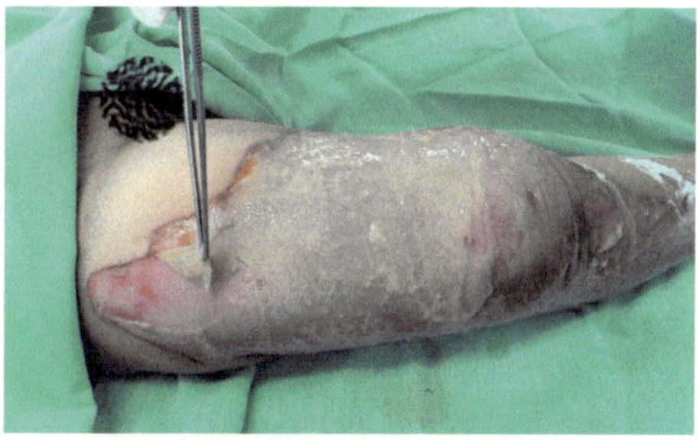

Fig. 30. Formed "pseudonecrosis" after the treatment with Dermazin

3.3 Bacteriological analysis

Acticoat is a dressing with a silver coating and unique physical structure of silver nanocrystalline, which in a moist environment provides a long-lasting and steady release of free silver ions and radicals on the surface of a burn wound. Although **Acticoat** releases 30 times less silver than 0.5 per cent solution of silver nitrate ($AgNO3$) and SSD, it has a much quicker and more powerful antibacterial effect. It is an effective agent against Gram-positive and Gram-negative microorganisms, including aerobic and facultative anaerobic organisms and fungi. It is effective against all pathogenic microorganisms isolated from burn wounds, especially Pseudomonas aeroginosa, Staphylococcus aureus - MRSA and VRE (Tredget et al., 1998). Its antiseptic effect is revealed within 30 minutes of the application and lasts up to 3 days (Wright et al., 1999). The Minimum Inhibitory Concentration (MIC) and the Minimum Bactericidal Concentration (MBC) of the three silver dressings (Acticoat, AgNO3 and SSD) have been spectrophotometrically studied, determined and compared using five bacterial strains, which are of clinical interest (Demling & DeSanti, 2002). **Acticoat** has the lowest MIC and MBC in comparison with the other two silver dressings. Due to these laboratory proven results, a preliminary in vitro analysis has not been carried out. The investigation of the results from the bacteriological analysis after the **Acticoat** application indicates that (Figures 31-35):

- The wounds of 96 children (86%) were without bacterial growth at the beginning of the treatment with **Acticoat** and remained unchanged in 95 children until the end of the treatment.
- A Gram-positive and Gram-negative flora was isolated in 16 children at the beginning of the treatment (5 with Staph.aureus-MRSA, 2 with Str.ß haemoliticus and 6 with Staph.epidermidis).
- In one child with uncontaminated wound at the beginning of the treatment, the wound became colonized by Ps. aeroginosa (microbial number was below the critical value of 10^3, 10^2) during the treatment course.
- Bacterial growth was not observed in 109 children (97%) at the end of the treatment. Contaminated wounds of two children at the beginning of the treatment remained unchanged even after the third dressing, but the microbial number was below the critical values (1 child with Ps. aeroginosa 10^3 and 1 child with Staph.aureus-MRSA 10^2).

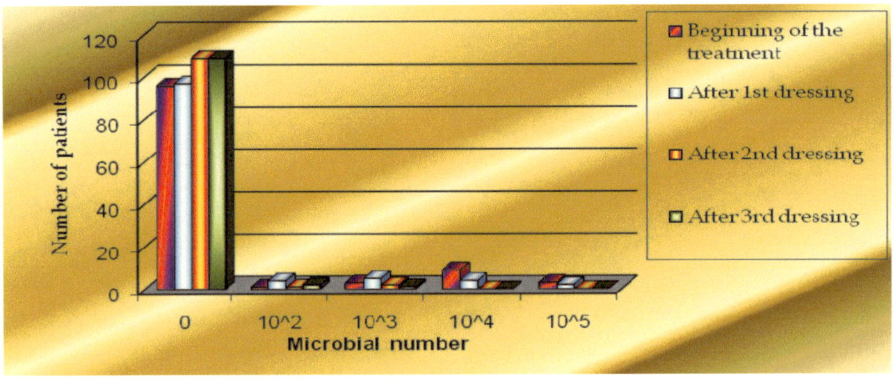

Fig. 31. Bacterial growth distribution during the treatment with Acticoat

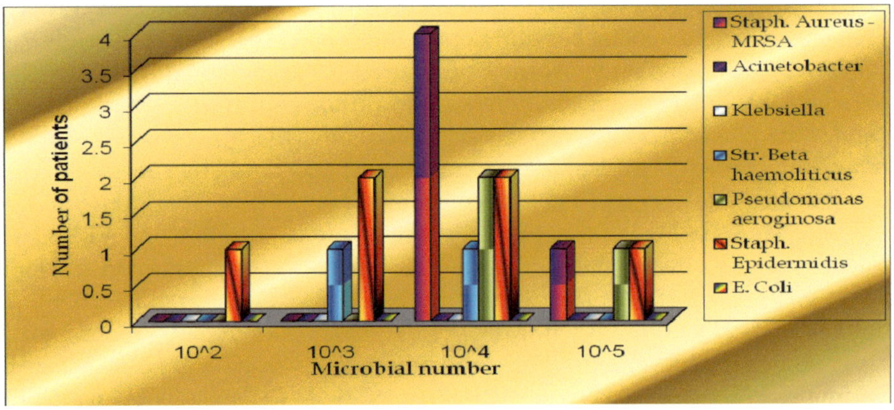

Fig. 32. Distribution of the bacteria and bacterial growth at the beginning of the treatment with Acticoat

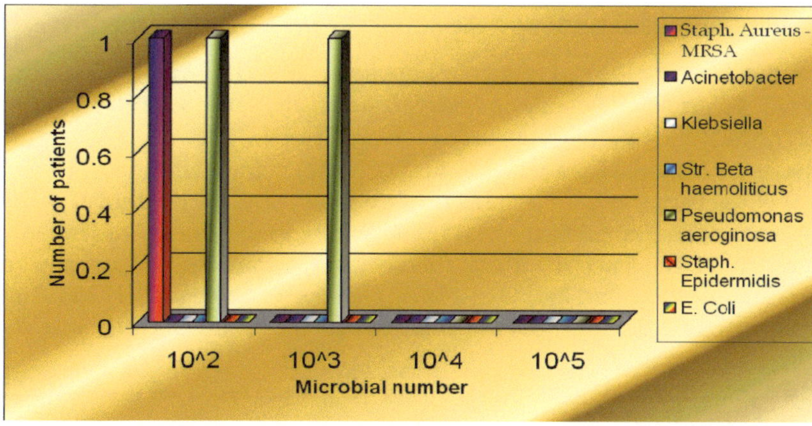

Fig. 33. Distribution of the bacteria and bacterial growth at the end of the treatment with Acticoat

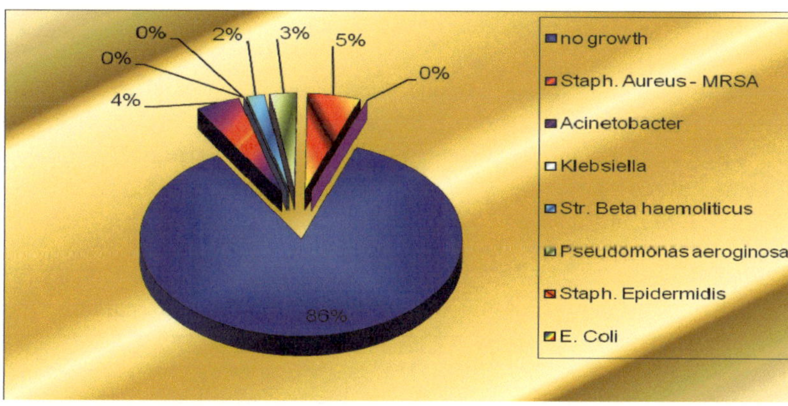

Fig. 34. Distribution of the bacteria at the beginning of the treatment with Acticoat

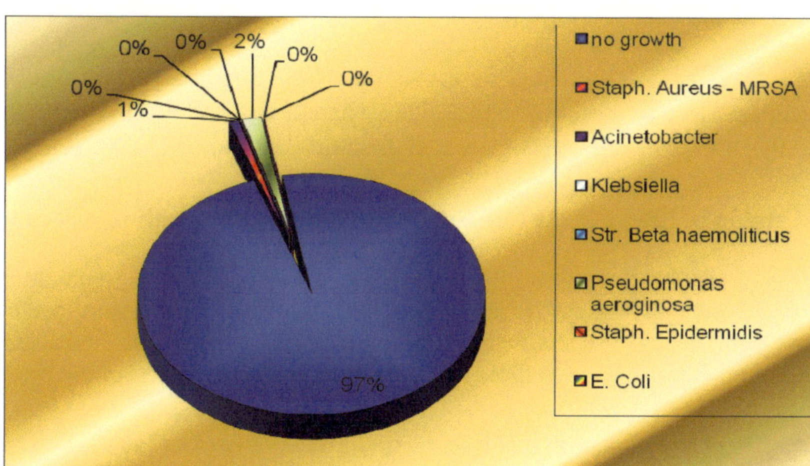

Fig. 35. Distribution of the bacteria at the end of the treatment with Acticoat

4. Comparative analysis between Acticoat™ and SSD (Dermazin)

4.1 Comparative bacteriological analysis between Acticoat™ and SSD (Dermazin)

A comparative bacteriological analysis between **Acticoat™** and **SSD** (**Dermazin**) has been carried out. The following parameters have been monitored:

- The type of the bacterial flora (wound surface swab) before the **Acticoat™** application;
- The type of the bacterial flora (wound surface swab) after each removal of the dressing. The dressings were changed every 3 days according to the already described way;
- The quantity of the bacterial flora (tissue biopsy samples) in gram wound tissue (microbial number), before and after the application of the agent. The critical value for development of a local and general infection of the wound is 10^5 bacteria per gram tissue (b/gr).

The performed prospective clinical study comprised 111 patients – 68 (61.26%) of them were treated with Acticoat™ and 43 (38.74%) with Dermazin. The gender distribution is: 67 males (60.36%) and 44 females (39.64%). The average age of these children was 4.78±4.38 years in the age range of 9 months – 18 years. The total number of the burns was 265: 151 (56.98%) of which were treated with Acticoat™ and 114 (43.02%) with Dermazin.

4.1.1 Results

It could be seen from Tables 1 and 2 that the patients included in the sample do not statistically differ with respect to age, burn area and burn depth. The further analysis shows that there is no significant difference of gender distribution. The initial similarity of the main confounding factors gives a good basis for the comparison of the outcome obtained from the treatments with the two agents.

Parameter	Treated with Acticoat™			Treated with Dermazin			p
	N	$\overline{X}$	SD	N	$\overline{X}$	SD	
Age	66	4.65	4.11	43	4.97	4.80	n.s.
Burn area	68	7.65	5.95	43	9.95	7.84	n.s.

Table 1. Comparative analysis of the age and burn area of the patients treated with the studied agents ($\overline{X}$ - mean value, SD- standard deviation, N- number, n.s. – not significant)

4.1.2 Initial status of the patients treated with the two agents with respect to bacterial flora

It is clear from Table 3 that bacterial flora is registered in 17.65% of the patients treated with **Acticoat™** and in 13.95% of those treated with **Dermazin**. The Fisher's exact test classifies the difference with respect to this parameter as non-significant. The ratio of the bacterial findings deep in the wound was identical to those on the surface at the beginning of the treatment.

4.1.3 The status of the bacterial flora on 4th day after the first dressing

The technology of treatment with the two agents allows comparison of impact only on the 4th day after the first dressing. The bacterial flora decreased from 17.65% at the beginning of

Degree	Statistics	Agent		Total
		Acticoat™	Dermazin	
II A	Number	54	38	92
	% w.r. degree	58.70	41.30	100.00
	% w.r. agent	40.91	43.18	41.82
II B	Number	62	40	102
	% w.r. degree	60.78	39.22	100.00
	% w.r. agent	46.97	45.45	46.36
III	Number	16	10	26
	% w.r. degree	61.54	38.46	100.00
	% w.r. agent	12.12	11.36	11.82
Total	Number	132	88	220
	% w.r. degree	60.00	40.00	100.00
	% w.r. agent	100.00	100.00	100.00

Table 2. The sample participants distribution with respect to the burn degree and agent (w.r. - with respect to)

Bacterial flora on the surface	**Statistics**	**Agent**		**Total**
		Acticoat™	**Dermazin**	
Absence	Number	56	37	93
	% w.r. flora	60.22	39.78	100.00
	% w.r. agent	82.35	86.05	83.78
Presence	Number	12	6	18
	% w.r. flora	66.67	33.33	100.00
	% w.r. agent	17.65	13.95	16.22
Total	Number	68	43	111
	% w.r. flora	61.26	38.74	100.00
	% w.r. agent	100.00	100.00	100.00

Table 3. The sample participants distribution with respect to the agent and existence of bacterial flora (w.r. - with respect to)

the treatment up to 16.18% on the 4th day for **Acticoat™**, while an increase from 13.95 up to 25.58% was observed in the patients treated with **Dermazin**. The change is significant, but it is in favour of the treatment with **Acticoat™**. On the 4th day of the treatment the ratio of the bacterial findings deep in the wound was completely identical to that on the surface. The dynamics of the change of the bacterial findings for the two agents on the 1st and 4th (Figure 36).

The dynamics of the change of the bacterial flora on the surface, treated with the two agents, showed that from 4 bacterial findings of Staph.aureus - MRSA at the beginning of the treatment with Acticoat™ only one was isolated on the 12th day, whereas from 3 bacterial findings of Pseudomonas aeroginosa two were present, while the other initial bacterial findings were killed.

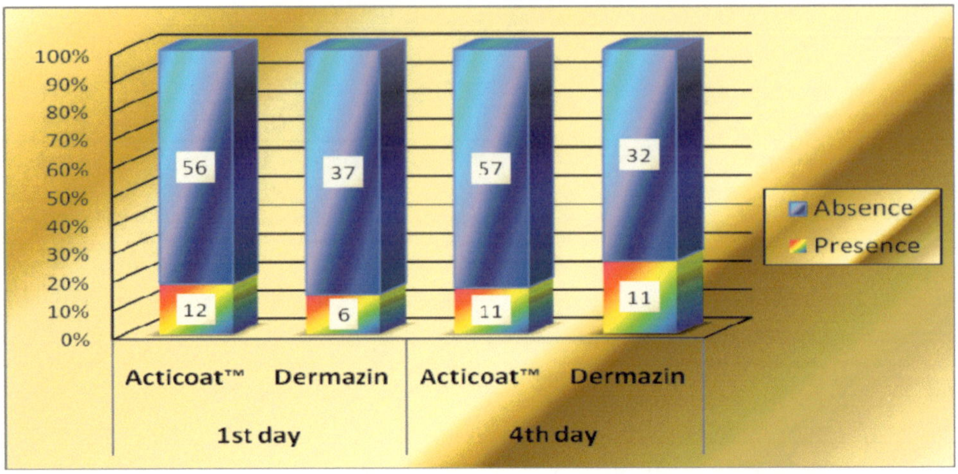

Fig. 36. The dynamics of the bacteria change for the two agents on the 1st and 4th day

In the treatment with Dermazin, an increase in the present bacterial findings or appearance of new ones in the course of treatment up to the 4th day were observed. This is most pronounced for Acinetobacter and Pseudomonas aeroginosa with respect to quantity. There was a decrease in Staph.aureus - MRSA from 5 to 3 findings and complete clearing of Str.beta haemoliticus (from 1 to 0), but the sterility as a whole aggravated for this agent on the 4th day (Figures 37-39).

The results of the deep analysis of the bacterial flora also showed the advantages of the treatment with Acticoat™ (Figures 40-42). The patients treated with Acticoat™ have worse bacteriological status in the beginning and significantly better dynamics on the 4th day of the treatment, while a worsening of the sterility in the deepness is observed for the patients treated with Dermazin. In one patient treated with Acticoat™, bacterial flora was observed only on the surface, but not in the deepness on the 8th and 12th day.

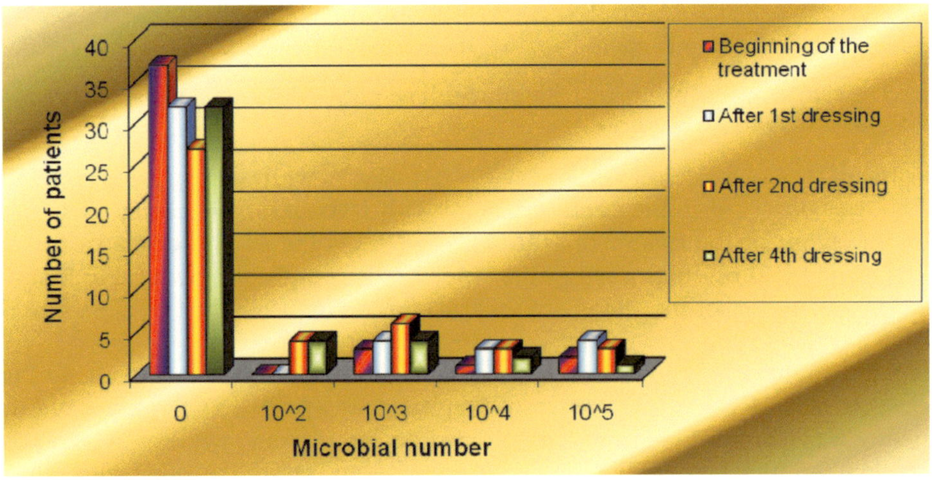

Fig. 37. Bacterial growth distribution during the treatment with Dermazin

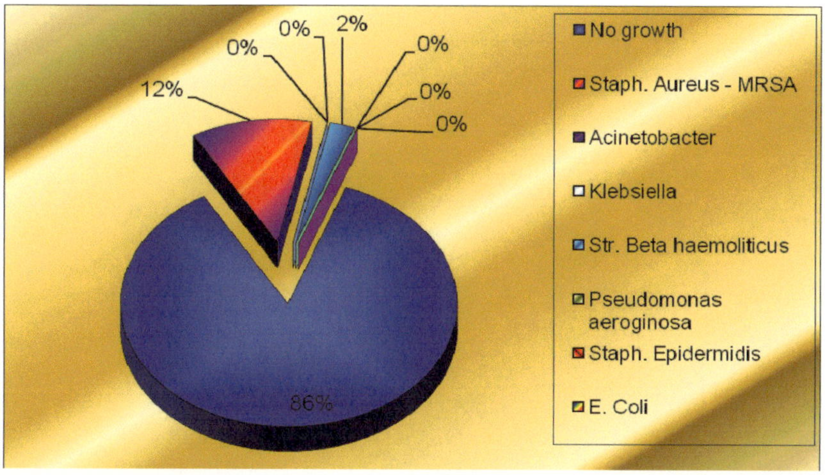

Fig. 38. Distribution of the bacteria at the beginning of the treatment with Dermazin

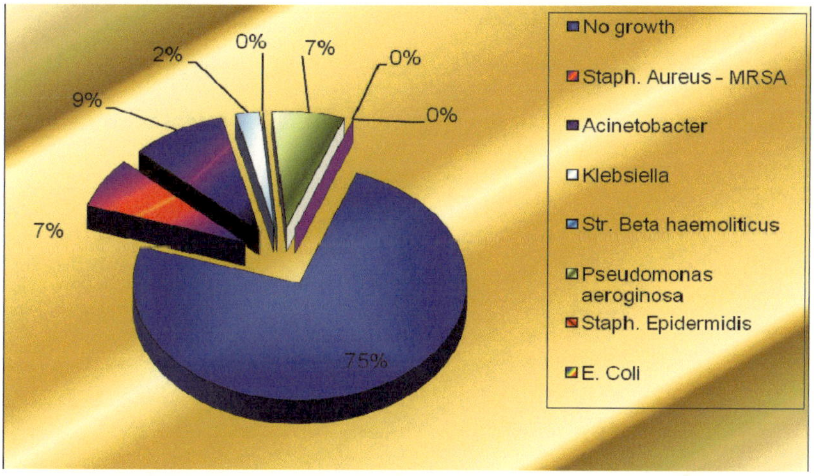

Fig. 39. Distribution of the bacteria at the end of the treatment with Dermazin

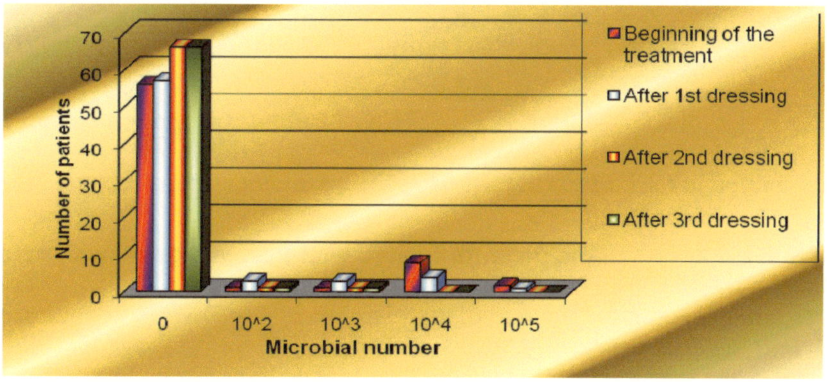

Fig. 40. Bacterial growth distribution during the treatment with Acticoat

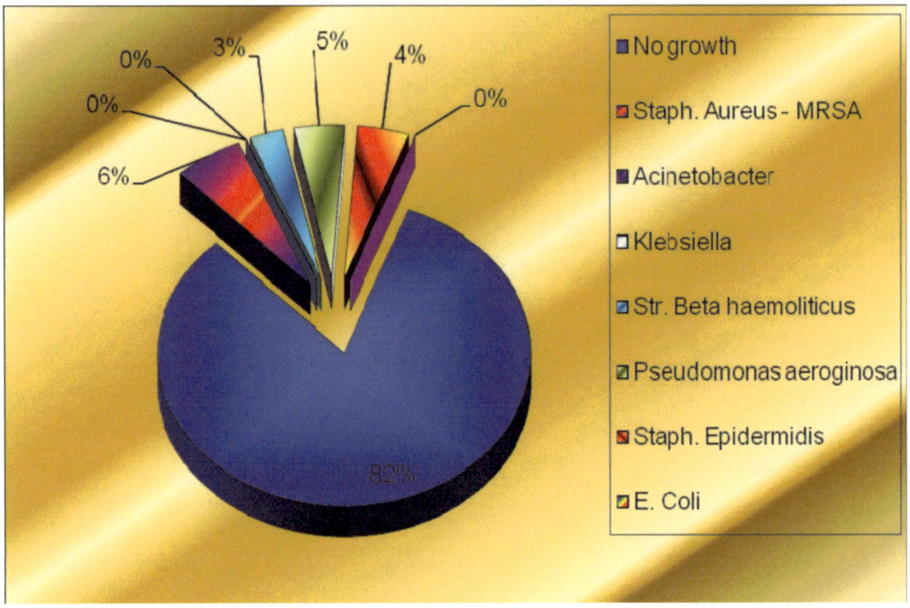

Fig. 41. Distribution of the bacteria at the beginning of the treatment with Acticoat

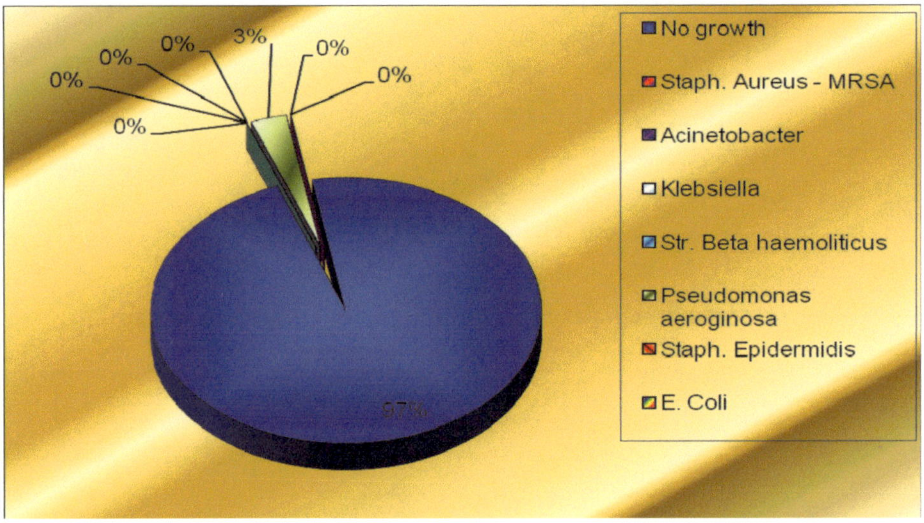

Fig. 42. Distribution of the bacteria at the end of the treatment with Acticoat

4.2 Comparative analysis of the patients treated with the two agents with respect to clearing time, epithelization and hospital stay

The results unambiguously illustrated that Acticoat™ possesses significantly better therapeutic effect in comparison with Dermazin (Figures 43-56; Table 4). It was clear that the burns treated with Acticoat™ had significantly shorter clearing/ epithelization time and hospital stay (Table 4).

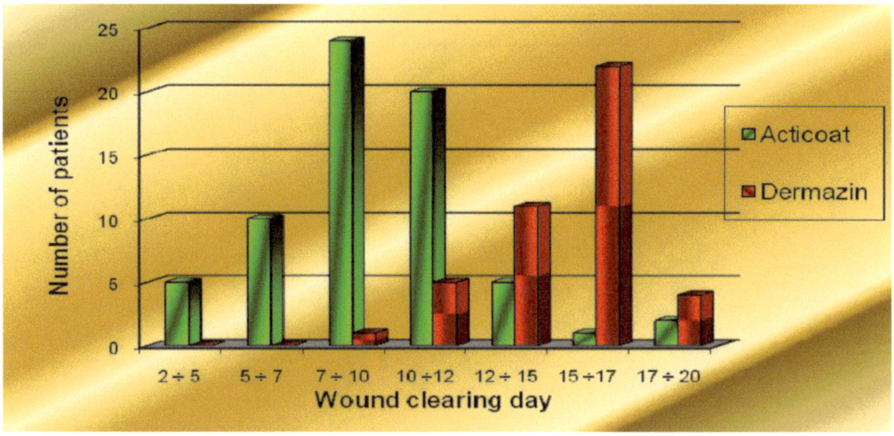

Fig. 43. Distribution of the wound clearing time

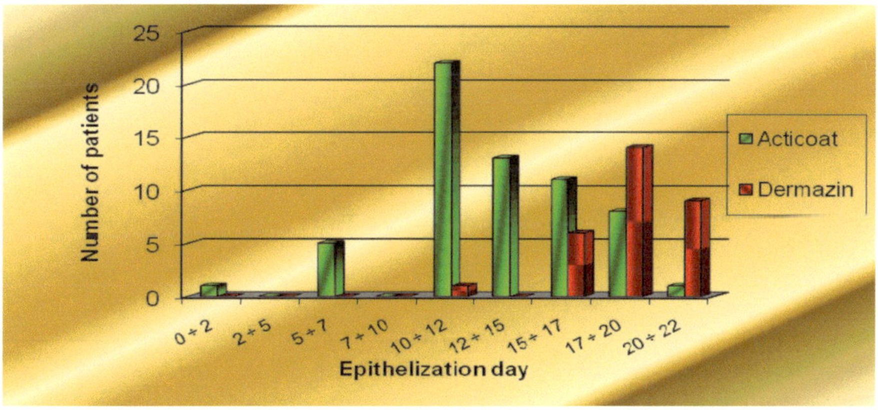

Fig. 44. Distribution of the wound epithelization time

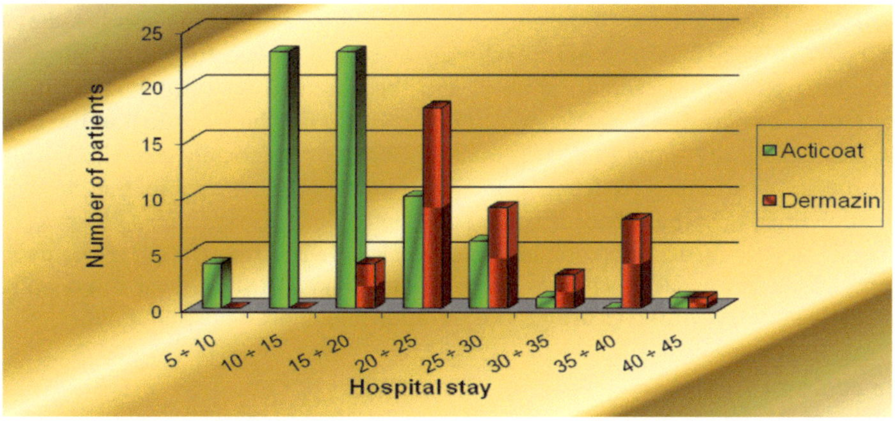

Fig. 45. Distribution of the hospital stay

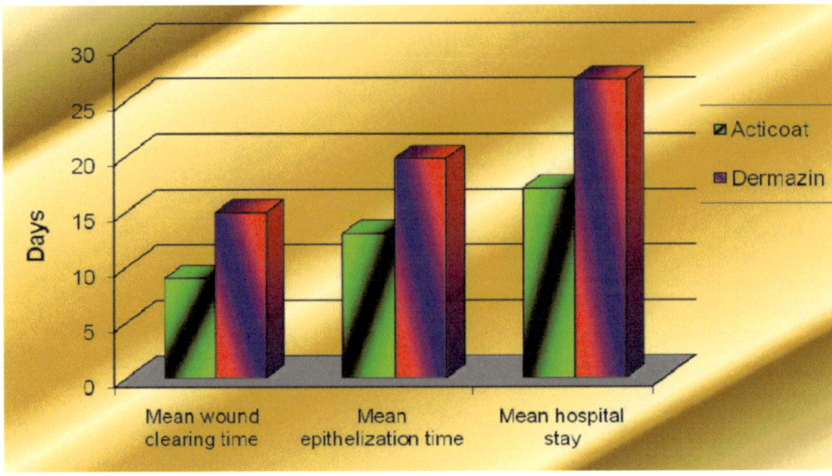

Fig. 46. Mean wound clearing time, mean epithelization time and mean hospital stay

Parameter	Treated with Acticoat™			Treated with Dermazin			p
	N	$\overline{X}$	SD	N	$\overline{X}$	SD	
Clearing day	66	8.92	3.16	43	14.93	2.20	<0.001
Epithelization time (days)	60	12.98	4.02	39	19.79	3.02	<0.001
Hospital stay (days)	66	16.95	6.19	42	26.90	6.91	<0.001

Table 4. Comparative analysis of the patients treated with the studied agents with respect to clearing time, epithelization time and hospital stay

The performed comparative statistical analysis (t-test) reveals that the differences of application of **Acticoat™** and **Dermazin** were statistically significant. The obtained p-value for the three tests (comparison of the clearing time, epithelization time and hospital stay for the two agents) was $p<0.01$. The Mann-Whitney test was applied for the statistical analysis of the bacterial growth (microbial number) and the obtained value ($p=<0.01$) implied that the difference of application of **Acticoat™** and **Dermazin** for the treatment of the monitored patients was statistically significant. This analysis showed statistically significant differences between the application of **Acticoat™** and **Dermazin** with respect to the clearing time, epithelization time, hospital stay and microbial growth.
The comparative clinical and microbiological analysis between the two silver agents revealed that treatment with **Acticoat™** achieves better efficacy in killing superficial and deep bacterial flora and yielded faster wound clearing, epithelization and shorter hospital stay.

4.3 Side effects

Three children of the observed contingent treated with **Acticoat™** developed rash, which was transient and faded quickly. The most probable reason for the rash was due to the occlusive effect of the dressing caused by the polyurethane foil. Toxic effects were not observed. The hyperpigmentation of the intact skin was transient and disappeared within 14 days after the end of the treatment or dressing change. In the children of the control group with **Dermazin** no toxic and allergic reactions were observed. Cases of argyria were not observed.

4.4 Comparative cost analysis between Acticoat™ and SSD (Dermazin)

The comparative cost analysis was based on the treatment of a burn wound of second degree (IIAB) with 2000 cm^2 area. One surgeon, one anaesthesiologist, one surgical nurse, one anaesthetic nurse and one hospital attendant were involved for application of both agents. Table 5 shows the cost comparison of both agents.

	Acticoat™	**Dermazin**
Labour cost per dressing (L)	€ 13.36	€ 13.36
Materials per dressing (M)	€ 311.65	€ 93.60
Total Cost per dressing (L+M)	**€ 325.01**	**€ 106.96**
Dressing numbers (n)	4	20
Total (Euros) - (L+M)*n	**€ 1300.04**	**€ 2139.20**

Table 5. Comparative cost (in Euros) analysis of the treatment of a burn (2000 sm^2) of second (IIAB) degree for both agents

The cost comparative analysis demonstrated that the treatment of a second degree (IIAB) burn wound (2000 cm^2 area) with Dermazin was more expensive by approximately € 839 (65% more expensive) than the treatment with Acticoat.

5. Discussion

General concepts and techniques for treatment of all wounds are applied regardless of the mechanism causing the wound. The key to high quality and proper local treatment is the correct and complete assessment of the burn wound. This includes etiology, localization, area (cm^2), depth, exudation (quantity, type, colour), smell, appearance of the wound surface, appearance of the intact skin, presence of pain, and prior treatment method. The treatment goals are determined on the basis of proper assessment preceding the treatment. The burn wound changes dynamically depending on inner (release inflammatory mediators, bacterial proliferation) and outer (dehydration, hypotension and cooling) factors. Thus, the applied local agent is subjected to permanent control (both objective and subjective). The perfect dressing for children should provide optimal protection, reparation and minimization of the pain (Khundkar et al. 2010).

Silver-impregnated Acticoat™ dressing has been used in the Clinic of Burns at the "Pirogov" Emergency Hospital since 2004 and has gradually prevailed as the standard dressing in the treatment of burn wounds and post-traumatic defects. The clinical studies, conducted in the Clinic of Burns in Children in the second half of 2009 and 2010, demonstrate the advantages of topical treatment with nanocrystalline silver and was concluded that the agent was efficient in all cases and was easily tolerated. The less frequent and atraumatic dressing changes make this agent a preferable one for children. The clinical observations of the use of Acticoat ™ and the comparative analysis with Dermazin show that the time of dressing changes is reduced by 50%, since the dressing change is every 3rd day, in contrast to the Dermazin dressing, which has to be changed every 12 hours. This yields a reduced use of sedative and narcotic agents applied in dressings as well as less stress in dressing change, respectively (Probert & Burston, 2005).

Prior to the development of this type of dressing, it was considered that moist environment contributes to increased risk of infection. The clinical observations of many authors (Ang et al., 2003; Fong & Wood, 2006; Wright, et al. 2002) as well as our own studies reject such concern. Dermazin and other types of SSD extract water from the wound surface as a result of the cream hyperosmolarity, which requires frequent change. All the advantages, which the moist environment has for the healing process, pose the question of maintaining the moisture (Fong, 2005). The moistening of Acticoat has double effect - to maintain the moist environment in the wound and to release the antimicrobial power of nanocrystalline silver. The results (clinical and bacteriological) of polyethylene foil application, as an instrument for moisture maintaining, are very good. Everyday moistening by irrigation or change of the upper gauze layers is unpractical and more difficult to control. Use of Intrasite gel and Allevyn is expensive and economically disadvantageous, therefore, semi-occlusive dressings are utilized. Each modern dressing should possess the property of moisture transmission and control. The complete occlusion may create an environment for the development of facultative pathogenic microorganisms, causing infection. For this reason, the Moisture Vapour Transmission Rate (MVTR) is an important parameter for each modern dressing. A value of MVTR = 600-3000 for the polyethylene foil is determined, and a complete occlusion occurs at value <500. Excellent moisture maintaining until the next dressing change was observed in the monitored clinical contingent and maceration was not observed. The typical imbibition was temporal and disappeared immediately after the change of the dressing type or after the treatment was discontinued. In cases of infected wounds with abundant exudation, an additional moistening is not necessary because the dressing has absorption property when it comes in contact with the wound exudates.

The clinical observations on the contingent studied confirm these properties of Acticoat. The comparative study carried out in the clinic shows that the mean time for the wound clearing is 8.92 days for Acticoat, whereas for Dermazin it is longer - 14.93 days. Correspondingly, the epithelization time is shorter for Acticoat (mean =12.98 days), while for Dermazin the mean epithelization time is 19.79 days. This parameter is particularly essential in the treatment of second-degree (IIA and IIB) burns, which epidemically have the highest incidence rate, and in the treatment of the so-called "mixed burns", in which the epidermis is completely damaged while the dermis is damaged at various levels of thickness. Contrary to deep burns, mixed burns have the capacity of spontaneous healing in case of proper treatment. The incidence rate of these burns (having in mind a total damaged body area) is high, although it has not specially been reported in the literature. While the treatment method for the first- and third-degree burns is clearly determined, the algorithm for this type of superficial burns is a dilemma (Storm-Versloot et al., 2010). In this case, the active surgical behaviour has some disadvantages, since there are not exact demarcations of the areas, which will epithelize in time and those which will not close non-operatively. Good and fast epithelization of these border burns is very important in widespread burns with vast areas of deep burn, where the shortened epithelization time contributes to the quicker decrease in the total burn area and to the increase in the area of possible donor sites (Wright et al., 2002). The shortened wound epithelization time diminishes the risk of development of bacteraemia and septic condition, which are a major cause of death in burns. Thus, the necessity of antibiotic therapy is reduced (Tonkin & Wood, 2005). Earlier wound clearing and closing diminishes the risk of development of hypertrophic scars and joint contractures on the one hand, and contributes to the child's faster recovery, on the other. An optimum microenvironment and absence of cytotoxic factors are essential for the phase of epithelization of the wound healing process. In-vitro studies show that Acticoat is toxic to both keratinocytes and fibroblasts, suppressing proliferation at the same time (Andrew et al., 2005; Burd et al., 2007; Paddle-Ledinek et al., 2006). The monitored patients' clinical results do not demonstrate such an in-vitro effect. This is confirmed by other in vivo studies. Apart from burn wounds, the anti-inflammatory, antibacterial and epithelotonic effect of the dressing is utilized in wounds covered with fresh autografts and donor sites (Demling & DeSanti, 2002; Olson et al., 2000; Silver, 2007). A faster stabilization and re- epithelization in comparison with other types of antiseptic and epithelotonic dressings was observed. Well-healed autografts and epithelization of the mesh splits (95%), in case of Acticoat application on 5 children with fresh autografts, was observed after the removing of the first dressing. In application on donor sites (5 children) almost full epithelization (96%) was detected in one child, and in the remaining 4 children full epithelization was observed on the 8th day. The donor sites were monitored up to six months and no signs of hypertrophic scarring appeared.

The bacteriological observations demonstrate the powerful antibacterial effect of Acticoat. The rate and degree of killing of microbes is higher than those of the other silver agents used so far, which is due to the specific physical-chemical structure (Dunn & Edwards-Jones, 2004). After 30 minutes, nanocrystalline silver reduces the number of viable bacteria to very low levels, while the other dressings achieve this effect after 2 hours (Wright et al., 1999; Yin, 2003; Burrell, 2003; Heggers et al., 2005; Lansdown, 2006). Pure silver ions and radicals have been shown to provide protection against a broad spectrum of bacteria (more than 150 types), viruses and fungi and especially antibiotic-resistant bacteria. This effect is prolonged and lasts up to 3 days after the dressing application. Acticoat has preventive antibacterial function, too. Applied on wounds, which have no bacterial growth, it prevents contamination. The dressing reduces the risk of wound contamination, being a highly efficient agent for the prevention of general bacterial infection, especially in widespread burns (Singh et al., 2007; Nadworny et al, 2010). This is confirmed by the microbiological studies carried out (Hadjiiski & Argirova, 2008). Wounds without bacterial growth at the beginning of the treatment remained uncontaminated until the end of the treatment, and only in one child local infection (below the critical values) was observed during the treatment course. From the initially contaminated wounds (in 16 children), bacterial flora with non-significant quantitative values was isolated only in 3 children at the end of the treatment. Wherever a local infection was isolated, regardless of its type, the microbial numbers remained below the critical values and signs of general infection were not observed (Figures 31-35). The antimicrobial preventive activity described is essential for the successful surgical treatment of widespread and deep burns. The bacterial monitoring of the children to whom Acticoat was applied on excised sites, autografts and donor sites (total - 15) showed a negative bacterial growth. The results of the microbiological analysis are assessed as very good in 97%, good in 2% and unsatisfactory in 1% of the cases. The use of Acticoat does not lead to the development of resistant bacterial strains. The distinct agent action -superficial and in depth - against Ps.aeroginosa and St.aureus MRSA, which is demonstrated by the obtained results, make the dressing preferable for burn wounds (Chae et al., 2010). Thus, the need of antibiotic therapy is reduced, leading to a decreased risk of the development of multi-resistant strains. A fungal infection was not isolated in the studied children. The Acticoat™ low adherent property allows a less painful dressing change, which makes it a preferable dressing for children (Tancheva, 2008). The long-lasting activity of the dressing reduces the total number of dressing changes. This yields better comfort, mobility and ability of the patients to participate in rehabilitation programmes. In the analysis of silver serum concentrations, haematological and biochemical parameters of the patients of the studied clinical contingent, treated with nanocrystalline silver, no indication for toxicity was observed (Moiemen et al., 2011; White, 2010). Due to lack of toxic effect, it is suitable for application even on very young children, unlike Dermazin (Rustogi et al., 2005). Side effects were not observed in the youngest patient, who was 9 months old. Silver is deposited mostly in the skin, oral mucosa, gums, kidneys, liver and cornea. Excretion is done mostly by biliary way. Monitoring of the plasma levels is recommended in burns over 10% and burns of second (IIB) and third (III) degree, and especially in patients with abnormal liver and kidney function (Landsdown, 2006).

6. Conclusion

The obtained clinical results, microbiologically and statistically verified, as well as the conducted comparative study between Acticoat and Dermazin, provide reasons to consider the Acticoat silver dressing as highly efficient for application in superficial burns of second (IIA and IIB) degree, pre-surgical treatment of patients, prophylaxis and treatment of infection in burns, treatment of donor sites, excised sites and autografts.

The presented properties of Acticoat allow us to define it as one of the leading agents for local treatment of burns. During the short time of its use in our clinic, it has been recognized as a preferable agent for wound treatment. The ease of use, powerful antibacterial effect, lower frequency of dressing change, variety of sizes, good moulding, shortened time of wound clearing and epithelization, and painless dressing change are the advantages of Acticoat™ over the other silver agents used so far. Acticoat™ is significantly more cost effective than the other frequently used agent Dermazin.

7. References

Andrew, P. et al. (2005). Evaluation of Cytotoxicity and Antimicrobial Activity of Acticoat® Burn Dressing for Management of Microbial Contamination in Cultured Skin Substitutes Grafted to Athymic Mice, *J Burn Care Rehabil*, 26, pp.238–246

Ang, E. et al. (2003). Pain Control in a Randomized, Controlled, Clinical Trial Comparing Moist Exposed Burn Ointment and Conventional Methods in Patients with Partial-Thickness Burns, *J Burn Care Rehabil*, 2003, Sep-Oct; 24(5), pp.289-96

Atiyeh, B.S.; Dibo, S.A. & Hayek, S.N. (2009). Wound Cleansing, Topical Antiseptics and Wound Healing, *International Wound Journal*, 6(6), pp.420-430

Burd, A. et al. (2007). A comparative Study of the Cytotoxicity of Silver-based Dressings in Monolayer Cell, Tissue Explant, and Animal Models, *Wound Repair Regen.*; 15(1), pp. 94-104

Burrell, R.E. (2003). A Scientific Perspective on the Use of Topical Silver Preparations. *Ostomy Wound Manage*, 49 (Suppl.): 19

Burrell, R.E.; Wright, J.B.; Heggers, J.P. & Davis,G.J. (1999). Efficacy of silver coated dressings as barriers in a rodent burn sepsis model. *Wounds*,11(4), pp.64-71

Cavanagh, M.H.; Burrell, R.E. & Nadworny, P.L. (2010). Evaluating Antimicrobial Efficacy of New Commercially Available Silver Dressings. *International Wound Journal*, Oct., 7(5), pp.394-405

Chae, J. et al. (2010). Comparison of the Efficacies of Silver-containing Dressing Materials for Treating a Full-thickness Rodent Wound Infected by Methicillin-resistant Staphylococcus Aureus: P1563, *Clinical Microbiology & Infection*, 16 Sup 2:S454, April 2010

Cuttle, L. et al. (2007). A Retrospective Cohort Study of Acticoat™ versus Silvazine™ in a Paediatric Population, *Burns*, Sep. 2007, 33 (6), pp.701-7

Demling, R.H. & De Santi, L.(2001). Effects of Silver on Wound Management, *Wounds*, 13 (Supp A), pp.5-15

Demling, R.H. & De Santi, L.(2002). The Rate of Re-epithelialization Across Meshed Skin Grafts is Increased With Exposure to Silver, *Burns*, 28(3), pp.264-6

Dunn, K. & Edwards-Jones, V. (2004). The Role of Acticoat™ with Nanocrystalline Silver in the Management of Burns, *Burns*, 30, Suppl. 1, SILS9, pp. S1-S9

Fong, J.; Wood, F. & Fowler, B. (2005). A Silver Coated Dressing Reduces the Incidence of Early Burn Wound Cellulites and Associated Costs of Inpatient Treatment: Comparative Patient Care Audits, *Burns*, 31, pp.562-567

Fong, J. & Wood, F. (2006). Nanocrystalline Silver Dressing in Wound Management: A Review, *International Journal of Nanomedicine*, 1(4), pp.441-449

Fong, J. (2005). The Use of Silver Products in the Management of Burn Wounds: Change in Practice for the Burn unit at Royal Perth Hospital, *Primary Intention*, 13(4), pp. S16-S22

Gravante, G. et al. (2009). Nanocrystalline Silver: A Systematic Review of Randomized Trials Conducted on Burned Patients and an Evidence-Based Assessment of Potential Advantages Over Older Silver Formulations, *Annals of Plastic Surgery*, 63(2), pp.201-205, August 2009

Hadjiiski, O. & Argirova, M. (2008). Antiseptic agents containing silver components, *Handbook on Surgery with Atlas*, Vol. VII - Burns and Frostbite (Hadjijski O. Editor), pp. 86-97 (in Bulgarian)

Heggers, J. et al. (2005). Therapeutic Efficacy of Three Silver Dressings in an Infected Animal Model, *J Burn Care Rehabil*,.26, pp. 53–56

Huang, Y. et al. (2007). A Randomized Comparative Trial between Acticoat and SD-Ag in the Treatment of Residual Burn Wounds, Including Safety Analysis, *Burns*, Vol. 33 (2), pp.161-166

Khundkar, R.; Malic, C. & Burge, T. (2010). Use of Acticoat Dressings in Burns: What Is the Evidence? *Burns*, 36(6), pp.751-8

Klasen, H. (2000). A Historical Review of the Use of Silver in the Treatment of Burns. II. Renewed Interest for Silver, *Burns*, 26, pp.131-138

Landsdown, A.B. (2006). Silver In Health Care: Antimicrobial Effects and Safety in Use, *Curr. Probl. Dermatol*, 33, pp.17-34

Leaper, D.J. (2006). Silver Dressings: Their Role in Wound Management, *Int Wound J.*, 2006, 3, pp.282-294

Moiemen, N.S. et al. (2011). Acticoat Dressings and Major Burns: Systemic Silver Absorption, *Burns*, 37 (1), pp.27-35

Nadworny, P.L. et al. (2010). Does Nanocrystalline Silver Have a Transferable Effect?, *Wound Repair Regen.*, 18(2), pp.254-65

Olson, M.E. et al. (2000). Healing of Porcine Donor Sites Covered With Silver-coated Dressings, *Eur. J. Surg*, 166(6), pp. 486-9

Orvington, L. (2001). Nanocrystalline Silver: Where the Old And Familiar Meets a New Frontier, *Wounds*, 13(Suppl B), pp.5-10

Orvington, L. (2001). The Role of Silver Technology in Wound Healing: Part 2 Why Is Nanocrystalline Silver Superior?, *Wounds, A Compendium Clinical Research and Practice*, 13(2)(Suppl.B), pp.5-10

Paddle-Ledinek, J.E.; Nasa, Z. & Cleland, H.J. (2006). Effect of Different Wound Dressings on Cell Viability and Proliferation, *Plast Reconstr Surg*, 117(7 Suppl), pp.110S-118S, discussion 119S-120S.

Probert, R. & Burston, S. (2005). Wounds with a Silver Lining, *Primary Intention*, 13(4), pp. 10-S14

Rustogi, R. et al. (2005). The Use of Acticoat™ in Neonatal Burns, *Burns*, 31(7), pp.878-882

Singh, V. et al. (2007). The Pathogenesis of Burn Wound Conversion, *Annals of Plastic Surgery*, 59(1), pp.109-115

Silver, G.M. et al. (2007). A Silver-Coated Antimicrobial Barrier Dressing Used Postoperatively on Meshed Autografts: A Dressing Comparison Study, *J Burn Care Res*, 28, pp.715-719.

Storm-Versloot, M.N. et al. (2010). Topical Silver for Preventing Wound Infection, *Cochrane Database Syst Rev*, 17;(3), CD006478.

Tancheva, D. (2008). Burns and Frostbite, In: *Handbook on Surgery with Atlas*, Vol. VII - Burns and Frostbite (Hadjijski O. Editor), pp.222-231, "Prof. M. Drinov" Academic Publishing House (in Bulgarian)

Tonkin, C. & Wood, F. (2005). Nanocrystalline Silver Reduces the Need for Antibiotic Therapy in Burn Wounds, *Primary Intention*, 13(4), pp.163-168

Tredget, E. et al. (1998). A Matched-Pair, Randomised Study Evaluating the Efficacy and Safety of Acticoat Silvercoated Dressing for the Treatment of Burn Wounds, *J Burn Care Rehabil*, 19(6), pp.531-537

White, R. (2010). Silver-containing Dressings: Availability Concerns, *Ostomy Wound Manage*, 56(8), pp.6-8

Wright, J.B. et al. (2002). Early Healing Events in a Porcine Model of Contaminated Wounds: Effects of Nanocrystalline Silver on Matrix Metalloproteinases, Cell Apoptosis, and Healing, *Wound Repair Regen*, 10, pp.141-51

Wright, J.B. et al. (1999). Efficacy of Topical Silver Against Fungal Burn Wound Pathogens, *Am J Inf Cont*, 27, pp.344-50.

Wright, J.B.; Hansen, C.E. & Burrell, R.E. (1998). The Comparative Efficacy of Two Antimicrobial Barrier Dressings: In-vitro Examination of Two Controlled Release of Silver Dressings, *Wounds*, 10, pp.179-188

Yin, H.G. (2003). Antimicrobial Effects of Acticoat Nanocrystalline Silver-Coated Dressing, *John A. Boswick - Burn and Wound Care Symposium*, Maul, Hawaii, February 2003.

Yin, H.Q.; Langford, R. & Burrell, R.E. (1999). Comparative Evaluation of the Antimicrobial Activity of Acticoat Antimicrobial Barrier Dressing, *J. Burn Care & Rehabil*, 20, pp.195-200

18

How Does Human Amniotic Membrane Help Major Burn Patients Who Need Skin Grafting: New Experiences

Ali Akbar Mohammadi[1] and
Mohammad Kazem Mohammadi[2]
[1]*Associate Professor of Surgery, Shiraz Burn Research Center, Division of Plastic Surgery, Department of Surgery, Shiraz University of Medical Sciences, Shiraz*
[2]*Faculty of Science, Ahvaz Branch, Islamic Azad University, Ahvaz*
Iran

1. Introduction

Burns are among the most common traumas in developing countries, which consume large amounts of medical resources. It is important to find an appropriate material for dressing of burn wounds that improves healing and is readily available, easily applicable, and economical and also be protective from infection and desiccation, and facilitate healing. [1]
Most burn injuries happen in people with lower socio-economic class. Therefore, reducing the expenses of burn treatment is an important goal alongside healing as the primary aim. [2]
Amniotic membrane has been used since 1910 with variable success as a material for burn injury coverage. [3] It has the following advantages:

- readily available in sufficient quantity
- application not associated with immunological problems
- large size
- simple to prepare and sterilize
- no allergic reactions
- up to 15% reduction of water losses in wounds
- histological structure similar to that of skin [4,5]

The disadvantage of the use of amniotic membrane is that there is some risk of viral infection transmission, e.g. hepatitis, syphilis and AIDS. [4]. Two varieties of amniotic membrane are mainly used:

- in Toto (amnion + chorion) on deep burns
- amnion alone (epithelium + basal membrane) on superficial burns[3]

The amnion is a thin semi-transparent tissue forming the innermost layer of the fetal membrane. As fresh amnion carries contamination risk and disease transmission, amnion is collected from placentae of selected and screened donors. Various preservation methods have been introduced, including cryopreservation in liquid nitrogen, preservation in silver nitrate, storage in antibiotics solution, glycerol-preserved sheets, dried sheets and gamma-irradiated sheets. [6]

It has been claimed to be one of the most effective biological skin substitutes used in burn wounds, with efficiency of maintaining low bacterial counts. It also has advantages of reducing loss of protein, electrolytes and fluids, decreasing the risk of infection, minimizing pain, acceleration of wound healing and good handling properties. [6]

Amniotic membrane is readily available and does not present immunological problems and allergic responses. It also reduces water loss.

The risk of the transmission of some viral infections has to be taken into account. Bacterial examinations performed in 20 patients with burn wounds covered with amniotic membrane showed low or no bacterial colonization of the burn surface. It is concluded that amniotic membrane should be more widely used in this particular aspect of burn treatment. [4]

Human amniotic membrane has several interesting physiologic and histologic characteristics which are the basis of its increased use in burn patients. It also has a unique combination of properties, including the facilitation of migration of epithelial cells, reinforcement of basal cellular adhesion and encouragement of epithelium differentiation.

Amniotic membrane is able to modulate stromal scarring and has anti-inflammatory activity and is primarily used for covering partial thickness burns until complete healing [7].

Amnion is primarily used for covering partial-thickness burns until complete healing.

The most important features of amniotic membrane can be divided to 4 categories:

- Rapid adherence to the wound bed.
- Increased angiogenesis.
- Inhibition of protease activity and PMN infiltration.
- Rapid re-epithelialization and promotion of wound healing.

These characteristics has guided researchers to use this magic & cheep membrane as an adjunct to burn patients management and there are numerous researches on its benefits in acute burn wound management. We want to explain our new experiences in amniotic membrane administration on skin graft taking and also their early & late advantages & disadvantages in this group of burn patients .

2. Amniotic membrane as a skin graft fixator, and graft take accelerator to Increase overall graft take in non-complicated wounds

Amniotic membrane immediately adheres to the grafted areas & fixes skin graft to their bed, which eliminates suturing on extremities and diminishes the need for suturing on other body parts. It also eliminates painful suture removal, accelerates graft take and decreases traumatic graft loss induced by suture removal.

The revascularization of a skin graft depends on immobilization of the graft on the wound bed. In cases where circular dressings are needed, the graft may be displaced under the dressing, leading to partial graft loss and several methods of graft fixation have been described [7,8,9]. A common technique is to use stitches but this is time consuming and the stitches need to be removed after graft take. Placing surgical drapes over the graft is another method but these must be removed on the second or third day when the grafts are still not well vascularised, and this can lead to graft failure. Fixation with skin staples was introduced as a fast and reliable method for graft fixation; [11]however it is expensive and stressful for the patient as these staples must be removed which can be painful and frightening, particularly for children. Forgotten staples are another troublesome complication. [12] (Fig 1a ,b)

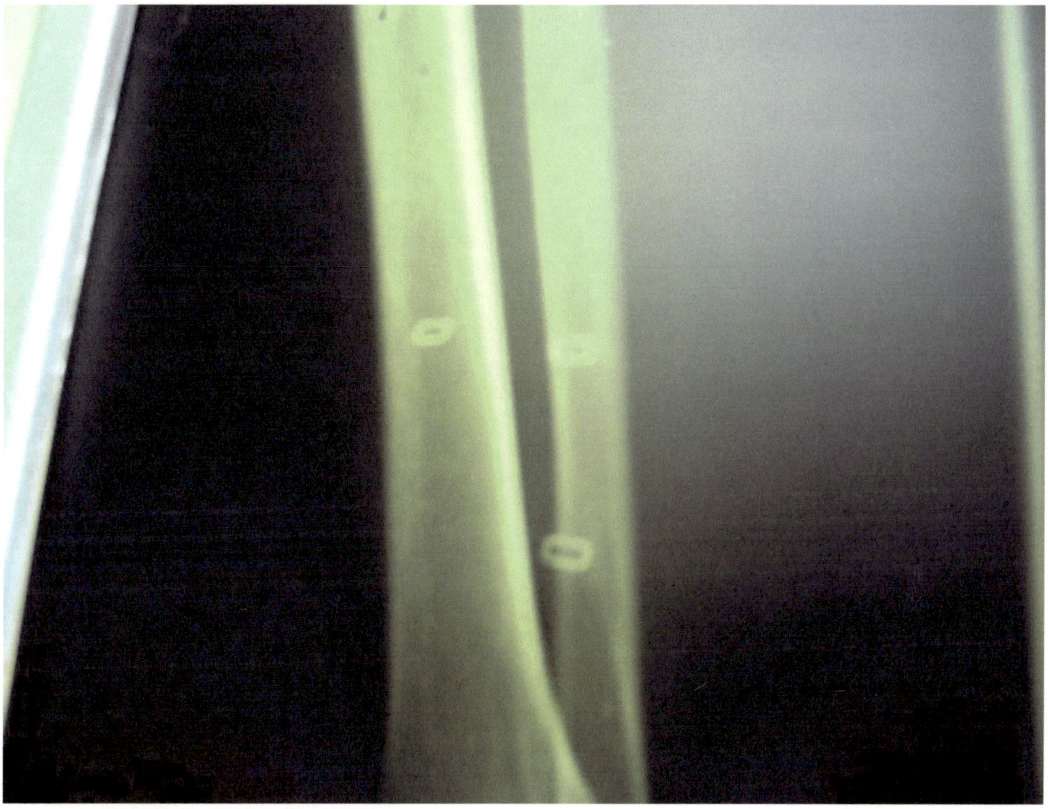

Fig. 1a. Incidental radiologic finding of multiple asymptomatic forgotten staples

Another technique uses steri-strip micro porous tapes for fixation, but the surrounding skin must be completely healthy to retain the tapes. [8] Other methods applying different materials such as honey [13] or cyanoacrylate [14] have been designed. We would like to present a method of graft fixation pioneered at our burn center and found convenient for both patient and surgeon, using amniotic membrane as fixator. This is particularly appropriate in children and also extremity burns. The skin graft is inserted on the wound bed, then covered with amniotic membrane (Fig. 2) and the dressing is applied.

The membrane adheres to the grafted area in a few minutes. There is no need for stitches or staples in extremities [15] or just a few anchoring sutures may be needed in some other body parts. [16]

Several studies have shown that the application of amniotic membrane as a graft fixator is accompanied by rapid re-epithelialization and healing [2,16,17] .Amniotic membrane has also been found an effective biological dressing for burns, as it diminishes the loss of plasma, fluid, protein and heat . [17], [18] ,[19] .

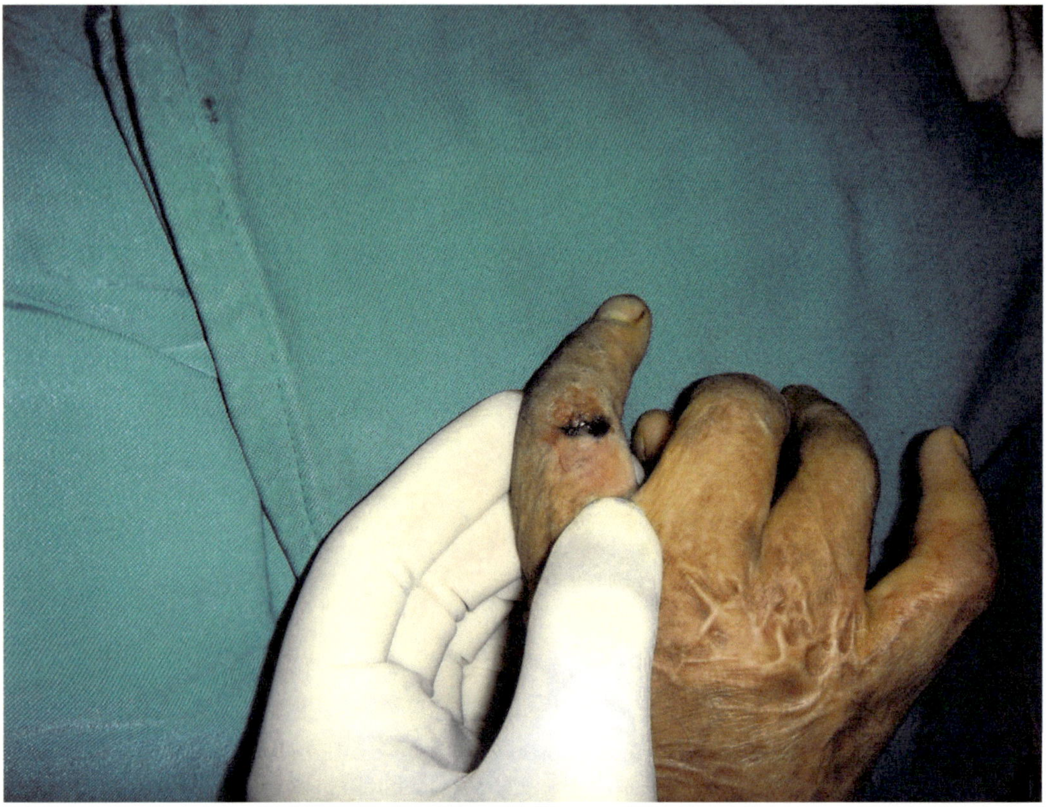

Fig. 1b. Painful forgotten staples removed 1 year after skin grafting.

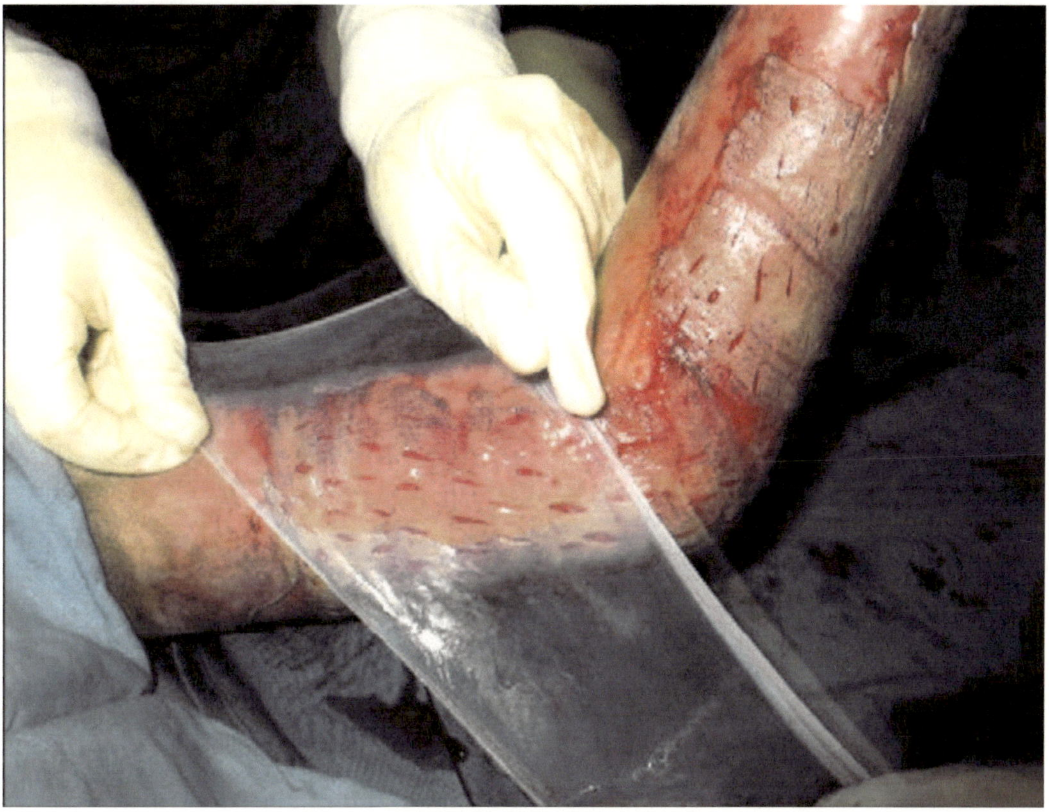

Fig. 2. Applying amniotic membrane for skin graft fixation.

In one study we evaluated the effect of amniotic membrane on rate of graft take. The patients were divided into two groups: 54 limbs in amnion group and 54 limbs in control group. The mean success rate of graft take was about 97 % and mean graft take duration was about 7 days in amnion group (Fig 3) versus 89 % and 14 days in control group respectively. Also this difference was statistically significant.

Our results show that amniotic membrane as skin graft fixator has no negative impact on graft take, but also significantly reduces the duration of complete graft take which is very important for both patient and health care system. Therefore, we recommend amniotic membrane as a skin graft fixator, and graft take accelerator to eliminate or diminish the need for painful and traumatizing postoperative dressing changes and thereby help to decrease the cost and also need for possible regrafting .

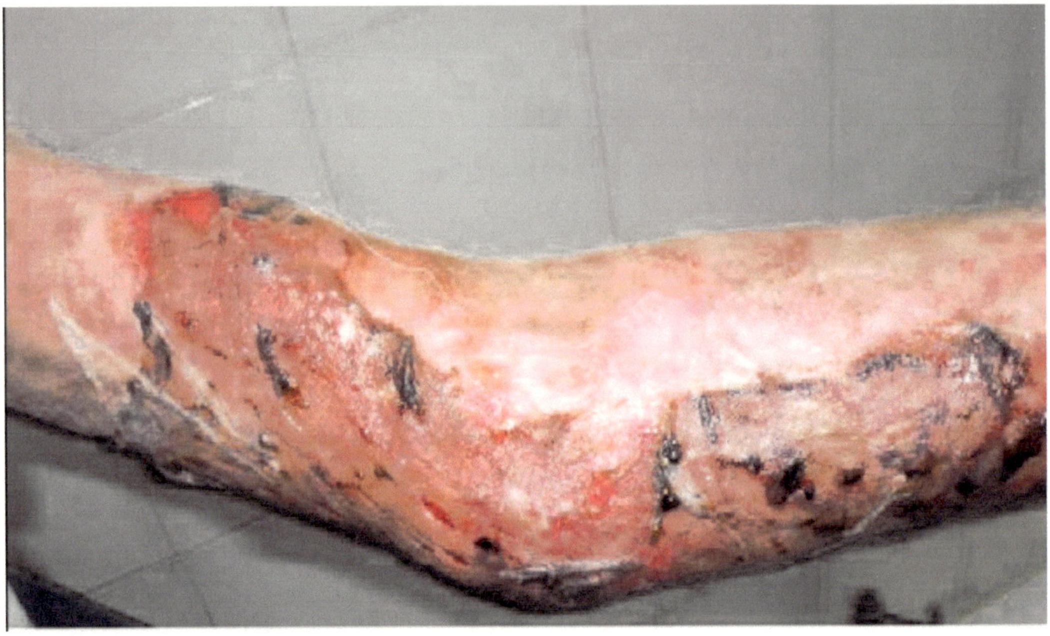

Fig. 3. The graft fixed with amniotic membrane, 5 days after procedure

3. Acceleration of donor site healing

Donor site morbidity including delayed and non-healing wounds and hypertrophic scar formation are major problems in skin grafted burn patients. Amniotic membrane dressing of skin graft donor sites ,accelerates epithelialization and results in early wound closure, thereby, significantly reducing the risk of complications and eliminates postoperative dressing change.

Amnion have been used to cover clean partial-thickness wounds and donor sites, and applied as a temporary dressing for freshly excised burns.

It has advantages such as pain relief, prevention of infection, maintenance of a moist environment to promote healing, good adherence to wounds, and simple handling [2, 11-14]. Laboratory investigations have revealed that the basement membrane (BM) of amnion shares major BM components with human skin, and the BM zone resembles human skin, morphologically [17]. The epithelial side of denuded amnion has been shown to support the proliferation, spreading, and differentiation of corneal, mucousa and bronchial epithelial cells [18-20]. Furthermore, the stroma of amnion can serve as a dermal matrix in which fibroblasts show good adherence and proliferation [21, 22].

After cleansing the donor bed of blood, the amniotic membrane is applied (Fig 4) & then covered with Vaseline gauze simple dressing. The amniotic membrane adheres to the wound bed and peels off, when the wound is completely epithelialized.

We studied 50 patients which had 2 similar donor sites of both lower exterimities. The mean healing time was about 6 days in amnion group and 13 days in control group, and pain was significantly lower in amnion group.

The desirable properties include rapid adherence, transparency, decreased patient discomfort and decrease in infection. One of the most important observations was that, amniotic membrane was used as a single application dressing. In all cases, it remained over the donor bed until healing was complete. This characteristic (single application) significantly reduces patient discomfort and costs by elimination the need for multiple dressing changes.

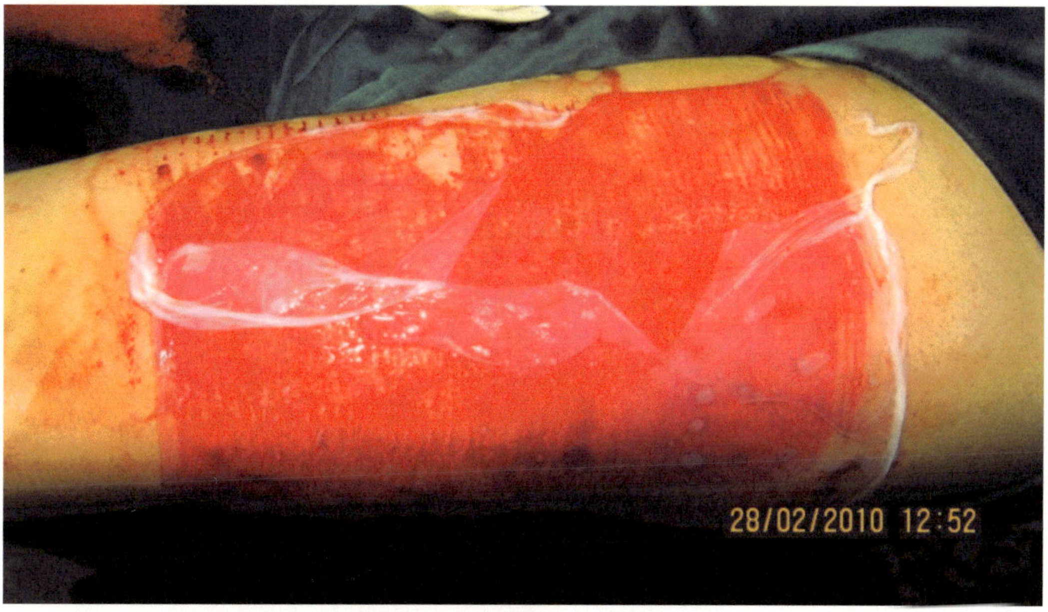

Fig. 4. Amniotic membrane dressing of donor site

Our clinical experience with amniotic membrane moved us to use this product widely for donor sites, especially in children.

4. Increased graft take in old infected granulation tissue

The standard treatment today for deep partial-thickness and full-thickness burns is early excision and grafting (E&G) but this technique may not be possible in centers with poor medical facilities. In these centers burn physicians should wait and see until the superficial burns heal primarily or granulation tissue appears in the base of the wound.

One problem in delayed grafting is the appearance of granulation tissue which, in addition to microbial colonization, reduces graft take and increases complications, mortality, hospital stay and costs. [20- 32]

Old granulation tissue is a prevalent problem in developing countries. Management of these wound is very difficult, the result of skin grafting is poor and still there is no consensus about the best treatment modality of these wounds.

The problem which now arises is how to apply skin grafts on chronic granulation tissue and controversy continues on the best management.

Some surgeons favor application of graft after removal of granulation tissue while others favor application of grafts directly on the granulation tissue. We used amniotic membrane to manage these wounds in a clinical randomized control trial and observed good results. (not published)

90 adult patients with old burn wounds (more than two weeks after granulation tissue appearance) and infected (according to the surgeon diagnosis and positive tissue cultures) were included in this study. (Fig 5).

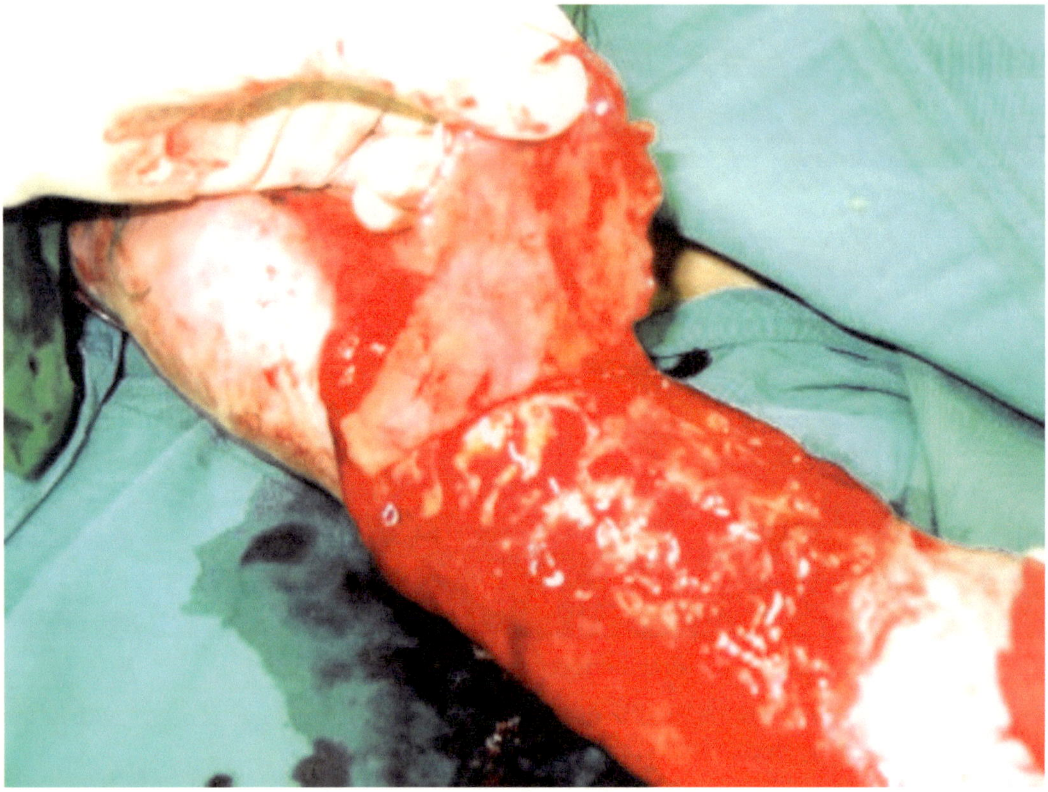

Fig. 5. Old granulation tissue in a burn patient (these wounds are shinny and easily removed with minimal digital pressure)

The most frequent bacterial isolate from burn wound culture was staphylococcus followed by pseudomonas. The most common cause of chronicity of burn wound was delay in referring of patient to burn center.

The extremities were randomly divided into two groups. Debridement of granulation tissue was performed in both groups. In group A, the graft surface was covered with amnion and in Group B(control group)skin grafting was performed in the conventional fashion.

Graft take was assessed on 14th post-grafting day.

The graft take was 90.13 % in amnion group and 65.61 % in control group that was statistically significant .(p value < 0.05)

5. Decreased hypertrophic scar and itching

Hypertrophic scar and itching are disabling complications in burn patients. We studied & saw interesting result with applying amniotic membrane on skin grafted areas in diminishing hypertrophic scar & itching. This may be explained by accelerated wound healing & epithelialization.

Hypertrophic scarring after injuries, and especially burns, is a great concerns for patients and a challenging problem for clinicians.
Hypertrophic scars may cause significant functional and cosmetic impairment, and pruritus causes discomfort for the patient, and is responsible for decrease in quality of life. Pruritus causes discomfort and decreases quality of life .Hypertrophic scars result from general failure of normal wound healing processes. After burn injury, hypertrophic scars typically, appear on the trunk and extremities. [33]
Many factors such as race, age, genetic factors, hormone levels, atopy and immunologic responses of the individual patient appear to play a role. The type of injury, wound size and depth, anatomic region and mechanical tension on the wound are important as well. Also, complicating factors such as bacterial colonization and infection of the wound seem to induce hypertrophic scarring [34]. To predict the development of a hypertrophic scar in a burn wound, the time interval between burn and and healing is the most important factor and is closely related to depth and size of the wound [35].
Treatment of the hypertrophic scar still is a challenging issue due to the lack of effective treatments. Various treatments are currently available including surgical excision, steroid injection, radiation, laser therapy, silicone gels, calcium channel blockers and pressure therapy. Although management of hypertrophic scars has advanced in the past years, the lesions remain difficult to prevent and treat. Burn hypertrophic scars are often widespread and not linear . Although extensive research has led to an increase of knowledge in the pathophysiologic processes of wound healing and the formation of scars, but still there is no consensus regarding the best treatment to reduce or prevent hypertrophic scarring. Recurrences remain common and patient satisfaction is variable .
Optimal treatment of the burn wound is of eminent importance for wound healing and the prevention of hypertrophic scar formation. Deitch et al demonstrated that wound closure should be achieved within three weeks to reduce the risk for hypertrophic scar development [36]. Timing of grafting is still under debate, both for survival of the patients as well as the incidence and quality of hypertrophic scar. Adequate topical wound treatment allows for wound healing with controlled inflammation and should be applied to obtain fast wound closure. The autologous split thickness skin graft is still the mainstay of burn wound surgery. Although autologous split thickness skin graft may result in faster wound closure, it may not prevent hypertrophic scar formation in the operated area.
Several studies have shown that the application of amniotic membrane as a biological dressing in the management of burns is accompanied by rapid re-epithelialization and healing. Amniotic membrane has been found an effective biological dressing for burns, as it diminishes the oozing of plasma, bacterial count, and fluid, protein and heat loss [15-17].
In another study, we evaluated the effect of amniotic membrane as an adjunct in split-thickness skin graft on itching and hypertrophic scar formation in burn patients.(not published) This double blind randomized clinical controlled trial showed 59.25 % decreased itching and 64.81 % less hypertrophic scar formation in the skin grafted area covered with amniotic membrane in comparison to areas which managed by conventional skin grafting method.
This study showed that using amniotic membrane as an adjunct in split-thickness skin grafting significantly reduces post-burn itching and hypertrophic scar formation. It seems that additional research still is required to determine the best possible treatments. Since there is no optimum treatment option at present, amniotic membrane can be used as a novel

modality in prevention rather than treatment of hypertrophic scar formation and itching in burn patients.

6. Conclusion

According to our experiences, amniotic membrane can strongly participate in skin grafted areas to improve skin graft take and decrease post graft complications.

7. Acknowledgment

I am grateful to the Shiraz burn research center staffs, ghotbeddin burn hospital physicians, caregivers and also countless burn patients for their invaluable helps, Hamed Ghoddusi Johari ,M.D for contribution in our research , (effect of amniotic membrane on skin graft take) and Mandana Kiasat Dolatabadi , M.D (effect of amniotic membrane on old infected granulation tissue) as their thesis for degree on general of surgery and Shima Eskandari (effect of amniotic membrane on hyper trophic scare formation and itching) as her thesis for degree of MD, Mr. Iman Ahrari ,medical student for their help in edition , Miss Zahra Moradi and Mrs. Masumeh Kherad for their special contribution in our researches, Mrs Zahra Jahedmah and Mrs. Mahbubeh Nazari for taking photographs .

8. References

[1] Mohammadi A.A, Sabet B, Riazi H, Tavakkolian A.R, Mohammadi M.K, Iranpak S. Amniotic Membrane Dressing: an Excellent Method for Outpatient Management of Burn Wounds. IJMS,Vol 34:1, 2009.1 61

[2] Ravishanker R, Bath A.S, Roy R. Amnion Bank- the use of long term glycerol preserved amniotic membranes in the management of superficial and superficial partial thickness burns. Burns 2003; 29: 369-74

[3] Robson MC, KrizekTJ, Koss N, Samburg JL. Amniotic membrane as a temporary wound dressing. Surg Gynaccol Obstet.1973; 136: 904-6.

[4] Hadjiiski O,Anatassov N. Amniotic membranes for temporary burn coverage. Annals of Burns and Fire Disasters. 1996; 10: 2-7

[5] Lorusso R, Geraci V, Masellis M. The treatment of superficial burns with biological and synthetic material: frozen amnion and biobrane . Annals of the MBC. 1989; 2: 2 -5

[6] SukariHalim A, Khoo T.L, Mohd. YussofSh.J.Biologic and synthetic skin substitutes: An overview .Indian J Plast Surg. 2010;43(Suppl): S23-S28

[7] Sangwan V.S, Burman S, Tejwani S, Mahesh S.P, Murthy R. Amniotic membrane transplantation: a review of current indications in the management of ophthalmic disorders. Indian J Ophthalmol. 2007; 55(4):251-60.

[8] Rudge R. An easy and safe method of split-thickness skin graft fixation. Burns 2007;33:1074-5

[9] Mah E, Morrison W.A. A stitch in time (Save Mines).Plast Reconstr Surg 2006;117:2535-6.

[10] Yenidu¨ nya MO, O¨ zdengill E, Emsen I. Split-thickness skingraft fixation with surgical drape. Plast Reconstr Surg, 2000;106:1429-30.

[11] Alexander G, Al-Rasheed A.A. Skin stapler removal by artery forceps: a hazardous practice? Burns, 2005;31:116.

[12] Mohammadi, AA , Ghoddusi johari, H . forgotten staples. Burns.2009; 35: 611

[13] Ilteris Murat E. A different and safe method of split thickness skin graft fixation: medical honey application. Burns 2007;33:782-7.
[14] Adler N, Nachumovsky S, Meshulam-Derazon S, Ad-El D.Skin graft fixation with cyanoacrylate tissue adhesive in burn patients. Burns 2007;33:803
[15] Mohammadi AA, Ghoddusi Johari H. Amniotic membrane: A skin graft fixator convenient for both patient and surgeon. Burns 2008;34:1051-1052
[16] Mohammadi AA, Ghoddusi Johari H.Anchoring sutures:useful adjuncts for amniotic membrane for skin graft fixation in extensive burns and near the joints. Burns 2010;36:1134-1141
[17] Antasov W, Mazalova J, Todorod R, Stereva K, Trencheva W. Use of amniotic membrane as biological dressing in contemporary treatment of burn. Ann Medit Burns Club.1994;7:202-5.
[18] Sawhney C.P. Amniotic membrane as a biological dressing in the management of burns. Burns 1989;15:339-42.
[19] Haberl M, Oner Z, Bayraktar U, Bilgin N. The use of silver nitrate-incorporated amniotic membrane as a temporary dressing. Burns, 1987;13:159-63.
[20] Morykwas M.J, Thornton J.W, Bartlett R.H. Zeta potential of synthetic and biological skin substitutes: effects on initial adherence. Plast Reconstr Surg ,1987;79:732-9.
[21] Yang L, Shirakata Y, Tokumaru S, Xiuju D, Tohyama M, Hanakawa Y, et al. Living skin equivalents constructed using human amnions as a matrix. J Dermatol Sci.2009;56(3):188-95.
[22] Gajiwala K, Gajiwala AL. Evaluation of lyophilised, gamma-irradiated amnion as a biological dressing. Cell Tissue Bank 2004;5:73-80.
[23] QuinbyJr W.C, Hoover H.C, Scheflan M, Walters P.T, Slavin S.A, Bondoc CC. Clinical trials of amniotic membranes in burn wound care. Plast Reconstr Surg 1982; 70:711-7.
[24] Park M, Kim S, Kim I.S, Son D. Healing of a porcine burn wound dressed with human and bovine amniotic membranes. Wound Repair Regen 2008;16:520- 8.
[25] Oyama N, Bhogal B.S, Carrington P, Gratian M.J, Black M.M. Human placental amnion is a novel substrate for detecting autoantibodies in autoimmune bullous diseases by immunoblotting. Br J Dermatol 2003;148:939-44.
[26] Koizumi N, Fullwood NJ, Bairaktaris G, Inatomi T, Kinoshita S, Quantock AJ. Cultivation of corneal epithelial cells on intact and denuded human amniotic membrane. Invest Ophthalmol Vis Sci ,2000;41:2506-13.
[27] Nakamura T, Endo K, Cooper L.J, Fullwood N.J, Tanifuji N, Tsuzuki M, et al. The successful culture and autologous transplantation of rabbit oral mucosal epithelial cells on amniotic membrane. Invest Ophthalmol Vis Sci 2003;44: 106-16.
[28] Sakamoto T, Hirano K, Morishima Y, Masuyama K, Ishii Y, Nomura A, et al. Maintenance of the differentiated type II cell characteristics by culture on an acellular human amnion membrane. In Vitro Cell Dev Biol Anim 2001;37:471-
[29] Solomon A, Wajngarten M, Alviano F, Anteby I, Elchalal U, Pe'er J, et al. Suppression of inflammatory and fibrotic responses in allergic inflammation by the amniotic membrane stromal matrix. Clin Exp Allergy 2005;35:941-8.
[30] Burman S, Tejwani S, Vemuganti G.K, Gopinathan U, Sangwan V.S. Ophthalmic applications of preserved human amniotic membrane: a review of current indications. Cell Tissue Bank 2004;5:161-75.

[31] Fred W. Endof and Nicole S. Gibran .In: Brunicardi FC, Anderson DK,Billiar TR, Dunn DL, Hunter JG, Pollock RE. editors Schwartz's principles of Surgery. New York: MacGraw - Hill; 2010.p.197- 207 .

[32] Sanjay D ,Rakesh D, Anand K and Bhavani R. Comparative study of skin grafting with and without surgical removal of granulation tissue in chronic burn wounds . Burns .2007; 33:872-878

[33] Ozbek S, Ozgenel Y, Etoz A, Akin S, Kahveci R, Heper Y, ErcanI, Ozcan M. The effect of delayed admission in burn centers on wound contamination and infection rates. Ulus Travma Acilcerrahi Derg. 2005; 11(3) : 230-7.

[34] Bloemen M.C, van der Veer W.M, Ulrich M.M, van Zuijlen P.P, Niessen F.B, Middelkoop E. Prevention and curative management of hypertrophic scar formation. Burns 2009; 35: 463-475.

[35] Niessen F.B, Spauwen P.H, Schalkwijk J, Kon M. On the nature of hypertrophic scars and keloids: a review. Plast Reconstr Surg 1999;104(5):1435-58.

[36] Cubison T.C, Pape S.A, Parkhouse N. Evidence for the link between healing time and the development of hypertrophic scars (HTS) in paediatric burns due to scald injury. Burns 2006;32(8):992-9.

19

Influence of Microorganisms on the Healing of Skin Grafts from Chronic Venous Leg Wounds

Tine Yding Wolff[1], Thomas Bjarnsholt[2,3],
Klaus Kirketerp-Møller[4] and Trine Rolighed Thomsen[1,5]
[1]*Life Science Division, The Danish Technological Institute*
[2]*University of Copenhagen, Faculty Of Health Sciences, Department of International Health, Immunology and Microbiology*
[3]*Rigshospitalet, Department for Clinical Microbiology*
[4]*Orthopedic Department, Hvidovre University Hospital*
[5]*Department of Biotechnology, Chemistry and Environmental EngineeringAalborg University*
Denmark

1. Introduction

Chronic wounds are associated with a significant morbidity and continue to affect an increasing number of patients. In developed countries an estimated 1-2% of the population will suffer from a chronic wound at some point in their lifetime. Chronic wound treatment is associated with considerable expenses and in the United States alone more than 25 billion dollars are spent on treatment annually (Percival et al., 2011).

Although it is well known that infection is involved in making the wound chronic and unable to heal, the process for identifying bacterial flora within wounds is not standardized (Frankel et al., 2009). The microorganisms associated with chronic wounds are usually investigated by traditional culture–dependent methods by taking a swab or biopsy from the wound and applying it as inoculate for various microbial cultures. The introduction of molecular biological methods and improved sampling techniques has illustrated that the culture-dependent methods presumably underestimate the microorganisms present in the wound. This is often due to a combination of inadequate growth conditions and colonization with slow, unculturable, fastidious or anaerobic bacteria growing in biofilms (Price et al., 2010).

It is well known that naked bacterial DNA can persist in a sample for a while after the infection has been eliminated, and the risk of detecting DNA from dead (non-viable) bacteria is a recognized bias when using molecular methods. The commercially available kit Molysis (Molzym, Bremen, Germany) degrades the naked bacterial DNA residing in a sample, thereby, improving the detection of viable and hence more clinically relevant bacteria in the subsequent molecular analysis. RNA has a much shorter half-life than DNA making it suitable as a measure of microbiological activity in a sample. RNA extracted from a sample can be converted into cDNA and used as a target in polymerase chain reaction (PCR) or the RNA can be targeted directly within the cell for instance by fluorescence in situ hybridization (FISH).

The exact role and function of microorganisms in chronic wounds is not fully understood, but bacteria seem to have an important influence on the prognosis of the wound. In a study by Høgsberg et al. (in press) the bacterial flora was examined in chronic wound beds determined for split-skin grafting using conventional culture methods. In the study the presence of *Pseudomonas aeruginosa* was found to be particularly important. If *P. aeruginosa* was present, only 33% of the grafted chronic wounds healed successfully in contrast to 77% when *P. aeruginosa* was not detected. This emphasizes the importance of a careful sampling technique, characterization of the wound and clinical correlation.

In this chapter we describe techniques to characterize the microorganisms from a swab or skin grafting biopsy from chronic wounds. New and previously obtained results are presented and discussed.

2. Molecular methods for studying the microbial flora in chronic wounds

Various methods have been applied for the study of microorganisms in chronic wounds and each method has its advantages and disadvantages. In most clinical settings the gold standard is traditional culture-based methods. The weakness of cultivation is that it can take several days to obtain a final identification, and that fastidious and slow-growing microorganisms in the sample might be overlooked. However, cultivation usually provides additional information such as phenotypic resistance patterns that are highly relevant from a clinical perspective. Molecular diagnostic approaches on the other hand offer a more rapid and deep identification but have other limitations. In the following section some of the well-established molecular techniques are described as well as a few of the latest methods in the field.

2.1 16S rDNA cycle

Culture-independent identification of bacteria can be carried out by performing a ribosomal RNA (rRNA) gene cycle e.g. (Nielsen et al., 2008; Thomsen et al., 2010). This method is based on the fact that the composition of the gene encoding the bacterial 16S rRNA (16S rDNA) is unique for each bacterial species. Total DNA is extracted from a sample and the 16S rDNA is amplified nearly in its full length by PCR using broad-range primers. If the sample is polymicrobial the resulting PCR product will consist of amplicons with varying sequences making it unsuitable for direct sequencing. The individual amplicons need to be separated before sequencing, and construction of clone libraries and denaturant gradient gel electrophoresis (DGGE) are two different ways of achieving that (Andersen et al., 2007; Muyzer et al., 1993; Thomsen et al., 2010).

To construct clone libraries the amplicons are ligated into plasmid vectors and cloned into *E. coli* cells. The cells are spread on agar plates and grown over night, and each colony appearing on the plate represents one amplicon. The vectors are then extracted from each individual colony, and the 16S rDNA amplicons are sequenced. By performing BLAST (Basic Local Alignment Search Tool) searches in public databases (Altschul, 1997), the obtained sequences can be assigned to specific bacteria, and an improved phylogenetic resolution can be obtained by performing a phylogenetic analysis on basis of the sequences.

In DGGE the amplicons are separated by providing them with a GC-rich primer tail and loading them on a polyacrylamide gel containing a gradually increasing concentration of chemical denaturant. The unique base composition of each amplicon results in individual melting points meaning that the amplicon can only move through the gel until a certain point, where the double stranded structure is fully melted and only held together by the GC tail. Upon staining, each band on the gel theoretically represents a unique 16S rDNA amplicon which can be excised and extracted from the gel and sequenced. Construction of clone libraries and DGGE are relatively labour-intensive methods with many individual steps and it takes several days to obtain the sequences that eventually reveal the bacteria present in a sample. This makes the methods unsuitable for diagnostic purposes where a rapid answer is required, whereas, they are more relevant as a research tool. The sequence information provided by the clone libraries and the DGGE can be used to make more specific analyses on the original sample, such as FISH or quantitative PCR (qPCR).

2.2 qPCR / RT-qPCR

qPCR is a culture-independent method for determining the number of a specific gene in a sample. qPCR basically proceeds like a regular PCR but has the advantage that the formation of PCR product can be followed as it progresses, making laborious post-PCR steps such as gel electrophoresis unnecessary. In qPCR the formation of PCR product is usually detected by one of two techniques: addition of a dye that fluoresces upon binding to double stranded DNA, or by application of a sequence-specific probe that fluoresces only when the target DNA is present. In both cases, the fluorescence is measured by a detector in the PCR machine after each PCR cycle. The intensity of the fluorescence progresses exponentially as does the PCR product formation because the increase in fluorescence is proportional to the increasing amount of target sequence. By analyzing standards with known concentrations of the target sequence, it is possible to quantify the initial amount of target DNA in the sample. In order to focus only on the active bacteria the RNA can be extracted from the sample, converted into cDNA and used as target in qPCR in a method called reverse transcriptase qPCR RT-qPCR).

2.3 FISH

DNA-FISH and peptide nucleic acid (PNA)-FISH rapidly identify microorganisms in complex samples and provide information about number, morphology and spatial distribution. The FISH technique is based on fluorescent probes of varying specificity that are complementary to a ribosomal RNA sequence, and the target cells can be visualized using fluorescence microscopy. A detailed procedure has been published by Amann (1995) and Stender (2003).

2.4 Pyrosequencing

Pyrosequencing is a method of DNA sequencing based on the "sequencing by synthesis" principle and it is likely to replace the relatively labour-intensive procedure of constructing clone libraries. It differs from the classic Sanger sequencing, in that it relies on the detection of pyrophosphate release upon nucleotide incorporation, rather than chain termination with dideoxynucleotides (Ronaghi et al., 1998). This deep sequencing technique has been used to evaluate the diversity of microbial populations where thousands of reads/sequences can be obtained from each sample (Andersson et al., 2007; Bogaert et al.; Dowd et al., 2008; Price et al., 2009; Price et al., 2010; Smith et al., 2010; Stewart et al., 2010; Wolcott et al., 2009).

2.5 Ibis T-5000

The Ibis T5000 Biosensor system combines automated sample preparation, PCR amplification, electrospray ionization mass spectrometry, and information management to rapidly characterize known and unknown organisms. The system is based on base ratios (not base sequences) and can provide test results in six to seven hours (Ecker et al., 2008). The method was recently identified as the molecular system most likely to fulfill the requirements of routine diagnosis in orthopedic surgery (Costerton et al., 2011).

2.6 Method evaluation

All the mentioned methods are somehow biased and application of multiple methods is generally recommended for research studies. For example, the nucleic acid extraction efficiency is crucial for all methods except FISH, where sample fixation is important. Primer specificity, differential amplification efficiency and incomplete databases for bioinformatic search are other possible biases. In addition, it is important to be critical to molecular findings based on DNA. Previous studies have shown that naked bacterial DNA can reside in a sample for a long time after an infection has been eradicated fx Pichlmaier et al. (2008). The PCR techniques cannot distinguish between DNA from active and dead bacteria and this raises the question of the clinical relevance of the findings. Targeting RNA instead of DNA (for instance using FISH or RT-qPCR) could help exclude irrelevant findings and focus only on the active bacteria.

3. Results

In a study by Thomsen and coworkers (2010) the bacterial flora in different types of wound material from 14 skin graft operations was examined. Routine cultivation as well as a panel of DNA-based methods were performed and the results compared. Cultivation showed polymicrobial growth in all but one wound, and *S. aureus*, *P. aeruginosa*, *K. oxytoca* and enterococci were identified most often, whereas no anaerobic species were found. In most of the samples the finding of *S. aureus* and *P. aeruginosa* by cultivation was confirmed by the molecular methods. However, for all samples DNA from additional species was identified, including anaerobic bacteria. Among others DNA from *Alcaligenes* sp., *Anaerococcus* sp., *E. faecalis* and *Stenotrophomonas* sp. was identified.

Furthermore, the study comprised an examination of the spatial location of *S. aureus* and *P. aeruginosa* within two wounds using species specific qPCR. This showed a great variation in the distribution of bacteria at different locations in the same wound. As an example, the number of *P. aeruginosa* varied with three orders of magnitude for two biopsies taken from the same wound indicating that the bacteria grow locally in micro colonies (biofilms) (Figure 1). This tendency to proliferate in biofilms is illustrated in Figure 2, where a biopsy from a skin graft operation is examined for the presence of *P. aeruginosa* using PNA-FISH. In a recent analysis we examined the bacterial diversity in four samples (referred to as A-D) taken from the same wound by standard cultivation techniques as well as construction of clone libraries, PNA FISH and qPCR on basis of DNA and RNA (Table 1). Cultivation identified three bacterial species: *Staphylococcus pettenkoferi*, *Enterobacter cloacae* and

Stentrophomonas maltophilia. These findings were confirmed in one or more of the clone libraries (*S. pettenkoferi* DNA was found in clone library A and C, *S. maltophilia* DNA in C and D and *E. cloacae* DNA in D). DNA from additional bacteria was found in all four clone libraries of which *Propionibacterium* sp., *Massilia timonae, Brevibacterium pityocampae, Streptococcus mitis, Achromobacter* sp. and *Acinetobacter* sp. were the most abundant. The presence of *Propionibacterium acnes*, a common inhabitant of the human skin, was confirmed and quantitated with species specific qPCR.

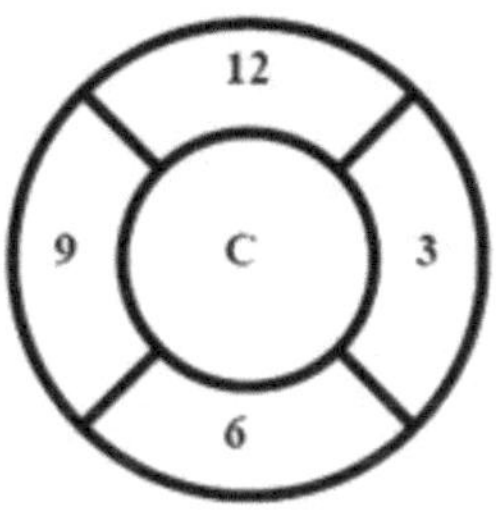

		S. aureus		*P. aeruginosa*	
	method	Wound E	Wound F	Wound E	Wound F
C	q-PCR	**89**±11%	**200**±13%	**510**±18%	**920**±9%
	cultivation			+	
	DGGE	+	+		
3	q-PCR	No sample	**86**±8%	No sample	**300**±13%
	cultivation				
	DGGE		+		
6	q-PCR	**240**±10%	**290**±8%	**760**±7%	**8200**±8%
	cultivation			+	
	DGGE	+	+		
9	q-PCR	**310**±13%	**80**±5%	**47**±9%	**800**±10%
	cultivation			+	
	DGGE	+	+		
12	q-PCR	**180**±8%	**93**±12%	**280**±3%	**15**±5%
	cultivation			+	
	DGGE	+	+		

Fig. 1. Quantitative PCR data obtained from two wounds (wound E and F, respectively) for *S. aureus* and *P. aeruginosa* (copies/ng DNA ±standard error of the mean, n=3). Cultivation and DGGE results are mentioned as well + : Samples were taken under skin graft operations at the center (C), and at approximately 3, 6, 9, and 12 o'clock around the wounds' periphery. From Thomsen (2010).

Some of the 16S rDNA sequences from clone library A, C and D matched *Staphylococcus* sp. upon BLAST search.

To further annotate these bacteria, RT-qPCR assays targeting *S. aureus femA* mRNA and *Staphylococcus* sp. 16S rRNA were applied. The *S. aureus* specific qPCR was negative for all four samples whereas the *Staphylococcus* sp. assay was positive, indicating that the clones matching *Staphylococcus* sp. originated from coagulase-negative staphylococci (CoNS).

mRNA from *P. acnes* and *Staphylococcus* sp. was detected in the four wound samples indicating that these bacteria were active at the time of sampling. This partially corresponds with the cultivation results where *Staphylococcus pettenkoferi* was observed, whereas *P. acnes* was not. *P. acnes* is considered to be a fastidious bacterium that requires anaerobic growth conditions and has a slow growth rate. This might explain why it was not detected by cultivation.

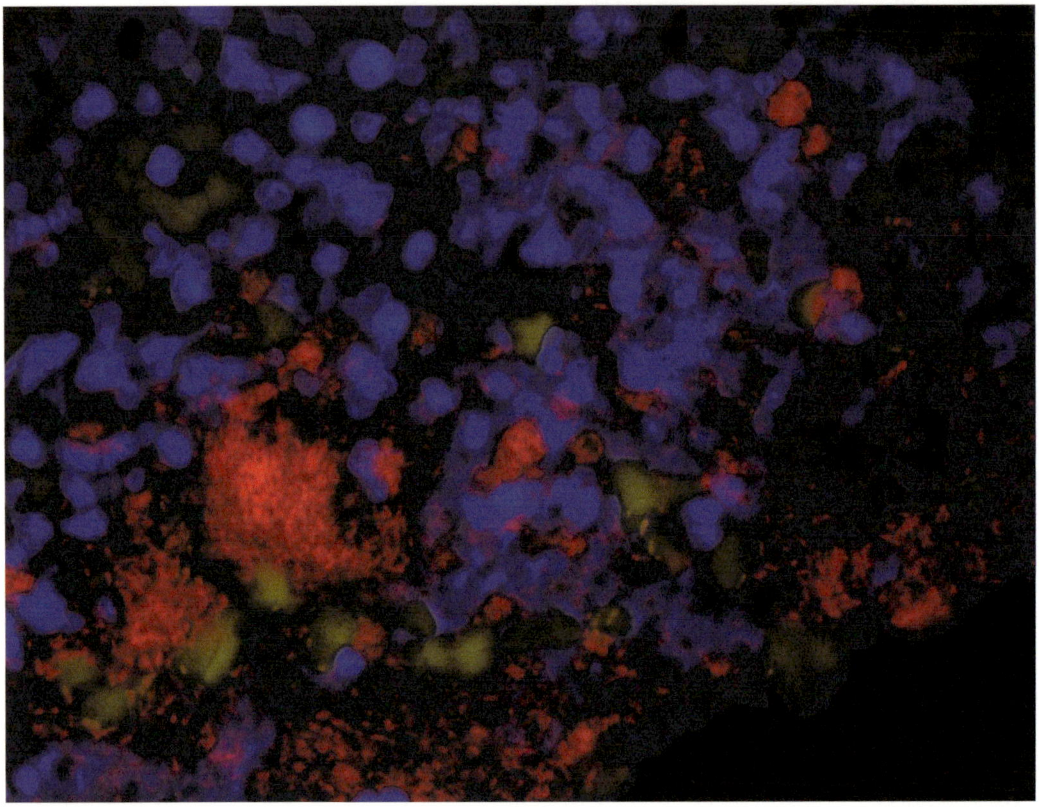

Fig. 2. *P. aeruginosa* identified in a biopsy from a skin graft operation by a specific PNA FISH probe (red stain). Host cells were stained with DAPI (blue).

P. aeruginosa and *S. aureus* are common in chronic wound infections but in this specifically examined case not found by cultivation, or in any of the clone libraries or by species specific qPCR. When comparing the results of our recent analysis to those obtained by Thomsen and coworkers (2010) it is seen that in both cases DNA from *Brevibacterium* sp., *Anaerococcus* sp., *Achromobacter* sp. and *Alcaligenes faecalis* was identified using the clone library approach but not by cultivation. Furthermore, both studies show that molecular methods identify additional bacteria compared to cultivation and that the bacterial composition differs depending on the location within the individual wound.

Sample	Cultivation	Clone libraries (genomic DNA) Parentheses numbers of clones	qPCR (genomic DNA)	RT-qPCR (cDNA)
A	*Staphylococcus pettenkoferi, Enterobacter cloacae, Stentrophomonas maltophilia*	*Brevibacterium pityocampae* (7), *Staphylococcus* sp. (8), *Propionibacterium* sp. (19), *Massilia timonae* (1), *Staphylococcus epidermidis* (1), *Xanthomonas* sp. (1), *Xanthomonadaceae* sp. (2), *Stenotrophomonas* sp. (3), *Herbaspirillum* sp. (1) and 12 uncultured bacteria best matching: *Ralstonia solanacearum* (1), *Massilia timonae* (5), *Propionibacterium* sp. (1), *Propionibacterium acnes* (3) and *Acidobacterium* sp. (2).	1200 *P. acnes* CFU/g tissue	Positive for *P. acnes* Positive for *Staphylococcus* sp.
B		*Propionibacterium* sp. (23), *Streptococcus mitis* (4), *Achromobacter* sp. (2), *Kocuria* sp. (3), *Micrococcus* sp. (2), 12 uncultured bacteria best matching: *Ralstonia solanacearum* (3), *Anaerococcus* sp. (2), *Kocuria* sp. (4), *Propionibacterium* sp. (1), *Achromobacter xylosoxidans* (1) and *Neisseriales* sp. (1).	1200 *P. acnes* CFU/g tissue	Positive for *P. acnes* Positive for *Staphylococcus* sp.
C		*Acinetobacter* sp. (4), *Staphylococcus* sp. (1), *Stenotrophomonas maltophilia* (4), *Stenotrophomonas* sp. (5), *Propionibacterium* sp. (4), *Alcaligenes faecalis* (1), *Micrococcus* sp. (2), *Mesorhizobium* sp. (1), *Enterobacter hormachei* (1) and 22 uncultured bacteria best matching: *Propionibacterium acnes* (3), *Enterbacter hormachei* (4), *Anaeromyxobacter* sp. (2), *Lactobacillus iners* (7), *Ralstonia solanacearum* (2), *Corynebacterium accolens* (3), *Bradhyrizobium* sp. (1).	1700 *P. acnes* CFU/g tissue	Positive for *P. acnes* Positive for *Staphylococcus* sp.
D		*Achromobacter denitrificans* (5), *Achromobacter* sp. (4), *Enterobacter hormachei* (7), *Stenotrophomonas maltophilia* (6), *Enterobacter* sp. (1), *Enterobacter cloacae* (1), *Propionibacterium* sp. (1), *Staphylococcus* sp. RNA (1) and 25 uncultured bacteria best matching: *Enterobacter hormachei* (12), *Enterobacter cloacae* (6), *Streptococcus alactolyticus* (4), *Enterococcus ludwigii* (2) and *Massilia* sp. (1).	1000 *P. acnes* RNA CFU/g tissue	No *P. acnes* detected Positive for *Staphylococcus* sp.

Table 1. Comparison of 4 separate biopsies from one wound investigated by cultivation, clone libraries, qPCR and RT-qPCR. Genomic DNA and RNA extracted from the four samples were examined using qPCR and RT-qPCR assays specific for *Propionibacterium acnes, Staphylococcus sp., P. aeruginosa* and *S. aureus.* RT-qPCR was only used to prove the presence of active bacteria and not to quantitate the bacteria.

4. Discussion

4.1 Microbial diversity

Over the years the microbial flora in chronic wounds has been target for thorough investigation and the advancing culture-independent techniques become more and more common as research tools. In such studies the molecular methods generally tend to reveal a much greater microbial diversity than the traditional cultivation methods. The study by Thomsen and coworkers (2010) is an example of this, where culture-independent methods revealed multiple species in each investigated wound. All of the wounds contained *S. aureus*, and *P. aeruginosa* was also frequently found, but aside from this, rather different floras were identified for the individual wounds. Furthermore, the molecular biological methods detected a varied anaerobic flora in some of the wounds and pathogenic species not found previously in chronic venous leg ulcers were identified. No anaerobes or new species were detected with culture methods. This corresponds well with the results of our recent examination of four biopsies taken from the same wound. Only aerobic bacteria were identified by cultivation whereas DNA and RNA from the anaerobic *P. acnes* were found by molecular methods. Furthermore, the molecular methods indicated varying polymicrobial communities in all four samples. Surprisingly, *S. aureus* and *P. aeruginosa* were not identified neither by cultivation or the cultivation independent methods in this specific wound.

The examination of wound flora has mainly focused on bacterial diversity, but a study from Dowd and collagues (2010) indicated that fungi might also be important in chronic wound infections. In their retrospective study, 915 chronic wounds were examined using molecular methods and fungal DNA was identified in 208 samples (corresponding to 23% of the investigated samples). DNA from a total of 48 different fungal species was identified of which yeasts of the *Candida* genus were the most abundant. In a retrospective analysis of the DNA resulting from the wounds included in the Thomsen (2010) study, qPCR with universal fungal primers and probe revealed fungal DNA in one of 14 samples.

In a recent study by Smith (2010) pyrosequencing was used to identify bacterial populations in 49 pressure ulcers. Diversity estimators were utilized and wound community compositions analyzed in relation to metadata such as age, race, gender, and comorbidities. Pressure ulcers are shown to be polymicrobial of nature with no single bacterium exclusively colonizing the wounds. The microbial community among such ulcers is highly variable and typically contains 3-10 primary populations. Up to hundreds of different species can be present in each wound; however, many in trace amounts only. There are no clearly significant differences in the microbial ecology of pressure ulcers in relation to metadata except when considering diabetes. The microbial populations and composition in the pressure ulcers of diabetics may be significantly different from the communities in non-diabetics. However in this particular work, the location of the pressure ulcer was not recorded. As diabetes tends to facilitate pressure ulcers on lower extremities due to neuropathy, the variability could reflect variations in location of the ulcer rather than diabetes itself.

The biofilm mode of growth seems important in chronic wounds with many different species present and it is generally accepted that the microbial composition of the entire wound is not represented in only one wound biopsy. Using FISH, we detected bacteria in biofilms in a biopsy from a skin graft operation (see Fig. 2) and this might explain how the bacteria survive inside the wound bed. In chronic wounds individual micro colonies might exist that only consist of single species, and it is very likely that mono- and polymicrobial biofilms can be found in the same ulcer, but the importance and relevance of this has yet to be established (Kirketerp-Moller et al., 2008; Burmølle et al., 2010). There are also biofilms in healing wounds, and other factors like host response, virulence and antibiotic resistance seem important for the fate of the wound.

4.2 Heterogeneous distribution

A chronic wound is a heterogeneous environment that varies at different locations with regard to the accessibility of oxygen and the flow of fluid. Furthermore, external influences such as the application of a wound dressing can cause local changes in the wound. This means that different microorganisms have more or less favorable growth conditions at different locations which often results in a heterogeneous microbiological distribution throughout the wound (Price et al., 2010). Wolcott (2009) concluded that individual wounds have distinct ecological footprints, and within the individual wounds there can be both significant site specific differences and relative uniformity in the bacterial ecology.

The heterogeneous distribution of microorganisms in chronic wounds has been described in several studies and the clinical relevance of this is discussed (e.g. by Fazli et al., 2009; Kirketerp-Moller et al., 2008¸Wolcott et al., 2009). Using qPCR and FISH it has been illustrated that the number of the pathogens *S. aureus* and *P. aeruginosa* varied depending on the location and depth of the wound examined (Fig. 1) (Thomsen et al., 2010). *S. aureus* was primarily located close to the wound surface while *P. aeruginosa* was primarily located deeper in the wound (Fazli et al., 2009). Some bacterial species were present all over the chronic venous leg ulcer while some were only present in parts of the wounds (Thomsen et al., 2010).

The macroscale spatial variation in wound microbiota was also investigated by Price et al. (2010). A total of 31 curette samples were collected at the leading edge, opposing leading edge, and/or center of 13 chronic wounds. Bacterial community composition was characterized using a combination of 16S rDNA-based pyrosequencing and various other methods. A total of 58 bacterial families and 91 bacterial genera were characterized among the 13 wounds. While substantial macroscale spatial variation was observed among the wounds, bacterial communities at different sites within individual wounds were significantly more similar than those in different wounds ($p=0.001$). Our recent study of four biopsies from one wound showed a similar tendency regarding the spatial heterogeneity. The clone libraries constructed for each sample had sequences in common, for instance *P. acnes* that appeared in all libraries, but also contained bacterial sequences that were unique to the particular location. Even though the results are based on only one wound they support the prevalent opinion that a careful adjustment of sample sites may improve the quality of wound microbiota studies. However, the significant similarity in bacterial communities from different sites within individual wounds indicates that studies failing to control for sampling site should not be disregarded based solely on this criterion. Ideally a composite sample from multiple sites across the surface and in the depth of individual wounds may provide the most robust characterization of wound microbiota (Price et al., 2010); however, this is often not possible clinically.

The introduction of next-generation sequencing methods such as pyrosequencing has made it possible to achieve huge amounts of information about the microbial composition in a sample in a relatively short time. However the large amount of data generated by the new methods gives rise to new challenges considering data handling and especially interpretation. As stated in the review by Rogers and coworkers (2010), different species in a polymicrobial infection can interact and thereby result in a different pathogenesis than the individual species would cause. This could mean that microorganisms that are usually considered non-pathogenic might play an important role in a polymicrobial community. For the time being it cannot be concluded if the new molecular methods are helpful to the clinicians or if all the extra information only complicates the overall picture. More studies have to be carried out to elucidate this.

The uneven distribution of bacteria in the wounds is highly relevant for the clinician and how and when the sample is taken highly influences the outcome of the diagnostic analysis. The ideal solution would be to examine the entire wound and identify every single pathogen, but again this is not possible nor does it provide the full answer. New questions would arise: Which bacterial strain or even subgroup is important and what influence do they have on the healing of the wound? Evaluating the result of a culture-independent analysis is after all still a paramount challenge for the clinician.

4.3 Consequences

4.3.1 Optimal sampling and diagnosis

No diagnostic methods can compensate for the three-dimensional uneven distribution of microorganisms in chronic ulcers. Several studies have indicated that the microbial flora varies at different locations in a wound (fx Kirketerp-Moller et al, 2008; Fazli et al, 2009, Thomsen et al., 2010), emphasizing the importance of adequate sampling techniques and ideally the use of multiple swabs or biopsies when examining wounds.

In situations where infected tissue is removed with the purpose of attaching a skin graft, instead of focusing on the microbial flora in the removed tissue it might be more relevant to focus on the remaining tissue on which the graft is to be attached (Bitsch et al., 2005). Microbial growth reduces the chance of the skin graft healing, and therefore examining the debrided wound before placing the graft, for instance by using a swab, might be of value. The surface of the chronic wound is likely to host commensal flora, and it is more likely that an in-depth residing bacterium is more pathogenic than a superficial one.

When designing a protocol for sampling we propose the following to be considered: 1. Revise the ulcer before sampling. 2: Swap a large area or take a big or multiple biopsies.

Melendez et al. (2009) developed a panel of qPCR assays targeting 14 common, clinically relevant pathogens for rapid identification of bacteria directly from tissue samples. Thirty-nine tissue samples from 29 chronic wounds were evaluated and the results compared with those obtained by culture. As revealed by culture and PCR, the most common organisms were methicillin-resistant *Staphylococcus aureus* (MRSA) followed by *Streptococcus agalactiae* (Group B *Streptococcus*) and *P. aeruginosa*. Under optimal conditions, the turnaround time for PCR results is only 4-6 h. Furthermore, qPCR is an inexpensive approach that easily can be introduced into clinical practice for detection of organisms directly from tissue samples. However, the downside to qPCR is that the primers and probe dictate the specificity and therefore there is a risk of overlooking species. For instance the qPCR assays reported by Melendez et al. (2009) only monitored aerobic pathogens but other studies have indicated that it is highly relevant to include assays for anaerobic pathogens and probably also fungi. The anaerobic and also slow-growing pathogen *P. acnes* was fx detected in the investigated wound presented in this study. In addition to the DNA identified in the clone libraries RNA from *P. acnes* was also identified indicating that the bacterium had been active very recently.

Which method is the optimal to examine the microbial flora of a chronic wound is a subject of discussion but in order to get as much information as possible the sample could be examined using a combination of traditional cultivation methods and molecular methods especially for research purposes.

4.3.3 The role of microorganisms in chronic wounds

Non-healing ulcers of mixed origin could heal if the underlying, but in many cases, still unknown cause was resolved. One of these factors is bacterial biofilm. But what is the difference between the biofilm in the healing group and in the non-healing group? Right now it is uncertain which microorganisms are the real important and truly pathogenic ones in chronic wounds, so should we treat for all of them? The most abundant microorganisms are not necessarily the most important in the wound from a clinical perspective. Furthermore, the pathogenicity between different strains and phenotypes differ, and they probably differ over time within the same phenotype. The most abundant bacteria found by traditional methods might just be the one with the most optimal growth conditions. Other factors like virulence genes, communication between the bacteria, the physical environment for the microorganisms and the host-biofilm interaction are also important. Hemolytic streptococci for instance are more virulent than certain other bacteria and a relatively small load of these are needed to initiate the infection of a wound. The beta-haemolytic *Streptococcus* and *Staphylococcus aureus* are examples of species that are highly virulent and co-exist very well with other species. So far it is unknown whether the virulence of a certain species is dependent upon another. Cell–cell communication in bacteria is accomplished through the exchange of chemical signal molecules called autoinducers. This process, called quorum sensing (QS), allows bacteria to monitor their environment for the presence of other bacteria and to respond to fluctuations in the number and/or species present by altering particular behaviors (Miller & Bassler, 2001). The N-acyl homoserine lactone QS signal molecule in *P. aeruginosa* will trigger the production of virulence factors such as rhamnolipids that have been shown to eliminate neutrophils in vitro (Van Gennip et al., 2009). Adding detection of known virulence genes to the molecular methods would be helpful in the process of interpretation.

Ideally, each wound should be carefully evaluated and in addition to traditional biofilm-based wound care strategies, an antimicrobial/antibiofilm treatment program with individualized therapeutic approaches should be identified for each patient's respective wound microflora (Smith et al., 2010; Wolcott et al., 2009). However, we do not have the tools for interpretation yet. First some questions should be asked when studying chronic wounds: What are the microorganisms doing to prevent healing of the wound? Can markers of the microbial community be identified that predict a change in infection dynamics and clinical outcomes? Would it be sufficient to search only for the presence of *Pseudomonas*? Can these new strategies directly characterize the impact of antimicrobial therapies, allowing treatment efficacy to be both assessed and optimized (Rogers et al., 2010)?

5. Conclusion

Longitudinal studies correlating multiple analyses of the microorganisms present in a chronic wound to patient metadata will increase our understanding of the problems that are caused by the microorganisms. The questions researchers should ask are: What role does every single bacterial and fungal species have in the ulcer? Which role does the biofilm formation play and is it the same for all species? Which virulence factors are the most important, and does QS play a role? The understanding of the exact function of the microorganisms in chronic wounds will make the use of molecular methods as a diagnostic tool highly relevant in the future. Only by obtaining thorough knowledge of this we will be able to develop sufficient treatment strategies for each individual ulcer. We find it premature to implement the new culture independent methods into daily clinical practice as it will drive the clinician to act on the results. The result of that could very well be the application of additional antibiotics because "if the bug is there, it must do harm". For now we do not know that, but we need to find out. Until then, the clinicians will have to rely on "Best-Practice Principals".

6. Acknowledgement

Bo Jørgensen is acknowledged for sampling; Vibeke Rudkjøbing, Masumeh Chavoshi, Martin Aasholm, Yijuan Xu and Per Halkjær Nielsen are acknowledged for scientific work and input.

7. References

Altschul, S. F., Madden, T. L., Schaffer, A. A., Zhang, J., Zhang, Z., Miller, W. & Lipman, D. J. (1997). Gapped BLAST and PSI-BLAST: a new generation of protein database search programs. *Nucleic Acids Research,* 25, 3389-3402.

Amann, R. I. (1995). In situ identification of microorganisms by whole cell hybridization with rRNA-targeted nucleic acid probes. In: *Molecular Microbial Ecology Manual* A. D. L. Akkermans, J. D. van Elsas & F. J. de Bruijn (Eds.), pp. MMEM-3.3.6/1-MMEM-3.3.6/15. London: Kluwer Academic Publications.

Andersen, A., Hill, K. E., Stephens, P., Thomas, D. W., Jorgensen, B., & Krogfelt, K. A. (2007). Bacterial profiling using skin grafting, standard culture and molecular bacteriological methods. *J Wound Care,* 16(4), 171-175.

Andersson, A., & mfl. (2007). Comparative analysis of human gut microbiota by barcoded pyrosequencing. *PLoS ONE, 3*(7), e2836.

Bitsch, M., Saunte, D. M., Lohmann, M., Holstein, P. E., Jorgensen, B., & Gottrup, F. (2005). Standardised method of surgical treatment of chronic leg ulcers. *Scand J Plast Reconstr Surg Hand Surg,* 39(3), 162-169.

Bogaert, D., Keijser, B., Huse, S., Rossen, J., Veenhoven, R., van Gils, E., et al. Variability and diversity of nasopharyngeal microbiota in children: a metagenomic analysis. *PLoS One,* 6(2), e17035.

Burmølle, M., Thomsen, T.R., Fazli, M., Dige, I., Christensen,L., Homøe, P. et al. (2010). Biofilms in chronic infections - a matter of opportunity - Monospecies biofilms in multispecies infections. *FEMS Immonol Med Micro,* 59(3), 324-336.

Costerton, J. W., Post, J. C., Ehrlich, G. D., Hu, F. Z., Kreft, R., Nistico, L., et al. (2011). New methods for the detection of orthopedic and other biofilm infections. *FEMS Immunol Med Microbiol,* 61(2), 133-140.

Dowd, S., Sun, Y., Secor, P., Rhoads, D., Wolcott, B., James, G., et al. (2008). Survey of bacterial diversity in chronic wounds using Pyrosequencing, DGGE, and full ribosome shotgun sequencing. *BMC Microbiology,* 8(1), 43.

Dowd, S. E., Delton Hanson, J., Rees, E., Wolcott, R. D., Zischau, A. M., Sun, Y., et al. (2010). Survey of fungi and yeast in polymicrobial infections in chronic wounds. *J Wound Care,* 20(1), 40-47.

Ecker, D. J., Sampath, R., Massire, C., Blyn, L. B., Hall, T. A., Eshoo, M. W., et al. (2008). Ibis T5000: a universal biosensor approach for microbiology. *Nat Rev Micro,* 6(7), 553-558.

Fazli, M., Bjarnsholt, T., Kirketerp-Moller, K., Jorgensen, B., Andersen, A., Krogfelt, K., et al. (2009). Nonrandom distribution of Pseudomonas aeruginosa and Staphylococcus aureus in chronic wounds. *J Clin Microbiol,* 47(12), 4084-4089.

Frankel, Y. M., Melendez, J. H., Wang, N.-Y., Price, L. B., Zenilman, J. M., & Lazarus, G. S. (2009). Defining Wound Microbial Flora: Molecular Microbiology Opening New Horizons. *Arch Dermatol,* 145(10), 1193-1195.

Kirketerp-Moller, K., Jensen, P., M, F., Madsen, K., Pedersen, J., Moser, C., et al. (2008). The distribution, organization and ecology of bacteria in chronic wounds. *J Clin Microbiol,* 46(8), 2717-2722.

Melendez, J. H., Frankel, Y. M., An, A. T., Williams, L., Price, L. B., Wang, N. Y., et al. (2009). Real-time PCR assays compared to culture-based approaches for identification of aerobic bacteria in chronic wounds. *Clin Microbiol Infect,* 16(12), 1762-1769.

Miller, M. B., & Bassler, B. L. (2001). Quorum sensing in bacteria. *Annu Rev Microbiol,* 55, 165-199.

Muyzer, G., De Waal, E. C., & Uitterlinden, A. G. (1993). Profiling of Complex Microbial Populations by Denaturing Gradient Gel Electrophoresis Analysis of Polymerase Chain Reaction-Amplified Genes Coding for 16S rRNA. App Env Micro, 59(3), 695-700.

Nielsen, M., Thomsen, T. R., Moser, C., Hoiby, N., & Nielsen, P. H. (2008). Use of cultivation-dependent and -independent techniques to assess contamination of central venous catheters: a pilot study. *BMC Clin Pathol,* 8(10).

Percival, S. L., Hill, K. E., Malic, S., Thomas, D. W., & Williams, D. W. (2011). Antimicrobial tolerance and the significance of persister cells in recalcitrant chronic wound biofilms. *Wound Repair Regen,* 19(1), 1-9.

Pichlmaier, M., Marwitz, V., Kühn, C., Niehaus, M., Klein, G., Bara, C., et al. (2008). High prevalence of asymptomatic bacterial colonization of rhythm management devices. *Europace,* 10(9), 1067-1072.

Price, L., Liu, C., Melendez, J., Frankel, Y., Engelthaler, D., Aziz, M., et al. (2009). Community analysis of chronic wound bacteria using 16S rRNA gene-based pyrosequencing: impact of diabetes and antibiotics on chronic wound microbiota. *PLoS ONE,* 4(7).

Price, L. B., Liu, C. M., Frankel, Y. M., Melendez, J. H., Aziz, M., Buchhagen, J., et al. (2010). Macroscale spatial variation in chronic wound microbiota: a cross-sectional study. *Wound Repair Regen,* 19(1), 80-88.

Rogers, G. B., Hoffman, L. R., Whiteley, M., Daniels, T. W., Carroll, M. P., & Bruce, K. D. (2010). Revealing the dynamics of polymicrobial infections: implications for antibiotic therapy. *Trends Microbiol,* 18(8), 357-364.

Ronaghi, M., Uhlen, M., & Nyren, P. (1998). A sequencing method based on real-time pyrophosphate. *Science,* 281(5375), 363, 365.

Smith, D. M., Snow, D. E., Rees, E., Zischkau, A. M., Hanson, J. D., Wolcott, R. D., et al. (2010). Evaluation of the bacterial diversity of pressure ulcers using bTEFAP pyrosequencing. *BMC Med Genomics,* 3, 41.

Stender, H. (2003). PNA FISH: an intelligent stain for rapid diagnosis of infectious diseases. *Expert Rev Mol Diagn,* 3(5), 649-655.

Stewart, F. J., Ottesen, E. A., & DeLong, E. F. (2010). Development and quantitative analyses of a universal rRNA-subtraction protocol for microbial metatranscriptomics. *ISME J,* 4(7), 896-907.

Thomsen, T. R., Aasholm, M. S., Rudkjøbing, V., Saunders, A., Bjarnsholt, T., Givskov, M., et al. (2010). The bacteriology of chronic venous leg ulcer examined by culture-independent molecular methods. Wound Repair and Regen 18(1), 38-49.

Van Gennip, M., Christensen, L. D., Alhede, M., Phipps, R., Jensen, P. O., Christophersen, L., et al. (2009). Inactivation of the rhlA gene in Pseudomonas aeruginosa prevents rhamnolipid production, disabling the protection against polymorphonuclear leukocytes. *Apmis,* 117(7), 537-546.

Wolcott, R., Gontcharova, V., Sun, Y., & Dowd, S. (2009). Evaluation of the bacterial diversity among and within individual venous leg ulcers using bacterial tag-encoded FLX and titanium amplicon pyrosequencing and metagenomic approaches. *BMC Microbiology,* 9(226).

20

Clinical Evaluation of Glyaderm, a Dermal Substitute Based on Glycerinized Donor Skin

Pirayesh A., Richters CD, Hoeksema H,
Verbelen J, Heyneman A and Monstrey S.
Burn centre, University Hospital, Gent
Euro Skin Bank, Beverwijk
Belgium
The Netherlands

1. Introduction

The main goal in burn management has always been increasing the survival of severely burned patients by rapid debridement and early closure of burn wounds, consequently reducing the risk of infection, sepsis and multi-organ failure. However, in the last decennia, surgical emphasis has shifted from survival to 'quality of survival', especially by improving the residual scars and preventing secondary contractures. Research and development of dermal skin substitutes has been directed towards improvement of scar quality by a bi-layered reconstruction of dermis and epidermis.

Allogeneic skin recovered from deceased donors is often used in the management of burns and other full thickness skin defects as a temporary coverage before definitive closure with autologous skin. Donor skin is used to improve the quality of the wound bed before grafting with autologous skin, as a biological dressing for partial thickness wounds (Hermans, 1989), or as overlay on widely expanded autograft (sandwich technique, Kreis et al., 1989). Excised full thickness defects treated with thin and widely expanded split thickness autografts often heal with an un-aesthetic, hypertrophic scar as final result as shown in figure 1.

In patients with extensive burns it is not possible to use thicker autografts with limited expansion because of increased donor site morbidity. These results may improve if a dermal subsitute is placed underneath the split thickness skin graft. This substitute can replace the dermal tissue that is lost and provide a scaffold to the cells infiltrating in the wound bed during the healing process. The scaffold must be designed in such a way the cells will produce the new collagen fibers in a random organized structure, replacing slowly the scaffold material instead of making the typical parallel oriented fibers of scars (Van der Veen et al., 2010). In the past decades, several dermal substitutes products have become available but the clinical evidence on the effectiveness is limited until now (Brusselaers et al., 2010). These commercially available products are based on animal derived collagen or human skin and associated with high costs (Jones et al., 2002).

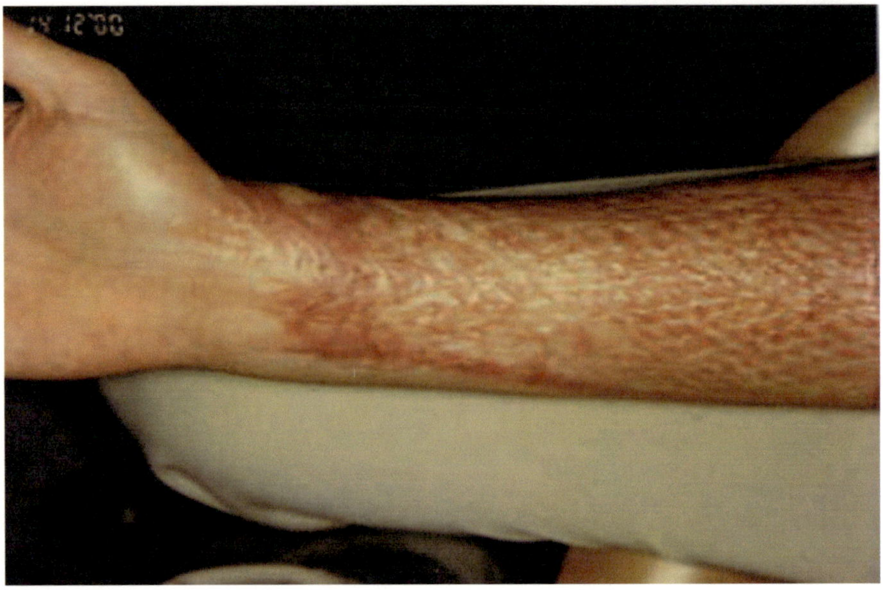

Fig. 1. Typical scar formation results after sandwich grafting, the mesh of the autologous skin graft pattern is still visible.

2. Development of dermal substitute

Dermal substitutes can be obtained from animal or human tissue as well as synthetic materials. The advantage of human skin is the presence of the natural collagen- elastin fibre network, providing the optimal three dimensional fibre structure for ingrowing fibroblast and blood vessels. Antigenic structures must be absent from the dermal substitute to avoid the induction of inflammatory processes that can worsen final scar quality. Human allogeneic skin has been applied to the wound as dermal substitute in the past as described by Cuono et al., 1987. In this method, the more immunogenic epidermis was removed several days after grafting the human donor skin and replaced by autogous cultured epithelial sheets. Technically, this method is difficult and in the allogeneic dermis cells of the donor remain present that can induce inflammation after wound closure. Therefore, several methods have been developed to remove the donor cells and hairs from the donor skin. This resulted in products known as Alloderm, Surederm, Graft jacket using enzymes and freeze drying techniques.

We have developed a cost-effective method to eliminate the antigenic structures by using low concentrations of sodium hydroxide (Richters et al. 2008). De-cellularization of glycerol 85% preserved skin starts by rinsing out the glycerol, thereafter the skin is incubated in 0.06M NaOH for 6 weeks. The NaOH solution is refreshed every week and finally neutralized. The acellular dermis is again preserved in glycerol 85%. This method avoids freezing which may damage the collagen and elastin fibers and, at the same time, it is very effective in washing out the donor cells and hairs. The prototypes, consisting of an intact, native collagen-elastin matrix obtained using the NaOH method were tested in a porcine model. Full thickness wounds of 4x4 cm were transplanted with the prototype and an autologous split skin graft meshed 1:3. Contraction of the wounds treated with this prototype was significantly lower compared to the control wounds, transplanted with only autologous skin (Richters et al., 2008, Pirayesh et al., 2007 and 2008). The six weeks treatment with NaOH showed the best results. Further experiments showed a two stage procedure was more optimal with the take rate of the autologous skin > 90% if the interval between application of the prototype and the autologous skin was 7 days. Final result with respect to contraction was comparable to Integra in this porcine model but the scar was more smooth (Pirayesh et al., 2011, manuscript in preparation). This encouraging results let to the first pilot of clinical experiments on burn patients.

3. Clinical application of Glyaderm

This novel dermal substitute is called Glyaderm, which is an abbreviation for Glycerol-preserved Acellular Dermis. Before application of Glyaderm, the wound bed must show viable granulation tissue. In most cases, woundbed preparation with allogeneic donor skin is needed; in burns this takes about 7 days after debridement. Glyaderm is preserved in

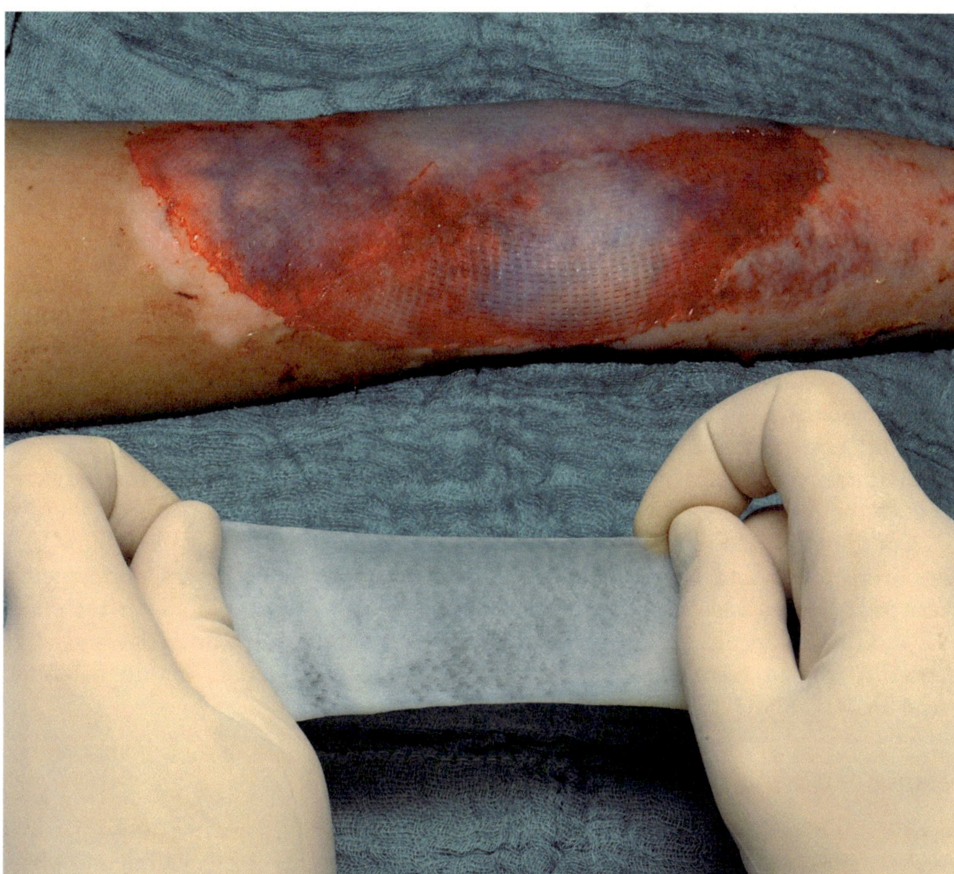

Fig. 2. Example of Glyaderm

85% glycerol and must be rinsed in sterile 0.9% NaCl before use on the patient. The Glyaderm is meshed 1:1 to allow drainage of wound fluid. Glyaderm was used on the patients also in a two stage procedure in clinical studies, approved by the local ethics committee of the University of Ghent, Belgium. A pilot study and a comparative study were performed sofar.

4. Pilot study

In the first non-randomized pilot experiments 15 patients with full thickness burns (TBSA < 40%) were selected to study the optimal wound dressing, to avoid dehydration and bacterial contamination of the Glyaderm during the first days before the autologous skin was applied. Then a group of 10 patients with full thickness wounds was selected (5 with burns and 5 with reconstructive wounds) and was treated to define the optimal time between the two operations using Laser Doppler Imaging. The depth of the burn wounds was first assessed using laser Doppler imaging (Monstrey et al., 2007) to assure the wounds were deep dermal. The patients were recruited and treated with Glyaderm and split thickness skin graft after wound bed preparation with glycerol preserved allografts. Patient demographics were recorded and Laser Doppler imaging was used to monitor the vascularization of glyaderm. We also discovered that Laser Doppler Imaging allows us to measure wound tissue perfusion and monitor daily ingrowth of blood vessels into the dermal substitute. This allows us to know the exact timeframe in which the dermal bed is vascularised enough and skin grafting can be carried out. This is typically after 5-7 days, much shorter than the period necessary for ingrowth of the currently most widely used commercial dermal substitute Integra (Dantzer et al., 2001)

4.1 Randomised, controlled, paired, intra-individual Comparative study in 30 patients

After completing the pilot studies, a comparative study was performed. Patients with full thickness burns or full thickness lower arm defects after free flap harvesting were recruited. Part of the wounds were treated with Glyadem and split thickness skin and the other part with split thickness skin only. This was done in anatomically related areas to allow paired, intra-individual comparison of the wound healing. Preferably, a left/right comparison was made and the experimental treatment was randomized. Patient demographics were recorded and at regular follow up time points of 1, 3, 6 and 12 months after wound closure biopsies were taken and objective and subjective scar assessment was performed. The dermatospectrometer was used to measure scar colour, Dermalab cutometer for pliability and the modified Vancouver scar scale as well as a contour scale (Brusselaers et al 2010) were used. All data were recorded in a purpose designed database and subjected to statistical analysis with SPSS software package.

5. Results of the pilot study

All recruited patients responded well to a dressing regimen of surfasoft, a semipermeable membrane, with betadine gel and paraffin gauze in terms of bacterial control and prevention from desiccation of Glyaderm with capital. Laser Doppler Imaging proved to show enhanced vascularization from day 1 to day 5 allowing to exactly delineate the optimal engraftment interval. This was found to be 6 days with a 1 day standard deviation.

The increase in blood vessel growth can be observed clearly in Figure 3, the areas with a red color represent blood vessel flow and these are larger on day 7 in this patient. The take of the Glyaderm was > 90% and the take of the autologous skin > 95%. The results with respect to scar formation in this pilot study were encouraging. Figure 4 shows pictures of the wound and final scar of the same patient as in Figure 3. The color of the scar is not red and the patient is able to move the head normally, indicating good elasticity.

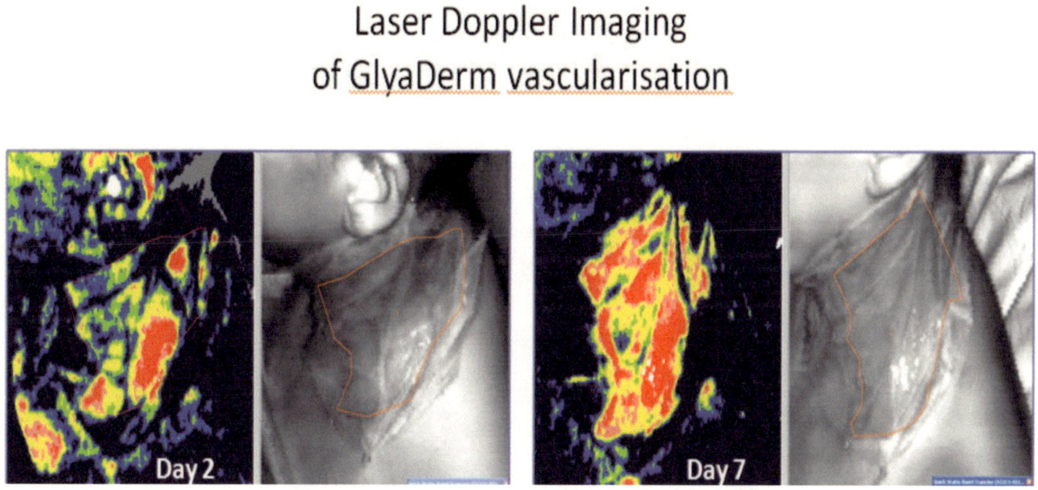

Fig. 3. Shows the growth of blood vessels in a deep burn wound treated with Glyaderm

6. Results of the comparative study

The take rates in the STSG on Glyaderm were comparable to the take rates in the wounds with a STSG alone (Wilcoxon Singed Ranks Test $Z = -0.823$, $p = .41$). Pliability and Visual Scores and contour scale assessment indicate a trend of improvement with Glyaderm treatments; however, follow-up times are currently too short with small numbers to be able to draw conclusions, we expect a necessary follow-up interval of two years. Comparing the Dermalab measurements for elasticity "Glyaderm + STSG" versus "STSG alone" statistics indicate that: Glyaderm + STSG" has significantly more elasticity when compared to "STSG alone" 1 month and 12 months after wound closure.

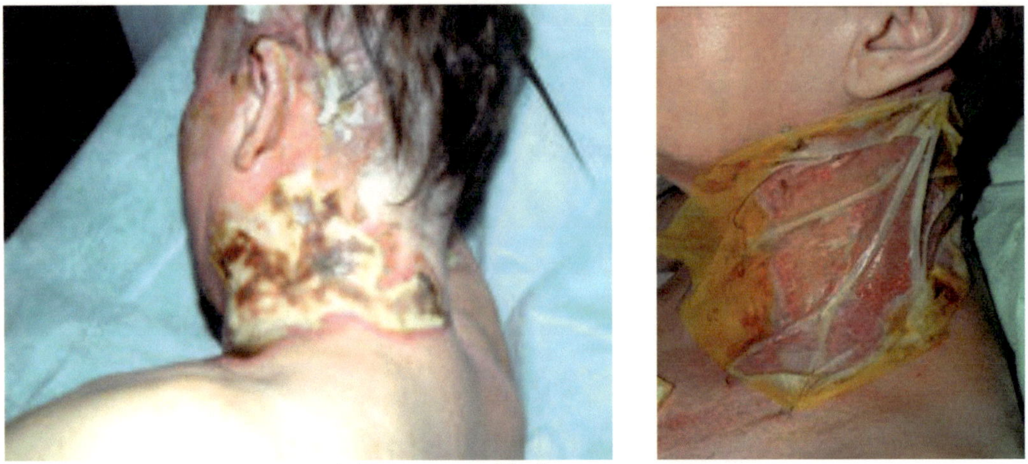

A: Burn wound before treatment

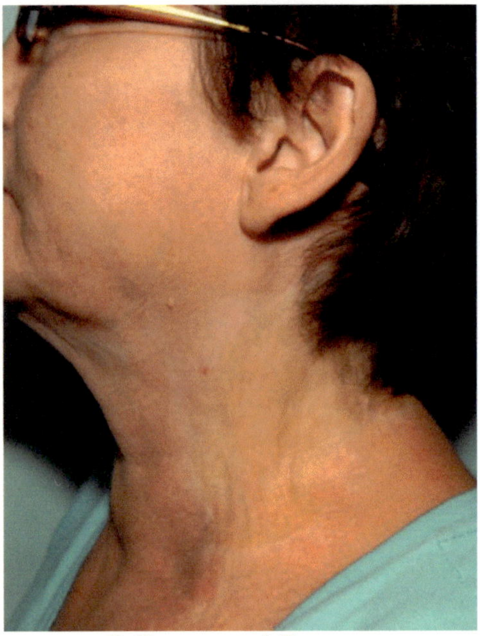

B: Two years follow-up

Fig. 4. Final results of this wound with respect to scar formation show a cosmetic good quality of the scar.

7. Conclusion

The results of the comparative, controlled, intra-individual clinical study show beneficial effects of a dermal substitute on the elasticity of the scar. The natural structure of the collagen and elastin fibers in glyaderm may have contributed to this effect. Glyaderm is the first non-commercial dermal substitute that can compete with all currently available dermal equivalents. Laser Doppler imaging allows monitoring of vascular ingrowth in dermal substitutes such as Glyaderm. Although most burn experts advocate the use of dermal substitutes, the challenge remains to objectively show the perceived benefit over split thickness skin grafting alone. The evolving evaluation with objective scar assessment tools within these studies may help to demonstrate this benefit in the near future.

Our next study with Glyaderm has started recently; a multi-centre clinical study in major European Burn centers. To allow also quality of life and cost-effectiveness studies, 60 patients will be treated with glyaderm + STSG and 60 patients with STSG alone.

Researchers continue their quest for the ideal skin substitute, and in the future it should be possible to create such an advanced skin substitute, containing melanocytes, hair follicles and sebaceous glands. The available products remain rather expensive, due to commercial incentives, high manufacturing costs, special shipment and storage conditions. Nevertheless, accelerated healing and closure of the wound will reduce the labour intensive dressing changes, hospital stay and the need for reconstructive surgery. Until the optimal off the shelve skin substitute becomes available, the burn surgeon can improve aesthetic and functional outcome by choosing from the gamut of currently available scaffolds for bilayered skin restoration. Glyaderm may well be an optimal cost-effective solution to bridge this gap in the near future.

8. References

Brusselaers N, Pirayesh A, Hoeksema H, Richters CD, Verbelen J, Beele H, Blot SI, Monstrey S. J Trauma 2010; 68: 490-501.

Brusselaers N, Pirayesh A, Hoeksema H, Verbelen J, Blot S, Monstrey S. Burn scar assessment: a systematic review of objective scar assessment tools. Burns 2010, 36:1157-1164.

Cuono CB, Langdon R, Birchall N, Barttelbart S, McGuire J. Composite autologous-allogeneic skin replacement: development and clinical application. Plast Recon Surg 1987, 80: 626-637.

Dantzer E, Braye FM. Reconstructive surgery using an artificial dermis (Integra): results with 39 grafts. Br J Plast Surg. 2001, 54: 659-664.

Hermans MHE. Clinical experience with glycerol preserved donor skin treatment in partial thickness burns. Burns 1989; 15: 57-60.

Jones I., Currie L., Martin P. A guide to biological skin substitutes. Br J Plast Surg 2002, 55: 185-193.

Kreis RW, Vloemans AFPM., Hoekstra MJ, Mackie DP, Hermans RP. The use of non-viable glycerol-preserved cadaver skin combined with widely expanded autografts in the treatment of extensive third-degree burns. J Trauma 1989; 29:51-55

Monstrey S, Hoeksema H, Verbelen J, Pirayesh A, Blondeel P. Assessment of burn depth and burn wound healing potential. Burns 2008; 34:761-769.

Pirayesh A, Monstrey S, Blondeel P, Hoekstra H, Vanoorbeek J, Hoeksema H, Richters CD. Development of a novel dermal substitute based on glycerinized allograft: Clinical (Phase I) and experimental evaluation. Burns 2007; 33:S13

Pirayesh A., Dur A.F.M., Paauw N.J., Monstrey S., Kreis R.W., Hoekstra M.J., Richters C.D. Evaluation of acellular dermis for closure of abdominal wall defects in a rat model. Eur Surg res 2008; 41 :345-352.

Pirayesh A., Hoeksema H, Richters CD, Monstrey S. Determination of the optimal time interval between application of a dermal substitute and grafting with autologous skin using Laser Doppler Imaging. Manuscript in preparation.

Richters C.D., Pirayesh A., Hoeksema H., Kamperdijk E.W.A., Kreis R.W., Dutrieux R.P., Monstrey S., Hoekstra M.J. Development of a dermal matrix from glycerol preserved allogeneic skin. Cell and Tissue Banking 2008; 9 : 309-315.

Van der Veen V, Van der Wal MB, Van Leeuwen MC, Ulrich MM. Midelkoop E. Biological background of dermal substitutes. Burns 2010; 36: 305-321.

21

External Wire Frame Fixation for Skin Grafts

Rei Ogawa and Hiko Hyakusoku
Department of Plastic, Reconstructive and Aesthetic Surgery, Nippon Medical School, Tokyo Japan

1. Introduction

Skin grafting has been used widely for various reconstructions. The complete survival of the skin graft is necessary for functional and aesthetic restoration, as incomplete survival delays wound healing and results in severe primary and secondary contraction of the graft and scar contractures. To promote successful skin grafting, bleeding of the recipient wound bed must be arrested during surgery and the graft must be appropriately compressed and completely fixed to prevent shearing against the wound bed. After the operation, it is necessary to maintain the compression force and fixation of the graft for at least 5–7 days.

One of the difficulties associated with skin grafting is differences in recipient site conditions. Areas that are difficult to graft are mobile areas such as the joints and the neck, and areas that have a free border, such as the eyelids and the perioral area. The authors currently use the external wire-frame fixation method[1-5] for reliable skin grafting, in particular when these areas are involved. This technique is useful for securing the graft to the wound bed and it prevents the graft edges from lifting. In addition, it can sometimes be used to fix joints at the same time. This technique is introduced and discussed in this chapter.

2. Technique and methods

During surgery, the skin graft is fixed with sutures as usual (Fig. 1-1). At the same time, a wire frame of 0.7–1.0 mm-diameter Kirschner wire that has the shape of the graft is created. In the case of digital skin grafts, the wire frame can be slightly larger than the recipient site so that the digital joint(s) can be fixed at the same time and results in a three-dimensional wire frame. To ensure that the frame edges do not stick out, the ends of the Kirschner wire meet each other in a thin plastic tube, such as the outer sheath of an indwelling needle. The wire frame shape should be adjusted finely to ensure that it does not induce a pressure ulcer.

The wire frame is placed onto the graft and attached with the same sutures that were used to stitch the graft (Figs. 1-2 – 1-7). Finally, tie-over fixation is performed in the usual manner with appropriate pressure (Figs. 1-8 – 1-11).

The tie-over and the wire frame are removed about seven days later in the case of full-thickness skin grafts, and five days later in the case of split-thickness skin grafts, prior to removing the grafted skin sutures. The patient can then begin rehabilitating the affected sites.

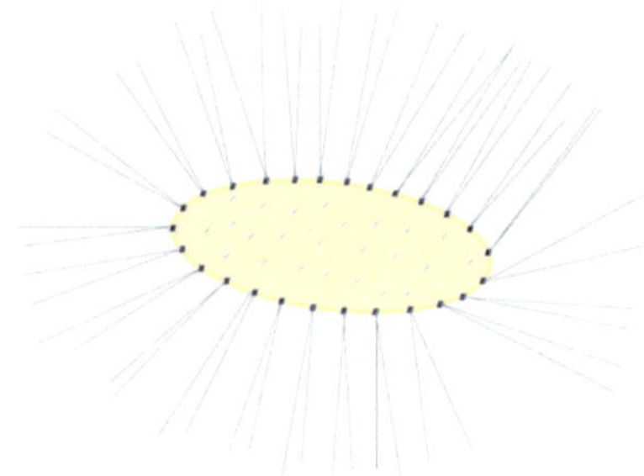

Fig. 1-1. The skin graft is sutured to the recipient site by 4-0 or 5-0 nylon or polypropylene sutures.

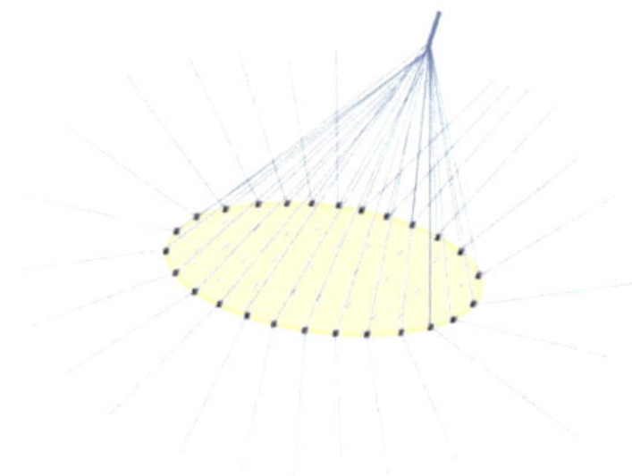

Fig. 1-2. One end of each suture is lifted and bound to the others, thus forming a hank.

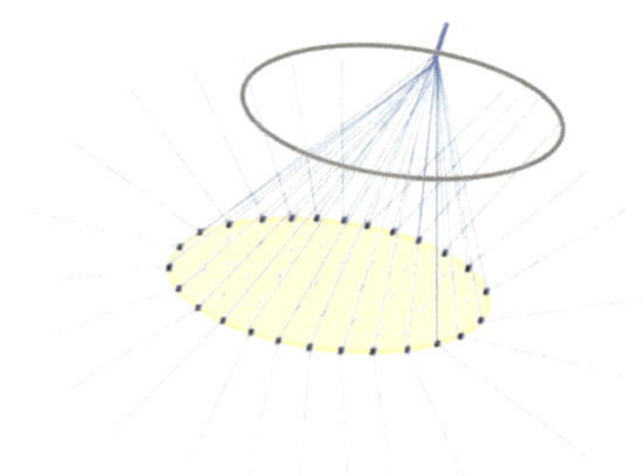

Fig. 1-3. The external wire frame is placed over the hank formed by the sutures.

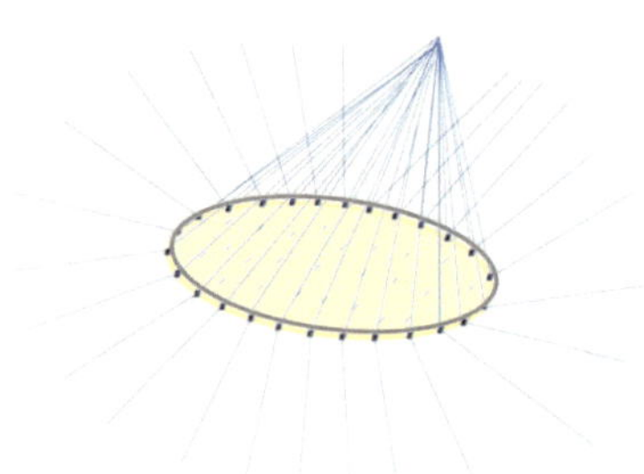

Fig. 1-4. The external wire frame is fitted onto the grafted skin.

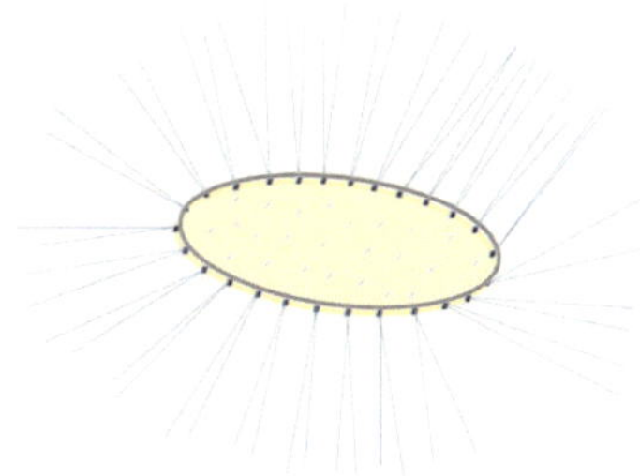

Fig. 1-5. The sutures are released from the hank.

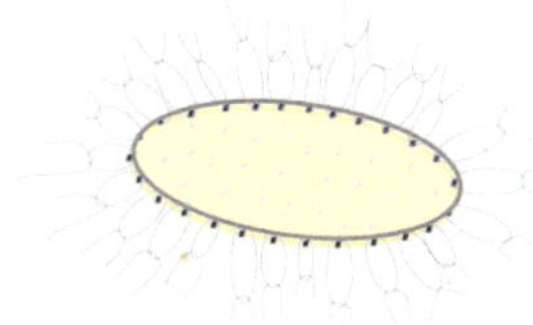

Fig. 1-6. To tie up and fix the external wire frame, the sutures are knotted.

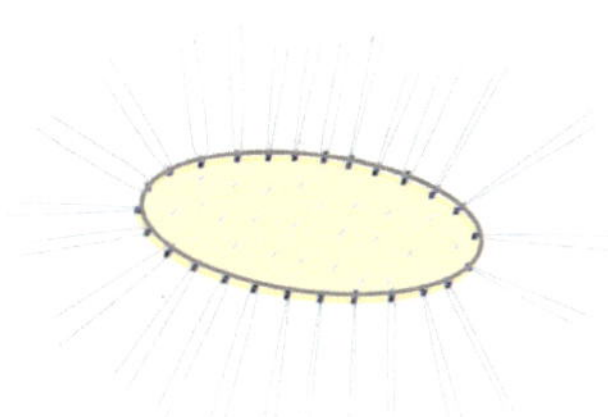

Fig. 1-7. The external wire frame is fixed tightly, with care taken to ensure that a pressure ulcer does not arise.

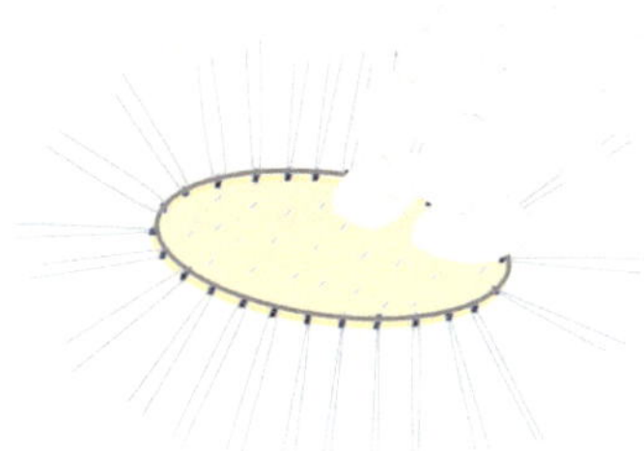

Fig. 1-8. Tie-over gauze is placed onto the grafted skin.

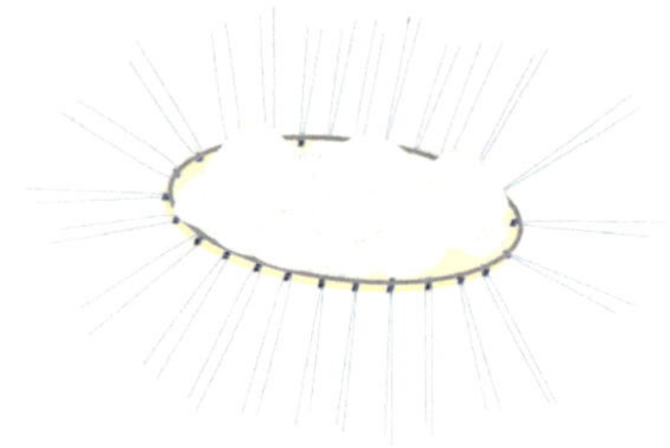

Fig. 1-9. The tie-over gauze is arranged so that its volume is distributed equally over the graft.

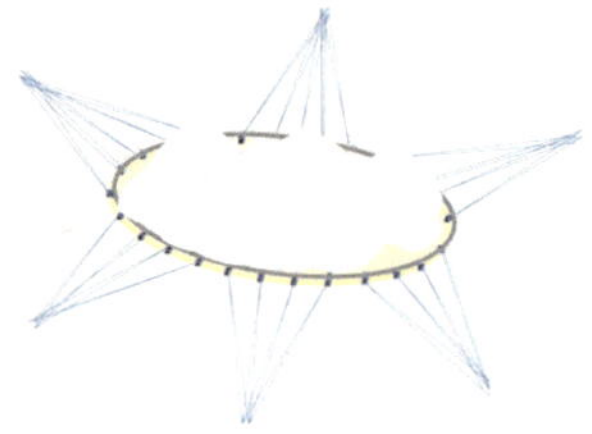

Fig. 1-10. The sutures are divided into 4–6 sets and bound into hanks.

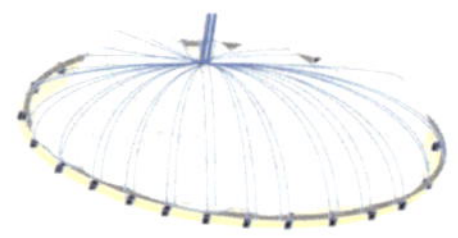

Fig. 1-11. The suture hanks that oppose each other diametrically are tied up, thus completing the tie-over fixation.

3. Discussion

With regard to eyelid skin grafts, the wire frame can eliminate the need for tarsorrhaphy, as an external wire frame allows the patient to open his or her eyes immediately after surgery without causing the skin grafts to move[2,5]. With regard to the perioral area, an external wire frame allows the patient to start eating immediately after surgery (Fig. 2-1 and 2-2). Moreover, the three-dimensional external wire frames[3] used with digits are useful for fixing the digital joint(s) as well as the skin graft (Fig. 3-1 and 3-2). If external fixation method is used for digital skin grafting, the digital joints do not need to be fixed by pinning the digit with Kirschner wire. Thus, external wire frames are particularly useful for the grafting of the palmar surfaces of the fingers.

In summary, external wire frame fixation can secure skin grafts to the wound bed with homogeneous pressure and reduce shear force at the periphery, thereby promoting skin graft take. It provides reliable but not excessive fixation that permits the early movement and rehabilitation that promotes functional and aesthetic restoration. It is a simple, cheap and individualized technique that is associated with easy perioperative management and nursing.

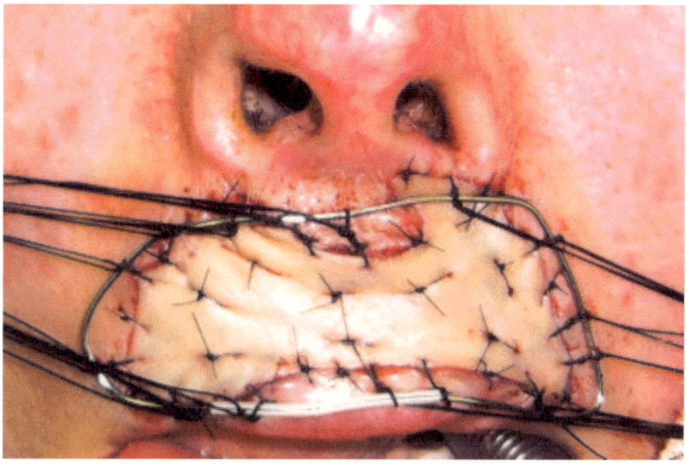

Fig. 2-1. Skin graft with external wire frame on the upper lip (intra-operative view)

Patient started to eatimmediately after surgery.

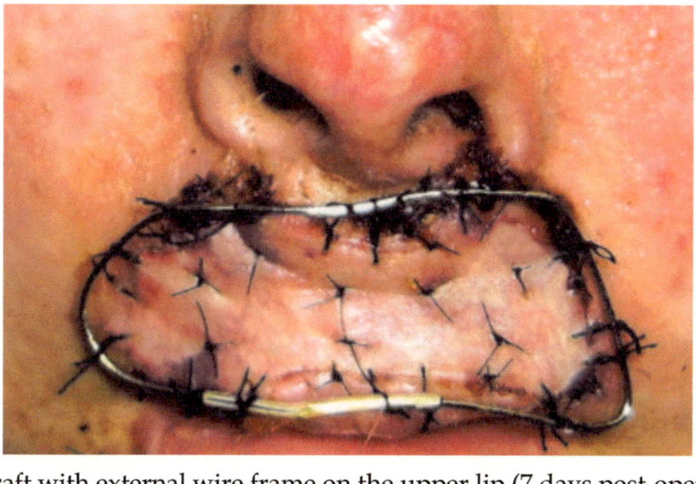

Fig. 2-2. Skin graft with external wire frame on the upper lip (7 days post-operative view)

Grafted skin survived completely.

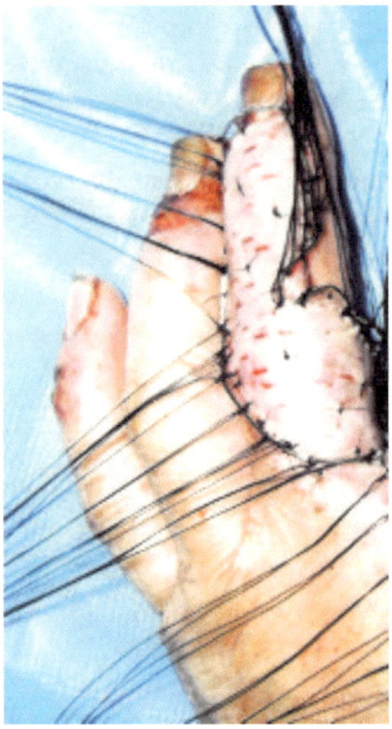

Fig. 3-1. Three-dimensional external wire frames used with digits (intra-operative view)

The digital joints did not need to be fixed by pinning using Kirschner wire.

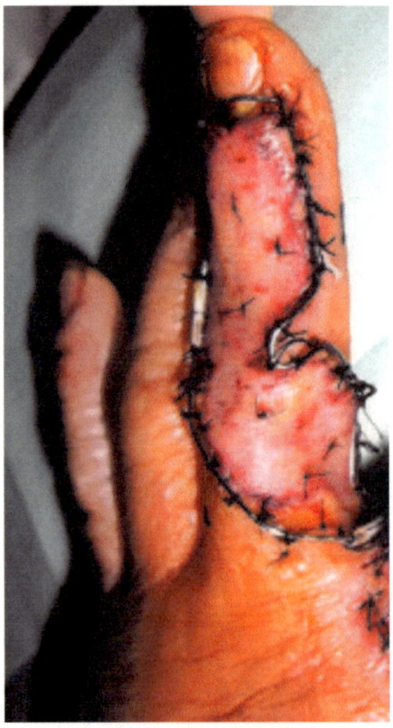

Fig. 3-2. Three-dimensional external wire frames used with digits (7 days post-operative view)

The grafted skin survived completely.

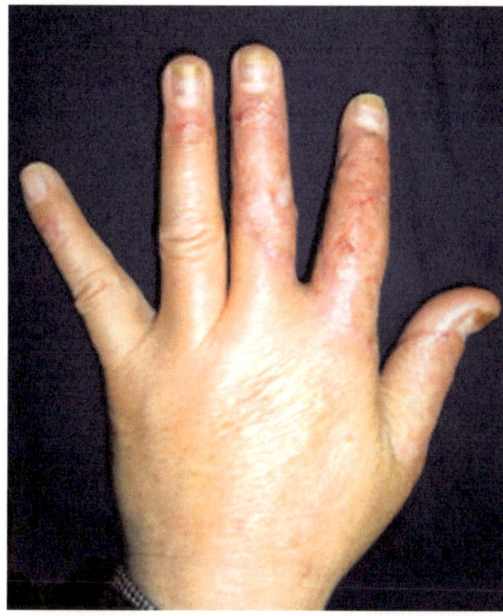

Fig. 3-3. Three-dimensional external wire frames used with digits (6 months post-operative view)

There were no functional limitation.

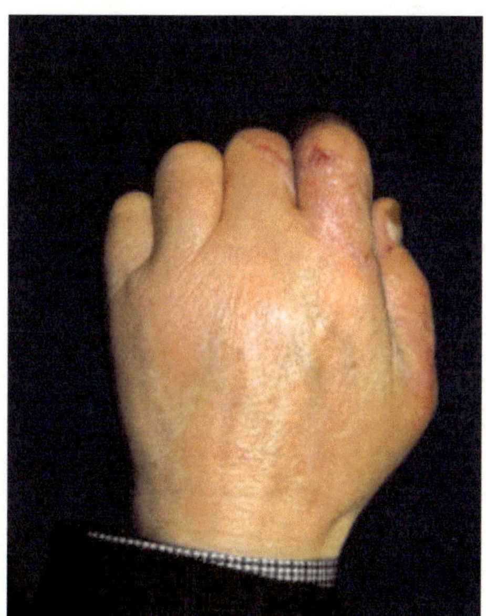

Fig. 3-4. Three-dimensional external wire frames used with digits (6 months post-operative view)

There were no functional limitation.

4. References

[1] Hirai T, Hyakusoku H, Fumiiri M. The use of a wire frame to fix grafts externally. Br J Plast Surg 1991; 44: 69-70.

[2] Murakami M, Hyakusoku H, Ishimaru S. External wire frame fixation of eyelid graft. Br J Plast Surg 2003; 56: 312-13.

[3] Ogawa R, Aoki S, Aoki M, Oki K, Hyakusoku H. Three-dimensional external skin graft fixation of digital skin graft. Plast Reconstr Surg. 2007 Jan;119(1):440-2.

[4] Ogawa R, Hyakusoku H, Ono S. Useful tips for successful skin grafting. J Nippon Med Sch 2007; 74: 386-92.

[5] Murakami M, Ogawa R, Hyakusoku H. Efficacy of 'rugby-ball shape' skin grafting using external wire frame fixation without tarsorrhaphy for lower eyelid reconstruction. J Plast Reconstr Aesthet Surg 2010; 63: e220-1.

22

Efficacy of Autogenous Dermis Graft for Wound Coverage

Seung-Kyu Han
Department of Plastic Surgery
Korea University College of Medicine Seoul,
Korea

1. Introduction

Skin grafting is the easiest and the most reliable way to obtain proper wound coverage. However, the two major concerns of skin grafting are the poor color match in the recipient sites and donor site morbidity including pain, discomfort, and hypertrophic scarring. Major pigment mismatches are common in split-thickness grafts particularly in darker skinned patients including Asians (Fig. 1). Several factors may play a role in the color mismatch of a regular skin graft. These include the amount of melanin, the degree of transfer of melanosomes to keratinocytes, and the number of melanocytes (Carlson et al., 2002; Velangi & Rees, 2001). Because the melanocytes are localized to the basal cell layer of the epidermis, the origin of the color mismatch has been assumed to be in the epidermal melanin (Tyack et al., 1997; Swope et al., 2002). Because regular skin grafts transferred to new locations maintain their epidermal specificity, a pigmentation difference with the surrounding skin is unavoidable.

To minimize the limitations of the classic skin graft, the author has developed a dermis graft, which is a deepithelialized split thickness skin graft, and have reported promising results of the method for coverage of small to medium sized wounds on the body (Han et al., 2007). The important aspects of this method involve the immediate return of the epidermis to the donor site in order to overcome the donor site morbidity and minimize the pigment mismatch between graft and surrounding skin by restoring the epidermal portion of the recipient site through inducing epithelization from the adjacent skin.

The purpose of this chapter is to present usefulness of the dermis graft in a wound coverage.

2. Surgical technique

After sharp debridement of the recipient site, skin and underlying subcutaneous tissue of the wound margin is undermined approximately 5mm in length along the periphery and meticulous hemostasis is obtained. The defect size of the recipient site measures. A thin epidermal flap is elevated on the gluteal area or the lateral thigh using a Zimmer dermatome, in which the thickness is set to 0.010 inches. The blade is then reset to 0.012 to 0.020 inches and the dermis to be grafted is cut from the same area. The previously elevated epidermal flap is replaced on the donor site and sutured with prolene. The harvested dermis is tailored to the size and shape of the defect including the undermined area and transferred

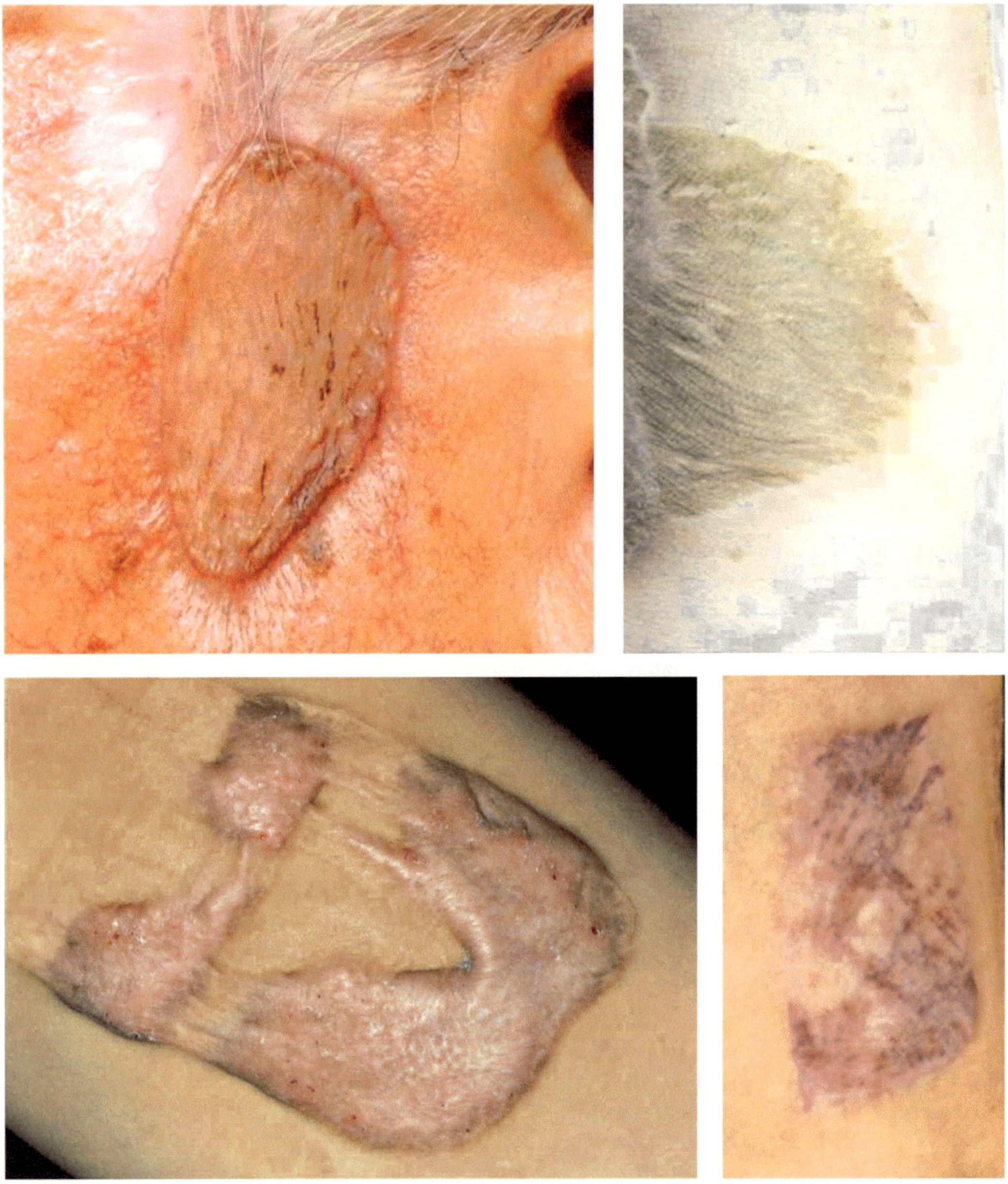

Fig. 1. Two major concerns of skin grafting. (*Above*) Poor color match in the recipient sites. (*Below*) Hypertrophic scar formation on the donor sites.

to the recipient site. The edge of the dermis graft is inserted into the undermined wound margin and fixed to the wound bed along the circumference of the defect using PDS sutures. The undermined marginal skin over the grafted dermis is then fixed to the underlying dermis using prolene sutures (Fig. 2). The skin sutures are removed after approximately 5 - 7 days in order to reduce the stitch marks. Sunshine is avoided for the first three to six months using sun-blocking agents.

3. Indication

The dermis graft is indicated in any cases with small to medium sized skin defect (smaller than 42.0 cm^2 based on the author's experience). Especially, a dermis graft is likely to have its greatest reconstructive role on the exposed areas such as the face, neck, forearms, and hands. In fairly large wounds (larger than 42.0 cm^2 based on the author's experience), the return of the patients to their normal daily activities is likely to be delayed because the epithelization of the graft takes a longer time. There is no data on the critical size or thickness of the dermis that can produce scar-free wound healing. Therefore, further study will be needed.

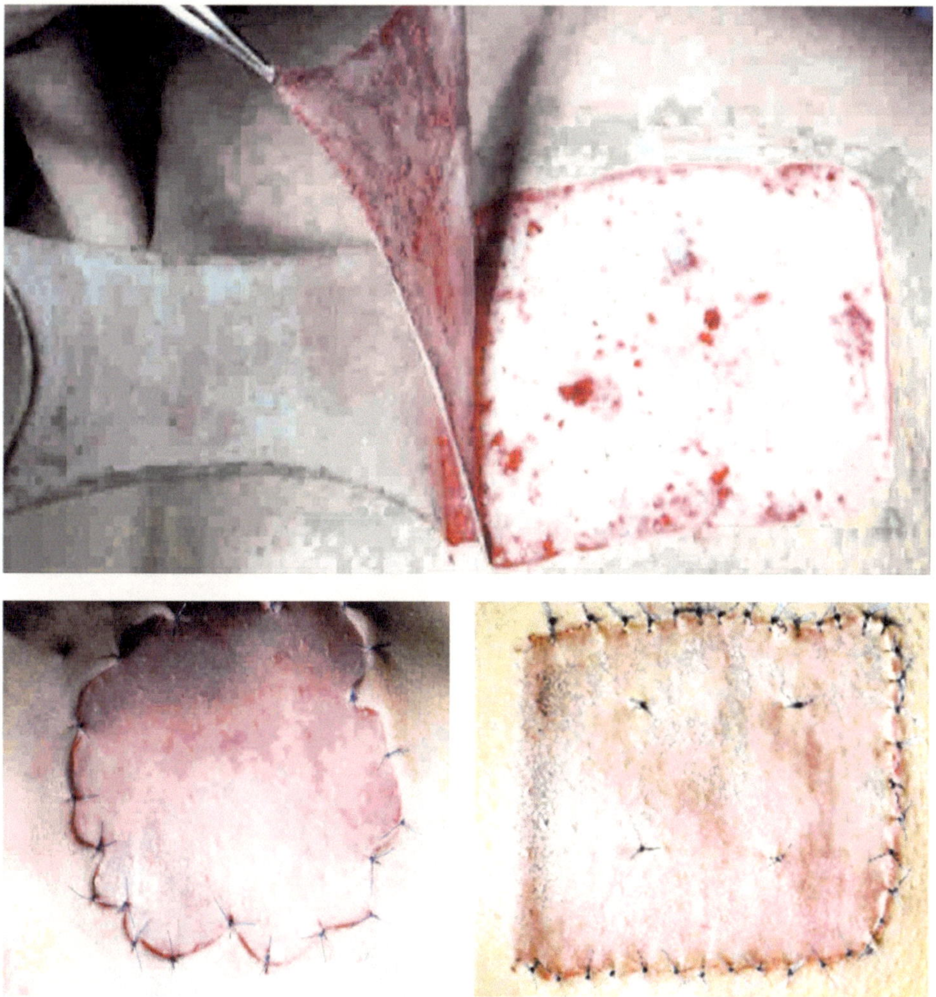

Fig. 2. (*Above*) The thin epidermal flap is elevated on the gluteal area, the dermis to be grafted is then cut on the same area. *(Below, left)* The edge of the dermis graft is inserted into the undermined wound margin and fixed to the wound bed along the circumference of the defect. (*Below, right*) The previously elevated epidermal flap is replaced on the donor site.

It was found that a full thickness small sized wound, which was left to heal by secondary intention, sometimes resulted in acceptable scarring in a concave area of the skin. In some wounds, however, a period of several weeks or months is required for complete healing, particularly in actinically damaged, fragile skin. Wounds on convex areas of the skin heal rather poorly (depressed scar) via secondary intention. The resultant wound contraction, which is an important clinical component, is not an uncommon problem (Fig. 3). Skin or dermal substitutes, which are currently produced by advanced technology, may replace the regular skin graft (Kuroyanagi et al., 2001; Terino et al., 2001). However, these procedures usually heal with a significantly conspicuous and unfavorable scar (Figs. 4 and 5). Further improvements are required in such technology to obtain a favorably aesthetic result as obtained with the dermis graft method.

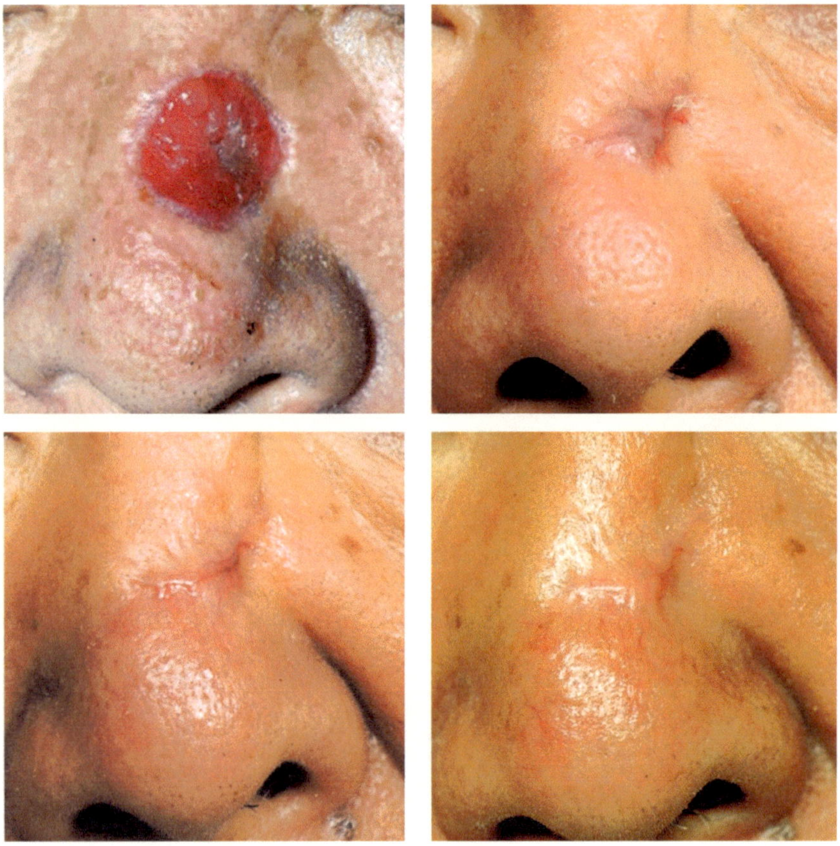

Fig. 3. An open wound on nasal dorsum, which was left to heal by secondary intention, resulted in a conspicuous wound contraction.

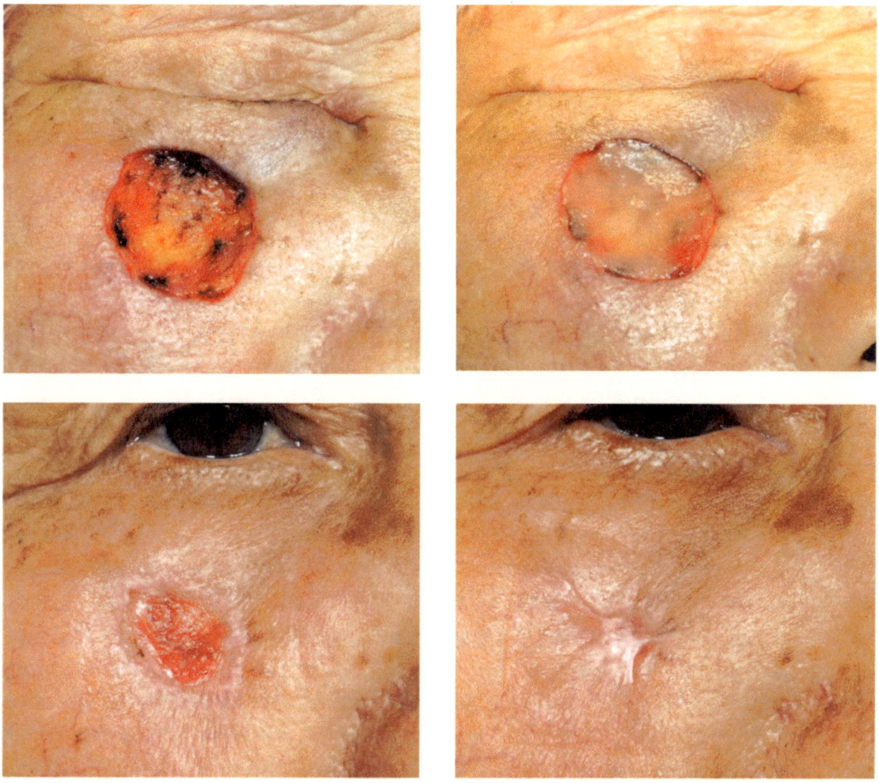

Fig. 4. A full thickness skin defect on a lower eyelid healed by grafting of an artificial dermis. The resultant scar was prominent with contraction.

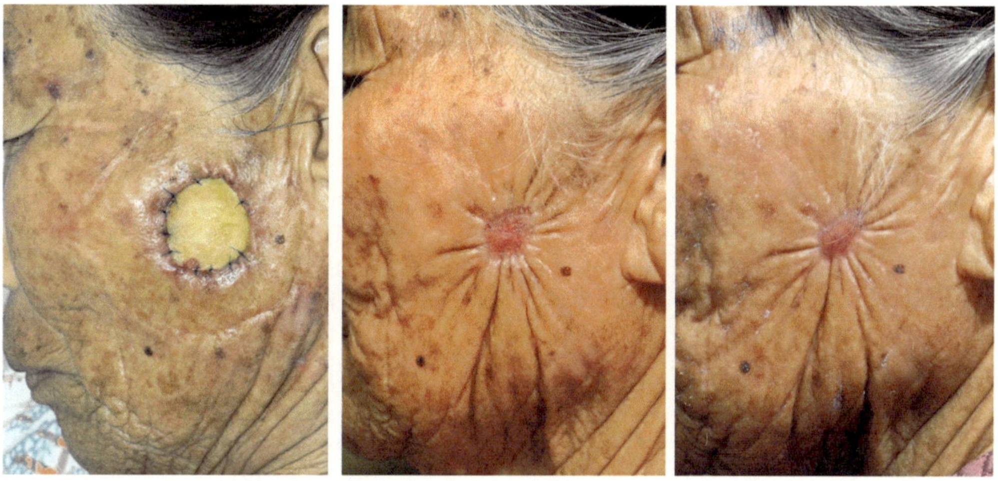

Fig. 5. A wound on cheek healed by grafting of an allogenic dermis. The resultant scar was unfavorable.

4. Author's experience

4.1 Clinical research

The author has evaluated the efficacy of the dermis graft used for wound coverage by comparing it with that of a regular skin graft (Han et al., 2007). The patients included in the study provided informed written consent for the study, but has not been registered in an official database of the institutional review board.

4.1.1 Patients and methods

From April of 2001 to March of 2004, the dermis graft was applied to 53 patients (17 male, 36 female), ranging in age from 6 to 61 years (average, 36.5 years). The size of the wound ranged from 2.7 to 42.0 cm^2, with a mean and a median size of 12.0 and 10.5 cm^2, respectively. The recipient sites were located as follows: 8 on the face, 6 on the forearm, 34 on the hand, 4 on the lower extremities, and 1 on the back. Simultaneously, a regular split thickness skin graft procedure was performed on the wounds of approximately the same size and location as the dermis graft in 33 patients. The size of the regular skin graft wound ranged from 2.3 to 42.0 cm^2, with a mean and a median size of 14.0 and 12.0 cm^2, respectively. The locations of the wound were as follows: 3 on the face, 6 on the forearm, 21 on the hand, and 3 on the lower extremities. This provided an opportunity to compare the results of the dermis graft with those of the regular skin graft. Prior to classifying the patients into the two treatment groups, detailed information of the new procedure (dermis graft), which included the surgical techniques, advantages, and disadvantages, was provided to each patient. The patients were classified according to their compliance. Compliant patients who fully understood and agreed to the new procedure underwent a dermis graft and noncompliant patients who did not want the new procedure underwent a regular skin graft.

The healing time for both groups was compared. The mean follow-up time was 12.4 months ranging from 3 months to 2 years. Twenty-six dermis graft patients and 20 regular skin graft patients had more than a 12-month follow-up period. The scar condition was evaluated in these long-term follow-up patients by two blind observers (plastic surgery residents in training at the author's institution) after a 12 to 24 month follow-up (average, 15.7 months for the dermis graft group and 15.0 months for the regular skin graft group) according to the Vancouver Scar Scale (VSS), which included pigmentation, scar height, pliability, and vascularity (Vloemans et al., 2003; Sullival et al., 1990). The averaged scores of the two observers were used as data for the analysis.

The patients' satisfaction for the donor and recipient site was also surveyed in the long-term follow-up patients. The patients' satisfaction was compared using a Visual Analogue Scale (VAS) with a score of 0 being the worst and 5 being the best. Statistical comparisons for the data of the VSS and the VAS were performed using a Mann-Whitney U-test. P values < 0.05 were considered significant.

4.1.2 Results

The graft take was complete in all patients in both groups. Refilling of the blood vessels and multiple pin point bleeding was observed on the grafted dermis within the first 2 to 3 days. Reepithelization occurred progressively from the periphery to the center of the grafted dermis.

The whole wound of the dermis graft had reepithelialized after grafting within 11 to 20 days (average 15.5±1.9 days). The skin grafted wounds had healed by 7 to 16 days (average 11.8±1.6 days). In the long-term follow-up, good quality skin characteristics were achieved in the dermis graft.

A comparison of the scars at the recipient site, as assessed by the VSS, showed that the dermis graft was superior to the regular skin graft in terms of pigmentation, height, and vascularity ($p<0.05$). No significant difference in pliability was detected. The overall average VSS scores of the dermis and skin graft were 1.0±1.1 and 1.6±1.1, respectively ($p<0.05$). The patients' satisfaction in the dermis graft group, as assessed by the VAS, was also better than that in skin graft group (4.2±0.9 and 3.4±1.1 each).

Regarding the donor sites, the results of the dermis graft were also satisfactory. All the donor sites of dermis graft healed within 9 days (average 7.5±0.8 days). In contrast, those of the regular skin graft required 11 to 16 days to heal (average 12.8±1.1 days). The donor sites of the dermis graft were also superior to those of the skin graft in terms of scar quality and patient satisfaction. The average of overall VSS scores for the donor sites of the dermis graft and regular skin graft were 0.7±0.9 and 1.3±0.7 each ($p<0.05$). The average VAS scores for the dermis and skin graft donors were 4.1±1.3 and 2.8±0.8 each ($p<0.05$). There were no significant complications and no functionally relevant scar in either group (Fig. 6).

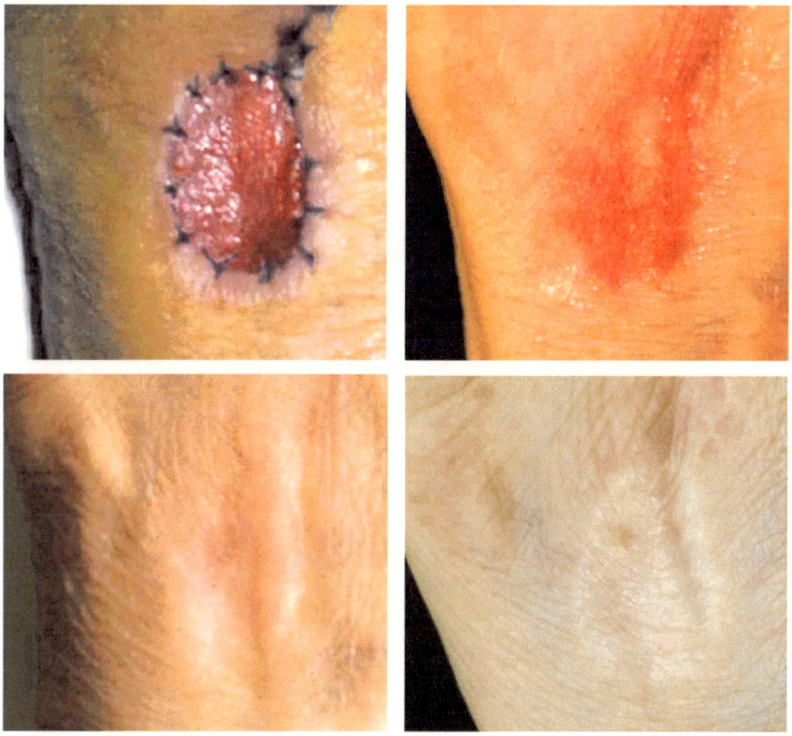

Fig. 6. A woman received a venous island flap coverage to reconstruct an amputated finger tip. *(Above, left)* The donor site was covered by a dermis graft harvested from her buttock. *(Above, right)* Two-month postoperative view. *(Below, left)* Eight-month postoperative view. *(Below, right)* Fourteen-month postoperative view, which demonstrated excellent color match with the adjacent skin.

4.2 Dermis graft on face after removal of skin cancer

The author has evaluated the reliability of the dermis graft for covering defects after removal of non-melanoma skin cancer on the face. Surgical excision of skin cancer leaves a soft tissue defect which requires reconstruction. Proper selection of reconstruction method is the key point to get a successful result on the face. In planning reconstruction for facial defects, reconstructive efforts should start from the safest and least invasive methods while achieving optimal functional and cosmetic outcomes. A variety of methods can be used to cover the defects; healing by secondary intention, a primary closure, a skin graft, and a local flap. Healing by secondary intention usually leaves a significantly conspicuous and unfavorable scar. Darker skin is more prone to hypertrophic scarring or keloids. The role of primary closure for reconstruction after complete eradication of skin cancer on the face is very limited because of defect size and shape. Only small defects with elliptical shapes yield satisfactory results after primary closure. A local flap may provide several advantages, including decreased scar contracture and satisfactory contour, color, and texture match. In some cases, however, a local flap is not feasible, mainly due to the limitation of size and arc of rotation, particularly in young patients. Poor flap design and inappropriate incisions may contribute to unacceptable scars, violation of aesthetic subunits, and resultant disfigurement on difficult-to-treat areas. In addition, compromise of flap vascularity and inadequate wound closure created by insufficient undermining, lack of deep closure, excessive tension, or inadequate approximation of wound edges predispose to unfavorable results.

4.2.1 Patients and methods

Thirty-eight patients (20 male, 18 female) were treated for the facial defects created by the resection of the non-melanoma skin cancer on the face from January 2006 and December 2008. The patients had more than 12-months of follow-up and the clinical records of all patients were reviewed. The patients' age ranged from 57 to 83 years (average, 68.7±6.3 years). The defect size ranged from 3.3 to 6.5 cm^2 with a mean of 5.1±0.9 cm^2. The location of the defect was as follows: 17 cases on the nose, 14 in the orbital area, 4 on the cheek, 2 on the temple area, and 1 on the forehead.

Functional and cosmetic outcomes, focusing on scar contracture, pain, itching, scar height, color, texture, and postoperative complications were assessed. The patients' satisfaction was also evaluated by using a VAS with a score of 0 being the worst and 10 being the best. The patients were followed up for 12 to 36 months (mean, 20.5±6.2 months).

4.2.2 Results

The graft was well taken by all patients. Reepithelization occurred progressively from the periphery to the center of the grafted dermis. The entire dermis graft reepithelialized after grafting within 17 to 27 days (mean, 25.1±2.4 days).

All patients had satisfactory results in both functional and cosmetic matters with high quality skin characteristics. No significant scar contracture was observed and none of the patients complained of pain or itching. In the scar height, 20 scars were flat and 18 scars were slightly depressed. Neither hypertrophic nor keloid scar was observed. In the color parameter, most of the scars (30 scars) showed favorable color match to the surrounding skin (Figs. 7 and 8) and 8 scars were hypopigmented (Fig. 9). Hyperpigmentation or redness was not observed. In terms of the skin texture, favorable smooth texture was obtained in 25 cases and shiny texture in 13 cases. Obviously conspicuous scar was not identified in all

cases and no revision procedure was needed to improve scar quality. There were no significant complications and no recurrences were observed during the follow-up. The patients' satisfaction with the dermis graft was also excellent (mean score 8.3±1.3).
Regarding the donor sites, the results of the dermis graft were also satisfactory. All the donor sites of dermis graft healed within 9 days (average 7.2±1.1 days). There were no significant complications and no functionally relevant scar (Fig. 10).

5. Advantages and disadvantages

The primary advantage of this method is to provide a graft that is similar to the surrounding skin, leaving minimal scars and color mismatch. Since the epidermal portion can be restored by epithelization, induced by the migration and proliferation of adjacent epidermal cells including melanocytes, the density and activity of the melanocytes as well as the precursor melanocytes of the epidermis of the graft become similar to those observed in the adjacent skin.

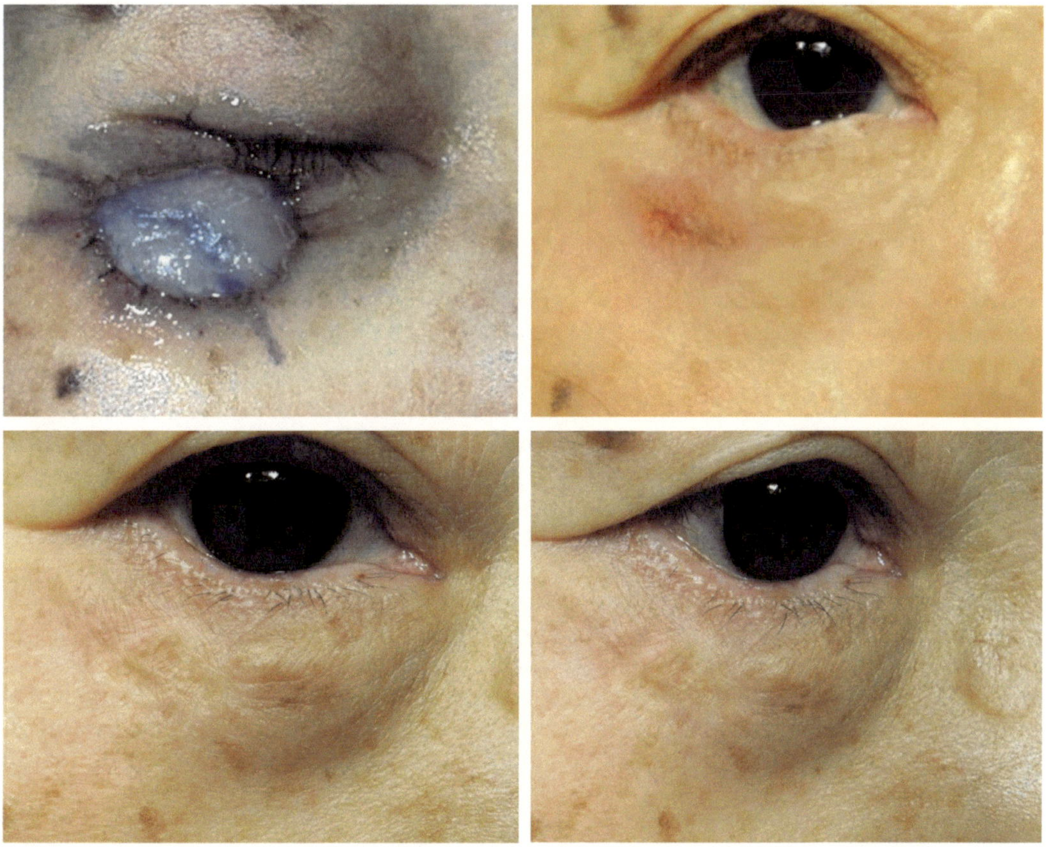

Fig. 7. A skin defect created by removal of basal cell carcinoma treated with the dermis graft. (*Above, left*) Immediate postoperative view. (*Above, right*) One-month postoperative view. (*Below*) Two-year postoperative view, which showed excellent results with minimal scar contraction.

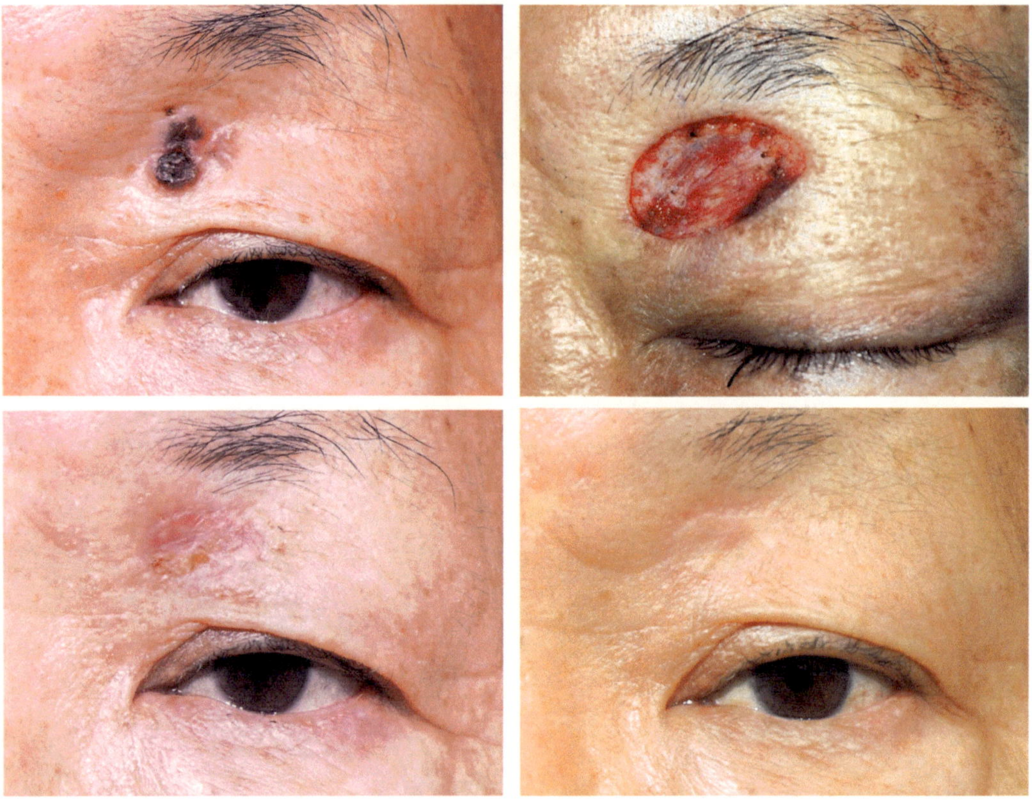

Fig. 8. A skin defect seen on a lower eyelid created by removal of basal cell carcinoma treated with the dermis graft. (*Above, left)* Preoperative view. (*Above, right)* After removal of the lesion. (*Below, left*) One-month postoperative view. (*Below, right*) One-year postoperative view. The resultant scar was acceptable.

Regarding wound contraction of the recipient site after dermis grafting, the contraction of myofibroblasts can be inhibited by grafting with a more dermal portion than a regular skin graft. In previous studies, the inhibition of scar contraction was attributed to the amount of dermal collagen rather than to the amount of epidermis (Chou et al., 2001; Rudolph, 1979; Brown et al., 1990). Another advantage of the dermis graft is the quick healing of the donor site without an obvious scar appearance because the epidermis can be replaced immediately to ensure the closure of the donor bed. Hypertrophic scarring is rare, and the level of pigmentation is less than that of the donor site in a regular skin graft. The patient has less donor site pain and discomfort, which is a very important component from the patient's point of view. Care of the donor site is also very simple. Dermis grafts are feasible for all wounds that are candidates for regular skin grafts including acute facial burns or post facial cancer excisions.

The only possible demerit with dermis grafting is the delay in complete healing of the recipient site. As previously described, there was a 3.7 day delay in graft healing of the recipient site (15.5 and 11.8 days in the dermis graft and the regular skin graft groups, respectively). However, it is believed that the 3.7 day delay would not cause significant trouble, and what ever problems there are can be overcome by selecting suitable sized wounds.

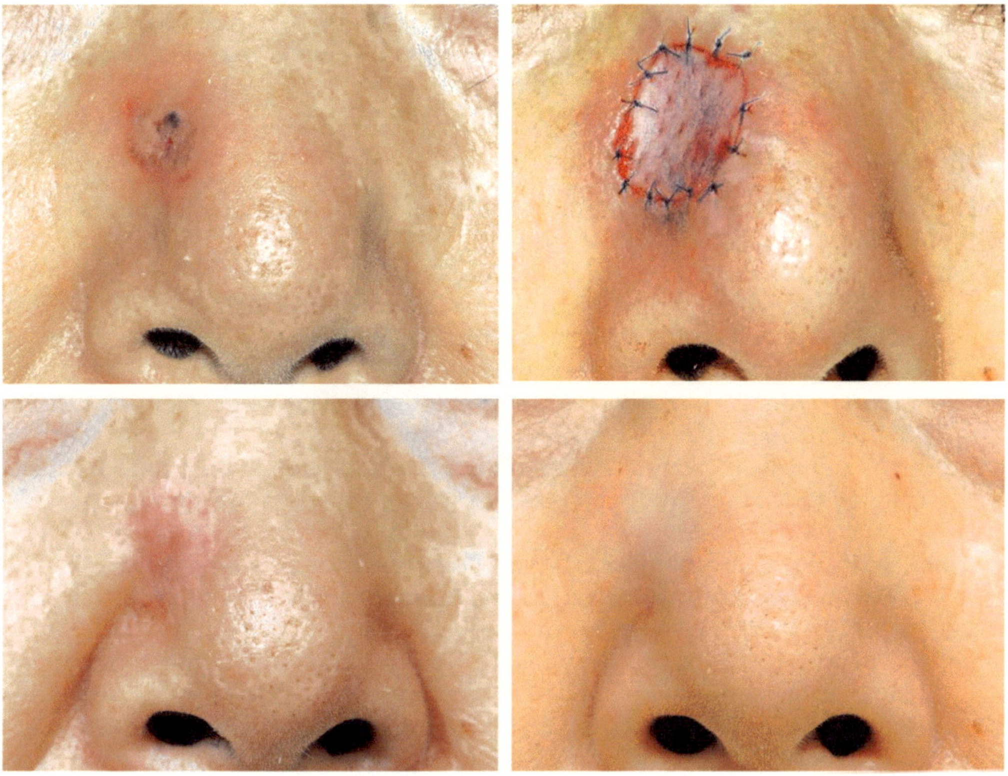

Fig. 9. A skin defect on a nose created by removal of basal cell carcinoma treated with the dermis graft. (*Above, left*) Preoperative view. (*Above, right*) Immediate postoperative view. (*Below, left*) One-month postoperative view. (*Below, right*) One-year postoperative view. Hypopigmentation of the grafted site was noted in this case.

Fig. 10. Healed donor sites of the dermis grafts demonstrate acceptable cosmetic results.

6. Conclusion

The dermis graft technique for wound coverage is superior to a regular skin graft technique in terms of the aesthetic results of both the recipient and donor sites. The donor site healing process is faster, and the patient's pain and discomfort can also be reduced significantly. The dermis graft can be used reliably for covering small to medium sized wounds on exposed areas and may be considered as the first choice.

7. References

Brown D, Garner W, Young L. Skin grafting: Dermal components in inhibition of wound contraction. *South Med J*. 1990;83:789-793.

Carlson JA., Grabowski R., Mu XC., Del Rosario A. Possible mechanisms of hypopigmentation in lichen sclerosus. *Am J Dermatopathol*. 2002;24:97-101

Chou TD., Chen SL., Lee TW., Chen SG. Reconstruction of burn scar of the upper extremities with artificial skin. *Plast Reconstr Surg*. 2001;108:378-384.

Han SK, Yoon TH, Kim JB, Kim WK. Dermis graft for wound coverage. *Plast Reconstr Surg*. 2007 ;120:166-172.

Kuroyanagi Y, Yamada N, Yamashita R, Uchinuma E. Tissue-engineered product: allogenic cultured dermal substitute composed of spongy collagen with fibroblasts. *Artificial Organs*. 2001;25:180-186.

Rudolph R. Inhibition of myofibroblasts by skin grafts. *Plast Reconstr Surg*. 1979;63:473-478.

Sullival, T., Smith, J., Kermode, J., McIver, E., and Courtermanche, D. J. Rating the burn scar. *J Burn Care Rehabil*. 1990;11:256-261.

Swope VB., Supp AP., Boyce ST. Regulation of cutaneous pigmentation by titration of human melanocytes in cultured skin substitutes grafted to athymic mice. *Wound Repair Regen*. 2002;10:378-385.

Terino EO. AlloDerm acellular dermal graft: applications in aesthetic soft tissue augmentation. *Clin Plast Surg*. 2001;28:83-90.

Tyack ZF., Pegg S., Ziviani J. Postburn dyspigmentation : Its assessment, management, and relationship to scarring. *J Burn Care Rehabil*. 1997;18:435-440.

Velangi SS., Rees JL. Why are scars pale? An immunohistochemical study indicating preservation of melanocyte number and function in surgical scars. *Acta Derm Venereol*. 2001;81:326-332.

Vloemans AF., Soesman AM., Suijker M., Kreis RW. Arandomised clinical trial comparing a hydrocolloid-derived dressing and glycerol preserved allograft skin in the management of partial thickness burns. *Burns*. 2003;29-34.

23

Cryopreservation of Skin Tissues for Skin Grafts

Suong-Hyu Hyon
Institute for Frontier Medical Sciences, Kyoto University 53 Kawahara-cho, Shogoin, Sakyo-ku, Kyoto Japan

1. Introduction

Preservation of living tissue and organs are very important to ensure successful transplantation. The storage of living tissue, from the time of removal of the donor tissue until transplantation, is one of the most important factors for successful tissue transplantation. The purpose of living tissue storage is to maintain the viability of the mammalian cells, and various methods have been developed to lengthen the time donor tissue can be stored without loss of cell integrity.

At present, low temperature is used as the major organ preservation method. Generally, cells are preserved in a frozen state at -196°C (1-3). The survival rate after such storage has been enhanced by controlled temperature freezing. However, cell survival after freezing can be low (namely, 20～40%), as with ES cells (embryonic stem cells),EG cells (embryonic genital cells) and induced pluripotent stem (iPS) cells. It would be of great advantage to researchers in the field of stem cell research to be able to preserve these cells more successfully. It would also be of benefit to be able to preserve other cells, such as platelets, over the long term without freezing. Likewise, research continues in our attempts to prolong the time for transplantation of solid organs, and in the development of optimal perfusion fluids that protect against ischemia remains an active subject of investigation. Various storage solutions for organ preservation, such as the UW solution developed at the University of Wisconsin (USA) are also in current clinical use. However, it is necessary to develop storage solutions that can maintain the viability of tissues and organs for longer periods because of the limitations of storage in UW solution.

After transplantation, many organs suffer from the generation of free radicals following reperfusion. The restoration of blood flow becomes a trigger for injury, with subsequent lipid peroxidation of the biomembrane leading to membrane failure and as a result, the transplanted organ fails. A logical goal would then be the development of a preservation fluid that would limit cell damage by preventing peroxylipid generation. Such a preservation fluid should limit cell division and multiplication. A room temperature storage state could also potentially prevent the injury to the small vessel endothelium seen with freezing and to delicate tissues, such as the cornea, which do not survive freezing well. Although these tissues can be held from 4 to 24 hours at 4°C, large organs impose a severe time limitation on the medical team (4-6). In addition, through advances in tissue engineering, cultured skin and cultured cartilage have reached the level of clinical application and demanded long term storage techniques for optimum utilization. Transplantation of xenogeneic organs from genetically prepared animal donors would likewise benefit from the possibility of longer periods of organ storage.

It has now been found that the polyphenols in green tea promote the preservation of tissues, such as blood vessels, cornea, nerves, islet tissues, articular cartilage and myocardium, at room temperature.(24) Furthermroe, in the case of hematopoetic stem cells, the polyphenols suppress the differentiation of the cells into erythrocytes, T cells and B cells. These findings suggest the possibility of a new method for tissue banking that does not require freezing.

We have been conducting the research on the applications of green tea polyphenol (epigallocatechin-3-0-gallate, EGCG) to the regenerative medicine (7-14). In the field of transplantation medicine, which is a subfield of regenerative medicine, we have faced challenging problems associated with graft tissues and organs, including loss of viability and function (15-18), hyperplasia and immunological rejection of grafted tissues after transplantation (19,20). To overcome these problems, we propose the use of a preservation medium containing EGCG, which has been shown to have anti-oxidative (22-34), anti-proliferative (8)and immunosuppresive properties (19).

Polyphenols have recently attracted attention as components of functional foods, and have been shown to have various bioactivities such as anticancer activity, antimicrobal and anti-virus activity since the 1980's.(7-11) Therefore, there are many papers and patents on the use of polyphenols for various applications. However, there has been no research which applies to the use of polyphenols for the preservation of various tissues and organs. We believe that such applications are possible, and we recently found an interesting phenomena related to the effects of polyphenols on mammalian cells and living tissues. We herein describe the effects of polyphenols on living cells and tissues, and present possible applications of polyphenols for their preservation.

2. Preservation solutions for organ and tissue transplantation

Polyphenols have a hydroxyl group attached to the 2nd carbon, and have properties completely different from other phenolic chemicals such as hydroxybenzene. The chemical structure of green tea polyphenol is shown in Figure 1. It is possible to classify these polyphenols into flavonoid hydrolysis type tannins and other polyphenols. Various chemical compounds are known within the polyphenol group. Representative members include catechin, which is mainly found in green tea and oolong tea, and anthocyanin, which is the red pigment in red wine The antioxidative effects of green tea polyphenol and catechin, as well as proanthocyanidin, are especially potent, and these agents are known to be associated with a lower morbidity from heart disease (35-37). It has also recently been reported in ***Nature*** that the proliferation of cancer cells was suppressed by polyphenols (38-39).

The success rate of organ transplantation has increased due to the improvements in surgical techniques and the development of new immunosuppressive agents in recent ten years. For instance, in the USA where transplantation is frequently practiced with organs or tissues from brain-dead donors, there were 4 million transplants performed in 2002.

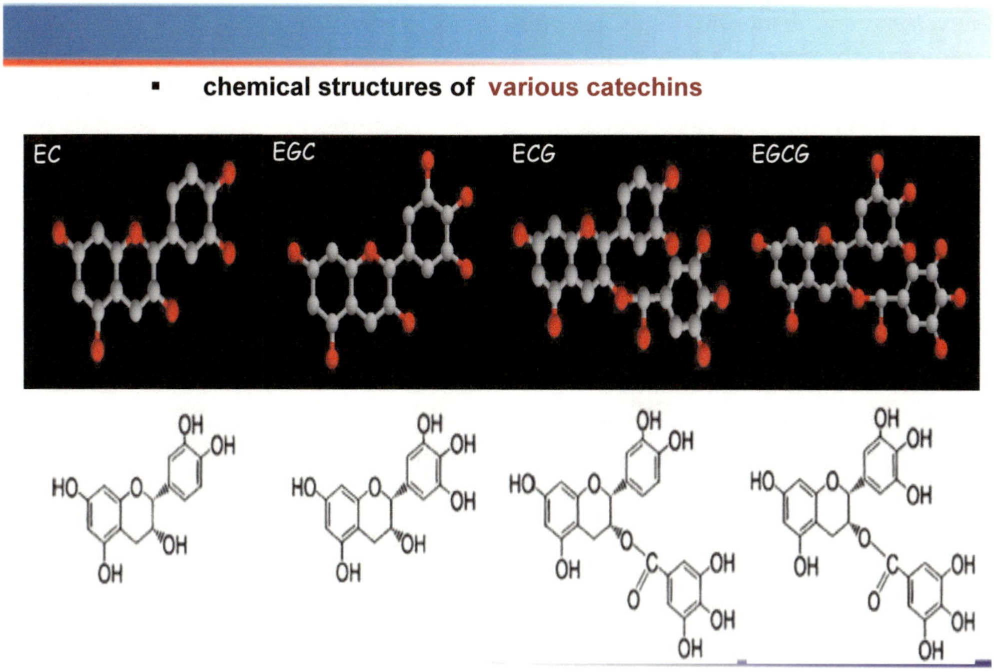

Fig. 1. The chemical structure of green tea polyphenol.

The donor organs or tissues are routinely transported in various preservation solutions. The UW (University of Wisconsin) solution and Euro-Collins solution are the first and the second most frequently used preservation solutions. These preservation solutions are mainly used for the transport of kidneys, liver, or pancreas. However, they cannot preserve the organs for longer than 24 hours at 4°C (40-44). In light of the increasing demand for donor organs and tissues, preservation solutions with better preserving abilities and the research and development of such solutions are urgently needed.

When organs or tissues are isolated from a donor, their blood circulation stops, and physiological activities rapidly decrease. Varying degrees of ischemia are commonly observed for these organs, and free radicals are generated upon the restart of blood flow, which leads to lipid peroxidation of the cell membrane, causing membrane damage and various dysfunctions of the transplanted organs. The development of a preservation solution that can minimize the oxidation and cell damage can solve this problem.

One of the traditional methods used to solve this problem has been freeze preservation (45-47). Although living tissues and cells are routinely preserved at -196°C, freezing and subsequent thawing cause some structural damage. For example, frozen blood vessels have damage that often make their transplantation difficult, and corneas cannot be preserved at 4°C for longer than one week without a significant degree of damage. Studies indicate that the cell damage is primarily caused by activated oxygen molecules emerging from the freezing and thawing processes, but also occurs even after exposing the living tissues and cells to ordinary temperatures after removal from the donor.

Recent advances in tissue engineering are now on the cusp of providing clinically useful cultured skin, cartilage and cornea specimens. However, these cultured tissues also require preservation, and better methods for long term preservation would be beneficial for ensuring that they can be successfully applied in the clinic field. To this end, we introduce the anti-oxidant polyphenol, EGCG, as a means to prevent the cell damage associated with organ and tissue preservation. Using EGCG, we can preserve living tissues and organs allowing for longer storage and more successful transplantation (13-34).

3. Control of mammalian cell proliferation

To study the effects of EGCG on cell proliferation, the rat fibroblast cell line, L-929, was cultivated in EMEM (with kanamycin 60mg/1) supplemented with 10% fetal bovine serum. A cell proliferation test was carried out at a cell density of 1.76×10^5 cells/ml. The polyphenol (250 μg/ml concentration) was added to another culture system as a control. The effects of the polyphenol in the rat fibroblast culture are shown in Figure 2. In the polyphenol system, the cells became round, although cell proliferation was still active, and the cell population was increased to 1×10^6 cells/ml on the fourth day after cultivation, but the proliferation decreased after 1 week of treatment, and resumed when the polyphenol was removed from the culture media.

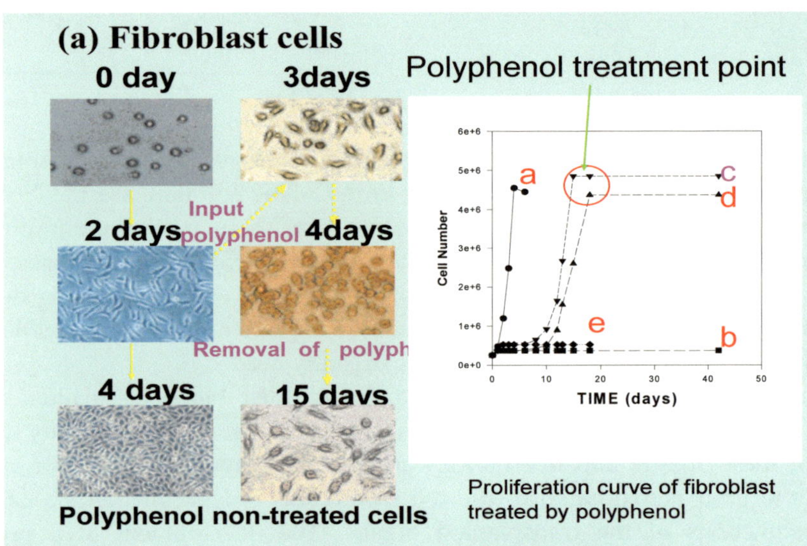

Fig. 2. The effect of polyphenols on the multiplication of the fibroblast.
(⟶) The polyphenol free. (- - ➔) The polyphenol addition.

We also assessed the effects of the polyphenol on the cell cycle. The results of treatment of the fibroblasts with the polyphenol as determined by flow cytometry are shown in Table 1. For the polyphenol-treated cells, the number of cells in the G0, G1 and G2/M-phases increased, although after 9 hours in culture, the number of cells in the S phase reached 0. A similar phenomenon was observed in porcine hepatocytes. In addition, the viable cell population did not decrease. Good results were also obtained for the protective effects of the green tea polyphenol against reactive oxygen species that induce oxidative stress in cultured rat calvarial osteoblasts.

Polyphenol	Cycle(%)	0	2	4	9	48*
Non-treated	G0G1	22.18	15.69	22.86	18.99	
	G2M	2.58	1.12	11.93	20.85	
	S	75.24	83.19	65.22	60.16	
Treated cells	G0G1	22.18	33.05	52.96	70.07	71.33
	G2M	2.58	11.00	13.83	29.93	20.54
	S	75.24	56.95	33.21	0	8.13

*Cell cycle fibroblasts cultured in medium only during 48hr after removal of p olyphenol from medium

Table 1. Time changes in cell cycle of untreated and polyphenol treated (250 mcg/ml) fibroblasts.

4. Green tea polyphenol affects the preservation of rats skin and improves the success rate of skin grafts

Although skin allografts are used in the treatment of serious burn injuries, skin disorders, and skin defects their use is limited because of the limited amount of normal skin that can be removed for such grafts (48). The best graft for the functional closure of wounds is the autograft. At the end of an autograft procedure, the remaining donor skin is routinely stored in a saline solution and applied to the open wound when graft loss or superficial wound breakdown occurs postoperatively. (49) However, long-time storage in saline leads to poor engraftment, and we were prompted to study other preservation media which would extend the storage time of skin grafts. Recently, it has been found that the polyphenols in green tea promote the preservation of tissues, such as the blood vessel, cornea, nerve, islet cells, articular cartilage and myocardium, at room temperature (12-34). These findings suggest the possibility of a new method for tissue banking without freezing.

As previously stated the dysfunction of transplants occurs as a result of free radicals due to ischemia, which triggers lipid peroxidation of the cell membrane when blood flow is restarted. It is reported that EGCG prevents peroxylipid generation. (50)

To determine whether the addition of EGCG to conventional cell culture medium could enhance the viability of stored skin grafts and also extend storage time, we performed a study using the skin from rats. The storage solution chosen for this study was Dulbecco's Modified Eagle Medium (Sigma, St. Louis, MO, USA) supplemented with 10% Fetal Calf Serum (FCS; Sigma), add and 1% antibiotic solution (including 10000U penicillin and 10 mg streptomycin, Sigma). EGCG was dissolved in the storage solution at a final concentration of

1 mg/ml. Transgenic Sprague-Dawley rats (8 weeks old, male) expressing the green fluorescent protein (GFP) (green 2 Kim et al., produced with the constructs used for the green mouse (51)), were a kind gift from Dr. Masaru Okabe (Genomic Information Research Center, Osaka, Japan).

For anesthesia, pentobarbital (50 mg/Kg) was administered intraperitoneally to the GFP transgenic rats. After shaving and depilating the backs of the rats, the back skins were biopsied. The muscular layers were immediately stripped from the skin biopsies. Skin samples measuring 1×1 cm were kept in sterile containers with 50ml preservation solution at 4°C and 37°C for up to 8 weeks. Periodically, some of preserved skin (30 min, 1, 2, 4, 6, 7, 8 weeks) were used for grafts in nude mice or were directly examined histologically.

From histological examinations of the 4°C preservation skin, it was noted that there was a decrease in the GFP value in the non-EGCG skin noted during the second week (Figure 3), as was a slight degeneration of the epidermal layer. The degeneration of the epidermal and dermal layers were noted beginning at 5 weeks in all 4°C groups (Figure 4).

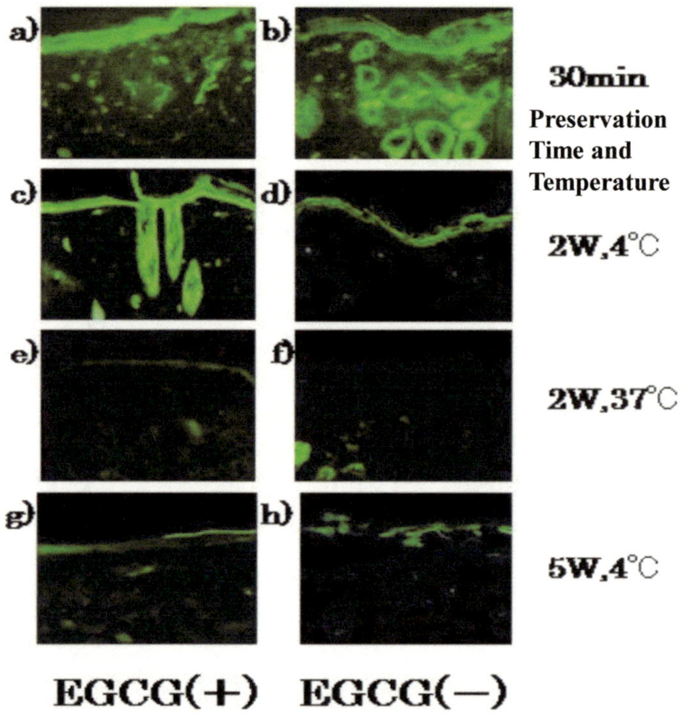

Fig. 3. Photographs showing cryosection of the preserved GFP rat skins. GFP value was slightly decreased according to preservation time.

In the 37°C preserved groups, degeneration and flakiness of the epidermal layer were noted beginning after one week of preservation, both with or without EGCG, and a decrease in the GFP value was observed, regardless of the presence of EGCG, at 2 weeks. Moreover, the epidermis was damaged in the tissue samples preserved without EGCG, although not in the EGCG group.

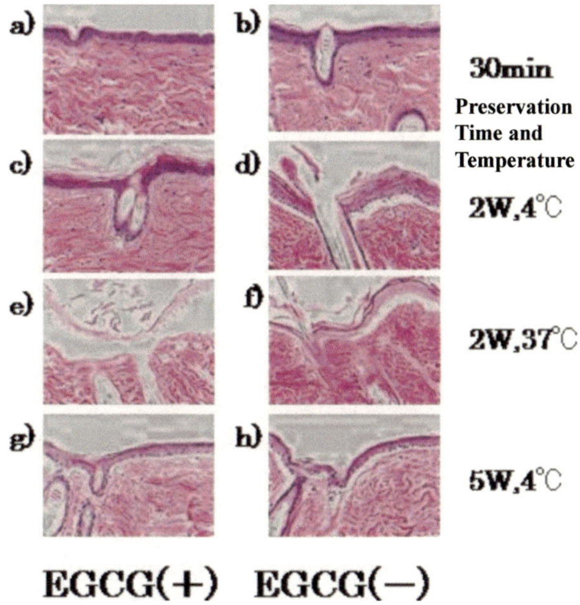

Fig. 4. Photographs showing H.E. stain of preservation GFP rat's skins. Degeneration of the epidermis and dermis was observed, according to preservation time. The degeneration is improved in EGCG groups compared to EGCG(-) groups.

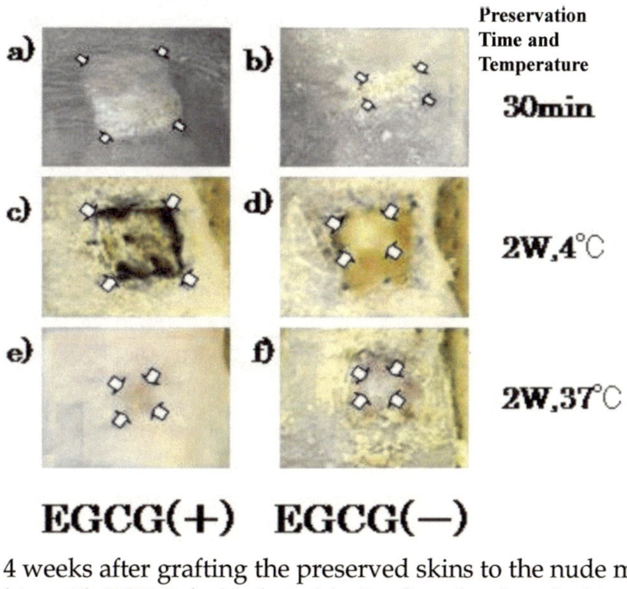

Fig. 5. Appearances 4 weeks after grafting the preserved skins to the nude mice. Thirty minutes preserved skin with EGCG, holds hair (a). On the other hand, skin without EGCG (b) has no hair and the graft size is smaller than that with EGCG groups (a). After 2 weeks preservation with EGCG at 4℃, grafts color were dark like necrosis, but it only remain EGCG. Grafts size were smaller or only scar were observed at all groups, except preservation under 4℃ with EGCG, after 2weeks preservation.

The rat skin grafted onto the nude mice after 30 minute preservation with EGCG showed a better condition than those implanted without EGCG, which showed loss of hair and shrinkage. In the EGCG-preserved groups, the skin color was dark and looked like there was necrosis superficially, however, the color was found to be due to the presence of the EGCG (Figure 5). After 2 to 7 weeks of preservation in EGCG at 4℃, there was good graft survival. In the other groups, the grafts shrunk or were only scar-like because of contracture or rejection.

In the histological analysis, grafts preserved at 4℃ with EGCG were found to have been completely accepted, with both epidermal and dermal layers remaining. On the other hand, grafts preserved at 4℃ without EGCG had no GFP positive keratinocytes or fibroblasts observed, and only phagocytes were observed in the dermal layer (likely targeting the GFP). In the 37℃ preserved groups, no GFP positive rat cells were observed, with or without EGCG (Figure 6). No grafts were successful from the 37℃ preserved groups (with or without EGCG). However, the 4℃ preserved grafts were accepted, and the success rate for the EGCG-treated grafts was 100% even after 4 weeks of preservation (Figure 7).

Wide skin defects caused by burns or trauma should be covered with skin grafts, but sometimes skin grafts fail due to various causes such as hematoma. When skin grafts are partially unsuccessful, small skin defects can be repaired, using the skin leftover from the primary grafting, if it is preserved. Moreover, injuries leading to complicated tears or small flap-like. In such cases, if the skin can be temporarily preserved, it can later be used as part of the graft after the wound condition is improved. Freeze-drying porcine skin, xenografts,

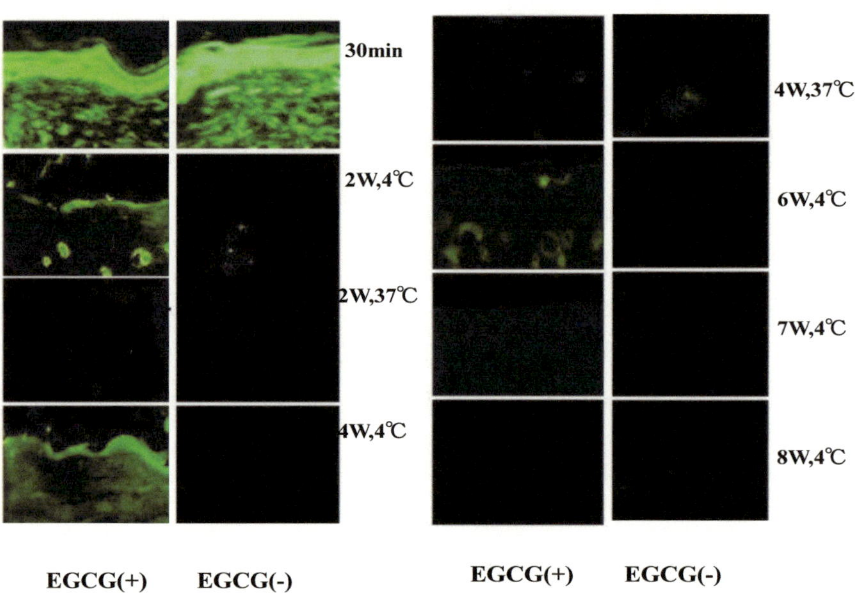

Fig. 6. Photographs showing cryosection of the GFP rat skins 28 days after grafting to nude mice (n=4-6). EGCG positive keratinocytes were observed only in the grafts preserved in 30 minutes preservation groups and 4℃ preservation groups with EGCG, 2weeks to 6 weeks (a, c, g, k). EGCG positive fibroblasts were seen only in grafts preserved at 4℃ with EGCG, 30 minutes to 7 weeks (a, c, g, k, m). In other groups, only phagocytes which ate the GFP were observed.

and frozen allografts are also used for wound coverage, but they are not usually permanently incorporated. Therefore, it is very useful to develop better technologies for the preservation of autografts.

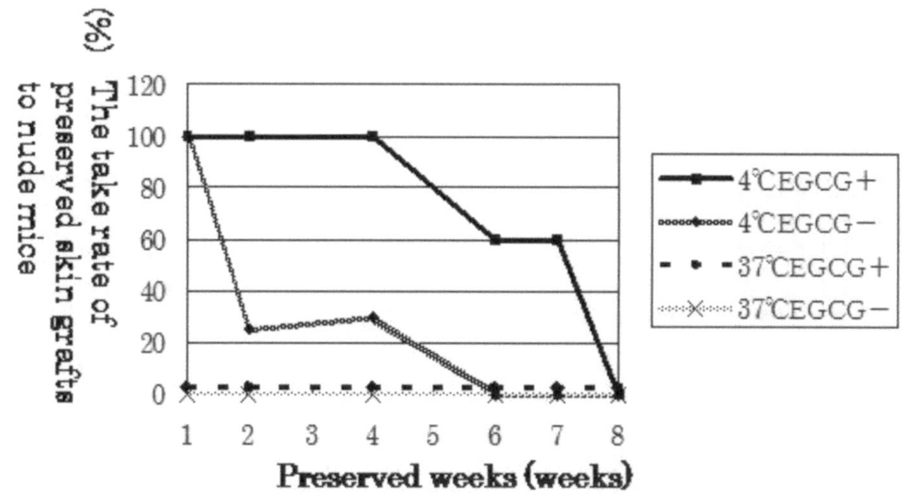

Fig. 7. The take rate of preserved skin grafts to nude mice, judged 28 days after surgery. No grafts took in 37℃ preserved groups with or without EGCG. Take rates were improved by addition of EGCG, at 4℃ preservation.

There have been a few reports on the preservation of the cornea, blood vessels, nerves, pancreatic islet cells, saphenous veins and peripheral nerves using EGCG. In the first reported experiment, histological examination revealed that EGCG improved the length of preservation time a skin sample. With time, skin samples start to degenerate from the epidermal layer to the dermal layer. Skins samples preserved at 4°C seem to undergo less degeneration than the ones at 37°C. However, it was difficult to judge the cell viabilities based on only histological examinations, because GFP was still present in all of the skin samples. Therefore, we investigated the viability of the skin specimens by examining whether the samples could lead to successful grafts. It has been reported that the dead tissue or skin is rejected by around two weeks after implantation. (52, 53)

We used immunodeficient mice as recipient animals and judged the success of skin grafts from GFP-Tg rats. The results indicated that the preservation of the skin with 37°C is not possible even if EGCG is added. Similarly, AE CRAM et al. reported that only 1/3 of their grafts were successful at ten days after transplanting skin samples preserved at 4°C for two weeks. In our study, at 4 weeks after transplantation of skins preserved for 4 weeks at 4°C with EGCG were successful, and one-third were still successful even after preservation for 7 weeks at 4°C with EGCG. We therefore concluded that EGCG was beneficial for the preservation of skin samples by decreasing the degeneration of the epidermal layer and suppressing the postoperative graft contraction.

There might be several reasons why EGCG improved the preservation of the skin. EGCG has strong anti-oxidative activities. The strong anti-oxidative activity of EGCG might inhibit the lipid peroxidation of cell membrane of the preserved skin. M. Kapoor et al. reported that

EGCG had anti-inflammatory and free radical scavenging effects *in vitro*. (54) EGCG was also reported to control cell division. We believe that a combination of these effects improved the condition of the preserved skin. In addition, the actions of EGCG, such as was strengthening the scaffold structure, and its antibacterial activity also seem to have contributed to its preserving effects. EGCG also improved the quality of scars after full thickness incisions in rats, likely because EGCG increases iNOS (inducible nitric oxide synthase), COX-2 (cyclooxygenase-2), and VEGF (vascular endothelial growth factor) expression, leading to the formation of new blood vessels. EGCG also has been shown to decrease arginase-I activity and protein levels. (54)
Our results suggest the possibility of the future clinical use of EGCG for skin preservation without freezing, although the mechanism underlying how EGCG exerts its beneficial effects on skin preservation still remains unclear.

5. Long term preservation of rat skin tissue by EGCG

EGCG enhances the viability of stored skin grafts and also extends the storage time for up to 7 week at 4°C. The addition of EGCG to conventional freezing medium, "Cell Banker" (CB), could enhance the viability of skin grafts stored at −196°C and also extend their storage time. Metabolic assays have been used as a surrogate measure of overall viability in the grafts. Skin tissue was transplanted from GFP transgenic rats into immunodeficient mice, and cell migration in graft tolerance of GFP positive cells was investigated after transplantation (55).
For anesthesia, pentobarbital (50 mg/kg) was administered intraperitoneally. After shaving and depilating the back of the rats, the back skin was elevated. After procurement, the muscular layer was immediately stripped from the skin biopsies. Skin samples from GFP rats measuring 1 × 1 cm were kept under sterile containers and refrigerated with PBS solution with or without EGCG for 1 night. Skin samples were then transferred to CB solution with or without EGCG and were stored in liquid nitrogen (-196°C) for up to about 24 weeks. Periodically, the preserved skin grafts of GFT rats were transplanted into nude mice (2, 8, and 24 weeks). Circular skin biopsies (8 mm in diameter) were also made using a sterile dermal biopsy punch (Kai Industries Co., Ltd. Gifu, Japan) and preserved in the same way for in vitro analysis.
A full-thickness excisional square wound (1 × 1 cm) was created on the dorsum of each nude mouse, and the GFP rat skin specimens were sutured to the adjacent normal skin with 6-0 ProleneTM thread. After surgery, the mice were housed in separate cages. Skin grafts were excised with 2–3 mm of the surrounding tissue, bisected, and processed for histology 14 days after transplantation (n =4–6).
The *in vitro* results showed that 1 mg/ml EGCG had the highest protective effect on skin samples when it was used at −196℃ for 2 weeks. At concentrations higher than 1.5 mg/ml, EGCG delayed the recovery of the metabolic activity of skin samples after thawing (Figure 8). Figure 9 shows that glucose consumption was gradually increased with time and the skin samples preserved with EGCG showed higher glucose consumption in all groups after preservation. The in vitro data showed decreased glucose consumption in the 8-week-preserved group in comparison to the 2-week-preserved group. By comparing Figures 8 and 9, We concluded that the presence of DMSO and EGCG in the freezing medium led to more effective maintenance of glucose consumption than freezing medium alone. Glucose

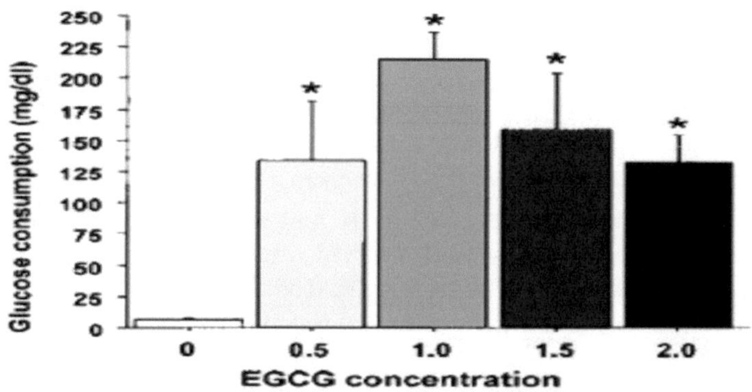

Fig. 8. The optimum concentration of EGCG for rat skin preservation was determined by measuring the metabolic activity. Skin biopsy samples were preserved in cell culture medium with various concentrations of EGCG and preserved at −196°C for 2 weeks. Glucose consumption was measured after 6 days of 37°C incubation after thawin.

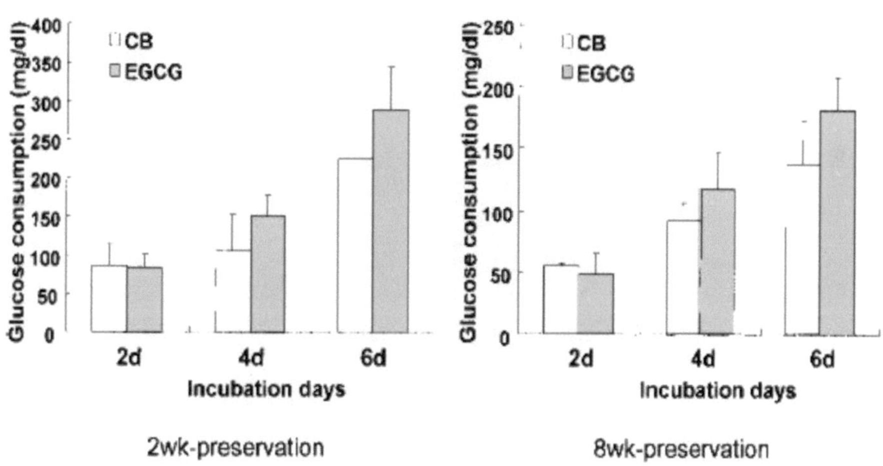

Fig. 9. Glucose consumption of the preserved skin biopsies after thawing. Skin biopsy samples were preserved in freezing medium (CB) with or without EGCG at −196°C for 4 and 8 weeks. There was no significant difference; however, the amount of glucose consumption in the EGCG groups showed faster metabolic recovery in comparison to the CB groups.

consumption by the 2-week-preserved skin samples treated with only EGCG after 6 days was about 220 mg/dl while the 4-week skin samples preserved with EGCG and DMSO was almost 300 mg/dl. After day 7 the possibility of bacterial contamination increased and false-positive data were obtained. All skin samples were washed with PBS containing antibiotics every 2 days. The GFP fluorescence appeared to be similar between the 2- and 8-week-preserved groups (Figure 10). The degradation of the epidermal layer to the dermal layer was observed in all groups, regardless of preservation. However, while the Skin grafts of GFP rats preserved in CB showed only green florescence around the dermis of the transplanted area in the 24-week-preserved group, the fluorescence of the epidermal layer and some viable cells were confirmed in the EGCG- preserved skin grafts. The degradation was therefore improved by EGCG in comparison to the CB group. An evaluation of the viability of the transplanted skin grafts was difficult with GFP confirmation only. The histology of the transplanted skin grafts of the GFP rats and nude mice was also therefore evaluated using H&E-stained sections (Figure 11). The grafts preserved with EGCG showed a dense dermal matrix and an intact epidermal layer, as shown in the GFP pictures. Micrographs of CB preserved skin grafts were not fully rejected; however, separation between the transplanted skin of the GFP rat and immunodeficient mouse was observed near the location of the original epidermal layer. The histological score was marked with micrographs of H&E-stained specimens based on the attached area of the transplanted skin graft and the condition of the surviving skin grafts (Figure 12). Dead and completely rejected skin grafts scored 0. The surviving skin grafts with a widely attached area, intact epidermis, and dermis with hair follicles and a dense matrix scored 5. Neither the survival rate of the skin grafts nor the histological scores indicated a clear difference between the 2-, 8-,and 24-week-preserved groups. However, both the survival rate of the skin grafts and the histological scores were increased by EGCG in all groups.

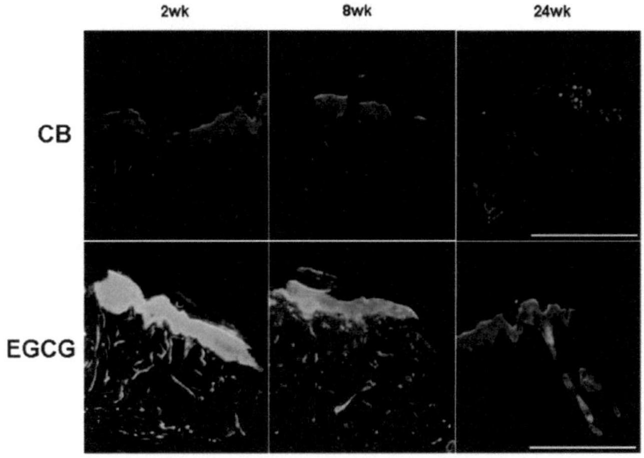

Fig. 10. Cryosections of GFP rat skin graft to a nude mouse (left: 2-week-preserved group, middle: 8-week-preserved group, fight: 24-week-preserved group). These micrographs are representative of four to six independent experiments, and showed similar results.

EGCG therefore enhances the viability of stored skin grafts and extends the storage time up to 7 weeks at 4°C. In this study, the storage time of the skin grafts was extended to 24 weeks by cryopreservation with both DMSO and EGCG. The survival rate of the transplanted skin grafts reached almost 100% in the 24-week-preserved group, indicating that long term storage is possible.(62)

Cryopreserved cells and tissues are increasingly being used for stem cell transplantation and tissue engineering. However, they are highly sensitive to freezing, storage, and thawing, which suggests the need for improved cryopreservation methods. When storing any living tissue, the destructive effects of hypoxic metabolism must be controlled. A tissue removed from its blood supply will die unless cellular metabolic activity is decreased or nutrients are provided. By reducing metabolism and providing nutrients, viability can be improved (56). EGCG was reported to control cell division, which causes the energy metabolism to decrease

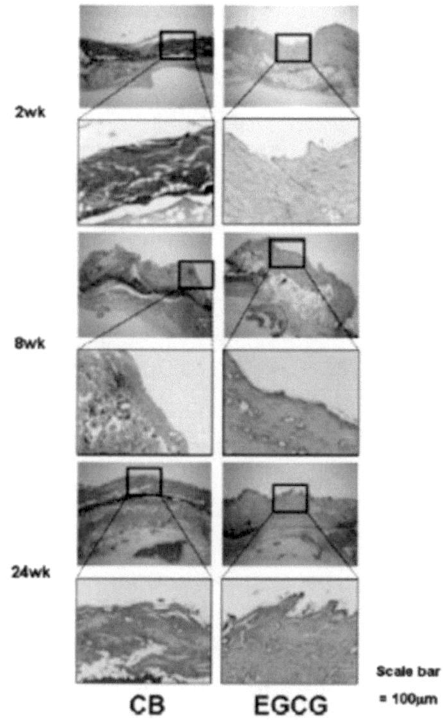

Fig. 11. Histological observation in skin grafts with H&E-stained micrographs (top: original magnification 5·, bottom: original magnification 20·). Degradation of the epidermal layer to the dermal layer was observed in the CB groups. The degradation was improved by EGCG in comparison to the CB groups. These photographs are representative of four to six independent experiments, and showed similar results.

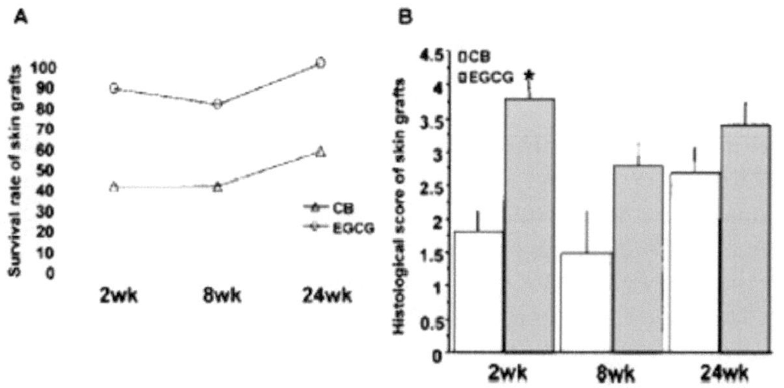

Fig. 12. (A) The survival rate of grafted GFP rat skin after 2 weeks. (B) Considering the epidermal morphology and dermal integrity of the transplanted grafts, a score was given from 0 to 5. A higher score indicates better condition of the skin grafts. The results are reported as the mean ± SE ($n = 4$–6) and analyzed by Fisher's PLSD test. The value marked with an asterisk is significantly ($p < 0.05$) different from the nontreatment groups.

by inhibiting the cell cycle. Therefore, the combination of such effects improves the condition of the preserved skin. In addition, EGCG reduces ischemia/reperfusion injury by attenuating nitric oxide synthase expression and activity, and improving hypoxic metabolism in preserved skin (57). Furthermore, other activities of EGCG, such as strengthening of the scaffold structure, immunomodulatory effects, and antibacterial activity, may also contribute to its preservative effects.

In the present study, the protection afforded by EGCG was similar for all three groups. EGCG and DMSO in the freezing medium were more effective for maintaining glucose consumption. These results suggest that oxygen radicals scavenged by EGCG may be responsible for damage at the membrane level, and thus, exogenous EGCG can protect cell membranes. These phenomena may be related to the intrinsic characteristics of polyphenol compounds, which readily penetrate cell membranes due to their amphipathic properties. These compounds are easily absorbed by lipid bilayers, extracellular matrices (e.g., collagen, fibronectin), and various cell membrane receptors. The absorption of polyphenolic compounds by such proteins is rapid, while the adsorption rates are slow. Consequently, the skin graft could be protected from freeze–thaw injuries due to absorption of EGCG by various membrane proteins and lipids (28). The glucose consumption of thawed tissues was assessed after 2, 4, and 6 days of incubation under tissue culture conditions. This post-thaw incubation period was selected to allow for recovery of the metabolic activity in damaged cells. These delayed measurements may be more characteristic of the actual viability of the skin allografts than measurements taken immediately after thawing and dilution. The cells may sustain lethal damage during the thawing and dilution process but have not yet completely disintegrated; thus, there may be residual metabolic activity in the lethally damaged cells immediately after thawing.

The viability of the preserved skin biopsy samples was investigated by examining whether skin specimens could be successfully grafted after preservation. It is reported that dead tissue or skin is rejected in around 2 weeks (58,59). Therefore, immunodeficient mice were used as recipient animals to judge the success of skin grafts from GFP rats (61). GFP fluorescent protein does not need any chemical substrate for visualization. By using a GFP transgenic animal, transplanted cells or tissues having GFP can be detected by direct visualization. Therefore, the GFP transgenic rat is thought to be a suitable skin donor for skin storage and transplantation studies.

A histological analysis demonstrated that the preserved skin began to degenerate from the epidermis to the dermis. The epidermis is easily degenerated during the preservation processes. Considering the histological data presented in previous studies, the results obtained after 2 weeks of preservation seem to be better for samples stored at 4°C than those with cryopreservation. However, the success of the 4°C preserved skin grafts was limited to a 7-week or shorter period, as the samples at 8 weeks no longer led to successful grafts.

EGCG therefore enhances the viability of stored skin grafts and extends the storage time up to 7 weeks at 4°C (61). In this study, the storage time of skin grafts was extended to 24 weeks by cryopreservation using EGCG, and the survival rate was almost 100% in the samples preserved for 24 weeks. These findings suggest that there may be future clinical applications for EGCG as an agent for skin preservation without freezing, although the mechanism by which EGCG promotes skin preservation remains to be elucidated (62).

6. Induction of hibernation of the cells and long term storage of living tissues

The control of cellular proliferation may be important for the prolonged storage of tissues in polyphenol solutions without freezing. Polyphenol is a kind of antioxidant that has similar antioxidant potential as vitamins C and E and superoxide dismutase (SOD). Because of its amphiphilic properties, it also dissolves well in both water and oil. It also has a very high affinity for protein, which allows it to combine with the protein, and yet dissociate with the progression of time, which is characteristic of a reversible adsorption. For the control of cell proliferation and tissue preservation, the latter characteristic is very important. Due to the high affinity between the polyphenol and proteins, the polyphenol can adsorb to a receptor on the cell surface that is integral to the process of cell division when cells are cultured, as shown in Figure 13. The signaling between cells is then blocked when the polyphenol bonds to this receptor, and the cell cycle is inhibited, resulting in no cells entering the S phase, inducing a type of hybernation. As the polyphenol reversibly leaves the cell membrane with the progression of time, the S phase of the cell cycle, and cell proliferation, can resume. The successful long-term storage in the unfrozen state is probably also due to the adsorption of the polyphenol to the collagen and proteoglycan of the extracellular matrix, where it may easily generate temporary cross-linking reactions. Basic research on the interaction between polyphenols and proteins have demonstrated interesting reversible absorption phenomena.(63)

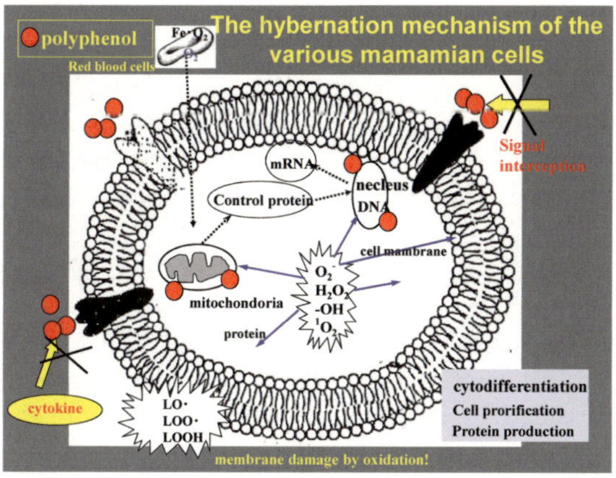

Fig. 13. The cell hibernation mechanism induced by the polyphenol.

7. Potential mechanisms for non-frozen preservation of mammalian tissues and organs by polyphenols

All of these studies were started based on the author's observation that polyphenols appeared to be useful for the physiological preservation of tissues or organs, particularly rat pancreatic islet cells [13]. Since then, evidence has been accumulating showing the beneficial effects of polyphenols on cell preservation. The extension of that observation to the preservation of tissues or even organs for transplantation will make it possible to store them for longer periods by regulating the concentration of polyphenols present in the storage solutions. Recently, it was reported that polyphenols can reduce the ischemia/reperfusion injury in rat lungs and preserve various types of tissues or organs including canine lungs,

rat aorta, rat peripheral nerves and mammalian pancreatic islet cells (12-34), supporting the author's hypothesis.
As shown in Figure 13, this non-frozen preservation of mammalian cells, tissues or organs might be mediated by hibernation, a reversible regulation of cell proliferation and survival through modulation of cell cycle-related genes by the polyphenols at the cellular level. With regard to this hypothesis, it has already been reported that the hibernation phenomenon triggered by polyphenols might be related to their intrinsic characteristics, including their bind with and penetration into the cell membrane or tissue matrix due to their amphipathic properties. The absorption of polyphenolic compounds to the proteins is generated early, but the desorption rate is very slow. Consequently, mammalian cells, tissues or organs could be physiologically preserved through adsorption of the compounds to membranous proteins and extracellular matrices, leading to both the reduction in structural deterioration and the prevention of oxidative damage (12-34).

8. Conclusion

As described above, the polyphenol was able to control the proliferation of various cell types, and was demonstrated to be very useful for the long term storage of various tissues, including islet cells, blood vessels, cartilage, corneas, nerves, and skin. Currently in the U.S.A., approximately 850,000 tissue allografts are transplanted into patients annually. Much of this tissue is stored frozen. The method of cryopreservation at -196°C was adopted at the University of Tokyo Hospital and the Osaka National Cardiovascular Center in April 1999. Cryopreservation methods are being used for the long term storage of blood vessel, cartilage and skin. However, current research is still being directed at improving the effectiveness of cryopreservation and of preservation fluids, such as the University of Wisconsin solution, for tissue transplantation. We have herein demonstrated that the preservation of various tissues for up to three months without freezing is now possible, with excellent maintenance of the histological and biomechanical characteristics of the tissue. The authors have also succeeded in preserving the rat sciatic nerve, guinea pig periodontal ligament and rat myocardium in a non-frozen condition for long term storage prior to preservation. This has been made possible by the development of a new preservation fluid with polyphenol as an additive antioxidant. Therefore, the cryopreservation of many tissues may eventually be superseded by their storage in the newly developed polyphenol tissue banking fluid. This method of cell and tissue preservation would be of great benefit, not only in Japan, but throughout the world, especially in developing countries where cryopreservation is often not possible.

9. References

[1] Karlsson, J.O.M., Cravalho, E.G., and Toner, M. (1993) Intracellular ice formation: Causes and consequences. Cryo-Letters 14: 323-336.
[2] Karlsson, J.O.M., and Toner, M.(1996) Long-term storage of tissues by cryopreservation: Critical issues. Biomaterials 17: 243-256.
[3] Armitage, W.J., and Juss, B.K.(1996) The influence of cooling rate on survival of frozen cells in monolayers and in suspension. Cryo-Letters 17: 213-218.

[4] Sandler, S., and Anderson, A. (1984) The significance of culture for successful cryopreservation of isolated pancreatic islats of Langerhans. Cryobilogy 21: 502-510.
[5] Rubinsky, B., Lee, C.Y., Bastacky. J., and Onik, G. (1990) The process of freezing and the mechanism of damage during hepatic cryosurgery. Cryobiology 27: 85-97.
[6] Wilkins, L.M., Watson, S.R., Prosky, S.J., Meunier, S.F., and Parenteau, N.L. (1994) Development of a bilayered living skin construct for clinical applcations. Biotechnol. Bioeng. 43: 747-756.
[7] 7.Nakayama M., K. Suzuki, M. Toda, S. Okubo, Y. Hara, and T. Shimamura(1993) Inhibition of the infectivity of influenza virus by tea polyphenols. Antiviral Reserch 21: 289-299.
[8] Yang, C. S. and Z. -Y. Wang(1993) Tea and cancer. J. Natil Canter Inst. 85: 1039-1049.
[9] Khan W. A., Z. Y. Wang, M. Athar, D. R. Bickers, and H. Mukhtar(1998) Inhibition of the skin tumorigenicity of (±)-7b, a8-dihydroxy-9a, 10a-epoxy-7,8,9,10-tetrahydro-benzo [a] pyrene by tannic acid, green tea polyphenols and quercetin in Sencar mice. Cancer Lett. 43: 7-12.
[10] Cao, Y. and R. Cao(1999) Angiogenesis inhibited by drinking tea. Nature398: 381.
[11] Yang, C. S. (1997) Inhibition of carcinogenesis by tea. Nature 389: 134-135.
[12] Hyon SH, Kim DH, Cui W, Inoue K, Tsutsumi S, : Long term preservation of rat's aorta under the unfrost condition and it's transplantation., Organ Biology 9, 61-69 (2002)
[13] Hyon S.-H. and Kim O.-J. "Long-term Preservation of The Rat Pancreatic Islets Hibernate under Physiologycal Conditions" J.Biotechnology, 85: 241-246 (2001)
[14] Hyon S.-H. and Kim O.-J. "Hibernation of Mammalian Cells at the Living Body Temperature" Biotechnology and Bioprocess Engineering, 6: 289-292 (2001)
[15] Han,D-W., Suh,H., Park,Y-H., Cho,B-K., Hyon,S-H., Park,J-C., :Preservation of Human Saphenous Vein against Resctive Oxygen Species-Induced Oxidative Stress by Green Tea Polyphenol Pre-treatment. Artificial Organ. 27(12) 1137-1142 (2003)
[16] Han,D-W., Park,Y-H., Kim.J-K., Lee.K-Y., Hyon.S-H., Suh,H., Park,J-C., : Effects of Green Tea Polyphenol on Preservation of Human Saphenous Vein. Journal of Biotechnology 110. 109-117 (2004)
[17] D-W.Han, Y-H Park, J-K Kim, T-G Jung, K-Y Lee, S-H Hyon, J-C Park : Long-term preservation of human saphenous vein by green tea polyphenol under physiological conditions. : Tissue Engineering, 11.(7-8).1054-1064(2005)
[18] D-W. Han, S-H.Hyon., J-C.Park., K-D.Park., Y-H.Park., H-K.Park.,: Non-frozen preservation of mammalian tissue using green tea polyphenolic compounds. : Biomedical Materials 1 R18-R29 (2006)
[19] D-W. Han., H-R.Lim., H-S. Baek., M-H.Lee., S-J. Lee., S-H.Hyon., J-C. Park., : Inhibitory effects of epigallocatechin-3-o-gallate on serum-stimulated rat aortic smooth muscle cells via nuclear factor-κB down-modulation. Biochemical and Biophysical Research Communications Vol,345 iss, 148-155 (2006)
[20] Matsumura, K., Tsutsumi, S., Hyon S-H.. : Epigallocatechin-3-O-gallate As a Novel Preservation Additive for Tooth Transplantation. J Oral Tissue Engin 3(3) 125-130 (2006)

[21] Omasa M., Fukuse,T., Matsuoka, K., Inui, K., Hyon,S.H., Wada, H.,: Effect of Green Tea Extracted Polyphenol on Ischemia / Reperfusion Injury After Cold Preservation of Rat Lung. Transplantation Proceedings.35: 138-139 (2003)

[22] Ikeguchi, R., Kakinoki, R, Okamoto, T., Matsumoto, T., Hyon,S.-H.,. Nakamura, T.,: Successful Storage of Peripheral Nerves using Green Tea Polyphenol : an Experimental Study in Rats. Experimental neurology 184 :688-696(2004)

[23] Zhang, C., Mastumoto, S., Hyon,S.-H.,.Qualley,SA., Upshaw, L., Strong, DM., Reems, JA.,Polyphenol, An Extract of Green Tea, Increases Culture Recovery Rates of Isolated Islets from Non-Human Primate Pancreata and Marginal Grade Human Pancreata.: Cell Transplantation、13,145-152,(2004)

[24] Hyon,S.-H., : A Non-Frozen Living Tissue Bank for Allotransplantation Using Green Tea Polyphenols : Yonsei Medical Journal. Vol.45, No.6 1025-1034 (2004)

[25] Ikeguchi.R, Kakinoki.R, Matsumoto.T, Hyon.S-H, Nakamura.T: Peripheral Nerve Allografts Stored in Green Tea Polyphenol Solution. Transplantation 79: 688-695 (2005)

[26] Matsumoto, T.Kakinoki, R.Ikeguchi, S-H,Hyon, T.Nakamura,.: Optimal conditions for peripheral nerve storage in green tea polyphenol: an experimental study in animals. Journal of Neuroscince Methods 145 255-266 (2005)

[27] D.-W.Han, H.H.Kim, H.J.Son, H.S.Baek, K.-Y.Lee, S.-H.Hyon, J.-C. Park : Protection of Human Fibroblasts from Reactive Oxygen Species by Green Tea Polyphenolic Compounds : Key Engineering Materials Vols.288-289 665-668 (2005)

[28] D.-W.Han, H.-H..Kim, M.-H.Lee, H.-S.Baek, K.-Y. Lee, S.-H.Hyon, J.-C. Park : Protection of osteoblastic cells from freeze/thaw cycle-induced oxidative stress by green tea polyphenol : Biotechnology Letters 27. 655-660 (2005)

[29] D-.K. Rah, D.-W. Han, H.-S. Hyon, J.-C. Park : Prevention of reactive oxygen species-induced oxidative stress in human microvascular endothelial cells by green tea polyphenol : Toxicol.Lett. 155: 269-275 (2005)

[30] Park,Y-H., Han,D-W., Suh.H., Ryu.G.H., Hyon.S-H., Cho,B-K., Park,J-C., ：Protective effects of green tea polyphenol against reactive oxygen speciesinduced oxidative stress in cultured rat calvarial osteoblast, Cell Biology and Toxicology, 19(5): 325-337 (2003)

[31] Nakayama, K., Kakinoki, R., Ikeguchi, R., Yamakawa,T., Ohta, S., Fujita, S., Noguchi, T., Duncan Scott FM, Hyon, S-H., Nakamura, T.：Storage and allogeneic transplantation of peripheral nerve using a green tea polyphenol solution in a canine model. Journal of Brachial Plexus and Peripheral Nerve Injury 2010, 5:17doi:10.1186/1749-7221-5-17

[32] Han, D-W., Jung, D-Y., Park, J-C., Cho, H-H., Hyon, S-H., Han. D- K.：Underlying mechanism for suppression of vascular smooth muscle cells by green tea polyphenol EGCG released from biodegradable polymers for stent application. JOURNAL OF BIOMEDICAL MATERIALS RESEARCH A Vol.95A 424-433 (2010)

[33] Han, D-W., Lee, M-H., Kwon, B-J., Kim, H-L., Hyon, S-H., Park, J-C.：Selective Inhibitory Effect of Epigallocatechin-3-gallate on Migration of Vascular Smooth Muscle Cells Molecules 2010, *15*(11), 8488-8500; doi:10.3390/molecules15118488 (2010)

[34] Lee, M-H., Han, D-W., Hyon, S-H., Park, J-C. : Apoptosis of human fibrosarcoma HT-1080 cells by epigallocatechin-3-O-gallate via induction of p53 and caspases as well as suppression of Bcl-2 and phosphorylated nuclear factor-κB" 、Apoptosis 、(in press)

[35] Nakayama M., K. Suzuki, M. Toda, S. Okubo, Y. Hara, and T. Shimamura(1993) Inhibition of the infectivity of influenza virus by tea polyphenols. Antiviral Reserch 21: 289-299.

[36] Yang, C. S. and Z. -Y. Wang(1993) Tea and cancer. J. Natil Canter Inst. 85: 1039-1049.

[37] Khan W. A., Z. Y. Wang, M. Athar, D. R. Bickers, and H. Mukhtar(1998) Inhibition of the skin tumorigenicity of (±)-7b, a8-dihydroxy-9a, 10a-epoxy-7,8,9,10-tetrahydro-benzo [a] pyrene by tannic acid, green tea polyphenols and quercetin in Sencar mice. Cancer Lett. 43: 7-12.

[38] Cao, Y. and R. Cao(1999) Angiogenesis inhibited by drinking tea. Nature398: 381.

[39] Yang, C. S. (1997) Inhibition of carcinogenesis by tea. Nature 389: 134-135.

[40] Bischof J, Hunt CJ, Rubinsky B, Burgess A, Pegg DE: Effect of cooling rate and glycerol concentration on the structure of the frozen kidney - assessment by cryoscanning electron- microscopy., Cryobiology, 27(3), 301-310 (1990).

[41] Wilkins L.M., , Watson SR, Prosky SJ, Meunier SF, Parenteau NL.: Development of a bilayered living skin construct for clinical-applications., Biotechnol. Bioeng., 43 (8), 747-756 (1994).

[42] Ploeg RJ, Goossens D, Sollinger HW, Southard JH, Belzer FO, : Efficacy of 48-hour pancreas preservation with UW solution in the dog allograft model., Transplant Proc 20, 1026-1028 (1988)

[43] Jamieson NV, Lindell S, Sundberg R, Southard JH, Belzer FO, : An analysis of the components in UW solution using the isolated perfused rabbit liver., Transplantation 46, 512-516 (1988)

[44] Hoffman B, Sollinger H, Kalayoglu M, Belzer FO, : Use of UW solution fro kidney transplantation., Transplantation 46, 338-339 (1988)

[45] Karlsson JOM, Cravalho EG, Toner M, : Intracellular ice formation : Causes and consequences., Cryo-Letters, 14, 323-336 (1993)

[46] Karlsson JOM, Toner M, : Long-term storage of tissues by cryopreservation : Critical issues, Biomaterials, 17, 243-256 (1996)

[47] Armitage WJ, Juss BK, : The influence of cooling rate on survival of frozen cells in monolayers and in suspension., Cryo-Letters, 17, 213-218 (1996)

[48] Hannah, B-B.; Performance and safety of skin allografts. Clin Dermatol. 23: 365-375, 2005.

[49] Cram, A.E.; Domayer, M.; Shelby, J.; Human skin storage techniques: a study utilizing a nude mouse recipient. J. Trauma. 23: 924-926, 1983.

[50] Aneja, R.; Hake, P.W.; Burroughs T.J.; Denenberg A.G.; Wong H.R.;Zingarelli B.; Epigallocatechin, a green tea polyphenol, attenuates myocardial ischemia reperfusion injury in rats. Mol Med. 10: 55-62, 2004

[51] Han, D-W.; Kim, H.H.; Lee, M.H.; Son, H.J.; Baek, H.S.; Kim, H.J.: Park, J-C.; Differential antiproliferative responses of green tea polyphenol for fibroblast cell line versus normal fibroblast. Biomater. Res. 9: 188-192, 2005.

[52] Cram, A.E.; Domayer, M.; Shelby, J.; Human skin storage techniques: a study utilizing a nude mouse recipient. J. Trauma. 23: 924-926, 1983.

[53] Rosenquist, M.D., Cram, A.E., Kealey, G.P.; Skin preservation at 4℃: a species comparison. Cryobiol. 25: 31-37, 1988.

[54] Kapoor, M., Howard, R., Hall, I., Appleton, I.; Effects of epicatechin gallate on wound healing and scar formation in a full thickness incisional wound healing model in rats. Am. J. Pathol. 165: 299-307, 2004.

[55] Hakamata, Y.; Tahara, K.; Uchida, H.; Sakuma, Y.; Nakamura, M.; Kume, A.; Murakami, T.; Takahashi, M.; Takahashi, R.; Hirabayashi, M.; Ueda, M.; Miyoshi, I.; Kasai, N.; Kobayashi, E. Green fluorescent protein-transgenic rat: A tool for organ transplantation research. Biochem. Biophys. Res. Commun. 286:779–785; 2001.

[56] Fahmy, F. S.; Navsaria, H. A.; Frame, J. D.; Jones, C. R.; Leigh, I. M. Skin graft storage and keratinocyte viability. Br. J. Plast. Surg. 46(4):292–295; 1993.

[57] Peng, P. H.; Ko, M. L.; Chen, C. F. Epigallocatechin-3-gallate reduces retinal ischemia/reperfusion injury by attenuating neuronal nitric oxide synthase expression and activity. Exp. Eye Res. 86(4):637–646; 2008.

[58] Cram, A. E.; Domayer, M.; Shelby, J. Human skin storage techniques: A study utilizing a nude mouse recipient. J. Trauma 23:924–926; 1983.

[59] Rosenquist, M. D.; Cram, A. E.; Kealey, G. P. Skin preservation at 4°C: A species comparison. Cryobiology 25:31–37; 1988.

[60] Hakamata, Y.; Tahara, K.; Uchida, H.; Sakuma, Y.; Nakamura, M.; Kume, A.; Murakami, T.; Takahashi, M.; Takahashi, R.; Hirabayashi, M.; Ueda, M.; Miyoshi, I.; Kasai, N.; Kobayashi, E. Green fluorescent protein-transgenic rat: A tool for organ transplantation research. Biochem. Biophys. Res. Commun. 286:779–785; 2001.

[61] Kawazoe, T.; Kim, H. H.; Tsuji, Y.; Morimoto, N.; Hyon, S.-H.; Suzuki, S. Green tea polyphenols effect skin preservation in rats and improved the rate of skin grafts. Cell Transplant. 17(1–2):203–209; 2008.

[62] HakHee Kim, Takeshi Kawazoe, Kazuaki Matsumura, Shigehiko Suzuki, Soung-Hyu Hyon: Long-Term preservation of rat skin tissue by Epigallocatechin-3-*0*-Gallate. Cell Transplantation Vol.18 pp.513-519 (2009)

[63] Suong-Hyu Hyon, unpublished data.

24

Sentinel Skin Allograft for Monitoring of Composite Tissue Transplants Rejection

Zamfirescu DG[1], Lascar I[1] and Lanzetta M[2]
[1]Carol Davila Bucharest Medical University
[2]University of Canberra
[1]Romania
[2]Australia

1. Introduction

In contrast to visceral solid-organ transplants, a vascularized composite tissue allograft (CTA) is not a single tissue, and is histologically heterogeneous. It is a neurovascularized module of nonvital tissues which include structural, functional and aesthetic units. CTAs are composed of a large spectrum of ectodermal tissues: epidermis and epidermal derivatives such as nails and hair, nerves and mesodermal tissues such as dermis, muscles, bones, articular cartilage, ligaments, tendons and paratenon and other supportive and connective tissues, adipose tissue, vessels. In addition there are hematopoietic tissues and cells from bone marrow and lymph nodes and these latter elements are immunocompetent. Each tissue has differing antigenicity, displays different antigen expression and presentation mechanisms. As a result, CTAs elicit nonsynchronized immune responses, of differing intensity, among their tissue components.

So far only 135 CTA transplantations were carried out on human patients: 68 hand transplantations (49 patients), 12 abdominal wall transplantations, 9 bone and vascularized articulations transplantations, 7 peripheral nerves, 2 tendons, 23 larynxes, 1 right abdominal muscle, 1 tongue, a lobe made of the cephalic cervical skin and 2 ears, and 11 faces.

The transplantation of a composite tissue allograft is only justified when excellent functional outcome can be achieved. This aim is more important for CTAs then for organ allografts as the procedure is not lifesaving and lifelong immunosuppressive therapy, with its associated risks and side effects, is difficult to justify. Even mild and reversible rejection episodes can decrease the chance of a favorable outcome.

Skin is an important component of a CTA and is the most immunogenic of the component tissues. The skin is more sensitive to rejection than any other tissues or visceral organ, and the primary reason is probably its unique immunologic defense function, with its special intrinsec antigenic and immunologic properties. Boss et al. identified these properties as "the skin immune system" and demonstrate, that the skin is not only the largest organ in the body but is itself an immunologic effector organ, with almost half its cells belonging or related to the immune system (especially the large quantity of dendritic cells within epidermis and dermis). For CTAs the best marker of rejection is by visual and histopathological examination of the skin, as it is the skin that is first involved in the rejection process.

Skin is an important component of a CTA and is the most immunogenic of the component tissues. The skin is more sensitive to rejection than any other tissues or visceral organ, and the primary reason is probably its unique immunologic defense function, with its special intrinsec antigenic and immunologic properties. Boss et al. identified these properties as "the skin immune system" and demonstrate, that the skin is not only the largest organ in the body but is itself an immunologic effector organ, with almost half its cells belonging or related to the immune system (especially the large quantity of dendritic cells within epidermis and dermis). For CTAs the best marker of rejection is by visual and histopathological examination of the skin, as it is the skin that is first involved in the rejection process.

Monitoring of CTA rejection is facilitated because the first tissue to be rejected is the skin, which is the outermost tissue of a CTA. Skin biopsy provides a more specific diagnosis to confirm the visual assessment but delays diagnosis. Repeated skin biopsies also lead to scarring that represents a considerable aesthetic problem in the case of a hand or face transplants. The ideal marker of CTA rejection should therefore obviate the need for biopsy of the transplant and provide easily warning of rejection of the graft itself. Early detection of the first stages of rejection enables advanced administration of salvage therapy, resulting in a rapid and efficient reversal of rejection.

2. Distant sentinel skin allograft (DSSG) - experimental study

Some studies report a more rapid rejection of isolated skin grafts compared to rejection of skin that is part of a CTA. This has led us to examine the use of distant sentinel skin allograft (DSSG) of donor origin transplanted simultaneously with a limb, as a marker of rejection.

In one of our studies, using a hind limb transplantation model in rats we demonstrated that the DSSG serves as a predictive marker for visual assessment, as well as a site for repeated biopsies that does not damage the CTA itself.

Sixty rats with hind limb transplants were included in this study. They were divided into two groups. Group 1 (n=15) received limb transplants and immunosuppressive therapy (control group). Group 2 (n=45) received a limb transplant and a simultaneous sentinel skin graft, plus immunosuppressive therapy.

Surgical procedure

Brown Norway (BN) rats served as donors and Lewis rats as recipients of orthotopic hind limb transplants and free skin flap allografts. The previously described surgical technique for limb replantation and transplantation was used.[7-11] A free full thickness skin graft 4 cm x 5 cm was obtain from the abdominal region of BN donors and transplanted to the inter

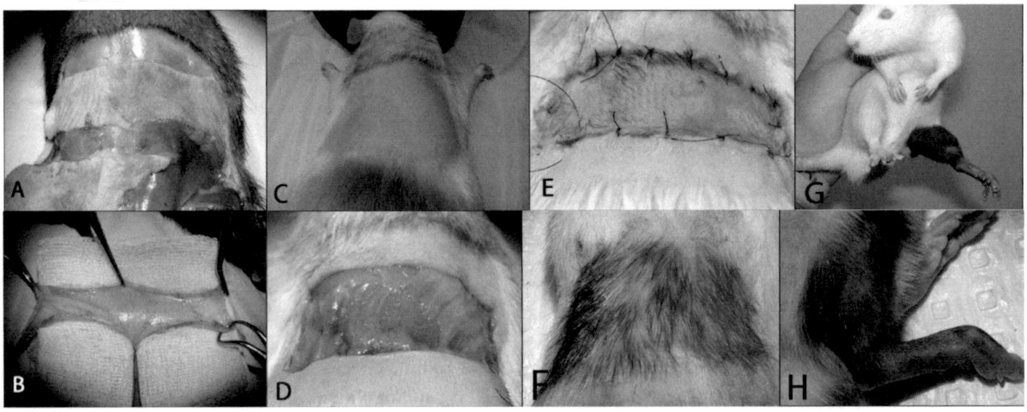

Fig. 1. Full thickness sentinel skin allograft and the hind limb transplantation

scapular region of LEW recipient rats. Special attention was given to preserve the panniculus carnosus and to apply the skin graft directly to this highly vascular tissue (**Fig 1**). **A-F** 4 x 5 cm full thickness skin graft harvested from the abdominal region of BN donor. DSSG transplanted to the inter-scapular region of LEW recipient rats. Special attention was given to preserve the **panniculus carnosus** (D) and to apply the skin graft on this highly vascular tissue. **G, H** The hind limb allotransplant

Immunosuppressive drug regime

All animals received standard immunosuppressive therapy, consisting of the triple drug combination with the first administration provided on the operative day. We used the standard regime consisting of FK506 (Prograf^R Janssen-Cilag) 2 mg/kg/ day; MMF (CellCept^R, Roche Products) 15 mg/kg/day and Prednisone (PredMix^R, oral liquid 5 mg/ml. Archpend) 0.5 mg/kg/day administered in 1 ml saline by oral gavage for 6 weeks. This time was sufficient to allow for complete healing of the skin graft and limb transplant, after which, all drugs were stopped. Salvage therapy was administered for early rejection episodes upon the first visual signs of rejection of the sentinel skin graft or of the transplanted limb skin. This consisted of FK506 10 mg/kg/day; MMF30 mg/kg/day and Prednisone 0.5 mg/kg/day. Salvage therapy was administered for 3 days, followed by the optimal drug regime until signs of rejection were reversed.

Visual monitoring of rejection

The skin of transplanted limbs and skin allografts was monitored twice a day for any signs of rejection, including erythema, changes in texture of the skin, desquamation, epidermolysis, edema, exudation and skin necrosis. After the withdrawal of immunosuppression rejection was assessed based on a new clinical (visual) and histologic grading system that was focused to more accurately describes the very early signs of skin rejection. Rejection was assigned visually, based on changes in color and texture of the skin in most clinically affected skin area.

Histological evaluation of the rejection

Tissue specimens were taken after withdrawal of immunosuppressive therapy, at the first signs of skin graft or limb skin rejection. Skin biopsies were fixed in 10% Neutral Buffered Formalin before transfer to 70% ethyl alcohol. Tissue samples were embedded in paraffin for routine light histological examination. Sections were stained with hematoxylin and eosin. A pathologist (CAL) read all the slides in a blinded fashion and scored the sections based on a proprietary histologic grading system. Rejection was assigned histologically, based on changes in the most immunoactive zone on the histological slides.

3. Results

One month post-operatively the skin grafts were well healed, with stable size and shape. To facilitate observation, hair from the skin graft and limb was removed with a depilatory cream at the end of the 6th postoperative week. This caused only a slight skin inflammation observed for one day in 3 rats.

Visual rejection episodes in controls

After the withdrawal of immunosuppression rejection was assessed based on a newly developed clinical (visual) and histologic grading system that was aimed to more accurately describes the very early signs of skin rejection. Rejection was assigned visually and histologically, based on changes in color and texture of the skin in most clinically affected skin area and in the most immunoactive zone on the histological slides. The details of this visual scoring system are shown in (**Table 1**).

Grade 0 No rejection	Normal epidermal and dermal appearance without evidence of rejection
Grade 1 Indeterminate/ supposed rejection	Very early visual signs of rejection Focal (<25% of limb or DSSG surface) inconspicuous changes in the skin color (pink/pinkish or slight red/reddish spots) and/or in the texture of the skin (dryness, fine scaling of epidermis)
Grade 2 Mild rejection	Clear visual signs of rejection Diffuse (25-50 % of DSSG or limb skin surface) clear changes in color and texture of skin, sometimes with slight limb edema, thickening of the skin
Grade 3 Moderate rejection	Extensive (more than 50% of DSSG or limb skin surface) and advances alteration of skin quality - desquamation, scabs, skin crusts
Grade 4 Severe rejection	Destruction of epidermis with intact dermis or complete destruction of the skin

Table 1. Visual grading system for assessment of rejection

Three animals (20%) showed early rejection and salvage therapy was successful in all cases. One of rats developed a second rejection episode, successfully treated with salvage therapy. In two of these three rats skin damage after resolution of rejection prevented assessment of grades 1 and 2 rejection do to incomplete or deficient healing. The remaining 12 rats (80%) were free of rejection during the treatment period.

The average time for the onset of grade 1 rejection in limb skin after immunosuppression ceased was 6.75 ± 1.42 days (median day 6.5) and 8.75 ± 2.38 days (median day 8) for grade 2. The mean interval between the onset of grade 1 and the development of grade 2 rejection in limb skin was 2 ± 1.35 days for rats free of early rejection (n= 12).

Visual rejection episodes in group 2 (rats with limb transplant and DSSG)

During the first 6 weeks 28 rats (62%) were rejection free. Seventeen rats (38%) developed early rejection. Thirteen rats (29%) were excluded from the study due to the poor quality of skin doe to incomplete or deficient healing after salvage therapy. In total, 32 rats, 28 without early rejection episodes and 4 rats with one episode of very early or early rejection, successfully reversed with salvage therapy, were evaluated after termination of immunosuppressive therapy (**Fig 2**).

The average onset grade 1 rejection was 5.06 days (median day 5) for DSSG, and 6.41 days (median day 6) for limb skin. The average interval between grade 1 rejection of the skin graft and grade 1 rejection of the limb skin was 1.35 days. Rats evaluated in group 2 displayed a strong statistic difference in the onset of grade 1 rejection of the skin graft and the limb skin ($p < 0.0005$).

The average onset grade 2 rejection was 8.28 days (median day 8) for DSSG, and day 9.21 7 (median day 9) for limb skin. The interval between grade 2 rejection of the skin graft and grade 2 rejection of the limb skin was 0.91 days. There was a small but statistically significant difference between the first day with visual signs of grade 2 rejection of the skin graft and the limb skin ($p < 0.05$).

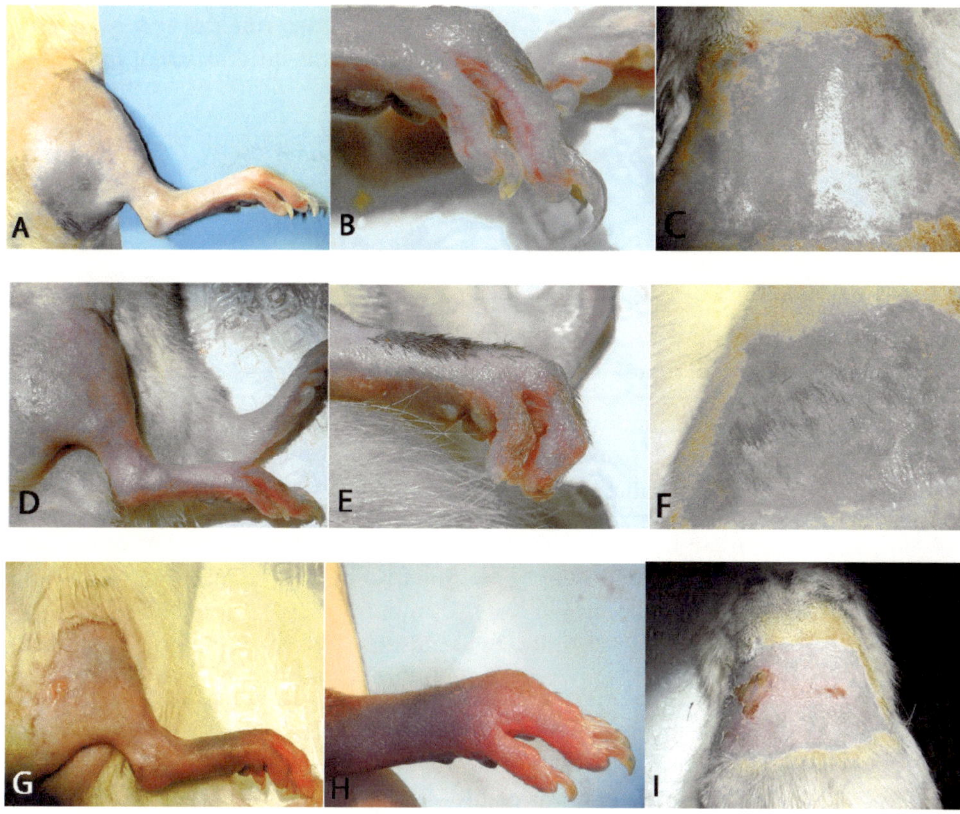

Fig. 2. Clinical (visual) aspect of rejection on the limb skin and on the DSSG in the earlier stages of rejection **A, B,C** *Grade 0 (No rejection)* - Normal epidermal and dermal appearance without evidence of rejection **D, E, F** *Grade 1 (Inconspicuous / indeterminate / supposed rejection)* - Very early visual signs of rejection; Focal (<25% of limb or DSSG surface) inconspicuous changes in the skin color (pink/pinkish or slight red/reddish spots) and/or in the texture of the skin (dryness, fine scaling of epidermis) **G, H, I** *Grade 2 (Mild rejection)* - Clear visual signs of rejection; Diffuse (25-50 % of DSSG or limb skin surface) clear changes in color and texture of skin, sometimes with slight limb edema, thickening of the skin

The time difference between the onset of grade 1 rejection and the development of grade 2 rejection was on average 3.4 days for DSSG and 2.9 days for limb skin. There was no significant difference between grades 1 or 2 rejection of the limb skin of control animals and rats with both a limb transplant and sentinel skin graft. As a result, we conclude that application of a skin allograft does not influence the rejection of a transplanted limb.

Histologic rejection results

161 biopsies from 45 animals were evaluated histologically for signs of rejection. Specimens were taken for suspected rejection or when the visual grade appeared to alter. Samples were

taken concurrently, from both the sentinel skin graft and limb allograft. Rejection was assigned histologically, based on changes in the most immunoactive zone on the histological slides. All slides were analyzed in a blinded fashion and scored based on a new histologic grading system. The new grading system was introduced to describe the very early changes in skin pathology observed during onset of rejection. The criteria used for histologic assessment of skin rejection are shown in **(Table 2, Fig 3)**.

Grade 0	Normal epidermal and dermal appearance without evidence of rejection Dermal mononuclear cell infiltration < 10 cells / 500X optic field
Grade 1 Indeterminate rejection	Dermal mononuclear cell infiltration 10-20 cells / 500X optic field Epidermal (especially on epidermo-dermal junction) mononuclear cells infiltration 1-3 cells / 200X optic field
Grade 2 Mild rejection	Diffuse intercellular edema (spongiosis) on basal layer of epidermis with normal continuity of epidermo-dermal junction Dermal mononuclear cell infiltration 10-20 cells / 500X optic field Epidermal (especially on epidermo-dermal junction) mononuclear cells infiltration > 3 cells / 200X optic field
Grade 3 Moderate rejection	Discontinuity of epidermo-dermal junction Focal basal cells vacuolization Dermal mononuclear cell infiltration more than 20 cells / 500X optic field Epidermal (especially on epidermo-dermal junction) mononuclear cells infiltration > 3 cells / 200X optic field Intercellular edema on basal layer of epidermis (spongiosis) Dyskeratosis of squamous cells in the epidermis or hair follicle epithelium
Grade 4 Severe rejection	Complete separation at the epidermo dermal junction Complete epidermal degeneration and necrosis Dense inflammatory infiltration in the dermis > 20 cells / 500X optic field

Table 2. Histology grading and scoring system for assessment of rejection

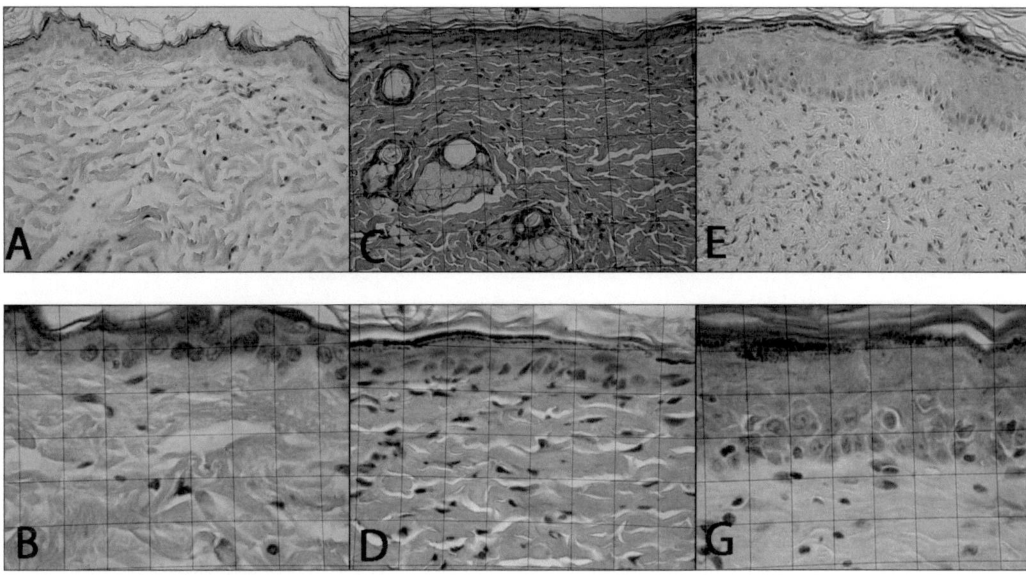

Fig. 3. Histological aspects of rejection in the earlier stages of skin rejection

A, B Grade 0 (H&E; 200x and 500x) *Normal epidermal and dermal appearance without evidence of rejection* - Dermal mononuclear cell infiltration < 10 cells / 500X optic field **C, D *Grade 1*** (H&E; 200x and 500x) *Indeterminate rejection* - Dermal mononuclear cell infiltration 10-20 cells / 500X optic field; Epidermal (especially on epidermo-dermal junction) mononuclear cells infiltration 1-3 cells / 200X optic field ***E, G. Grade*** 2 (H&E; 200x and 500x) *Mild rejection* - Diffuse intercellular edema (spongiosis) on basal layer of epidermis with normal continuity of epidermo-dermal junction; Dermal mononuclear cell infiltration 10-20 cells / 500X optic field; Epidermal (especially on epidermo-dermal junction) mononuclear cells infiltration > 3 cells / 200X optic field

The average grade of limb rejection noted in 35 samples harvested from 13 control rats was 1.57. In group 2, 126 samples from 32 rats were analyzed. Analyzing the early stages of rejection (grade 0 - 2), for corresponding skin graft and limb skin samples, the average grade of rejection observed for limb skin was 1.08 compared with 1.46 for the skin grafts. The difference in severity of rejection was found to be significant using a paired t test at $p < 0.005$. The higher average grade of rejection seen in sentinel skin infers that rejection develops sooner at this site. This finding confirms the hypothesis that a distant sentinel skin graft rejects before limb skin.

There was no significant difference using an unpaired t-test (p value = 0.86) between the onset of limb skin rejection in groups 1 and 2. The mean rejection grade was 1.57 for group 1 and 1.42 for group 2. This result confirmed visual analysis, and demonstrated that the sentinel skin graft did not influence the rejection of limb allografts when transplanted simultaneously.

4. Conclusions

In conclusion, these findings confirm a small, but significant delay in rejection of limb skin compared to a DSSG. Skin grafts transplanted simultaneously with a hind limb are thus a useful marker of rejection by providing advanced waning of an impending episode. This allows earlier intervention with salvage therapy and the consequent rapid initiation of therapy that is of benefit in a clinical setting. The DSSG can be placed on a site usually covered by clothing and may obviate the need for biopsies of the transplanted limb, with their associated scarring, functional and aesthetic consequences. The skin DSSG did not appear to significantly alter the incidence of severity of rejection and appear to be safe in this animal model. Modifications of the current visual and histopathological criteria for diagnosis of rejection were introduced to allow early detection.

The concept of DSSG is already applied in clinical settings. A series of three hand transplants performed where patients received an additional simultaneous full-thickness donor skin graft transplanted to the left hip area. This skin was used as a source for skin biopsies and as an additional area for monitoring rejection (distant sentinel skin graft, DSSG). The DSSG used in all three patients proved to be of benefit, allowing prediction of rejection of the hand by as much as 7 days. This allowed appropriate treatment to be started immediately. In one patient, salvage therapy (systemic and topical) was delayed until the hand showed the same clinical and histological signs of rejection. The skin changes resolved completely within 5 days at both locations. In the other two patients salvage therapy was started immediately DSSG showed the onset of rejection and rejection of the hand was not observed. However, the DSSG was of value only in the early postoperative phases. With time DSSG cells were replaced by "creeping substitution" of recipient skin and monitoring value was lost.

In our study, we found that the DSSG showed the first signs of rejection (grade 1), with a delay of 1.35 days before the limb skin detection. Sensitivity was reduced to 0.91 days for grade 2 rejection. The 7 days interval noted in Italian clinical cases, may be explain by a gradual taper of immunosuppressive therapy, rather than the complete withdrawal used in this study.

In the case of the first face transplantation a sentinel radial forearm flap harvested from the donor's left upper limb was transferred to the recipient's left submammary fold and suture end-to-end to the thoracodorsal vessels. This vascularized composite tissue flap, hidden under the hanging breast, was used to monitor indirectly the immunological behavior of the graft, aiming to avoid damage to the reconstructed face by repeated skin biopsies.

5. References

Andrew Lee W. P., Yaremchuk M J, Pan YC, Randolph MA, Tan CM, Weiland AJ. Relative Antigenicity of Components of a Vascularized Limb Allograft. Plast Reconstr Surgery, March 1991, Volume 87, Issue 3

Askenasy N Localized Bone Marrow Transplantation Leads to Skin Allograft Acceptance in Nonmyeloablated Recipients: Comparison of Intra-Bone Marrow and Isolated Limb Perfusion. *Stem Cells* 2002; 20: 86-93

Black KS., Hewitt CW., Aniel M., Grisham GR., Caiozzo VJ., Achauer BM. Neuromuscular capabilities in long-term composite tissue allografts. Transplant Proc 1988;20:369

Bos JD, Das PK, Kapsenberg ML. The skin immune system (SIS), 2nd Ed. Boca Raton: CRC Press, 1997

Buttemeyer R., Jones NJ., Min Z., Rao U. Rejection of the Component Tissues of Limb Allografts in Rats Immunosuppressed with FK506 and Cyclosporine. Plast Reconst Surg 1996;97:139

Doi K. Homotransplantation of limbs in rats. A preliminary report on an experimental study with nonspecific immunosuppressive drugs. Plast Reconstr Surgery 1979 Nov;64(5):613-21

Guzman-Stein A, Shons AR. Functional recovery in the rat limb transplant model: a preliminary study. Transplant Proc. 1987 Feb;19(1 Pt 2):1115-7.

Hewitt CW, Black KS, Fraser LA, Howard EB, Martin DC, Achauer BM, Furnas DW. Composite tissue (limb) allografts in rats. I. Dose-dependent increase in survival with cyclosporine. Transplantation. 1985 Apr; 39(4):360-4.

Hewitt CW, Black KS, Fraser LA, Howard EB, Martin DC, Achauer BM, Furnas DW. Composite tissue (limb) allografts in rats. I. Dose-dependent increase in survival with cyclosporine. Transplantation. 1985 Apr; 39(4):365-8.

Hewitt CW., Black KS., Aguinaldo AMA., Lin SS., Howard EB. Pathologic alterations in the skin component of composite tissue and skin allografts treated with Cyclosporine. Transplant Proc 1988;20:1003

Jones NF., Heberbraud D., Buttemeyer R., Zhao M., Benhaim P., Rao U. Comparison of Long-Term Immunosuppression for Limb Transplantation Using Cyclosporine, Tacrolimus and Mycophenolate Mofetil: Implications for Clinical Composite Tissue Transplantation. Plast Reconstr Surg 2001;107:777

Kim SK, Aziz S, Oyer P, Hentz VR. Use of cyclosporine-A in allotransplantation of rat limbs. Ann Plast Surg 1984; 12: 249-255

Lanzetta M, Dubernard JM. Hand Transplantation. Springer Milan 2007, 263-268

Lanzetta M, Dubernard JM. Hand Transplantation. Springer Milan 2007, 425-433

Llull R. An open proposal for clinical composite tissue allotransplantation. Transplant Proc Volume 30, Issue 6, September 1998, 2692-2696

Press BHJ, Sibley RK, Shons AR. Limb allotransplantation in the rat: extended survival and return of nerve function with continuous cyclosporine/prednisone immunosuppression. Ann Plast Surg 1986 1986 Apr;16(4):313-21.

Scott A. Gruber, Mansour V. Shirbacheh, Jon W. Jones, John H. Barker, Warren C. Breidenbach. Local drug delivery to composite tissue allografts (p 407-411). Microsurgery Volume 20 Issue 8 , 357 - 469 (2000)

Shapiro RI, Cerra FB. A model for reimplantation and transplantation of a complex organ: the rat hind limb. J Surg Res 1978;24:501–506

Zamfirescu DG, Owen E, Lascar I, Molitor M, Zegrea I, Popescu M, Bishop GA, Lauer CA, Simionescu M, Climov M, Lanzetta M., Sentinel skin allograft-a reliable marker for monitoring of composite tissue transplant rejection. Transplant Proc. 2009 Mar;41(2):503-8.

Zdichavsky M, Jones J, Ustuner TE, Ren X, Edelstein J, Maldonado C, Breidenbach WC, Gruber SA, Ray M, Barker JH. Scoring of skin rejection in a swine composite tissue allograft model. J Surg Res 1999;85:1–8

25

Immunological Considerations for Inducing Skin Graft Tolerance

Ethel J. Gordon
North Carolina Agricultural & Technical State University
United States of America

1. Introduction

While the first uses of skin transplantation may be found in anecdotal images involving the use of foreign tissue to cover burns and damaged skin, the modern era of skin grafting attempts to understand the phenomenon scientifically. One well documented case describes Joseph E. Murray's surgical procedure to use skin from a recently deceased person to cover the skin of a pilot who suffered disfiguring burns in 1944 (Murray, 1992) The transplanted skin survived for more than thirty days, despite any predictions of rejection that might have destroyed the tissue in two weeks or less. Murray hypothesized that the procedure was successful because of the weakened state of the recipient's immune system. Murray continued his interest in transplantation immunology, and ten years later his team was the first to engraft an organ from a living donor, (Murray, 1992).

In 1944 Medawar described rejection of allografts, that is, organs or tissues exchanged between individuals of the same species (Medawar, 1944). His pioneering work described the consequences of allograft and autograft transplantation in exquisite detail. He used the rabbit skin model to show differences in acceptance of autografts, using the same individual or same strain as the tissue source, vs. allografts that exchanged skin between different animals of the same species. He further used meticulously measured tissue size as a surrogate marker for skin antigen dose and documented the process of healing for autographs opposed to the "actively acquired immune reactions" that resulted in the necrosis of allografts. R. E. Billingham (1959) reviewed the fate of engrafted tissue that is rejected by the host in light of the then recently discovered major histocompatibility complex in the mouse (MHC). The MHC genes encode cell surface proteins that allow the immune system to discriminate between its own cells and foreign cells. Billingham referenced the use of isogenic mouse strains wherein each animal of the strain has identical MHC genes, and these animal models facilitated the understanding of graft versus host disease, rejection mediated by immunocompetent cells within a graft (Billingham, 1959).

Billingham, Brent, and Medawar (1953) described immunological tolerance that is actively acquired following prenatal exposure to foreign tissue in a mouse model. This phenomenon described the survival of engrafted tissue, whereas the same tissue generated immunity resulting in graft destruction when transplanted in the adult. After eight weeks, the tolerant mice were challenged with adult skin of the same donor origin as the primary transplant, in order to evaluate the persistence of tolerance. These experiments documented the utility of mouse models as a practical means to help us understand immunological processes. Five years later, Billingham and Silvers (1958) induced specific tolerance to the male chromosome associated Y antigen in neonatal female mice, again using the skin graft model. Researchers continue to use these basic methods to uncover the underlying mechanism of tolerance and immunity.

Skin grafts, with their enhanced antigenicity and abundant supplies of antigen presenting cells, remain a vigorous test of any tolerance induction system (Murray, 1971, Nasir et al., 2009, Tobin et al., 2009, Akdis, 2010, van den Berg et al., 2011, Kaplan, 2010, del Rio et al., 2010). Some of the skin associated antigens include autoantigens found on keratinocytes and appear to induce T lymphocyte reactivity that results in skin eruptions (Jackman et al., 2002). Antigenicity of skin has remained a concern for those promoting translational medicine, including those who promote the use of composite tissue allografts (Swearingen et al., 2008). The grafting of composite tissue is often used in limb replacement surgery. These grafts consist of complex combinations of multiple tissue types, including skin, adipose tissue, bone and others (Siemionow et al., 2009). The complexity of these composite tissue allografts is such that a new classification system was devised in order to accurately describe their attributes. Tissue antigenicity is one of the criteria on which the classification system is based (Gordon et al., 2009). These historical experiments helped to usher in the era of modern skin transplantation.

2. Generalized Immunosuppression to facilitate skin graft acceptance

Medical science has pursued a multiplicity of scientific directions in order to utilize solid organ transplantation as a potential cure for life-threatening diseases and as a treatment for sever disfigurement. Organ transplantation has been referred to as "One of the most remarkable achievements of medicine during the 20th century" (Goldstein, 2011). Scientific advances gleaned from the use of skin grafts and other tissue and organ grafts have restored tissue function, extended the life, and promoted the general well-being of the graft host. The spoken or unspoken hypothesis behind the use of generalized immunosuppression may be stated as follows: If the immune system in an otherwise healthy individual is capable of recognizing foreign tissue and mounting an attack against it, then significantly reducing all such recognition may allow for engrafted tissue to remain intact and functional. Many of these procedures required protracted or life-long treatments with unanticipated or negative sequelae (Ingvar et al., 2010, Berardinelli et al., 2009). The goal of these broad-based protocols was to protect the viability of the graft in order to protect the life of the host. Some notable examples of the use of generalized immunosuppressive agents are described below.

2.1 Three categories of drugs targeting lymphocytes have been described

Information gleaned from reviews in major journals describes three general categories of immunosuppressive agents (Halloran, 2004, Lindenfeld et al., 2004, Gonzalez Posada, 2006, 1970). These include antibodies directed against lymphocytes, steroids, and agents that interfere with metabolism or that have toxic effects on cells. The first category is often referred to as antilymphocyte or antithymocyte globulin (ALG or ATG). ALG in combination with an intrathymic dose of donor spleen cells was shown to induce graft survival in a rat model (Shen et al., 1996). Lewis-Brown Norway cardiac allografts showed extensive survival in Lewis rats; whereas skin grafts from the same donor strain were rejected at a similar rate as third party grafts, that is, grafts bearing transplantation antigens different from those of the donor or host. These experiments demonstrated further the increased antigenicity of skin in relation to other tissues. The author hypothesizes that additional non-MHC skin antigens may be responsible for the rejection. Additional aspects of skin antigenicity are described above (Murray, 1971, Nasir et al., 2009, Tobin et al., 2009, Akdis, 2010, van den Berg et al., 2011, Kaplan, 2010, del Rio et al., 2010).

Adding ALG to a protocol that includes azathioprine and prednisolone may reduce the toxic effects of ALG. Corticosteroids such as prednisolone reduce the inflammatory response, interfere with protein synthesis and are cytotoxic for lymphocytes. Despite the lymphocyte toxicity, these reagents were not found to prolong skin graft survival. The cytotoxic and antimetabolite drugs appeared to target DNA function, activity, or synthesis. Cyclophosphamide is a strong DNA cross-linker and alkylating agent. Methotrexate is a folic acid inhibitor that blocks DNA synthesis, and therefore interferes with cell division in lymphocytes. Azathioprine and 6-mercaptopurine are two related purine analogs that have been show to delay graft rejection. The effect of all of these drugs was variable depending on the species treated and the regimen used. Optimum regimen included using the drugs in combination with the specific antigen in order to have a more prolonged graft-protecting effect rather than a temporary dampening of the body's ability to mount an immune response.

2.2 Protection of rabbit skin by phenothiazine derivatives

Eyal and associates (1965) used phenothiazine related products to suppress immune responses to rabbit skin allografts. The team focused their attention on the action of three different compounds: chlorpromazine, perphenazine, or promethazine. They chose these reagents because of reports that these compounds could minimize cell death and tissue necrosis, albeit a protective effect was not witnessed with the engraftment of guinea pig skin. Eyal and colleagues hypothesized that an optimal dose and specific compound combination would be protective. These compounds produced different degrees of graft protection in controlled experiments where they were tested against normal saline in otherwise untreated animals. Both treatment and control groups of rabbits were given ear skin allografts of approximately equal sizes. They found that the most beneficial compound was promethazine, followed by perphenazine; and that the least protective was chlorpromazine. They attribute the extended skin graft survival of treated animals to a membrane protective effect of the drugs on graft recipient cells and to a reduced loss of donor antigen from the graft itself.

2.3 Prolongation of graft survival mediated by methylhydrazine derivatives

Floersheim (1967) used methylhydrazine derivatives to induce tolerance in MHC disparate adult mice and reported significant improvement in graft prolongation when the treatment was combined with an infusion of donor specific cells derived from spleen or from kidneys and liver. Graft survival was increased to at least twenty percent when this combined therapeutic approach was used. According to the US Environmental Protection Agency (EPA) these drugs may have a negative impact on liver and kidney primarily, and on blood and spleen secondarily (EPA, 2007). Acute but not chronic effects have been reported for humans (EPA, 2007). Thus despite some benefits in terms of graft survival, potentially harmful side effects limited more widespread use.

2.4 The use of urethane in combination with X-irradiation to protect skin grafts

Cole and Davis (1962) used a reagent known as a DNA antagonist and an inhibitor of mitosis in order to prolong survival of skin grafts in sub-lethally X-irradiated mice. They were aware of studies that demonstrating that high doses of radiation could protect a graft by suppressing an immune response. Cole and Davis hypothesized that a lower radiation dose in combination with urethane treatment would be immunoprotective and showed that sixty percent of the mice had significant skin graft survival. Mean graft survival in the treated animals was 40 days vs. 18 days for untreated mice of the same strain. Their study included an early attempt to develop irradiation bone marrow chimeric mice. A subsequent study induced skin graft tolerance that endured for more than 130 days and was specific for transplantation antigens of the bone marrow donor, as third party grafts were rejected (Davis and Cole, 1963). In such experiments, the native bone marrow is ablated, in whole or in part, by radiation, and specific donor derive bone marrow is used to replace the ablated cells of the host. Additional examples of irradiation bone marrow chimerism appear below.

More recently, urethane or polyurethane has been used as a dressing to promote wound healing of split thickness skin graft donors (Cigna et al., 2009), and as a component of negative pressure dressings for young burn patients who receive skin grafts (Psoinos et al., 2009).

2.5 Calcineurin inhibitors

Calcineurin is a protein phosphatase found in eukaryotic cells whose activity is significantly blocked by cyclosporine A and Fk506, now referred to as tacrolimus (Rusnak and Mertz, 2000). The once-popular calcineurin inhibitors (CNI) fell out of favor due to their observed nephrotoxicity (Groetzner et al., 2004). Additional complications of the use of CNI drugs include associated malignancies. Doesch et al. (2010) studied the development of neoplasias in cardiac patients treated with immunosuppressive drugs. They found a strong correlation between the use of CNIs or the drug azathioprine and the development of malignancies. These drug-associated malignancies include multiple forms of skin cancer, including squamous cell carcinoma (Wu et al., 2010), but exclusive of melanoma (Signorell et al., 2010). In contrast, the rate of malignancies was reduced in patients treated with non-CNI based agents such as mammalian target of rapamycin (m-TOR) inhibitors (Doesch et al., 2010).

3. Pre-engraftment reduction of tissue antigenicity

3.1 Cultured tissues and antibodies

Jacobs and Uphoff (1974) reviewed a variety of methodologies used to reduce the potential immune reaction between the donated tissue or organ and the graft recipient and reported that phenotypic changes including reduced antigenicity may be observed in cultured cells. These changes vary with species. The advantage of using these techniques may be a reduced dependence on the use of immunosuppressive agents. Antibodies may be used to treat the graft donor or the tissue itself. They summarized the experiments of Hellman and Duke (1967) who used a skin allograft model to demonstrate the reversal of tolerance to syngeneic skin when the tissue was incubated with skin of a MHC disparate donor. Unpredictably, pre-incubating donor and recipient skin together did not result in prolonged skin allograft survival.

3.2 Preconditioning with allogeneic RNA or DNA

In agreement with this data, the benefits of altering donor skin antigenicity was further demonstrated when Guttman et al. (1964) prevented acceptance of syngeneic skin grafts by pretreating mouse skin in vitro with allogeneic RNA. In contrast to these results, Lemperle et al. (1968) demonstrated that pre-treating donor tissue with RNA or DNA facilitated extended skin graft survival in MHC disparate donor and host combinations.

4. The use of chimerism to protect engrafted tissues

4.1 Bone marrow chimerism induced by whole body Irradiation

An early model of irradiation induced bone marrow chimerism was developed by two scientist working at the National Institute of Allergy and Infectious Disease (Liacopoulos and Goode, 1964). Liacopoulos and Goode were aware that overwhelming the immune system of potential tissue donors with a bolus of strong antigens from different sources may block reactivity to a specific unrelated antigen. This procedure is known as protein overloading and is directed towards the graft donor. The group tested the hypothesis that spleen cells, bone marrow or skin from animal models given a large dose of antigen would be tolerated in another animal. The graft recipients were irradiated and pretreated with donor strain derived cells prior to skin grafting. Rabbit gamma globulin or Limulus hemocyanin served as the strong antigens. The authors used both a mouse allograft model and a concordant rat-to-mouse xenograft model (Liacopoulos and Goode, 1964).

Owen et al. (1945) had observed earlier that naturally occurring tolerance could develop between dizygotic calves in utero. Since these calves each had a different immunological makeup, the prenatal exposure to each other's disparate antigenic makeup was undoubtedly the source of the immunological unresponsiveness. Stone et al. (1965) expanded the initial findings by engrafting skin between dizygotic twins known to be chimeric at the erythrocyte level. The discovery of chimerism in these calves provided the scientific basis for adapting this concept to the development of irradiation bone marrow chimerism as a model for the induction of transplantation tolerance.

Following these discoveries, a series of studies tested the hypothesis that the phenomenon of chimerism could be experimentally induced in order to prolong allograft survival (Mathe' et al., 1963, Seller, 1967, Lubaroff and Silvers, 1973, Buckley, 1975). Mathe' et al. (1965) applied this concept in order to protect a patient from leukemia. The patient was given whole body irradiation followed by a bone marrow transplant comprised of tissues from six different male and female donors, all of whom were related to the host. The bone marrow graft restored the myeloid and erythroid compartments. A skin graft from one of the male bone marrow donors remained intact and viable for more than seven months, while skin grafts from other donors were rejected. These results implied that the donor and the host were more histocompatible. More recent applications of irradiation bone marrow chimerism are discussed below.

Tolerance to allografts following whole body irradiation has been reviewed (Strober et al., 1979, Slavin et al., 1985, Sprent et al., 1993, Monaco, 2004). A potential mechanism to explain the success of these grafts was suggested by Okada and Strober (1982)who used a mixed lymphocyte reaction (MLR) to demonstrate that spleen cells from animals given whole body irradiation induced the proliferation of large numbers of cells directed against specific antigenic targets. This work extended earlier studies that identified two distinct populations of suppressor cells induced by these methods. One population responded specifically to bovine serum albumin (BSA) as an antigen, while the other responded non-specifically (Slavin and Strober, 1979).

4.2 The induction of chimerism without myeloablation

Several investigators have reported the induction of allogeneic bone marrow chimerism without myeloablation (Sykes, 1996, Pan et al., 2003, Fuchimoto et al., 2000, Shapira et al., 2003, Matthews et al., 2004, Ciurea and Andersson, 2009, Przepiorka et al., 1999). Myeloablation refers to the massive radiation induced destruction of the host's bone marrow cells, especially the T cell lineages, and the use of allogeneic bone marrow to replace the destroyed cells. Because of the radiation, with or without other treatments, the host is unable to reject the donated bone marrow cells. The major side effects associated with lethal whole body irradiation, have caused some investigators to develop non-myeloablative procedures (Sykes, 1996).

4.2.1 Chimerism to induce tolerance to allografts and xenografts

Sykes used low dose (3 Gy) whole body irradiation in combination with a higher dose (7 Gy) irradiation of the thymus and antibodies that deplete $CD4^+$ and $CD8^+$ T cells to generate specific tolerance to the cells and tissues of the donor (Sykes, 1996). Sykes used this protocol to show tolerance to allografts in the mouse, and tolerance of rat skin in murine hosts. She used the swine-to-mouse model to show that the protocol could be expanded to a discordant model, that is, one involving hyperacute reactions between widely disparate host and donor species. She depleted T cells and natural killer cells (NK) in thymectomized mice, then engrafted the thymus of a fetal pig. These mice were shown to accept a skin graft from the same donor strain as the thymus graft. Despite being described as "non-myeloablative, the procedure combines low dose total body irradiation with focused high level irradiation targeted to the thymus.

4.2.2 Irradiation-free chimerism in a murine allograft model

Pan et al. (2003) used a combination of costimulation blockade and a metabolism antagonist to reduce the donor T cell population in donor bone marrow to induce chimerism in mice. Depletion of donor T cells reduced the risk of graft vs. host disease (GVDH) wherein donor T cells initiate an immune response against the new host. Pan and colleagues used a combination of fludarabine, described below, the immunosuppressive drug cyclophosphamide, and interruption of the CD40/CD154 T cell activation pathway to facilitate donor bone marrow engraftment. The protocol resulted in mixed chimerism in the host and allowed donor origin skin grafts to survive.

4.2.3 Irradiation-free chimerism in a swine animal model

Fuchimoto and colleagues (2000) developed a technique to create a hematopoietic system composed of both donor origin and host origin cells, referred to as "mixed chimerism" to distinguish the results from full chimerism that often occurs when the host is given lethal irradiation followed by an allogeneic bone marrow transplant. They used high doses of stem cells separated from peripheral blood to induce mixed chimerism. The chimeric host accepted skin grafts from a donor whose transplantation antigens (swine leukocyte antigens, SLA) matched those of the bone marrow, but did not accept skin grafts from a third party donor, one that matched neither the bone marrow donor nor the new host.

4.2.4 Irradiation-free chimerism in humans

Shapira et al. (2003) reported an attempt to induce chimerism with no radiation in high risk patients who were not able to tolerate whole body radiation. The use of the drugs fludarabine and busulfan had a myeloablative effect on the host bone marrow cells. Fludarabine has been reported to minimize the development of neoplasias as well as to suppress metabolism (Matthews et al., 2004). Busulfan has been described as a myeloablation agonist that has been used to engraft bone marrow and stem cells (Ciurea and Andersson, 2009, Przepiorka et al., 1999). Eight percent of the patients developed full chimerism as evidence by donor origin hematopoietic cells. Regrettably, graft-versus-host disease (GVHD) was identified in most patients despite a brief low dose treatment of cyclosporine-A, and mortality was high.

5. Costimulation blockade to interrupt the process of T cell activation

If the events reported by Stone's group represent naturally occurring prenatal tolerance (Stone et al., 1965), how then may we induce tolerance in an adult? One answer may be found by dissecting the pathway for the development of immunity. These experiments tested the hypothesis that interference with one of the key steps leading to an immunological response would prevent the downstream events from occurring. This type of tolerance is referred to as peripheral tolerance as it leaves the host with the ability to respond to other immunological perturbans. Exposure of untreated animal models to a source of foreign antigen initiates the process of immunity and may provide the stimulus to recruit potentially alloreactive or xenoreactive cells from their histological sites. Subsequent interference with the reaction between CD40 and CD40L (CD154) or the reaction between B7 molecules and cytotoxic T lymphocyte-associated antigen (CTLA)-4 provides a scenario wherein cells that recognize the foreign antigen receive the initiating signal that recruits them to the site of antigen deposit, but not the required secondary signals. Costimulation blockade may be mediated by monoclonal antibodies directed against specific cell surface molecules, by the use of agonistic monoclonal antibodies to prevent reactivity induced by donor origin cells within the graft, referred to as graft-versus-host disease, (Albert et al., 2005, Yu et al., 2003, Yu et al., 2000) by the use of anti-sense RNA to facilitate apoptosis (Yu et al., 2004), or by deletion of cellular components expressing costimulation molecules. In systems where CD4 cells are important, graft survival may be accompanied by the expansion of $CD4^{+}$ CD25 Foxp3 regulatory cells.

When the elements of one's own immune system come into contact with particles, agents, cells or tissues not belonging to the host, those foreign agents are recognized as non-self. Immunity is the complex process of activating the body's adaptive immune defenses in order to protect the body from these specific invading elements. T cells are components of the adaptive immune system, and as such may be geared up to protect the body from foreign invaders, including pathogenic organism and transplanted cell and tissue grafts. They are increasingly protective upon re-exposure of the organism to the same antigen (Janeway C.A. et al., 2001).

An important feature of immunity is the activation of thymus derived lymphocytes or T cells. Grakoui et al. (1999) provided a detailed study of the environment and the molecular interactions required for T lymphocyte activation. In a host with an intact immune system, immunity would result in the destruction of engrafted tissue or organs from another individual who is not an identical twin. T cell activation is an essential feature of immunity, and thus a significant player in the acceptance or rejection of a graft. A hypothesis utilizing this information might be stated as follows: If T cell activation is important for immunity and graft rejection, then interruption of the T cell activation cascade will prevent or delay graft rejection. Preventing an immune reaction between graft and host would provide an environment conducive to transplantation tolerance. In particular, preventing an immune response to the specific graft-associated antigens, often described as anergy, would be more beneficial than a generalized immunosuppressive response because the host immune system would still be capable of protecting the body from other invaders.

Modern transplantation immunology owes a great debt to the pioneering work of Jenkins and Schwartz (1987) who demonstrated that antigen presentation devoid of a MHC context failed to stimulate T cell clones in vitro or T cells in vivo. They used a chemical crosslinking agent to affix pigeon cytochrome peptides to the surface of spleen cells. If properly presented with the cell's MHC surface molecules, the process would have resulted in T cell proliferation, IL-2 production (Jenkins et al., 1987) and antigen recognition (Jenkins and Schwartz, 1987). The inappropriate antigen presentation resulted in T cells unresponsive to their cognate (recognizable) antigen; and thus the authors concluded that the mechanism involved was the deletion of antigen-specific T cells (Jenkins and Schwartz, 2009). Their in vitro blockade of T cell activation was reproduced in the mouse model.

In 1993, Boussiotis et al. (1993) published their research implicating the costimulatory molecule B7 as a contributor to allograft immunity. Using a transfection model, the authors showed that interrupting the B7:CD28/CTLA4 pathway was consistent with an anergy model of immune unresponsiveness to one specific human derived transplantation antigen, HLA-DR7. In contrast, blocking the reaction between the intercellular adhesion molecule 1 (ICAM1) and lymphocyte function antigen 1 (LFA1) appeared to be associated with immunosuppression. Important contributors to T cell activation have been reviewed by Wingren et al. (1995) and include the work of Ford and Larsen (2009). The work of Jenkins, Schwartz, and colleagues has shown antigen specific T cell unresponsiveness (Jenkins et al., 1987, Jenkins and Schwartz, 1987, Jenkins and Schwartz, 2009). Further research led to clarification of the mechanisms of T cell signaling and activation. One set of stimulatory reactions was a consequence of the binding of B7 (CD80 or CD86) with CD28; while a different cascade of events followed the binding of CD40 with CD154 (CD40L). Many features of these pathways were elaborated by Bluestone et al. (1995) and have been reviewed by Lenschow et al. (1996). The three main pathways of T cell activation have been described by ML Ford and CP Larsen (2009).

Larsen et al. (1996) showed the importance of interrupting CD40/CD28 binding in skin and cardiac allografts, although mechanistic details remained for future investigations. Some mechanisms may include the induction of anergy, as mentioned above, the reduction of alloreactive T cell populations (Iwakoshi et al., 2000), the induction of regulatory T cells and the interactions of other cells with regulatory functions (Gordon and Kelkar, 2009), as discussed below, or diverting the proliferation of a specific T cell type (Li et al., 2009). Pree et al. have been advocates of the translational aspect of costimulation blockade. In a clinical setting, these protocols may facilitate mixed chimerism and prevent a GVH reaction that may otherwise ensue (Pree et al., 2009, Pan et al., 2003).

5.1 The B7/CD28 pathway and skin grafts

Preventing binding of B7 molecules on B cells to their ligands, CD28 on T cells has been shown to be effective for interrupting T cell activation. Shiao et al. (2007) used a humanized antibody directed against the T cell CD28 molecule to prevent the expansion of alloreactive T cells. The experiments were done in beige/SCID mice bearing human skin grafts and infused with peripheral blood cells expressing different human transplantation antigens (HLA) than those of the skin donor. Liu et al. (2007) used a gene therapy model to infuse antisense B7.1 in order to suppress alloreactivity to rat spleen cells. This model was not associated with GVHD as measured by examination of intestines, liver, skin, or other tissues(Liu et al., 2007). Rulifson et al. (2002) demonstrated that Langerhans cells resident in the skin of the donor were such effective antigen presenting cells (APCs) that they could prime T cells for activation independently of either the B7 or CD40 activation pathways. In their hands, the strength of this direct antigen presentation reaction limited the success of tolerance induction mediated through the interruption of either B7-CD28 or CD40-CD154 pathway. These findings are consistent with the work of Tao et al. (1997) who concluded that weak T cell receptor (TCR) signaling primed $CD4^{+}$cells in a CD28/B7 dependent manner. Early experiments using the skin allograft model were important for demonstrating that additional costimulatory molecules must be important for completing the T cell activation cascade (Kawai et al., 1996). Their report demonstrated suppressed proliferation and cytokine production by CD28 depleted T cells, nonetheless, these cells were capable of initiating skin allograft rejection.

5.2 Interrupting CD40 and B7 ligation

The combined effect of blocking the CD28 and CTLA4 ligation reactions was tested in a murine skin graft model (Li et al., 2006). The combined treatment was delivered via a replication incompetent adenovirus vector. Significant skin graft survival was demonstrated in the treated mice in contrast to rapid rejection of skin grafts in mice that were untreated or given non-expressing vectors. A detailed study outlining the efficacy of CTLA4Ig produced by different sources as an efficient tool for interrupting costimulatory signals produced by the ligation of B7/CD28 molecules was completed (Najafian and Sayegh, 2000). CTLA4Ig's higher affinity for B7 competitively inhibits B7/CD28 ligation, therefore interfering with the delivery of costimulatory signals. Other investigators found that CTLA4 signaling facilitated allograft survival of skin and islet grafts in mice treated with an infusion of donor derived antigen plus ant-CD154 monoclonal antibody (mAb) (Zheng et al., 1999). Tung et al. (2008) showed the combined effect of blockading both the B7 and CD40 pathways in a series of limb graft experiments. Balb/c male mice were donors of limbs engrafted onto C57Bl/6 female mice heterotopically. Costimulation blockade was mediated by anti-CD154 antibody with or without CTLA4-Ig. Anti-CD154 alone resulted in limb survival of 75 days, but graft survival was extended to 120 days by the combined therapy. Larsen et al. (1996) demonstrated the advantage of blocking both of these costimulatory pathways in order to facilitate the engraftment of skin and cardiac tissue. Both in vivo and in vitro confirmation of the effect was discussed.

Protracted survival of murine skin allografts in thymectomized mice treated with an infusion of donor derived spleen cells and anti-CD154 mAb was achieved only in mice expressing $CD4^{+}$ T cells, gamma interferon, and CTLA4 (Markees et al., 1998). In contrast, the studies by Gordon et al. (1998) using the concordant rat-to-mouse xenotransplantation model, showed no requirement of $CD4^{+}$ T cells or for gamma interferon for prolonging the survival of rat skin and islets in mice. The role of B7/CD28 ligation in providing costimulatory signals to effect T cell activation was confirmed by the studies of Onodera et al. (1997). They pre-sensitized Lewis rats with Brown-Norway skin grafts and evaluated the survival of cardiac grafts when recipients were treated with CTLA4Ig with or without an infusion of donor antigen. They hypothesized that graft survival was mediated by either clonal anergy or the deletion of alloreactive $CD8^+$ cells.

5.3 Interfering with CD40/CD154 ligation

Although the first study of the CD40/CD154 pathway to promote graft survival utilized a concordant rat-to-mouse islet xenograft model (Markees et al., 1996), the first use of this system to facilitate skin graft acceptance was reported by Larsen at al. (1996), and described aspects of the costimulatory process related to both CD28-B7 ligation and CD40-gp39 ligations. The "gp39" designation was later changed to CD154 in keeping with the system for naming cell surface molecules. In their hands, each set of costimulatory molecules provides necessary but not identical signals resulting in fully activated T lymphocytes. Interrupting both of these pathways provided conditions for prolonged survival of heart tissue and skin allografts.

Interrupting the reaction between CD40 and CD154 has been confirmed as an effective method for limiting T cell costimulation. This pathway is required for the generation of T cells that are fully activated against alloantigen (Yamada and Sayegh, 2002), and interruption of this pathway promotes graft survival or tolerance. Moodycliffe et al. showed that the binding of these molecules encouraged the migration of dendritic cells from the skin to the lymph nodes for effective antigen presentation (Moodycliffe et al., 2000). Their model assessed dendritic cell (DC) function in wild type C57Bl/6 mice or those devoid of CD154 molecules. A combined therapy consisting of a bolus infusion of donor derived spleen cells and a brief course of treatment with anti-CD154 mAb resulted in prolonged survival of rat skin grafts in mice. Graft survival was enhanced significantly in mice devoid of $CD4^+$ T cells (Gordon et al., 2001).

Nikolic et al. used a skin graft model to differentiate between models that blocked immunity to alloantigens vs. those that interrupted autoimmunity (Nikolic et al., 2010). They used normoglycemic non obese diabetic mice (NOD) that received whole body irradiation, T cell depletion, and anti-CD154 mAbs with or without bone marrow cells from C57Bl/6 mice. The treatment delayed or prevented hypoglycemia, but only prevented isletitis in mice that received bone marrow cells as well as the other conditioning treatments.

Xu et al. (2010) studied the role of minor histocompatibility antigens in bone marrow grafts. They found that when they used B10.BR skin to sensitize AKR mice to alloantigens, donor origin cells were cleared more rapidly than in unsensitized mice of the same strain. Recipient mice treated with antibodies to CD154 did not produce antibodies to minor histocompatibility antigens of the donor. These studies suggest that blockade of CD40-CD154 ligation may facilitate bone marrow transplantation and reduce the risk of reactivity to minor histocompatibility antigens.

Although blockade of CD40 and CD28 activation pathways did not produce the vasculopathy shown with other methods, translating this method into a clinical protocol was unexpectedly problematic because of the development of thromboembolisms (Yamada and Sayegh, 2002). Scientists have since analyzed the cause for the pathophysiological problems identified clinically. Their reports help to identify platelets as a source for soluble CD154 or CD40 ligand and demonstrate a correlation between increased circulating levels of this molecule and increased thrombus formation (Yacoub et al., 2010, Yuan et al., 2010). These studies show further that CD154's concentration is increased in hypertensive patients included non-diabetic and pre-diabetic persons with metabolic syndrome (Unek et al., 2010).

In an effort to overcome these complications, Gilson et al. (2009) compared two different isotypes of anti-CD40 monoclonal antibodies. Isotypes are any one of the five main structurally and functionally distinct categories of antibodies (Janeway C.A. et al., 2001). Gilson et al. (2009) found that the IgG2b, but not the IgG1 antibody had a synergistic effect on graft survival when combined with CTLA-4-Ig, and hypothesized that the use of alternative antibody isotypes may encourage the development of new reagents that are as effective as anti-CD154 antibodies, but without harmful clinical effects.

6. The induction of regulatory T cells (Tregs)

In 1975, Gelfand and Paul (1975) used an anti-thy1.2 antibody to facilitate C57Bl/6 skin grafts on Balb/c mice. The antibody, which was directed against thymocytes, resulted in prolonged skin graft survival in comparison to untreated mice. The study demonstrated infectious tolerance as the effect could be transferred to new hosts given cells of the treated mice. The authors thus hypothesized that the treatment generated a population of suppressor cells that regulated the processes responsible for graft survival. In the same year, Gershon hypothesized the existence of suppressor T cells that down modulated immune responses and detailed predominant requirements for their functionality (Gershon, 1975). These concepts were controversial at the time that they were advanced.

During the 1980's, the concept began to take hold that there existed a specific population of regulatory T lymphocytes with the capacity to specifically suppress immune responses. Maki et al. showed that B6AF1 mice pretreated with ALS and given both BMC and skin grafts from CH3 donor mice had suppressed reactivity against donor antigen as demonstrated by in vitro assays (Maki et al., 1981a, Maki et al., 1981b). Streilein and Niederkorn (1985) described the induction of a suppressor T cell population that helps to explain the phenomenon of the anterior chamber of the eye functioning as an immunologically privileged site. The suppressor activity was associated with improved skin graft survival and other host responses. The suppressor cells were described as Thy1.2 and L3T4 expressing $CD4^+$ T lymphocytes.

Subsequent studies by Subba and Grogan (1986) using rat skin allografts implanted in the anterior eye chamber resulted in minimal alloreactivity as measured in vitro. Treatment with cyclophosphamide or removal of the allograft reversed the immunosuppression seen in mixed lymphocyte reactions (MLR), thus implicating the involvement of suppressor cells.

Based on a wealth of more recently generated data, the scientific community no longer needs to be convinced that a regulatory cell population exists or can be induced. Regulatory T cells have been identified or induced by some of the methods shown in Table 1 below. We now accept the description of the predominant category of regulatory cells responsible for allograft survival, the generation of chimerism and mixed chimerism, protection from autoimmunity and reduced risk of graft vs. host disease (GVHD) and host vs. graft disease (HVG) as being $CD4^+$ $CD25^+$$Foxp3^+$ regulatory T lymphocytes. These Tregs may be naturally occurring in the thymus or adaptively induced in response to foreign antigen and costimulation blockade (Guo et al., 2008, Schwartz, 2005, Sakaguchi, 2005, Coenen et al.,

2005, von Boehmer, 2005). The Tregs express the forkhead transcription factor Foxp3 (Fontenot and Rudensky, 2005), and there is some evidence that the expression level of this transcription factor may be a key indicator of the level of immunosuppression potential (Chauhan et al., 2009) The immunosuppressive effect of these cells has been shown by in vivo and in vitro experiments.

Graft or Target	Authors	Method of Induction
Skin grafts Autoimmunity	(Oderup et al., 2006)	Il2Rbeta-/- recipients
Heart	(Oderup et al., 2006)	Rag 1 -/- given anti-154 and anti-B7
Chimerism	(Iudaev et al., 1975)	Sublethal WBI and BMC
Hy antigen and HVG	(Weng et al., 2007)	Sublethal WBI
Chimerism Skin allografts	(Yamazaki et al., 2007)	BMC, DST and anti-CD154
Skin graft	(Chai et al., 2005)	Foxp3 transduced expression in naïve $CD4^+$ $CD25^-$
Skin graft	(Banuelos et al., 2004)	DST and anti-CD154 in CD4, CD8, or CD25 depleted skin and islet graft recipients
Skin graft	(Sanchez-Fueyo et al., 2007)	Wt or Class II - mice
Skin graft Mixed chimerism	(Pilat et al., 2010)	Rapamyacin and costimulation blockade;
Skin graft	(Kim et al., 2011)	Anti-CD154, Non cytolytic anti-CD4
Composite tissue allograft	(Bozulic et al., 2011)	Anti-TCR, WBI

Legend: Table 1 describes some milestones in the history of regulatory T cell recognition. Abbreviations: WBI, whole body irradiation, BMC, bone marrow cells; HVG, host vs. graft reaction; Hy, male specific antigen; DST, donor specific antigen; wt, wild type; TCR, T cell Receptor

Table 1. The Induction of $CD4^+$ $CD25^+$ Regulatory T Cells

7. Other cells with regulatory functions

7.1 Double negative T cells

Double negative T cells, described as $CD3^+$ T lymphocytes bearing typical αβT cell receptors, but expressing no CD4, CD8, or NK1.1 surface molecules. These cells use the process of trogocytosis to gain access to the alloantigen, xenoantigen, or self peptides that are then expressed on their cells surfaces (Ford McIntyre et al., 2008). Trogocytosis is the process of utilizing broken pieces of plasma membrane as an antigen capture mechanism (Hudrisier et al., 2007). B and T cell receptors as well as some costimulatory co-receptors appear to be involved in this process.

7.2 $CD8^+$ T cells

$CD8^+$ T cells have been shown to promote skin allograft survival in fully mismatch donor-host combinations. Graft survival was initiated by rapamycin treatment of graft hosts (El Essawy et al., 2011). El Essawy and colleagues found that C57Bl/6 mice devoid of CD4 molecules handily rejected DBA mouse skin allografts, but showed prolonged (median survival, >100 days) survival of these grafts following rapamycin treatment of the grafts hosts. These regulatory/suppressor T cells were $CD28^+$ but showed low levels of IFN-γ, IL-2, and IL-10.

7.3 Natural Killer T (NKT) cells

Natural Killer T (NKT) cells are lymphocytes bearing TCR T cell receptors. A regulatory role for these cells was described in mice devoid of the Jα18 segment of the TCR and in mice lacking the CD1 restricting element associated with NKT cells following costimulation blockade mediated by a transfusion of donor antigen and a short course of anti-CD154 mAb (Gordon and Kelkar, 2009). Graft survival was abbreviated in the Jα18 and in the CD1 deficient mice as compared to wild type mice of the same strain (Gordon and Kelkar, 2009).

7.4 Induction of tolerogenic dendritic cells

Adorini and Penna (2009) report on the use of vitamin D receptor (VDR) agonist as a means of inducing tolerogenic dendritic cells (DCs). These DC are associated with an immunosuppressive effect. The use of secosteroid hormones that function as VDR agonist help to induce DCs that then facilitate the induction of CD4(+) CD25(+) Foxp3(+) regulatory T cells.

8. The humanized mouse as a model for the study of the human immune system

The humanized mouse model takes advantage of the existence of basic cellular deficiencies in non-obese diabetic (NOD) and CB-17 *scid/scid* strains of mice. Some strains are crosses between the two and bear the deficiencies of each parental type. The severe combined immunodeficient substrain lacking a functional IL-2 receptor gamma gene has become a more advanced mouse model. These mice may be infused with human hematopoietic stem cells that reconstitute a functional human immune system in the murine environment. These genetically altered mice provide important tools for studying autoimmunity, cellular and molecular interactions of the human immune system, solid tumors and other forms of cancer, and may provide models for studying human retroviruses or other infections where no appropriate animal model exists. Many of these strains have been developed by Lenny Schultz and others at Jackson Laboratories (Bar Harbor, ME). Some phenotypic characteristics of the most recent strain include the lack of T cells, B cells, and NK cells. There is no IL-2R γ chain, both the innate and adaptive compartments of the immune system are defective, and most antibody responses are very low. Salient features of these mice including timelines for their development have been reviewed recently (Van Duyne et al., 2009, Ishikawa et al., 2008, Hill et al., 1991). In the section below, we review the use of this important model for investigation in several areas of biomedical research.

8.1 Humanized mouse system for the study of skin grafts and wound healing

Racki et al. (2010) compared usage of NOD-scid IL2rgamma(null) mouse (NSG) vs. the CB17-scid bg (SCID.bg) mouse to study skin allograft survival vs. rejection. They found that components of the human immune successfully engrafted into the NSG mouse, but that skin graft survival was poor. In contrast, the SCID.bg mouse was less successful in engrafting human cells, but showed improved skin graft survival over the NSG model. Their results showed that infiltration of transplanted human skin by glucocorticoid receptor isoform 1 (GR-1$^+$) cells impaired graft survival. GR-1$^+$ cells are immature myeloid cells that may differentiate into dendritic cells, have been identified in human bone marrow recipient, and are characterized as having an immunosuppressive effect (Li et al., 2004). When Racki's team treated NSG mice with antibodies to GR1, the cellular infiltrate decreased and skin graft survival was improved. Additional studies that impact skin graft survival and wound healing used an alternative model, the nude mouse (Escamez et al., 2004). This mouse lacks a thymus, and therefore has no mature T lymphocytes. They found that treating laboratory engineered "skin equivalent" with keratinocyte growth factor improved wound healing.

Gilet et al. (2009) used SCID mice reconstituted with human PBLs and engrafted with human skin to study T cell subset recruitment mediated by the cytokine CCL17. Erdage and Morgan (2004) used the same animal model (huPBMC-SCID) to study the differences in allo- and xenoreacivity to bioengineered skin modified with or without keratinocyte growth factor. The team used the same model to study the survival of human fetal vs. neonatal skin grafts. They found that the lower MHC Class I and Class II expression in fetal skin was associated with longer graft survival than that of neonatal skin (Erdag and Morgan, 2002). Issa et al. (2010) separated regulatory T cells from human PBLs and used them to control immune responses to skin allografts in a humanized mouse model.

8.2 The humanized mouse system and autoimmunity

The humanized mouse model has become an important research tool for the study of type 1 diabetes and psoriasis. Pearson et al. (Pearson et al., 2008) described the NOD-Rag1null Prf1null Ins2Akita spontaneously hyperglycemic mouse model. This model has no autoimmune defect, but may be used to study type 1 diabetes in an environment that avoids any toxicity associated with chemically induced diabetes models. King et al. (2008) describe the engraftment of peripheral blood mononuclear cells (PBMC) vs. human stem cells. They induced diabetes and showed that an infusion of allo-PBMCs leads to islet graft rejection, thus they proposed the use of this model to study mechanisms of human islet allograft rejection. Other aspects involving the use of these animal models to study diabetes have been reviewed (King et al., 2008, Shultz et al., 2007).

Humanized mouse models of psoriasis have been developed that use bioengineered skin derived from biopsies and from patients with psoriasis (Guerrero-Aspizua et al., 2010). A psoriasis pathology was duplicated by injecting cultivated T cell populations along with IL-17and IL-22, and depriving the skin of its stratum corneum. This model will be used to assess the pathophysiology of the disease and to suggest alternative therapeutic targets, and to test new hypothesis related to patient outcomes in pre-clinical investigations.

Bhagavathula et al. (2005) used the severe combined immunodeficient (SCID) mouse to demonstrate the effectiveness of humanized neutralizing mAbs directed against transduced amphiregulin as a therapeutic agent reversing some phenotypic characteristics of psoriasis in transplanted skin. The mAb decreased epidermal thickness in vivo and reduced keratinocyte growth in vitro.

Because TNFα antagonists have been used to counter the effects of psoriasis, Gordon et al. (2005) used a humanized mAb directed against TNFα to dissect the mechanism of action of these reagents. They injected the reagent into otherwise unaffected skin engrafted onto the SCID-HU mouse model and they injected highly activated T cells in order to simulate an acute psoriasis phenotype. The concentration of epidermal Langerhans cells (LCs) in the plaques began to increase within one week of the mAb treatment, and thus the loss of LCs was associated with plaque development. These studies help to clarify the method of action of the TNFα antagonist and suggest a method for reversing the course of this disease in patients.

8.3 The humanized mouse system and immunity: Graft vs. Host Disease (GVHD)

This model has been used to study GVHD. Soluble FasL was used to treat graft recipients in order to prevent alloreactivity of immunocompetent donor T cells that recognize the host antigens (Bohana-Kashtan et al., 2009). Pinot et al. (2010) describe the development of the NSG mouse model and its use in studying xeno-GVHD. Vlad et al. (2009) used this mode to demonstrate the prevention of GVHD through the use of an immunoglobulin component, the immunoglobulin-like transcript 3-Fc protein, that induces $CD8^+$ suppressor cells.

8.4 The humanized mouse system as a source for induced pluripotent stem cells

Hanna et al. (2007) used a humanized mouse model of sickle cell anemia to describe the benefits of using induced pluripotent stem cells (IPS) derive from adult fibroblast cells. This "knock-in" model replaced mouse globin genes with mutated human Aγ and β^S globin genes. The homozygous mutant developed many phenotypic characteristics of the sickle cell disease. Tail snips from these mice were used as a source of fibroblast cultures. Retroviral vectors were used to transduce expression of the four transcription factors needed to reprogram the adult mouse cells or to express selectable markers. The investigators used homologous recombination to repair the genetic defect responsible for sickle cell disease. The investigators anticipate future studies that eliminate the use of retroviral vectors and oncogenes in applications of IPS for human use.

9. Conclusions

The modern world of skin grafting, arising from its historical roots to new depths of scientific understanding, will help to advance translational science and medicine. Skin grafts allow us to understand specific immunological functions, help dissect the mechanisms responsible for tissue and organ specific tolerance, identify additional regulatory cells or functions required for transplantation tolerance, test the development of mouse models of the human immune system and help answer fundamental questions related to the use of stem cells as curative agents for human disease.

10. References

1970. Immunosuppressive drugs. I. *Br Med J,* 4, 663-5.

Adorini, L. & Penna, G. 2009. Induction of tolerogenic dendritic cells by vitamin D receptor agonists. *Handb Exp Pharmacol*, 251-73.

Akdis, M. 2010. The cellular orchestra in skin allergy; are differences to lung and nose relevant? *Curr Opin Allergy Clin Immunol,* 10, 443-51.

Albert, M. H., Yu, X. Z., Martin, P. J. & Anasetti, C. 2005. Prevention of lethal acute GVHD with an agonistic CD28 antibody and rapamycin. *Blood,* 105, 1355-61.

Banuelos, S. J., Markees, T. G., Phillips, N. E., Appel, M. C., Cuthbert, A., Leif, J., Mordes, J. P., Shultz, L. D., Rossini, A. A. & Greiner, D. L. 2004. Regulation of skin and islet allograft survival in mice treated with costimulation blockade is mediated by different CD4+ cell subsets and different mechanisms. *Transplantation,* 78, 660-7.

Berardinelli, L., Messa, P. G., Pozzoli, E., Beretta, C. & Montagnino, G. 2009. Malignancies in 2,753 kidney recipients transplanted during a 39-year experience. *Transplant Proc,* 41, 1231-2.

Bhagavathula, N., Nerusu, K. C., Fisher, G. J., Liu, G., Thakur, A. B., Gemmell, L., Kumar, S., Xu, Z. H., Hinton, P., Tsurushita, N., Landolfi, N. F., Voorhees, J. J. & Varani, J. 2005. Amphiregulin and epidermal hyperplasia: amphiregulin is required to maintain the psoriatic phenotype of human skin grafts on severe combined immunodeficient mice. *Am J Pathol,* 166, 1009-16.

Billingham, R. E. 1959. Reactions of grafts against their hosts. *Science,* 130, 947-53.

Billingham, R. E., Brent, L. & Medawar, P. B. 1953. Actively acquired tolerance of foreign cells. *Nature,* 172, 603-6.

Billingham, R. E. & Silvers, W. K. 1958. Induction of tolerance of skin isografts from male donors in female mice. *Science,* 128, 780-1.

Bluestone, J. A. 1995. New perspectives of CD28-B7-mediated T cell costimulation. *Immunity,* 2, 555-9.

Bohana-Kashtan, O., Morisot, S., Hildreth, R., Brayton, C., Levitsky, H. I. & Civin, C. I. 2009. Selective reduction of graft-versus-host disease-mediating human T cells by ex vivo treatment with soluble Fas ligand. *J Immunol,* 183, 696-705.

Boussiotis, V. A., Freeman, G. J., Gray, G., Gribben, J. & Nadler, L. M. 1993. B7 but not intercellular adhesion molecule-1 costimulation prevents the induction of human alloantigen-specific tolerance. *J Exp Med,* 178, 1753-63.

Bozulic, L. D., Wen, Y., Xu, H. & Ildstad, S. T. 2011. Evidence That FoxP3+ Regulatory T Cells May Play a Role in Promoting Long-Term Acceptance of Composite Tissue Allotransplants. *Transplantation,* 91, 908-15.

Buckley, R. H. 1975. Bone marrow and thymus transplantation in ataxia-telangiectasia. *Birth Defects Orig Artic Ser,* 11, 421-4.

Chai, J. G., Xue, S. A., Coe, D., Addey, C., Bartok, I., Scott, D., Simpson, E., Stauss, H. J., Hori, S., Sakaguchi, S. & Dyson, J. 2005. Regulatory T cells, derived from naive CD4+CD25- T cells by in vitro Foxp3 gene transfer, can induce transplantation tolerance. *Transplantation,* 79, 1310-6.

Chauhan, S. K., Saban, D. R., Lee, H. K. & Dana, R. 2009. Levels of Foxp3 in regulatory T cells reflect their functional status in transplantation. *J Immunol,* 182, 148-53.

Cigna, E., Tarallo, M., Bistoni, G., Anniboletti, T., Trignano, E., Tortorelli, G. & Scuderi, N. 2009. Evaluation of polyurethane dressing with ibuprofen in the management of split-thickness skin graft donor sites. *In Vivo,* 23, 983-6.

Ciurea, S. O. & Andersson, B. S. 2009. Busulfan in hematopoietic stem cell transplantation. *Biol Blood Marrow Transplant,* 15, 523-36.

Coenen, J. J., Koenen, H. J., Van Rijssen, E., Hilbrands, L. B. & Joosten, I. 2005. Tolerizing effects of co-stimulation blockade rest on functional dominance of CD4+CD25+ regulatory T cells. *Transplantation,* 79, 147-56.

Cole, L. J. & Davis, W. E., JR. 1962. Homograft reaction in mice: effect of urethane and sublethal x-radiation. *Science,* 135, 792-3.

Davis, W. E., Jr. & Cole, L. J. 1963. Homograft tolerance in mice: use of urethan and sublethal irradiation. *Science,* 140, 483-4.

Del Rio, M. L., Bernhardt, G., Rodriguez-Barbosa, J. I. & Forster, R. 2010. Development and functional specialization of CD103+ dendritic cells. *Immunol Rev,* 234, 268-81.

Doesch, A. O., Muller, S., Konstandin, M., Celik, S., Kristen, A., Frankenstein, L., Ehlermann, P., Sack, F. U., Katus, H. A. & Dengler, T. J. 2010. Malignancies after heart transplantation: incidence, risk factors, and effects of calcineurin inhibitor withdrawal. *Transplant Proc,* 42, 3694-9.

El Essawy, B., Putheti, P., Gao, W. & Strom, T. B. 2011. Rapamycin Generates Graft-Homing Murine Suppressor CD8(+) T Cells That Confer Donor-Specific Graft Protection. *Cell Transplant.*

Epa, E. P. A. 2007. Methylhydrazine. 60-34-4.

Erdag, G. & Morgan, J. R. 2002. Survival of fetal skin grafts is prolonged on the human peripheral blood lymphocyte reconstituted-severe combined immunodeficient mouse/skin allograft model. *Transplantation,* 73, 519-28.

Erdag, G. & Morgan, J. R. 2004. Allogeneic versus xenogeneic immune reaction to bioengineered skin grafts. *Cell Transplant,* 13, 701-12.

Escamez, M. J., Garcia, M., Larcher, F., Meana, A., Munoz, E., Jorcano, J. L. & Del Rio, M. 2004. An in vivo model of wound healing in genetically modified skin-humanized mice. *J Invest Dermatol,* 123, 1182-91.

Eyal, Z., Warwick, W. J., Mayo, C. H., 2nd & Lillehei, R. C. 1965. Homograft Rabbit Skin Protection by Phenothiazine Derivatives. *Science,* 148, 1468-9.

Floersheim, G. L. 1967. Drug-induced tolerance for skin allografts across the H-2 barrier in adult mice. *Science,* 156, 951-4.

Fontenot, J. D. & Rudensky, A. Y. 2005. A well adapted regulatory contrivance: regulatory T cell development and the forkhead family transcription factor Foxp3. *Nat Immunol,* 6, 331-7.

Ford Mcintyre, M. S., Young, K. J., Gao, J., Joe, B. & Zhang, L. 2008. Cutting edge: in vivo trogocytosis as a mechanism of double negative regulatory T cell-mediated antigen-specific suppression. *J Immunol,* 181, 2271-5.

Ford, M. L. & Larsen, C. P. 2009. Translating costimulation blockade to the clinic: lessons learned from three pathways. *Immunol Rev,* 229, 294-306.

Fuchimoto, Y., Huang, C. A., Yamada, K., Shimizu, A., Kitamura, H., Colvin, R. B., Ferrara, V., Murphy, M. C., Sykes, M., White-Scharf, M., Neville, D. M., Jr. & Sachs, D. H. 2000. Mixed chimerism and tolerance without whole body irradiation in a large animal model. *J Clin Invest,* 105, 1779-89.

Gelfand, M. C. & Paul, W. E. 1975. Prolongation of allograft survival in mice by administration of anti-Thy 1 serum. I. Mediation by in vivo activation of regulatory T cells. *J Immunol,* 115, 1-4.

Gershon, R. K. 1975. A disquisition on suppressor T cells. *Transplant Rev,* 26, 170-85.

Gilet, J., Chang, Y., Chenivesse, C., Legendre, B., Vorng, H., Duez, C., Wallaert, B., Porte, H., Senechal, S. & Tsicopoulos, A. 2009. Role of CCL17 in the generation of cutaneous inflammatory reactions in Hu-PBMC-SCID mice grafted with human skin. *J Invest Dermatol,* 129, 879-90.

Gilson, C. R., Milas, Z., Gangappa, S., Hollenbaugh, D., Pearson, T. C., Ford, M. L. & Larsen, C. P. 2009. Anti-CD40 monoclonal antibody synergizes with CTLA4-Ig in promoting long-term graft survival in murine models of transplantation. *J Immunol,* 183, 1625-35.

Goldstein, D. R. 2011. T cell costimulation blockade and organ transplantation: a change of philosophy for transplant immunologists? *J Immunol,* 186, 2691-2.

Gonzalez Posada, J. M. 2006. Current trends in immunosuppression. *Nefrologia,* 26 Suppl 2, 3-8.

Gordon, C. R., Siemionow, M. & Zins, J. 2009. Composite tissue allotransplantation: a proposed classification system based on relative complexity. *Transplant Proc,* 41, 481-4.

Gordon, E. J. & Kelkar, V. 2009. Natural killer T cell facilitated engraftment of rat skin but not islet xenografts in mice. *Xenotransplantation,* 16, 135-44.

Gordon, E. J., Markees, T. G., Phillips, N. E., Noelle, R. J., Shultz, L. D., Mordes, J. P., Rossini, A. A. & Greiner, D. L. 1998. Prolonged survival of rat islet and skin xenografts in mice treated with donor splenocytes and anti-CD154 monoclonal antibody. *Diabetes,* 47, 1199-206.

Gordon, E. J., Woda, B. A., Shultz, L. D., Rossini, A. A., Greiner, D. L. & Mordes, J. P. 2001. Rat xenograft survival in mice treated with donor-specific transfusion and anti-CD154 antibody is enhanced by elimination of host CD4+ cells. *Transplantation,* 71, 319-27.

Gordon, K. B., Bonish, B. K., Patel, T., Leonardi, C. L. & Nickoloff, B. J. 2005. The tumour necrosis factor-alpha inhibitor adalimumab rapidly reverses the decrease in epidermal Langerhans cell density in psoriatic plaques. *Br J Dermatol,* 153, 945-53.

Grakoui, A., Bromley, S. K., Sumen, C., Davis, M. M., Shaw, A. S., Allen, P. M. & Dustin, M. L. 1999. The immunological synapse: a molecular machine controlling T cell activation. *Science,* 285, 221-7.

Groetzner, J., Meiser, B., Landwehr, P., Buehse, L., Mueller, M., Kaczmarek, I., Vogeser, M., Daebritz, S., Ueberfuhr, P. & Reichart, B. 2004. Mycophenolate mofetil and sirolimus as calcineurin inhibitor-free immunosuppression for late cardiac-transplant recipients with chronic renal failure. *Transplantation,* 77, 568-74.

Guerrero-Aspizua, S., Garcia, M., Murillas, R., Retamosa, L., Illera, N., Duarte, B., Holguin, A., Puig, S., Hernandez, M. I., Meana, A., Jorcano, J. L., Larcher, F., Carretero, M. & Del Rio, M. 2010. Development of a bioengineered skin-humanized mouse model for psoriasis: dissecting epidermal-lymphocyte interacting pathways. *Am J Pathol,* 177, 3112-24.

Guo, F., Iclozan, C., Suh, W. K., Anasetti, C. & Yu, X. Z. 2008. CD28 controls differentiation of regulatory T cells from naive CD4 T cells. *J Immunol,* 181, 2285-91.

Guttmann, R. D., Kraus, E. D. & Dolan, M. F. 1964. Rejection of Isogeneic Murine Skin Grafts Following Exposure to Allogeneic Ribonucleic Acid. *Nature,* 203, 196-8.

Halloran, P. F. 2004. Immunosuppressive drugs for kidney transplantation. *N Engl J Med,* 351, 2715-29.

Hanna, J., Wernig, M., Markoulaki, S., Sun, C. W., Meissner, A., Cassady, J. P., Beard, C., Brambrink, T., Wu, L. C., Townes, T. M. & Jaenisch, R. 2007. Treatment of sickle cell anemia mouse model with iPS cells generated from autologous skin. *Science,* 318, 1920-3.

Hellmann, K. & Duke, D. I. 1967. In Vitro Alteration of Skin Graft Antigenicity. *Transplantation,* 5.

Hill, B. T., Whelan, R. D., Hosking, L. K., Shellard, S. A., Hinds, M. D., Mayes, J. & Zwelling, L. A. 1991. A lack of detectable modification of topoisomerase II activity in a series of human tumor cell lines expressing only low levels of etoposide resistance. *Int J Cancer,* 47, 899-902.

Hudrisier, D., Aucher, A., Puaux, A. L., Bordier, C. & Joly, E. 2007. Capture of target cell membrane components via trogocytosis is triggered by a selected set of surface molecules on T or B cells. *J Immunol,* 178, 3637-47.

Ingvar, A., Smedby, K. E., Lindelof, B., Fernberg, P., Bellocco, R., Tufveson, G., Hoglund, P. & Adami, J. 2010. Immunosuppressive treatment after solid organ transplantation and risk of post-transplant cutaneous squamous cell carcinoma. *Nephrol Dial Transplant,* 25, 2764-71.

Ishikawa, F., Saito, Y., Yoshida, S., Harada, M. & Shultz, L. D. 2008. The differentiative and regenerative properties of human hematopoietic stem/progenitor cells in NOD-SCID/IL2rgamma(null) mice. *Curr Top Microbiol Immunol,* 324, 87-94.

Issa, F., Hester, J., Goto, R., Nadig, S. N., Goodacre, T. E. & Wood, K. 2010. Ex vivo-expanded human regulatory T cells prevent the rejection of skin allografts in a humanized mouse model. *Transplantation,* 90, 1321-7.

Iudaev, N. A., Pokrovskii, B. V., Asreibekova, M. K. & Mal'tsev, A. V. 1975. [Characteristics of testosterone-binding cytoplasmic components in the human endometrium and their interaction with chromatin]. *Biokhimiia,* 40, 1123-30.

Iwakoshi, N. N., Mordes, J. P., Markees, T. G., Phillips, N. E., Rossini, A. A. & Greiner, D. L. 2000. Treatment of allograft recipients with donor-specific transfusion and anti-CD154 antibody leads to deletion of alloreactive CD8+ T cells and prolonged graft survival in a CTLA4-dependent manner. *J Immunol,* 164, 512-21.

Jackman, S. H., Keerthy, S. & Perry, G. 2002. Murine epidermal cell antigen (Skn)-directed autoimmunity induced by transfer of CD4+ T cells. *Ann Clin Lab Sci,* 32, 171-80.

Jacobs, B. B. & Uphoff, D. E. 1974. Immunologic modification: a basic survival mechanism. *Science,* 185, 582-7.

Janeway C.A., Travers P., Walport M. & AL., E. 2001. Immunobiology: The Immune System in Health and Disease.

Jenkins, M. K., Pardoll, D. M., Mizuguchi, J., Chused, T. M. & Schwartz, R. H. 1987. Molecular events in the induction of a nonresponsive state in interleukin 2-producing helper T-lymphocyte clones. *Proc Natl Acad Sci U S A,* 84, 5409-13.

Jenkins, M. K. & Schwartz, R. H. 1987. Antigen presentation by chemically modified splenocytes induces antigen-specific T cell unresponsiveness in vitro and in vivo. *J Exp Med,* 165, 302-19.

Jenkins, M. K. & Schwartz, R. H. 2009. Pillars article: antigen presentation by chemically modified splenocytes induces antigen-specific T cell unresponsiveness in vitro and in vivo. J. Exp. Med. 1987. 165: 302-319. *J Immunol,* 183, 4150-67.

Kaplan, D. H. 2010. In vivo function of Langerhans cells and dermal dendritic cells. *Trends Immunol,* 31, 446-51.

Kawai, K., Shahinian, A., Mak, T. W. & Ohashi, P. S. 1996. Skin allograft rejection in CD28-deficient mice. *Transplantation,* 61, 352-5.

Kim, J. I., O'connor M, R., Duff, P. E., Zhao, G., Lee, K. M., Eliades, P., Deng, S., Yeh, H., Caton, A. J. & Markmann, J. F. 2011. Generation of adaptive regulatory T cells by alloantigen is required for some but not all transplant tolerance protocols. *Transplantation,* 91, 707-13.

King, M., Pearson, T., Rossini, A. A., Shultz, L. D. & Greiner, D. L. 2008. Humanized mice for the study of type 1 diabetes and beta cell function. *Ann N Y Acad Sci,* 1150, 46-53.

Larsen, C. P., Elwood, E. T., Alexander, D. Z., Ritchie, S. C., Hendrix, R., Tucker-Burden, C., Cho, H. R., Aruffo, A., Hollenbaugh, D., Linsley, P. S., Winn, K. J. & Pearson, T. C. 1996. Long-term acceptance of skin and cardiac allografts after blocking CD40 and CD28 pathways. *Nature,* 381, 434-8.

Lemperle, G. 1968. Prolonged survival of skin allografts after incubation with recipient DNA or RNA. *J Surg Res,* 8, 511-21.

Lenschow, D. J., Walunas, T. L. & Bluestone, J. A. 1996. CD28/B7 system of T cell costimulation. *Annu Rev Immunol,* 14, 233-58.

Li, Q., Pan, P. Y., Gu, P., Xu, D. & Chen, S. H. 2004. Role of immature myeloid Gr-1+ cells in the development of antitumor immunity. *Cancer Res,* 64, 1130-9.

Li, X. C., Rothstein, D. M. & Sayegh, M. H. 2009. Costimulatory pathways in transplantation: challenges and new developments. *Immunol Rev,* 229, 271-93.

Li, Z. L., Tian, P. X., Xue, W. J. & Wu, J. 2006. Co-expression of sCD40LIg and CTLA4Ig mediated by adenovirus prolonged mouse skin allograft survival. *J Zhejiang Univ Sci B,* 7, 436-44.

Liacopoulos, P. & Goode, J. H. 1964. Transplantation Tolerance Induced in Adult Mice by Protein Overloading of Donors. *Science,* 146, 1305-7.

Lindenfeld, J., Miller, G. G., Shakar, S. F., Zolty, R., Lowes, B. D., Wolfel, E. E., Mestroni, L., Page, R. L., Ii & Kobashigawa, J. 2004. Drug Therapy in the Heart Transplant Recipient: Part I: Cardiac Rejection and Immunosuppressive Drugs. *Circulation,* 110, 3734-3740.

Liu, C., Pan, S., Jiang, H. & Sun, X. 2007. Gene transfer of antisense B7.1 attenuates acute rejection against splenic allografts in rats. *Transplant Proc,* 39, 3391-5.

Lubaroff, D. M. & Silvers, W. K. 1973. Importance of chimerism in maintaining tolerance of skin allografts in mice. *J Immunol,* 111, 65-71.

Maki, T., Gottschalk, R., Wood, M. L. & Monaco, A. P. 1981a. Specific unresponsiveness to skin allografts in anti-lymphocyte serum-treated, marrow-injected mice: participation of donor marrow-derived suppressor T cells. *J Immunol,* 127, 1433-8.

Maki, T., Okazaki, H., Wood, M. L. & Monaco, A. P. 1981b. Suppressor cells in mice bearing intact skin allografts after blood transfusions. *Transplantation,* 32, 463-6.

Markees, T. G., Appel, M. C., Noelle, R. J., Mordes, J. P., Greiner, D. L. & Rossini, A. A. 1996. Tolerance to islet xenografts induced by dual manipulation of antigen presentation and co-stimulation. *Transplant Proc,* 28, 814-5.

Markees, T. G., Phillips, N. E., Gordon, E. J., Noelle, R. J., Shultz, L. D., Mordes, J. P., Greiner, D. L. & Rossini, A. A. 1998. Long-term survival of skin allografts induced by donor splenocytes and anti-CD154 antibody in thymectomized mice requires CD4(+) T cells, interferon-gamma, and CTLA4. *J Clin Invest,* 101, 2446-55.

Mathe, G., Amiel, J. L., Schwarzenberg, L., Cattan, A. & Schneider, M. 1963. Haematopoietic Chimera in Man after Allogenic (Homologous) Bone-Marrow Transplantation. (Control of the Secondary Syndrome. Specific Tolerance Due to the Chimerism). *Br Med J,* 2, 1633-5.

Mathe, G., Amiel, J. L., Schwarzenberg, L., Cattan, A., Schneider, M., Devries, M. J., Tubiana, M., Lalanne, C., Binet, J. L., Papiernik, M., Seman, G., Matsukura, M., Mery, A. M., Schwarzmann, V. & Flaisler, A. 1965. Successful Allogenic Bone Marrow Transplantation in Man: Chimerism, Induced Specific Tolerance and Possible Anti-Leukemic Effects. *Blood,* 25, 179-96.

Matthews, E. J., Kruhlak, N. L., Benz, R. D. & Contrera, J. F. 2004. Assessment of the health effects of chemicals in humans: I. QSAR estimation of the maximum recommended therapeutic dose (MRTD) and no effect level (NOEL) of organic chemicals based on clinical trial data. *Curr Drug Discov Technol,* 1, 61-76.

Medawar, P. B. 1944. The behaviour and fate of skin autografts and skin homografts in rabbits: A report to the War Wounds Committee of the Medical Research Council. *J Anat,* 78, 176-99.

Monaco, A. P. 2004. The beginning of clinical tolerance in solid organ allografts. *Exp Clin Transplant,* 2, 153-61.

Moodycliffe, A. M., Shreedhar, V., Ullrich, S. E., Walterscheid, J., Bucana, C., Kripke, M. L. & Flores-Romo, L. 2000. CD40-CD40 ligand interactions in vivo regulate migration of antigen-bearing dendritic cells from the skin to draining lymph nodes. *J Exp Med,* 191, 2011-20.

Murray, J. E. 1971. Organ transplantation (skin, kidney, heart) and the plastic surgeon. *Plast Reconstr Surg,* 47, 425-31.

Murray, J. E. 1992. Human organ transplantation: background and consequences. *Science,* 256, 1411-6.

Najafian, N. & Sayegh, M. H. 2000. CTLA4-Ig: a novel immunosuppressive agent. *Expert Opin Investig Drugs,* 9, 2147-57.

Nasir, S., Bozkurt, M., Krokowicz, L., Klimczak, A. & Siemionow, M. 2009. Correlation of chimerism with graft size and revascularization in vascularized and nonvascularized skin allografts. *Ann Plast Surg,* 62, 430-8.

Nikolic, B., Onoe, T., Takeuchi, Y., Khalpey, Z., Primo, V., Leykin, I., Smith, R. N. & Sykes, M. 2010. Distinct requirements for achievement of allotolerance versus reversal of autoimmunity via nonmyeloablative mixed chimerism induction in NOD mice. *Transplantation,* 89, 23-32.

Oderup, C., Malm, H., Ekberg, H., Qi, Z., Veress, B., Ivars, F. & Corbascio, M. 2006. Costimulation blockade-induced cardiac allograft tolerance: inhibition of T cell expansion and accumulation of intragraft cD4(+)Foxp3(+) T cells. *Transplantation,* 82, 1493-500.

Okada, S. & Strober, S. 1982. Spleen cells from adult mice given total lymphoid irradiation or from newborn mice have similar regulatory effects in the mixed leukocyte reaction. I. Generation of antigen-specific suppressor cells in the mixed leukocyte reaction after the addition of spleen cells from adult mice given total lymphoid irradiation. *J Exp Med,* 156, 522-38.

Onodera, K., Chandraker, A., Schaub, M., Stadlbauer, T. H., Korom, S., Peach, R., Linsley, P. S., Sayegh, M. H. & Kupiec-Weglinski, J. W. 1997. CD28-B7 T cell costimulatory blockade by CTLA4Ig in sensitized rat recipients: induction of transplantation tolerance in association with depressed cell-mediated and humoral immune responses. *J Immunol,* 159, 1711-7.

Owen, R. D. 1945. Immunogenetic Consequences of Vascular Anastomoses between Bovine Twins. *Science,* 102, 400-1.

Pan, Y., Luo, B., Sozen, H., Kalscheuer, H., Blazar, B. R., Sutherland, D. E., Hering, B. J. & Guo, Z. 2003. Blockade of the CD40/CD154 pathway enhances T-cell-depleted allogeneic bone marrow engraftment under nonmyeloablative and irradiation-free conditioning therapy. *Transplantation,* 76, 216-24.

Pearson, T., Shultz, L. D., Lief, J., Burzenski, L., Gott, B., Chase, T., Foreman, O., Rossini, A. A., Bottino, R., Trucco, M. & Greiner, D. L. 2008. A new immunodeficient hyperglycaemic mouse model based on the Ins2Akita mutation for analyses of human islet and beta stem and progenitor cell function. *Diabetologia,* 51, 1449-56.

Pilat, N., Baranyi, U., Klaus, C., Jaeckel, E., Mpofu, N., Wrba, F., Golshayan, D., Muehlbacher, F. & Wekerle, T. 2010. Treg-therapy allows mixed chimerism and transplantation tolerance without cytoreductive conditioning. *Am J Transplant,* 10, 751-62.

Pino, S., Brehm, M. A., Covassin-Barberis, L., King, M., Gott, B., Chase, T. H., Wagner, J., Burzenski, L., Foreman, O., Greiner, D. L. & Shultz, L. D. 2010. Development of novel major histocompatibility complex class I and class II-deficient NOD-SCID IL2R gamma chain knockout mice for modeling human xenogeneic graft-versus-host disease. *Methods Mol Biol,* 602, 105-17.

Pree, I., Pilat, N. & Wekerle, T. 2009. Bone marrow transplantation as a strategy for tolerance induction in the clinic. *Front Biosci,* 14, 611-20.

Przepiorka, D., Khouri, I., Thall, P., Mehra, R., Lee, M. S., Ippoliti, C., Giralt, S., Gajewski, J., Van Besien, K., Andersson, B., Korbling, M., Deisseroth, A. B. & Champlin, R. 1999. Thiotepa, busulfan and cyclophosphamide as a preparative regimen for allogeneic transplantation for advanced chronic myelogenous leukemia. *Bone Marrow Transplant,* 23, 977-81.

Psoinos, C. M., Ignotz, R. A., Lalikos, J. F., Fudem, G., Savoie, P. & Dunn, R. M. 2009. Use of gauze-based negative pressure wound therapy in a pediatric burn patient. *J Pediatr Surg,* 44, e23-6.

Racki, W. J., Covassin, L., Brehm, M., Pino, S., Ignotz, R., Dunn, R., Laning, J., Graves, S. K., Rossini, A. A., Shultz, L. D. & Greiner, D. L. 2010. NOD-scid IL2rgamma(null) mouse model of human skin transplantation and allograft rejection. *Transplantation,* 89, 527-36.

Rulifson, I. C., Szot, G. L., Palmer, E. & Bluestone, J. A. 2002. Inability to induce tolerance through direct antigen presentation. *Am J Transplant,* 2, 510-9.

Rusnak, F. & Mertz, P. 2000. Calcineurin: form and function. *Physiol Rev,* 80, 1483-521.

Sakaguchi, S. 2005. Naturally arising Foxp3-expressing CD25+CD4+ regulatory T cells in immunological tolerance to self and non-self. *Nat Immunol,* 6, 345-52.

Sanchez-Fueyo, A., Domenig, C. M., Mariat, C., Alexopoulos, S., Zheng, X. X. & Strom, T. B. 2007. Influence of direct and indirect allorecognition pathways on CD4+CD25+ regulatory T-cell function in transplantation. *Transpl Int,* 20, 534-41.

Schwartz, R. H. 2005. Natural regulatory T cells and self-tolerance. *Nat Immunol,* 6, 327-30.

Seller, M. J. 1967. Erythrocyte chimerism after injection of spleen cells into anemic mice of the W-series. *Science,* 155, 90-1.

Shapira, M. Y., Or, R., Resnick, I. B., Bitan, M., Ackerstein, A., Samuel, S., Elad, S., Zilberman, I., Miron, S. & Slavin, S. 2003. A new minimally ablative stem cell transplantation procedure in high-risk patients not eligible for nonmyeloablative allogeneic bone marrow transplantation. *Bone Marrow Transplant,* 32, 557-61.

Shen, Z., Mohiuddin, M., Goldstein, C., Yokoyama, H. & Disesa, V. J. 1996. Durability of donor-specific and organ-specific heart transplant tolerance induced by intrathymic pretreatment with allogeneic spleen cells. *J Thorac Cardiovasc Surg,* 111, 429-31.

Shiao, S. L., Mcniff, J. M., Masunaga, T., Tamura, K., Kubo, K. & Pober, J. S. 2007. Immunomodulatory properties of FK734, a humanized anti-CD28 monoclonal antibody with agonistic and antagonistic activities. *Transplantation,* 83, 304-13.

Shultz, L. D., Pearson, T., King, M., Giassi, L., Carney, L., Gott, B., Lyons, B., Rossini, A. A. & Greiner, D. L. 2007. Humanized NOD/LtSz-scid IL2 receptor common gamma chain knockout mice in diabetes research. *Ann N Y Acad Sci,* 1103, 77-89.

Siemionow, M. Z., Kulahci, Y. & Bozkurt, M. 2009. Composite tissue allotransplantation. *Plast Reconstr Surg,* 124, e327-39.

Signorell, J., Hunziker, T., Martinelli, M., Koestner, S. C. & Mohacsi, P. J. 2010. Recurrent non-melanoma skin cancer: remission of field cancerization after conversion from calcineurin inhibitor- to proliferation signal inhibitor-based immunosuppression in a cardiac transplant recipient. *Transplant Proc,* 42, 3871-5.

Slavin, S., Or, R., Weshler, Z., Fuks, Z., Morecki, S., Weigensberg, M., Bar, S. & Weiss, L. 1985. The use of total lymphoid irradiation for allogeneic bone marrow transplantation in animals and man. *Surv Immunol Res,* 4, 238-52.

Slavin, S. & Strober, S. 1979. Induction of allograft tolerance after total lymphoid irradiation (TLI): development of suppressor cells of the mixed leukocyte reaction (MLR). *J Immunol,* 123, 942-6.

Sprent, J., Kosaka, H., Gao, E. K., Surh, C. D. & Webb, S. R. 1993. Intrathymic and extrathymic tolerance in bone marrow chimeras. *Immunol Rev,* 133, 151-76.

Stone, W. H., Cragle, R. G., Swanson, E. W. & Brown, D. G. 1965. Skin Grafts: Delayed Rejection between Pairs of Cattle Twins Showing Erythrocyte Chimerism. *Science,* 148, 1335-6.

Streilein, J. W. & Niederkorn, J. Y. 1985. Characterization of the suppressor cell(s) responsible for anterior chamber-associated immune deviation (ACAID) induced in BALB/c mice by P815 cells. *J Immunol,* 134, 1381-7.

Strober, S., Slavin, S., Gottlieb, M., Zan-Bar, I., King, D. P., Hoppe, R. T., Fuks, Z., Grumet, F. C. & Kaplan, H. S. 1979. Allograft tolerance after total lymphoid irradiation (TLI). *Immunol Rev,* 46, 87-112.

Subba Rao, D. S. & Grogan, J. B. 1986. Depressed host response to skin implants in the anterior chamber of the eye. *J Surg Res,* 41, 636-44.

Swearingen, B., Ravindra, K., Xu, H., Wu, S., Breidenbach, W. C. & Ildstad, S. T. 2008. Science of composite tissue allotransplantation. *Transplantation,* 86, 627-35.

Sykes, M. 1996. Hematopoietic cell transplantation for the induction of allo- and xenotolerance. *Clin Transplant,* 10, 357-63.

Tao, X., Constant, S., Jorritsma, P. & Bottomly, K. 1997. Strength of TCR signal determines the costimulatory requirements for Th1 and Th2 CD4+ T cell differentiation. *J Immunol,* 159, 5956-63.

Tobin, G. R., Breidenbach, W. C., 3rd, Ildstad, S. T., Marvin, M. M., Buell, J. F. & Ravindra, K. V. 2009. The history of human composite tissue allotransplantation. *Transplant Proc,* 41, 466-71.

Tung, T. H., Mackinnon, S. E. & Mohanakumar, T. 2008. Costimulation blockade of CD40 and CD28 pathways in limb transplantation. *Transplant Proc,* 40, 3723-4.

Unek, I. T., Bayraktar, F., Solmaz, D., Ellidokuz, H., Yuksel, F., Sisman, A. R. & Yesil, S. 2010. Enhanced levels of soluble CD40 ligand and C-reactive protein in a total of 312 patients with metabolic syndrome. *Metabolism,* 59, 305-13.

Van Den Berg, L. M., De Jong, M. A., Witte, L., Ulrich, M. M. & Geijtenbeek, T. B. 2011. Burn injury suppresses human dermal dendritic cell and Langerhans cell function. *Cell Immunol,* 268, 29-36.

Van Duyne, R., Pedati, C., Guendel, I., Carpio, L., Kehn-Hall, K., Saifuddin, M. & Kashanchi, F. 2009. The utilization of humanized mouse models for the study of human retroviral infections. *Retrovirology,* 6, 76.

Vlad, G., Stokes, M. B., Liu, Z., Chang, C. C., Sondermeijer, H., Vasilescu, E. R., Colovai, A. I., Berloco, P., D'agati, V. D., Ratner, L., Cortesini, R. & Suciu-Foca, N. 2009. Suppression of xenogeneic graft-versus-host disease by treatment with immunoglobulin-like transcript 3-Fc. *Hum Immunol,* 70, 663-9.

Von Boehmer, H. 2005. Mechanisms of suppression by suppressor T cells. *Nat Immunol,* 6, 338-44.

Weng, L., Dyson, J. & Dazzi, F. 2007. Low-intensity transplant regimens facilitate recruitment of donor-specific regulatory T cells that promote hematopoietic engraftment. *Proc Natl Acad Sci U S A,* 104, 8415-20.

Wingren, A. G., Parra, E., Varga, M., Kalland, T., Sjogren, H. O., Hedlund, G. & Dohlsten, M. 1995. T cell activation pathways: B7, LFA-3, and ICAM-1 shape unique T cell profiles. *Crit Rev Immunol,* 15, 235-53.

Wu, X., Nguyen, B. C., Dziunycz, P., Chang, S., Brooks, Y., Lefort, K., Hofbauer, G. F. & Dotto, G. P. 2010. Opposing roles for calcineurin and ATF3 in squamous skin cancer. *Nature,* 465, 368-72.

Xu, H., Huang, Y., Hussain, L. R., Zhu, Z., Bozulic, L. D., Ding, C., Yan, J. & Ildstad, S. T. 2010. Sensitization to minor antigens is a significant barrier in bone marrow transplantation and is prevented by CD154:CD40 blockade. *Am J Transplant,* 10, 1569-79.

Yacoub, D., Hachem, A., Theoret, J. F., Gillis, M. A., Mourad, W. & Merhi, Y. 2010. Enhanced levels of soluble CD40 ligand exacerbate platelet aggregation and thrombus formation through a CD40-dependent tumor necrosis factor receptor-associated factor-2/Rac1/p38 mitogen-activated protein kinase signaling pathway. *Arterioscler Thromb Vasc Biol,* 30, 2424-33.

Yamada & Sayegh, M. H. 2002. The CD154-CD40 costimulatory pathway in transplantation. *Transplantation,* 73, S36-9.

Yamazaki, M., Pearson, T., Brehm, M. A., Miller, D. M., Mangada, J. A., Markees, T. G., Shultz, L. D., Mordes, J. P., Rossini, A. A. & Greiner, D. L. 2007. Different mechanisms control peripheral and central tolerance in hematopoietic chimeric mice. *Am J Transplant,* 7, 1710-21.

Yu, X. Z., Albert, M. H., Martin, P. J. & Anasetti, C. 2004. CD28 ligation induces transplantation tolerance by IFN-gamma-dependent depletion of T cells that recognize alloantigens. *J Clin Invest,* 113, 1624-30.

Yu, X. Z., Bidwell, S. J., Martin, P. J. & Anasetti, C. 2000. CD28-specific antibody prevents graft-versus-host disease in mice. *J Immunol,* 164, 4564-8.

Yu, X. Z., Martin, P. J. & Anasetti, C. 2003. CD28 signal enhances apoptosis of CD8 T cells after strong TCR ligation. *J Immunol,* 170, 3002-6.

Yuan, M., Ohishi, M., Wang, L., Raguki, H., Wang, H., Tao, L. & Ren, J. 2010. Association between serum levels of soluble CD40/CD40 ligand and organ damage in hypertensive patients. *Clin Exp Pharmacol Physiol,* 37**,** 848-51.

Zheng, X. X., Markees, T. G., Hancock, W. W., Li, Y., Greiner, D. L., Li, X. C., Mordes, J. P., Sayegh, M. H., Rossini, A. A. & Strom, T. B. 1999. CTLA4 signals are required to optimally induce allograft tolerance with combined donor-specific transfusion and anti-CD154 monoclonal antibody treatment. *J Immunol,* 162**,** 4983-90.